D1358487

Handbook of
OTOACOUSTIC
EMISSIONS

A Singular Audiology Text
Jeffrey L. Danhauer, Ph.D.
Audiology Editor

Handbook of
OTOACOUSTIC
EMISSIONS

JAMES W. HALL, III, Ph.D.

Department of Communicative Disorders
College of Health Professions
University of Florida Health Sciences Center
Gainesville, Florida

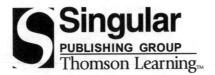

Singular
PUBLISHING GROUP
Thomson Learning™

Singular Publishing Group
Thomson Learning
401 West A Street, Suite 325
San Diego, California 92101-7904

Singular Publishing Group, Inc., publishes textbooks, clinical manuals, clinical reference books, journals, videos, and multimedia materials on speech-language pathology, audiology, otorhino-laryngology, special education, early childhood, aging, occupational therapy, physical therapy, reha-bilitation, counseling, mental health, and voice. For your convenience, our entire catalog can be accessed on our website at *http://www.singpub.com.* Our mission to provide you with materials to meet the daily challenges of the ever-changing health care/educational environment will remain on course if we are in touch with you. In that spirit, we welcome your feedback on our products. Please telephone (**1-800-521-8545**), fax (**1-800-774-8398**), or e-mail (*singpub@singpub.com*) your comments and requests to us.

© 2000, by Singular Publishing Group

Typeset in 10/12 Palatino by SoCal Graphics
Printed in Canada by Transcontinental Printing

All rights, including that of translation, reserved. No part of this publication may be reproduced, stored in a retrieval system or transmitted in any form or by any means, electronic, mechanical, recording, or other-wise, without the prior written permission of the publisher.

Library of Congress Cataloging-in-Publication Data

Hall, James W., audiologist
   Handbook of otoacoustic emissions/James W. Hall, III.
       p. cm.
   Includes bibliographic references and index.
   ISBN 1-56938-873-9 (softcover : alk. Paper)
   1. Otoacoustic emissions—Handbooks, manuals, etc. I. Title.

RF294.5.O76 H34 1999
617.8'4—dc21

                                                 99-047212
                                                    CIP

CONTENTS

6 Distortion Product and Transient Evoked OAEs: Effect of Peripheral Auditory Dysfunction and Hearing Loss — 223

7 Manufacturers' Forum — 271

8 Clinical Applications of OAEs in Children — 389

9 Clinical Applications of OAEs in Adults — 481

PREFACE

The clinical application of otoacoustic emissions (OAEs) with children and adults has profoundly altered audiology. During their graduate education, however, the vast majority of clinical audiologists received neither didactic instruction nor practical experience with OAEs. These professionals, and a new generation of audiology students, need a practical guide for recording, analyzing, and interpreting OAEs—a book covering both distortion product and transient evoked OAEs and incorporating the latest discoveries in cochlear anatomy and physiology. The *Handbook of Otoacoustic Emissions* was written by a clinical audiologist to meet this objective. For the budding or practicing audiologists, handy features include test protocols, normative data, troubleshooting tips, numerous interesting pediatric and adult case reports, and the rationale and test strategies for a variety of clinical applications of OAE from newborn hearing screening and diagnostic pediatric assessment (encompassing a review of auditory neuropathy) to monitoring ototoxicity. OAEs cannot be recorded, of course, without equipment designed specifically for presentation of stimuli to the ear and detection of responses (OAEs) from the ear. For the convenience of the busy clinician, the handbook also includes multiple manufacturers' introductions to OAE devices. Professionals in the clinic and laboratory will appreciate the extensive up-to-date references. Whatever your professional interests or preferences—from pediatrics to geriatrics—OAEs are likely to contribute to your clinical practice and allow you to better serve your patients. This book is written for you.

James W. (Jay) Hall, III, Ph.D.
October 1999

ACKNOWLEDGMENTS

This book is dedicated **Larry Mauldin** — an always kind, highly intelligent, and ever fun-loving person who gave generously and willingly to the profession of audiology. Larry was born in Bonham, Texas to Robert Woodrow and Allene Hasten Mauldin. In 1968, he graduated as valedictorian from Bonham High School. Larry went on to earn a degree in Biology from Rice University, located across the street from The Methodist Hospital and Baylor College of Medicine in Houston, Texas. While he was a Rice student, and after graduation in the early 1970s, Larry was employed as a research assistant and technical utility man in the auditory research laboratories of James Jerger at Baylor College of Medicine. The amazing research productivity of those halcyon years was possible largely because of Larry's creativity and efforts in periodically reconfiguring laboratory and clinical instrumentation for new studies, and in reliably keeping cantankerous devices (e.g., the impetuous DEC-8 computer) up and running. Larry's contribution to this unusually prolific period in Dr. Jerger's audiologic research at Baylor College of Medicine is documented by his co-authorship on a host of pace-setting papers on tympanometry and acoustic reflexes, and the auditory brainstem response.

My career was similarly advanced by Larry's talents as a classroom instructor and his technical expertise. The Acknowledgments of my dissertation in 1979 included the statement: "I am grateful to . . . Larry Mauldin for kindly assisting in the construction and maintenance of the instrument used in this study." (The "instrument" was the aforementioned infamous DEC computer.) For a number of years during this era, Larry was enrolled as a Ph.D. student at BCM. Later, as he moved on to work for a variety of manufacturers of audiologic equipment and hearing instruments, Larry similarly influenced other generations of audiologists. Larry was invariably generous with his time and talents, always given with a ready smile and lively spirit. He leaves behind his wife Cheryl Mauldin, a son Geoffrey, a stepson Aaron, a daughter Jennifer, and a granddaugher Taylor.

With pleasure I acknowledge my faithful and incomparable secretarial assistant **Melba Carpenter** at the Vanderbilt Balance and Hearing Center, and the irreplaceable staff of the audiology clinics of Vanderbilt University Medical Center—**Ann Byrn, Susan Lytle, Stacy McDaniel, Jennifer Dillard, Lisa Hamstead, Paige Harden,** and **Georgette Smiley, R.N.**

I once again gladly express gratitude for support and patience to my wife **Missy** and the two children still at home—**Austin** and **Victoria**—while this book was written who saw far too little of their husband/father.

★★★★★

This book was prepared entirely while I was affiliated with the Department of Hearing and Speech Sciences and Department of Otolaryngology in the Vanderbilt Bill Wilkerson Center for Otolaryngology and Communicative Disorders at **Vanderbilt University** in Nashville, Tennessee.

DEDICATION

In memory of

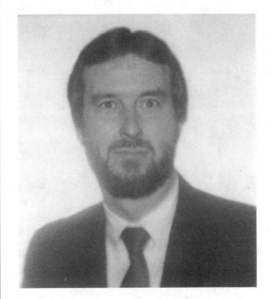

Larry Mauldin

September 2, 1949 – May 17, 1998

CHAPTER

1

Otoacoustic Emissions: Then and Now

Read Me First!

HISTORICAL OVERVIEW

As clinical audiology developed during the 20th century, each decade seemed to be dominated by specific procedures for auditory assessment, or certain types of tests (Figure 1–1). Although commercially available equipment for measuring hearing thresholds for tonal signals was introduced as early as the 1920s, pure tone audiometry really came into clincal practice during the 1940s (Bunch, 1943). Toward the end of the 1940s, a collection of eminent researchers at the Psychoacoustic Laboratory (PAL) at Harvard (e.g., Egan, 1948; Hudgins, Hawkins, Karlin, & Stevens, 1947) and the Father of Audiology himself, Raymond Carhart at Northwestern University (Carhart, 1946), published classic papers describing the development of materials for clinical assessment of speech threshold and word recognition. Routine clinical application of these materials began during the 1950s (Hirsh et al., 1952).

During the 1960s, audiologists enthusiastically performed tone decay tests, Békésy audiometry, the alternate binaural loudness balance (ABLB), and short increment sensitivity index (SISI) procedures within a test battery for differential diagnosis of sensorineural hearing loss, site-of-lesion determination, and the identification of retrocochlear auditory dysfunction (e.g., Johnson, 1965).

The classic paper on aural impedance, now termed immittance, measurement was published at the start of the 1970s (e.g., Jerger, 1970). Within a few short years audiologists everywhere were signing up for impedance workshops and then proudly recording tympanometry and acoustic reflexes on patients young and old. Although "discovered" in the early 1970s (Jewett & Williston, 1971), ABR really became incorporated into clinical practice during the 1980s with the commercial availability of instrumentation, and hundreds of papers describing fundamental findings, such as the generators of the response in humans (Møller, Jannetta, & Moller, 1981), documenting the value of its multiple clinical applications in children and adults (see Hall, 1992).

OAE similarly dominated the curiosity and clinical interests of audiologists toward the end of the decade of the 1990s. With the introduction of a clinical device for measurement of transient evoked OAEs in 1988, and even more so as at least a half dozen FDA-approved devices for measurement of distortion product OAEs were introduced by the mid-1990s, audiologists scrambled to learn more about this new-to-them procedure and to discover for themselves how OAE might contribute to the detection and assessment of auditory function in their pediatric and adults patients. The final word on the contribution of OAE to clin-

The foundations of audiology were established in the late 1940s. Raymond Carhart was educating the first generation of audiologists at Northwestern University. At the Psychoacoustic Laboratory at Harvard a collection of hearing scientists with names like Hirsh, Egan, Hudgins, and Hawkins were developing speech audiometry materials. Otto Metz in Germany was applying aural impedance measures in the clinical assessment middle ear pathology. In England, clinical researchers Dix, Hallpike and Hood introduced one of the first diagnostic audiologic procedures — the ABLB. During the same time period, another British scientist — Thomas Gold — was discovering the anatomic underpinnings of OAEs in a laboratory at Cambridge University.

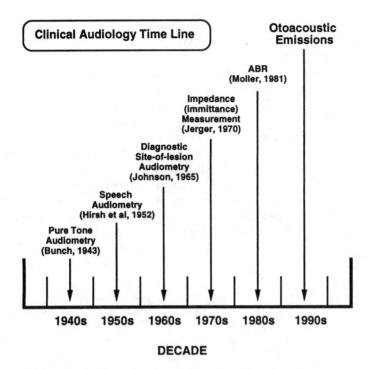

Figure 1–1. Time line for major clinical audiologic procedures showing OAE measurement as the "test of the 1990s."

ical audiology is, of course, not yet in. Indeed, even basic questions about measurement and analysis strategies remain unanswered. Nonetheless, it is patently clear that OAEs provide valuable information on auditory function and can make an important and unique contribution to early detection of cochlear impairment and to diagnostic audiologic assessment. OAEs are certainly not a passing fad. Rather, OAEs are now an essential, and permanent, component of the clinical audiology test battery. Every minute invested in the systematic study (or review) of cochlear anatomy and physiology and the principles of OAE generation and measurement and in developing the technical expertise required for recording, analyzing, and interpreting OAE in various patient populations will be returned with interest many times over in the clinical setting. Without a doubt, OAEs are here to stay!

von Békésy Versus Gold

In the 19th century von Helmholtz suspected that the cochlea consisted from base to apex of structural units (comparable to piano strings) that were individually tuned to different frequencies. This *resonance theory* was not, however, endorsed by the most famous cochlear investigator in the first half of the 20th century. Georg von Békésy instead systematically developed with an extensive series of elegant experiments the well-known *place*, and *traveling wave*, *theory* to explain hearing, in particular frequency coding and pitch perception. During the 1940s alone, von Békésy published his experimental findings in no less than 19 scientific articles. As summarized in the obituary written by Zwislocki, von Békésy published what was, at that time, the definitive word on how the cochlea functioned. In a word, the cochlea functioned "passively." In 1948, a British auditory scientist Thomas Gold (Figure 1–2) proposed, based on a series of investigations of the cochlea as a frequency analzyer with his colleague Sir R. J. Pumphrey in The Zoological Laboratory at Cambridge University, that the cochlea was characterized by "active processes." Gold summarized his observations as follows:

> It is shown that the assumption of a "passive" cochlea, where elements are brought into mechanical oscillation solely by means of the incident sound, is not tenable. The degree of resonance of the elements of the cochlea can be measured, and the results are not compatible with the very heavy damping which must arise from

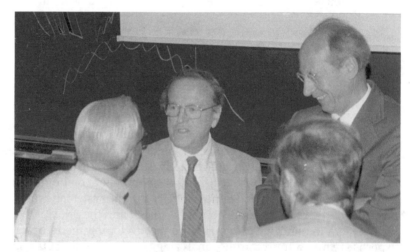

Figure 1–2. Dr. Thomas Gold (center facing camera), an Englishman who at Cambridge University in the late 1940s conducted basic auditory research suggesting the presence of "mechanical resonators" within the cochlea. Dr. Gold's work laid the foundation for later investigations that demonstrated outer hair cell motility and otoacoustic emissions. This photograph was taken in 1988, toward the end of Dr. Gold's illustrious career as a cosmologist. Dr. J. J. Zwislocki is to his left, Dr. E. Zwicker is to his right, and Dr. David Kemp has his back to the camera.

the viscosity of the liquid. For this reason the "regeneration hypothesis" is put forward, and it is suggested that an electromechanical action takes place whereby a supply of electrical energy is employed to conteract the damping. (Gold, 1948, p. 492)

The interposition of a feedback stage . . . makes a construction possible where the nerve ending abstracts much energy from a mechanical resonator. (Gold, 1948, p. 498)

Given the prominence of von Békésy, the respect within the hearing science community for his meticulous experimental techniques, and the general acceptance of his theories on hearing, it is not at all surprising that Gold's apparently unorthodox viewpoints were not immediately adopted. Dr. Gold's thesis would certainly not be heartily defended by von Békésy. Quite the contrary. Over 40 years after his prophetic papers were written, Gold (1989) recounted:

A brief biographical sketch of Dr. Thomas Gold can be found in Chapter 10 (Future Directions).

I started to think—in my capacity as a tame physicist—I started to think "well what could such a mechanism—the hardware of the ear —what could it do? And I concluded very quickly that the degree of resonance that could be acheived in a passive system was of course limited. (p. 300)

Well, I puzzled very much about that for some time, and then one day when I was sitting for a colloquium in the Cavendish—listening to an extremely dull physics colloquium—nothing to do with the subject—and my mind strayed, and I said to myself—'Boy! If the thing only had a positive feedback in it, all these problems would disappear wouldn't they (p. 300)

We had written in the 1948 paper on the physical basis of the action of the cochlea and we clearly spelled out that when you observed it on a live cochlea the frequency response curve you would see would be a curve that rises steeply and cuts off very steeply. I had discussed at length in 1948 with von Békésy at Harvard, that the observations that he made on the dead cochlea were unrepresentative. But he wouldn't have that! He thought that there must have been some cunning neural mechanism that somehow steepens up the subjective response. (p. 301)

So I returned from my meeting with Békésy even more convinced that I was correct because, before I met him, I may have had the viewpoint that well, maybe these great men they have something up their sleeve that we don't know about that I don't understand. (p. 302)

Although von Békésy addressed such topics as resonance in the cochlear partition, his mechanical perspective was very different from Thomas Gold's. For example, in his monumental text *Experiments in Hearing* (1960), von Békésy stated,

> The appearance of disturbing resonances and the difficulty with which they were avoided . . . only by a painstaking cementing of openings leading to the semicircular canals . . . raised the following question. Why is the natural stapes located on that side of the cochlear partition that leads to the semicircular canals? . . . How much more expedient it would be, from the physical standpoint, if the stapes were attached at the round window. (p. 451)

In retrospect, it is easy to conclude that, due to his fondness for conducting investigations in cadavers, the brilliant von Bekesy would never have discoved active processes within the cochlea, nor even imagined the possibility of otoacoustic emissions. To be blunt, dead men (and women) don't have OAEs.

Thomas Gold: The Rest of the Story

Professor Thomas Gold, a physicist by training, was during World War II contributing to the valiant British military effort in the Admiralty Signals Establishment where he headed a laboratory for the development of radar devices. Immediately after the war, he took a job in the Cavendish where the world's largest magnetron was being built. Then, he decided to join his friend R. J. Pumphrey at the Zoology Laboratory at Cambrige. Dr. Pumphrey was a biologist by training who had also been involved in radar research during the war. Having limited previous experience in hearing science probably served Gold well. His open-minded and innovative approach to cochlear investigation, coupled with concepts borrowed from his work in radio technology (especially transduction of frequency information by receivers), no doubt contributed importantly to the mechanical resonator theory. After this productive foray into hearing science, Dr. Gold left this field of endeavor and subsequently developed a reputation for work in astronomy and cosmology, and an apparently "controversial nonbiological hypothesis for the origin of oil" (Gold, 1989, p. 299).

Kemp's Echoes

Thirty years later, another British physicist picked up the work that Gold had left undone. David Kemp (see Biographical Sketch 1–1) in his Auditory Perception Research Laboratory at the Royal National Throat, Nose, and Ear Hospital in London, as early as 1975, was accumulating psychoacoustic evidence suggesting the possibility of distortion products within the ear. Preliminary recordings of SOAE and DPOAE were made 2 years later. This work led to the official report of the discovery of OAE by Kemp in 1978 and within the next year more detailed descriptions of this exciting new phenomenon (Anderson & Kemp, 1979; Kemp, 1979a, 1979b, 1980) . Examples of "stimulated

Biographical Sketch

David T. Kemp, Discoverer of Evoked Otoacoustic Emissions

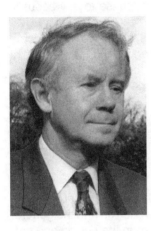

Dr. David Kemp, an Englishman, who discovered OAEs and reported his exciting findings in a 1978 paper.

Dr. Kemp studied physics, electronics, and atmospheric physics before moving into industrial noise control and, finally, into audiology in 1972. He joined a clinical research team at the Nuffield Hearing and Speech Centre in London England, which was committed to the improved assessment of auditory ability of hearing-impaired children. Dr. Kemp became interested in the basic mechanisms of hearing and particularly in the minute anomalies observable in perfectly healthy ears during psychoacoustical experiments. Like Gold 30 years earlier, he came to the conclusion that mechanically active mechanisms must exist in the ear, mechanisms that could, under some circumstances, oscillate spontaneously. Kemp went on to develop an integrated hypothesis in which auditory combination tones, threshold fine structure, and mild tonal tinnitus, were all related (Kemp & Martin, 1976).

Kemp's hypothesis contradicted established cochlear theories at that time. It required that waves travelling along the cochlea travelled without attenuation, that they could be reflected and reversed by nonlinear processes and thereafter could reverberate along with distortions inside the cochlea for a considerable time. To confirm this hypothesis, Kemp demonstrated that sound could be recovered from the cochlea using an ear canal microphone following stimulation by either tones or clicks. Referring to these sounds as "evoked acoustic emissions," he presented his discovery of distortion product otoacoustic emissions first in 1978 at the Inner Ear Biology Conference in Seefeld (Kemp, 1979), whereas his discovery of transient evoked otoacoustic emissions

(continued)

(TEOAEs) was published in the seminal paper "Stimulated Acoustic Emissions From Within the Human Auditory System" (Kemp, 1964).

As a state-funded researcher into the assessment of children's hearing function, he patented the generic technique of using sound emission from the ear in response to any acoustic stimulus for the purpose of the early detection of auditory dysfunction, particularly in children, to promote a source of income for the Royal National ENT Hospital. Disappointed at the failure of the audiological instrument industry to recognize the importance of this new development over a 10-year period, Dr. Kemp formed his own company (Otodynamics, Ltd.) in 1988 to manufacture transient and distortion product OAE systems for screening and research use. His ILO 88 TEOAE system played a major role in demonstrating the viability of universal hearing screening for neonates.

Dr. Kemp is currently Professor of Auditory Biophysics at the ILO, University College of London, where he continues to be active studying basic mechanisms of the cochlea and the generation of OAEs. He also plays an active part in the design and production of Otodynamics OAE instruments (see Chapter 7).

---

acoustic emissions" described in this paper are illustrated in Figure 1–3. Dr. Kemp, in this classic paper in the *Journal of the Acoustical Society of America* (Kemp, 1978), stated,

A new auditory phenomenon has been identified in the acoustic impulse of the human ear. Using a signal averaging technique, a study has been made of the response of the closed external acoustic meatus to acoustic impulses near to the threshold of audibility. . . . This component of the response appears to have its origin in some nonlinear mechanism probably located in the cochlea, responding mechanically to auditory stimulation, and dependent upon the normal functioning of the cochlea transduction process. (p. 1386)

No defect in or spurious behavior of the instrumentation has been found which in any way mimics phenomenon seen in the normal ears . . . It has not been possible to formulate a purely acoustic explanation. . . . An origin in the middle ear itself is strongly counterindicated by the acoustic analyses performed by Zwislocki and others. (p. 1389)

Various physiological possibilities have been examined. Sound generation during acoustic reflex contractions of either the stapedius or post auricular muscles, cannot, for several reasons, account for the phenomenon . . .The possibility that electrophysio-

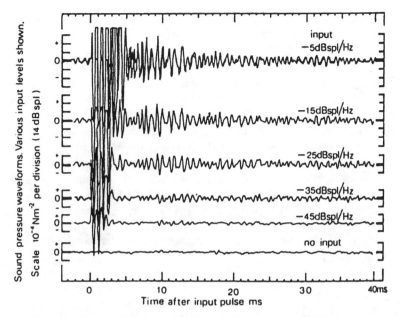

Figure 1–3. An example of the earliest reported OAE waveform recorded from the 1978 article (p. 1388) by David Kemp (Reprinted with permission from Kemp, D T. Stimulated Acoustic Emissions From Within the Human Auditory System. *Journal of the Acoustical Society of America 64*(5) 1386–1391, 1978). TEOAE waveforms are shown for a single normal subject at descending stimulus intensity levels. Most of the TEOAE energy appears within the initial 20 ms after the stimulus "input pulse." Note the high degree of replicability among waveforms.

logical signals of cochlear microphonic, neurogenic, or myogenic origin, where received and mistaken for acoustic signal was also rejected.

To summarize, the cochlear reflection hypothesis receives support from the new evidence here and from existing psychoacoustical evidence. (p. 1390)

In the absence of a complete understanding of the mode of action of the sensory cells in the cochlea, it is tempting to suggest that one of the functions of the outer hair cell population is the generation of this mechanical energy. If a cochlear origin is confirmed by experiments currently in progress, the technique developed in this study will provide a new avenue for investigation of the auditory system, with applications in both research and audiological medicine. (p. 1391)

In later publications, Kemp used the terms "evoked cochlear mechanical responses" and "echoes" to describe OAEs. The next logical term coined for OAE was "Kemp's echoes" (Wit, Langevoort, & Ritsma,

1981). OAEs, however, are clearly not simple, passive echoes of the stimulus reflected back from the inner ear.

Although clinical audiologists were, for the most part, oblivious of Kemp's discovery, word of OAE spread rapidly within the basic science community. Within a few years, an international collection of authors had independently published accounts of OAE . The excitement extended far beyond the isolated finding that sound produced by the ear could be measured in the human ear canal. The significance of OAE to the understanding of the principles of cochlear function, and hearing in general, was appreciated. Soon, there were other related breakthroughs in thinking on cochlear mechanics and physiology, on the dynamic role of outer hair cells in hearing, and even on function of the efferent auditory system. One of the best known authors of these publications was Hallowell Davis who described (Davis, 1983) the presence of a "cochlear amplifier":

> In the proposed overall model the organ of Corti acts at low levels as a sharply tuned amplifier to enhance the vibration of a narrow segment of the basilar membrane. This segment acts as a high-Q acoustic resonator. The inner hair cells clearly increase the discharge of nerve impulses in their afferent fibers when the amplitude of the movement of the basilar membrane, with or without the assistance of the cochlear amplifier (CA) reaches a constant value of about 3×10^{-10} m. At middle frequencies the gain in sensitivity provided at threshold by a healthy CA is about 45 dB, which is the length of the 'tips' of the tuning curves of both neural output and mechanical vibration. The CA is vulnerable to mechanical insult, as by noise or experimental operative procedures, to anoxia, and to certain drugs. The outer hair cells are necessary for CA and their cochlear microphonic (CM), acting in a controlled positive feedback relation is a possible source of the energy needed for "negative damping." (p. 81)

> What is the source of the energy for the CA? The best hint that we have is the requirement that the outer hair cells (OHC) be intact . . . This suggest[s] a motor function for OHC, with the efferent innervation providing a modulating influence, and perhaps a trophic function also . . . The large number of OHCs, three rows instead of one, may be an expression of the need for a large source of power. (p. 88)

Outer Hair Cells Can Move

As Hallowell Davis was describing the cochlear amplifier, William Brownell (see Biographical Sketch 1–2) and colleagues in the United States (Brownell, 1983; Brownell et al., 1985) and Flock in Sweden (Flock, 1980) were demonstrating that outer hair cells were capable of movement. The details on this remarkable capability of the inner ear, and cochlear anatomy and physiology in general, are reviewed in Chapter 2. von Békésy had extensively, but exclusively, studied a

Biographical Sketch

William Brownell and The Discovery of Outer Hair Cell Electromotility

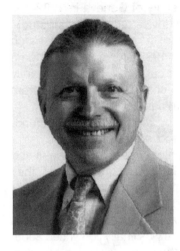

Dr. William "Bill" Brownell, one of the first auditory scientists to confirm that outer hair cells are capable of motility, the cochlear energy contributing to OAEs we record in the external ear canal.

Dr. William Brownell's interest in hearing began as early as high school, when he constructed a "working" model of the ear for a science fair project. After finishing his undergraduate studies in physics at the University of Chicago, Bill joined the Peace Corps and spent 2 years in Nigeria teaching high school science and mathematics. In the course of reading several science textbooks he had brought with him to the jungle, Bill discovered that his interests were in the neurosciences. Accordingly, when he returned from Africa, Brownell enrolled in the physiology graduate program at the University of Chicago and was awarded a Ph.D. in 1973 for work he did on central auditory pathways.

Bill took a faculty position at the University of Florida directly out of graduate school and began a career as an independent investigator. After setting up a laboratory to continue his studies of central auditory pathways, he began a remarkable series of studies on the inner ear. Bill felt that the hearing sciences—which at that time were dominated by engineering concepts—would profit enormously from an approach based on cell biology. Inspired by work being done on the retina, specifically a 10-minute report on photoreceptor synaptic activity at the 1976 Society for Neuroscience meeting, he began a study of synaptic vesicle recycling in cochlear hair cells.

During the next 5 years, Brownell's laboratory made a number of observations on cochlear function. One that was highly relevant to his later discovery of outer hair cell electro-

(continued)

motility was the first measure of the cochlear silent current (Brownell, Manis, Zidanic, & Spirou, 1983), the power supply for electromotility and otoacoustic emissions. While in Florida, Brownell also wrote a speculative review of cochlear transduction (Brownell, 1982) that presaged much of his later work. Bill took sabbatical leave at the University of Geneva in 1982–83, where his colleagues helped him devise techniques for studying solitary hair cells dissociated from the cochlea. This research took on a life of its own when late in 1982 Brownell and his team observed electromotility. Even though it could be readily observed, the conspicuous length changes that resulted from electrical stimulation were extraordinarily difficult to accept.

Electromotility violated common wisdom on cochlear function which, despite the recent discovery of otoacoustic emissions, viewed hair cells as mechanically passive. Brownell had suspected the cells would move, but the manner in which they were moving was inconsistent with the mechanism he thought might be at work. Bill required more than 6 months of evoking the same response before he was able to accept the movements as originating in the outer hair cell. He was finally convinced about its cellular origin when he found the cells responded by alternately lengthening and shortening as the voltage field was reversed.

A paper summarizing Dr. Brownell's observations was published in 1985 (Brownell, Bader, Bertrand, & de Ribaupierre, 1985) and may well be the single most important contribution to the hearing sciences in the last 15 years. It reported how the cell's cytoplasm was pressurized and that the movements appeared to originate in the cell's lateral wall. Brownell's experiments revealed that electromotility had a frequency response extending into the acoustic range and was nonlinear. His experiments also demonstrated that iontophoretic application of the efferent neurotransmitter acetylcholine resulted in length changes. Although his observations were largely qualitative, each has been replicated, extended, and further quantified.

Bill's "dancing" hair cells are now widely accepted as the cochlear amplifier and the origin of otoacoustic emissions. Subsequent experiments in his lab showed that salicylate blocked electromotility in isolated outer hair cells (Brownell, 1990; Shehata, Brownell, & Dieler, 1991). These studies were motivated by the observation that aspirin reversibly blocks otoacoustic emissions in humans. Realizing this new phenomena needed to be verified by other investigators, Brownell traveled to laboratories in Bethesda, Bristol, Houston, Montpellier, Omaha, and elsewhere, to demonstrate how to isolate the outer hair cells and in some cases participating in experiments.

Two years after his return to the United States, Bill joined the faculty of the Johns Hopkins Medical School. In 1994, he moved to the Baylor College of Medicine, where he holds the Jake and Nina Kamin Chair of Otolaryngology. Brownell has been principal investigator on research grants from the federal government for over 20 years. He is the recipient of a Fulbright and a Claude Pepper Award from NIH and has also received research awards from the Deafness Research Foundation, The Roche Research Foundation, INSERM, the Hasselblad Foundation, and the Max Kade Foundation. Brownell has been awarded the Kresge/Mirmelstein Award of Scientific Merit, the Self Help for the Hard of Hearing Special Friends of People with Hearing Loss Award, and a Distinguished Service Award from University of Chicago Medical and Biological Sciences Division.

Brownell's greatest recognition undoubtedly derives from the relatively large international community of scientists and clinicians now examining outer hair cell function. Work done in several laboratories, including his own, has established hair-cell motility as a key mechanism in active cochlear tuning and has tentatively identified the structural basis for motility. The molecular basis remains a mystery. It is a motor response that is thought to extend to the upper limit of hearing, which approaches 20,000 Hz in man and 100,000 Hz in bats. No other known motor response extends even up to 1000 Hz. Does hair-cell motility involve a truly novel biological mechanism? This question guides Bill's current research.

Ever wonder why we have three to four rows of outer hair cells and only a single row of inner hair cells? Were you even more perplexed in graduate school to learn that almost all (95%) of the important afferent eighth nerve fibers synapse with the minority inner hair cells? Read on to Chapter 2 to find peace of mind.

mechanically passive and functionally linear cochlea. The cochlea was capable of receiving and transducing energy. That was a fact proven repeatedly by numerous investigators. The unique structural (mechanical) properties of the basilar membrane, such as the differences in stiffness from base to apex, contribute importantly to the frequency analyzing capability of the cochlea. However, this mechanism predicted a broadly, or shallowly, tuned ear. In fact, the ear is finely tuned and capable of frequency selectivity performance that is far superior to what would be possible with a passive cochlea. Stated simply, when the living ear is stimulated with sound, the resulting basilar membrane movement and response exceed the energy of the sound minus the inevitable damping and subsequent loss of energy characteristic of the basilar membrane within the fluid-filled cochlea. The energy gain is greatest, of course, on the basilar membrane in the region corresponding to the frequency(ies) of the stimulus (stimuli). What structures and functions contribute to this cochlear amplifier, and where are they located within the cochlea?

Other observations on auditory anatomy prior to about 1980 were also curious. For example, Spoendlin in 1969 showed that most (90 to 95%)

afferent neurons innervate the inner hair cells, suggesting strongly that inner hair cells were the most important or maybe even the only sensory receptor in the cochlea. Then, why are there three rows of outer hair cells yet only one row of these important inner hair cells? What are we doing with all these outer hair cells? Hints as to the role of outer hair cells in cochlear function, especially threshold sensitivity and frequency selectivity, began to accumulate during the 1970s. Normal outer hair cell function certainly was needed for normal hearing sensitivity (e.g., Dallos et al., 1972), but that was quite puzzling since the outer hair cells had such sparse afferent innervation. Also, the work of Helmholtz in the 1800s, a few others before him, and more investigators in the 1960s and 1970s (e.g., Wegel & Lane, 1924; Goldstein, 1967; Goldstein & Kiang, 1968; Smoorenburg, 1972; Humes, 1980; Wilson, 1980; Zwicker, 1979, 1980, 1981) produced psychoacoustic (perceptual) suggestion, and later evidence, of extra, nonstimulus, sounds (i.e., distortion products) within the normally functioning cochlea. Where did this distortion come from? And what about the distinct differences in inner versus outer hair cell innervation by the efferent or descending auditory system? Efferent fibers synapse directly on the outer hair cells, whereas efferent fibers reach the inner hair cells only indirectly by making a synapse on radial auditory nerve fibers (e.g., Smith, 1961; Kimura & Wersall, 1962; Spoendlin, 1966).

In the creative tradition of OAE pioneers, such as Thomas Gold, Bill Brownell and David Kemp, several researchers at the Eaton-Peabody Laboratory of Auditory Physiology at Mass Eye and Ear Infirmary and Harvard Universty — Christopher Shera and John Guinan — are proposing a conceptually new system for categorizing OAEs. This new taxonomy for mammalian OAEs is summarized in a discussion of Future Directions (Chapter 10).

The many clues that something unusual (for a von Békésy-style passive and linear model) was happening in the cochlea became impossible to ignore by 1980. No doubt prompted by Kemp's discovery of OAE in 1978, a series of critical discoveries was reported during the early 1980s. What we would now describe as spontaneous OAEs were recorded in the ear canal (Wilson, 1980). And, Mountain (1980) showed that electrical stimulation of efferent auditory fiber influenced cochlear mechanics. Application of new experimental techniques confirmed nonlinear, and highly sensitive and tuned, basilar membrane vibration (Khanna & Leonard, 1982; Sellick, Patuzzi, & Johnstone, 1982). Clear evidence of outer hair cell motility to electrical stimulation in vitro (a living cochlea) by Brownell and colleagues (1983, 1985) provided probably the biggest missing piece to the puzzle of cochlear functioning. Immediately, the attention and intensive research efforts of many eminent basic auditory scientists were diverted to this new line of research (detailed in Chapter 2). Investigative efforts to better understand cochlear micromechanics and hair cell physiology, including outer hair cell motility, continue unabated even today.

CLASSIFICATION OF OAEs

According to conventional nomenclature, there are two general categories of OAE—spontaneous and evoked (Table 1–1). All OAE reflect cochlear processes. The conventional terminology and classification system for describing OAE is somewhat arbitrary. A new and very

Table 1–1. Traditional categories of otoacoustic emissions.

Type	Stimulus	Prevalence in Normal Ears*	Clinical Value?
Spontaneous	No stimulus required	Approximately 60% (less in males and in left ear)	Limited
Evoked			
Transient	Click or tone burst	99+%	Yes
Distortion product	Two pure tones	99+%	Yes
Stimulus frequency	Continuous pure tone	Unknown	No

*No cochlear pathology and hearing thresholds of 15 dB HL or better.

different system for classifying OAEs, recently developed by Shera and Guinan of M.I.T. (Shera & Guinan, 1999), is described in Chapter 10. For evoked OAE, the type of OAE is largely determined by the characteristics of the stimulus. In addition, an ear may simultaneously produce more than one type of OAE. Components of instrumentation common to the measurement of all OAE, illustrated in Figure 1–4, are a sensitive and low-noise microphone, a computer, and a processing system for extraction of the OAE from noise. As illustrated in Figure 1–4, *measurement of OAEs in the external ear canal, regardless of the type of OAE, is dependent on the integrity of the middle ear system, as well as the cochlea.* In the following discussion, we will assume entirely normal middle ear function. One must always keep in mind, however, that middle ear status must always be considered in the clinical measurement, analysis, and interpretation of OAE.

Spontaneous OAEs (SOAEs), as the term indicates, occur without external acoustic stimulation. They consist of energy at one or more frequencies emitted by the normal ear and recorded in the ear canal with a very sensitive microphone. The clinical value of SOAEs is limited, as they are not invariably produced by normal ears. That is, the absence of SOAE does not imply cochlear dysfunction. Also, the likelihood of SOAE even in normal ears is much higher for females than for males.

Three types of OAE are elicited or evoked with some kind of acoustic stimulus. *Stimulus frequency OAEs* (SFOAEs) are evoked with a constant pure-tone stimulus presented at a low intensity level and generally swept or changed slowly across a region of frequencies. SFOAEs are, by far, the least studied experimentally and clinically. There are no commercially available devices for recording SFOAE. For these reasons, SFOAEs are not discussed further in this book.

The two types of OAE applied clinically are the *transient evoked OAE* (TEOAE) and the *distortion product OAE* (DPOAE). The most common stimuli for the transient evoked OAE (TEOAE) are clicks, although TEOAEs can also be recorded with tone burst stimuli. Click stimula-

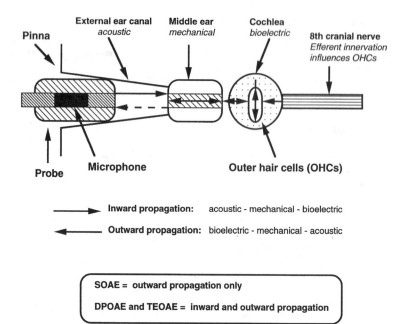

SOAE = outward propagation only

DPOAE and TEOAE = inward and outward propagation

Thinking of hopping on the OAE bandwagon? Don't forget to get a round-trip ticket. Measurement of OAEs depends on energy flow (stimulation) from the external ear canal to the cochlea, and then back along the same route from the cochlea (response) to the external ear canal. The ins and outs of OAE measurment are described in detail in Chapter 4.

Figure 1–4. A schematic diagram of the general instrumentation used to record OAEs. In addition to a computer, the major components are a transducer, a microphone, and a probe assembly for delivering the signal(s) and recording the responses (OAEs), plus software for generation of the signal(s), detecting and processing the response, and reducing noise also detected in the ear canal. Four distinct regions of the auditory system involved in measurement of OAEs are the external ear canal, middle ear, cochlea, and selected efferent auditory pathways. Importantly, OAE measurement requires inward propagaton of the stimulus (stimuli) to the cochlea and outward propagaton of the response (the OAEs) from the cochlea.

tion includes a broad band of frequencies and activates the cochlea simultaneously from basal to apical regions of the basilar membrane. The exact prevalence of TEOAE is unknown. Although TEOAEs were, in early reviews, described as always present in normally functioning cochleas, clinical experience has confirmed that a small number of persons with completely normal hearing sensitivity and otologic status may inexplicably have no recordable TEOAE. The prevalence of TEOAE is therefore slightly less than 100%.

DPOAEs, sometimes referred to simply as DPs, are elicited by the simultaneous presentation of two pure tones, closely spaced in frequency. The two frequencies (known as primaries) activate the cochlea in the same region of the basilar membrane. The lower frequency portion of the traveling wave for the higher frequency stimulus actually overlaps with the higher frequency portion of the traveling wave for lower frequency stimulus. One or more additional frequency components, the DP(s), is (are) produced at another frequency (or frequencies). As with the TEOAE, the prevalence for DPOAE in normally functioning cochlea is close to, but slightly less than, 100%.

Measurement, analysis, and interpretation of SOAE, DPOAE, and TEOAE are described in detail in Chapters 3, 4, and 5. What follows is an overview and an introduction to OAE measurement.

Spontaneous OAE

Among the different categories of OAE, spontaneous OAEs were the first type to be reported. Gold's (1948) observations on cochlear function were consistent with the likelihood that sounds could be emitted by the ear in the absence of any acoustic stimulation. As early as 1970, Kumpf and Hoke (1970, cited in Probst, Lonsbury-Martin, & Martin, 1991) reported that spectral analysis of acoustic energy within the ear canal contained frequency components (very narrow bands of energy) well above the noise floor. Since Kemp's classic description of OAE in 1978, SOAEs have been studied extensively in normal and pathologic ears of infants, children, and adults. Several commercially available OAE devices now permit clinical measurement of SOAE.

Spontaneous OAEs will never be relied on as a clinical procedure because they're always recorded from normal ears. SOAEs can, however, influence the clinical measurement and interpretation of transient evoked and distortion product OAEs.

A typical SOAE recorded from a young, normal-hearing female is illustrated in Figure 1–5. A probe containing a sensitive microphone, with low internal noise, is placed in the ear canal. While the patient is sitting quietly, sound in the ear canal is sampled and averaged over a brief time period. Ambient environmental noise, and physiologic noise, is always present in the ear canal, more so for the frequency region below about 1500 Hz. The measurement device performs a spectral analysis of this acoustic energy in the ear canal. The presence of SOAE is confirmed by the appearance of spikes, typically reaching amplitudes of 10 or 15 dB, at one or more frequencies. Selected features of SOAEs are summarized in Table 1–2. SOAEs are clearly more common in females than males. There also seems to be a greater likelihood of recording SOAE in the right than the left ear. SOAEs are characteristic of normal cochlear (and of course middle ear) function, and are not recorded at frequency regions with sensory impairment. The SOAE literature is reviewed in detail in Chapter 3.

Transient OAE

TEOAE recordings from humans were described in the classic 1978 article by David Kemp. Transient evoked OAEs (TEOAEs) are recorded in response to a very abrupt (click or tone burst) stimulus. There is

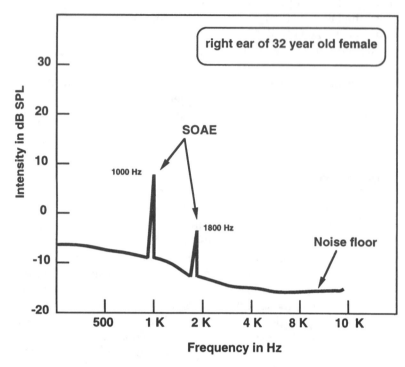

Spontaneous Otoacoustic Emission (SOAE)

Figure 1–5. A typical spontaneous OAE (SOAE) recorded in the external ear canal with no stimulus.

Table 1–2. Selected features of spontaneous otoacoustic emissions (SOAEs). SOAEs are described in detail in Chapter 3.

■ Present in no more than 60% of normal hearers

■ More common in females than in males

■ No clear effect of aging on SOAE if hearing sensitivity is normal (≤15 dB HL)

■ Comparable prevalence in infants, children, and young adults

■ Frequencies of SOAE are stable for long periods of time

■ Amplitudes of SOAE may fluctuate over time.

■ Most often present in the 1000 to 2000 Hz region

■ Multiple SOAE frequencies are common in individuals.

■ If present in an individual, likely to be present in both ears

■ There is no positive association between SOAE and tinnitus.

■ SOAE are not consistent with "objective tinnitus."

a well-appreciated tradeoff, or inverse relationship, between the duration and frequency content of acoustic stimuli. The shorter the stimulus, the broader the frequency range of the stimulus. Thus, a click (usually on the order of 0.1 ms or 100 μs in total duration) has a broad spectrum, whereas the spectrum for a relatively long-duration (e.g., 500 ms) pure tone (as used in pure tone audiometry) is limited to a single frequency. The transient stimulus used with TEOAE activates the cochlea simultaneously across a wide frequency region. If the cochlea, specifically the outer hair cells, is normal from the basal end of the basilar membrane to the apical end (and middle ear function is likewise normal), then robust and normal-amplitude TEOAE should be recorded from low frequencies up to about 5000 Hz.

Selected TEOAE stimulus and response parameters are illustrated in Figure 1–6. This discussion will be limited to an overview of generic characteristics of TEOAE, rather than measurement and analysis with a specific brand and model of equipment. A comprehensive review of TEOAE measurement and analysis is provided in Chapter 4. The first step in TEOAE measurement is the delivery of an optimal stimulus, which is typically a series of clicks. Clinically, two response properties of TEOAE are quantified and described. One is a display of the response in the time domain (see "5" in Figure 1–6). This temporal display of the response is invariably shown as one or two waveforms beginning about 2 to 3 ms after the stimulus and continuing out usually to about 20 ms. The earliest portions of the temporal waveform reflect TEOAE activity produced by the basal regions of the basilar membrane, whereas later portions of the waveform arise from more apical regions. Visual inspection of TEOAE temporal waveform fails to capture much clinically valuable information, especially regarding the status of the TEOAE at various audiometric frequencies. Spectral analysis of the TEOAE waveforms provides additional frequency information (see "6" in the Figure 1–6). This TEOAE display in the frequency domain clearly reveals the presence of TEOAE activity, above the noise floor, across the frequency region of 0 to 5000 Hz. These visual displays may be quantified, for more precise analysis. TEOAE absolute amplitude, or the TEOAE amplitude-noise difference, is calculated at individual frequencies, or summarized for bands of frequencies (see "7" in the Figure 1–6). Assuming normal middle ear status and that stimulus intensity was at or close to the target level and the spectrum was flat, then any reduction in the TEOAE signal-to-noise ratio, or lower correlation in any frequency region, would reflect cochlear (outer hair cell) dysfunction. Normative data can be derived for interpretation of these quantified TEOAE data. Finally, it is important to keep in mind that a variety of subject factors (nonpathologic and pathologic) may influence TEOAE. These factors must routinely be taken into account when TEOAE are interpreted clinically, as reviewed comprehensively in Chapter 5.

There are at least 10 different manufacturers of DPOAE systems. More devices for recording TEOAEs will probably be entering the marketplace soon as license requirements for manfacturers change at the beginning of the year 2000.

TRANSIENT EVOKED OTOACOUSTIC EMISSIONS (TEOAE)

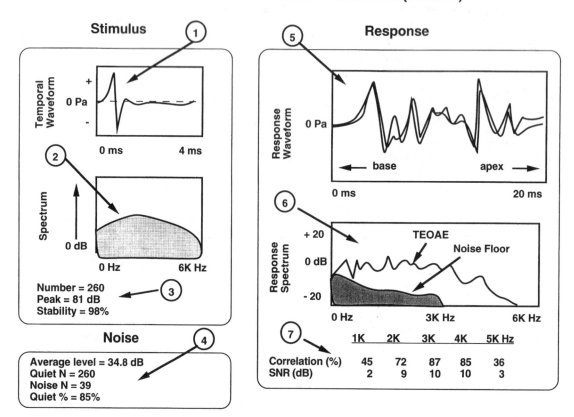

Figure 1–6. Stimulus and response parameters in the clinical measurement of transient OAEs (TEOAEs), including: (1) the temporal waveform of the stimuli (usually acoustic clicks), (2) the spectral waveform (frequency response) of the stimuli (a flat spectrum is desirable), (3) stimulus intensity level (in dB SPL) and the stability (in %) of the series of stimulus repetitions (260 in this example) over the duration of OAE measurement, (4) noise characteristics at quantified in the external ear canal during OAE measurement (e.g., average noise level in dB SPL and the proportion of the 260 stimuli presented when noise was lower versus higher than some predefined rejection level), (5) the temporal waveform of the TEOAEs measured in the external ear canal (two separate waveforms are shown), (6) spectrum for the TEOAE response and for noise measured concomitantly within the exernal ear canal (shaded area), and (7) examples of how the TEOAE response is quantified as a correlation in percent (e.g., reproducibility) between the two different TEOAE waveforms and as the ratio or difference between the amplitude of the TEOAE versus noise within certain frequency regions, such as octave frequency bands as shown here.

Distortion Products

Psychoacoustic studies of cochlear distortion products were reported consistently during the years before the initial studies of DPOAE were reported (e.g., Plomp, 1965; Goldstein, 1967; Wenner, 1968; Hall, 1972; Smoorenberg, 1972; Weber & Mellert, 1975; Zurek &

Clinical Concept

Sources of Noise in OAE Measurement

With OAE measurement, as with auditory evoked response measurement, the fundamental task is the detection of a signal embedded in noise. AERs are bio-electrical signals generated by the auditory pathways and nuclei in response to the stimulus, whereas the noise is background bio-electrical activity or myogenic activity, such as the ongoing EEG or muscle potentials, that is unrelated, or at least not directly related, to the stimulus.

In OAE measurement, our goal is to detect within the external ear canal sounds produced by the inner ear (the signal). This is complicated by other sounds (noise) that are inevitably also in the external ear canal. The two general types of noise are environmental and body noise, both of which are greatest in the low frequency region (below about 1000 Hz). It is impossible to avoid the noise, especially in clinical measurement of OAE. Fortunately, there are a number of technologic features in OAE instrumentation and testing strategies that usually allow the clinician to distinguish the different types of OAE (SOAE, TEOAE, and DPOAE) from the noise, as detailed elsewhere in this book.

The most common sources of noise in OAE measurement are:

■ Noise inherent to the microphone used to record OAE
■ Ambient test setting acoustic energy that enters the ear canal around or through the probe tip
■ Breathing
■ Rubbing of the probe tubing with clothing
■ Jaw movements
■ Muscle movements
■ Blood flow.

Still a little unclear about how TEOAEs and DPOAEs are recorded, analyzed, and interpreted? Don't get discouraged — that's what this book is all about. You'll find detailed discussions of OAE measurement and clinical application throughout Chapters 4 to 9.

Leshowitz, 1976; Humes, 1980; Allen & Fahey, 1992), and this line of research continues to be taken in studies of cochlear nonlinearity (Hicks & Bacon, 1999). Using stimulus parameters similar to those that generate DPOAE, these investigators assessed the perception of tones (distortion products) at f_2-f_1 and $2f_1-f_2$ by normal hearing subjects. During the same time period, evidence of these distortion products to primary frequency stimuli at appropriate f_2/f_1 ratios was also demonstrated in eighth nerve activity recorded electrophysiological-ly in animal experiments (Goldstein & Kiang, 1968; Pfeiffer & Molnar, 1974; Kim, 1980). More recently, evidence of difference tones (f_2-f_1) and cubic difference tones ($2f_1-f_2$) was recorded also as auditory evoked potentials from rostral regions (inferior colliculus) of the auditory brain stem in chinchilla (Arnold & Burkard, 1998). Clinical measurement of DP otoacoustic emissions evolved in the early 1990s as experimental instrumentation designed several years earlier was modified and then manufactured and marketed commercially (Fahey & Allen, 1985; Lonsbury-Martin et al., 1990a, 1990b; Rasmussen & Osterhammel, 1992; Rasmussen, Osterhammel, & Nielsen, 1992). The stimuli for DPOAE measurement are two closely spaced pure tones, referred to as primaries or f_1 and f_2. As illustrated in Figure 1–7, f_2 is the higher frequency and f_1 is the lower. The separation between the two frequencies is defined by the ratio of the higher to lower frequency, or f_2/f_1. A DPOAE will not be generated if these two frequencies are too far apart or too close together. Based on substantial research, it is clear that an f_2/f_1 ratio of about 1.22 produces a robust DPOAE in most normal ears and for most stimulus intensity and frequency combinations. The most appropriate stimulus intensity for evoking DPOAE in most clinical applications is in the range of 50 to 70 dB SPL. With higher stimulus intensities, there is a chance that passive (versus active) responses will be recorded, responses that do not always reflect outer hair cell activity. On the other hand, lower intensities often fail to generate a detectable DPOAE, even from persons with reasonably normal hearing sensitivity. There is now clear experimental evidence that DPOAE amplitude is slightly larger and, more importantly, sensitivity to cochlear dysfunction is enhanced, when the intensity of the f_2 primary (referred to as L_2) is lower in intensity than the f_1 primary (L_1). An appropriate overall stimulus intensity level for generating DPOAE clinically is about 55 to 65 dB, and an appropriate relative intensity difference is 10 to 15 dB. Therefore a DPOAE intensity arrangement of $L_1 = 65$ and $L_2 = 55$ dB is typically used clinically, at least initially.

The rationale underlying the DPOAE measurement strategy discussed here, including the selection of appropriate stimulus and acquisition parameters is thoroughly reviewed in Chapter 4.

The DPOAE response is the actual intermodulation distortion product (DP) produced by the ear when stimulated by these two closely spaced tones. In human ears, the prominant DP appears at the frequency defined by the simple equation $2f_1-f_2$, although DPs at other frequencies are possible (refer again to Figure 9). A clinical DPOAE device performs a spectral analysis of energy in the ear canal following stimulus presentation, and specifically searches for a peak in energy around this frequency. That energy is calculated in dB and compared to noise in the same frequency region. Noise is always present in the ear canal during DPOAE (or TEOAE) measurement, but more so for frequencies below about 1500 Hz. Sources of the noise are both ambient (environmental) and physiologic (patient). The results of animal experiments and clinical studies confirm that the region of the cochlea that is activated with this stimulus arrangement, that is, a frequency ratio of f_2/f_1 and intensities of $L_1 = 65$ and $L_2 = 55$ dB, is near the f_2 place.

DPOAEs are plotted in one of two ways. The most common format is the DPgram, illustrated in Figure 1–8. The DPgram is a graph of DPOAE amplitude as a function of the stimulus frequency. The stimulus frequency, usually as the f_2 primary in Hz, is plotted along the horizontal axis. The DP amplitude is plotted in dB SPL on the verti-

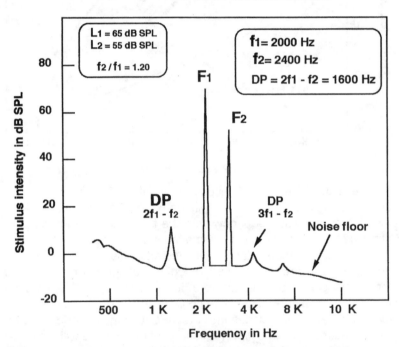

DPOAE Measurement

Figure 1–7. Major stimulus parameters in the measurement of distortion product OAEs (DPOAEs). The stimuli, or primaries, are labeled f_1 (lower frequency) and f_2 (higher frequency). The intensity level of these stimuli is indicated by the label L (i.e., L_1 and L_2). In this typical example, $L_1 = 65$ dB SPL and $L_2 = 55$ dB SPL. The relation or spacing between the two frequencies is described as the f2/f1 ratio (typically about 1.20). The distortion product (DP) recorded from the cochlea with presentation of these stimuli appears at other frequencies. The prominant DP in humans is at the frequency defined by the equation $2f_1 - f_2$, although DPs at other frequency regions are not uncommon. The noise levels or floors are always measured during OAE recording. Noise invariably is progressively greater for the lower frequency regions.

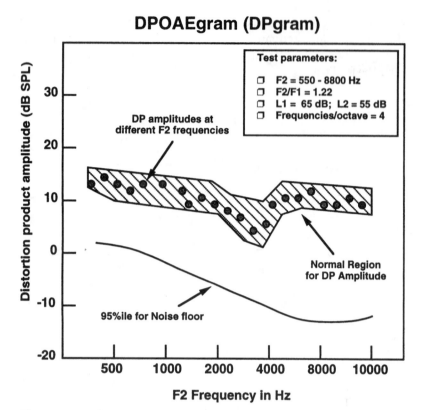

Figure 1-8. Schematic depiction of a DPOAEgram, sometimes abbreviated as DPgram. DP amplitude (vertical axis) is plotted as a function of stimulus frequency, here the f_2 stimulus. The number of stimulus frequencies per octave and the number of octaves included in the test can be manipulated by the tester. In this example of a diagnostic test, DPOAEs are plotted for four frequencies per octave, and for frequencies over a range from 500 to 10,000 Hz. The hatched region reflects a normal range for DPOAE amplitudes in an adult population, whereas the circles indicate DPOAE amplitude for an individual patient. The upper limit (95th percentile) for noise within the ear canal of adults (in the same test setting) is shown as a solid line. The DPOAE data shown in this figure are interpreted as normal.

cal axis. Each data point in the figure is the DP amplitude averaged for a number of presentations for the corresponding frequency. For each stimulus frequency, the noise floor in the region of the DP frequency $(2f_1 - f_2)$ is also plotted. To be considered a valid DPOAE, the DP amplitude must exceed the noise floor value by at least 3 dB. Normal DP amplitudes fall within an appropriate normative region (shaded in this figure). In recording DPOAE, the clinician can select a number of test parameters, including the stimulus intensity, the frequency region over which the recording will be done (maximum is

500 to about 8000 or 10,000 Hz), and the number of stimulus frequencies per octave (e.g., 1, 3, 6, etc.). DPOAE measurement and analysis are reviewed comprehensively in Chapter 4.

RELATION BETWEEN OAEs AND HEARING SENSITIVITY

OAEs are a very sensitive, clinically feasible measure of cochlear (outer hair cell) function. Already, OAEs are an integral part of the audiologic test battery. They can play an important role in the early identification and diagnosis of auditory dysfunction in varied pediatric and adult populations. OAEs can also be applied as an efficient and generally accurate tool for newborn hearing screening. However, neither TEOAE nor DPOAE are tests of hearing. In fact, there are a number of reasons why OAE will never replace the audiogram in hearing assessment. Selected important reasons are summarized in Table 1–3. Despite this lack of correlation between OAE and conventional audiometry, or really because of it, OAE makes a truly unique contri-

OAEs complement — rather than supplement — the audiogram. Think about this everytime OAE findings don't seem to fit with pure tone audiometry for a patient. The discrepancies are good because interpreted together they more fully describe the patient's auditory function.

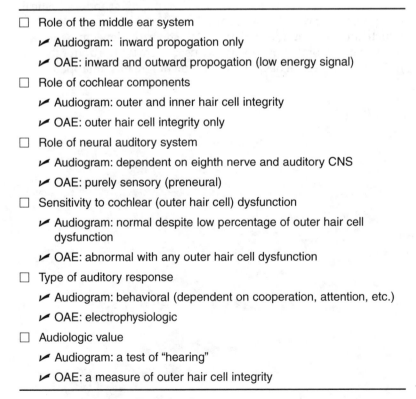

Table 1–3. Reasons why OAE will never replace the audiogram in estimating degree of hearing sensitivity loss.

☐ Role of the middle ear system

   ✔ Audiogram: inward propogation only

   ✔ OAE: inward and outward propogation (low energy signal)

☐ Role of cochlear components

   ✔ Audiogram: outer and inner hair cell integrity

   ✔ OAE: outer hair cell integrity only

☐ Role of neural auditory system

   ✔ Audiogram: dependent on eighth nerve and auditory CNS

   ✔ OAE: purely sensory (preneural)

☐ Sensitivity to cochlear (outer hair cell) dysfunction

   ✔ Audiogram: normal despite low percentage of outer hair cell dysfunction

   ✔ OAE: abnormal with any outer hair cell dysfunction

☐ Type of auditory response

   ✔ Audiogram: behavioral (dependent on cooperation, attention, etc.)

   ✔ OAE: electrophysiologic

☐ Audiologic value

   ✔ Audiogram: a test of "hearing"

   ✔ OAE: a measure of outer hair cell integrity

bution to clinical audiology. How and why OAEs are used in clinical audiology is the subject of this *Handbook of Otoacoustic Emissions*.

CLINICAL APPLICATIONS OF OAEs

Our appreciation and understanding of how OAEs can be exploited clinically is by no means complete. The list of clinical applications of OAEs is sure to grow longer in years to come.

Major clinical applications of OAEs in children and adults are summarized in Table 1–4. OAE are now an indispensable component in the pediatric diagnostic test battery (see Chapter 8 for details). With very young or difficult-to-test children, measurement of OAEs is rapidly becoming the standard-of-care. Another popular pediatric application of OAEs is newborn hearing screening. One of the most valuable and powerful uses of OAEs, especially DPOAEs with high-frequency stimuli, is monitoring ill patients for ototoxicity. There are a variety of OAE applications in adult patient populations, most deriving from the high sensitivity of OAEs to cochlear dysfunction even when the audiogram is unaffected.

CONCLUDING COMMENTS

Given the numerous clinical advantages offered by OAEs, additional useful roles in the audiologic assessment of children and adults are sure to be discovered in the new millenium. Also, within the next few years, a number of technical advances in equipment and sophisticated strategies and techniques for stimulating and recording OAEs, which are now at the experimental stage of development, will become incorporated into everyday use. There is little doubt that the full clinical potential of OAE measurement remains untapped.

Table 1–4. Clinical applications of OAEs and their rationale.

Application	Rationale
Newborn hearing screening	✓ OAEs can be recorded reliably from newborn infants
	✓ OAE recording can be performed in nursery setting (test performance may be affected by noise)
	✓ Normal OAEs are recorded in persons with normal sensory (cochlear) function
	✓ OAEs are abnormal in persons with even mild degrees of sensory hearing loss; the main objective of screening is to detect sensory hearing impairment
	✓ OAE recording may require relatively brief test time
	✓ OAE measurement may be performed by nonaudiologic personnel (e.g., at reduced cost)
Pediatric audiometry	✓ OAE recording is electrophysiologic and not dependent on patient behavioral response
	✓ OAEs assess cochlear function specifically (behavioral audiometry and ABR are also dependent on the status of the central auditory nervous system)
	✓ OAEs can be recorded from sleeping or sedated children
	✓ OAE recording requires relatively short test time
	✓ OAEs provide ear specific audiologic information
	✓ OAEs provide frequency specific audiologic information
	✓ OAEs are a valuable contribution to the "crosscheck principle"
Diagnosis of CAPD	✓ OAE recording is electrophysiologic and not dependent on patient behavioral response
	✓ OAEs are a sensitive means of ruling out cochlear (outer hair cell) dysfunction
Assessment in suspected functional hearing loss	✓ OAE recording is electrophysiologic, and not dependent on patient behavioral response
	✓ Normal OAEs usually imply normal sensory function
	✓ OAEs provide frequency-specific audiologic information
Differentiation of cochlear vs. retrocochlear auditory dysfunction	✓ OAEs are site-specific for cochlear (sensory) auditory dysfunction
	✓ In combination with ABR, OAEs can clearly distinguish sensory from neural auditory disorders
Monitoring ototoxicity	✓ OAEs are site-specific for cochlear (sensory) auditory dysfunction
	✓ Ototoxic drugs exert their effect on outer hair cell function; OAEs are dependent on outer hair cell integrity

(continued)

Table 1–4. *(continued)*

Application	Rationale
Monitoring ototoxicity *(continued)*	✔ OAE recording is electrophysiologic and not dependent on patient behavioral response; can be recorded from patients who, due to their medical condition, are unable to perform behavioral audiometry tasks or from infants and young children
	✔ OAEs can detect cochlear dysfunction before it is evident by pure tone audiometry
	✔ OAEs provide frequency-specific audiologic information
Tinnitus	✔ OAEs are site-specific for cochlear (sensory) auditory dysfunction
	✔ OAEs can provide objective confirmation of cochlear dysfunction in patients with tinnitus and normal audiograms
	✔ OAEs provide frequency-specific audiologic information which may be associated with the frequency region of tinnitus
Noise/music exposure	✔ OAEs are site-specific for cochlear (sensory) auditory dysfunction
	✔ Excessive noise/music intensity levels affect outer hair cell function; OAEs are dependent on outer hair cell integrity
	✔ OAEs can provide objective confirmation of cochlear dysfunction in patients with normal audiograms
	✔ OAE findings are associated with cochlear frequency specificity, i.e., "tuning"; musician complaints of auditory dyfunction can be confirmed by OAE findings, even with a normal audiogram
	✔ OAEs can provide an early and reliable "warning sign" of cochlear dysfunction due to noise/music exposure before any problem is evident in the audiogram

CHAPTER

2

Anatomy and Physiology

The four regions of the auditory system that either contribute to the generation of OAEs, or can influence OAE recording, are the: (1) external ear canal, (2) middle ear system, (3) cochlea, and (4) efferent auditory system (see Figure 2–1). The clinician must have a clear understanding of the anatomy and physiology of these auditory regions. This information is not merely esoteric and of interest only to serious, advanced graduate audiology students. Rather, the information is practical and directly applicable daily in successfully recording, accurately analyzing, and meaningfully interpreting OAE in varied patient populations. Time spent studying current basic research findings from the laboratory on, for example, outer hair cell morphology and physiology will pay off as one measures OAEs in the clinic. The following review highlights some of the more important principles of anatomy and physiology. It is by no means all inclusive, and new findings are being reported at an ever increasing rate. Also, the clinician performing OAE procedures is encouraged to read the references cited throughout and listed at the conclusion, of the chapter.

EXTERNAL EAR

The external ear canal is of critical importance in OAE recordings. It's the place where OAE measurement begins and ends. Take a few moments to inspect the external ear canal before inserting the OAE probe, and always consider this anatomic region whenever OAE findings are abnormal.

For almost all audiologic measurements, the stimulus is presented to the patient via the external ear canal, either directly with some type of earphone or remotely via a loudspeaker in the sound field. The exceptions to this general principle are, of course, procedures utilizing bone-conduction stimulation. The external ear canal typically functions, therefore, as a conduit for delivering an acoustic stimulus—tones,

AUDITORY SYSTEM PATHWAYS

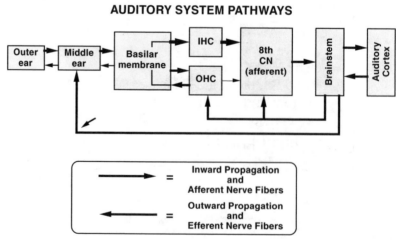

Figure 2–1. Flowchart summarizing major regions involved in the afferent and efferent auditory pathways. At several levels there is "motor feedback" that influences sensory auditory function.

speech, clicks—to the inner ear. The response is then usually recorded proximal to the external ear canal, that is, from the middle ear (e.g., immittance measures), the inner ear (e.g., ECochG), the eighth cranial nerve and brain stem (e.g., ABR), or more rostral auditory regions, including the highest levels of auditory cortex (e.g., AMLR or speech audiometry).

For OAEs, in contrast, the stimulus—a sound—is presented via the external ear canal and the response—the OAEs, also a sound—are recorded in the external ear canal. Thus, the external ear canal plays a dual, and really critical, role in OAE measurement. It is important to rule out, or at the least carefully document, pathology of the external ear canal prior to OAE measurement. But even nonpathologic conditions involving the external ear canal, such as cerumen, debris, foreign objects, or vernix casseosa in neonates, must be taken into account and considered whenever OAE findings are not entirely normal. Some of the more common problems associated with the probe in the external canal are summarized in Table 2–1. With TEOAE measurement, the probe contains one opening for presentation of the single stimulus (usually an acoustic click) and another for the OAEs, which leads to the microphone within the probe. The probe used for DPOAE measurement has three openings, or ports. One for each of the two primary frequency stimuli (f_1 and f_2) and the third for the DPOAE signal (typically at the frequency $2f_1-f_2$), leading again to the microphone within the probe. For both TEOAEs and DPOAEs, even a miniscule particle of cerumen or debris may partially or totally occlude these small-diameter openings, as illustrated schematically in Figure 2–2. The result may be a reduction in stimulus intensity, or possibly total absence of a stimulus in the ear canal. In either case, OAE data are invalid. Even if the stimulus openings in the probe are open and the stimulus is presented at the desired (target) intensity levels, partial or complete blockage of the microphone opening will either reduce measurable OAE activity or entirely eliminate detection of the OAEs.

Finally, in the absence of any pathologic or nonpathologic conditions, the natural and normal acoustics of the external ear canal can affect clinical OAE measurements. There are well-known differences in ear canal resonances and acoustics among children versus adults, and as a function of gender, that are related to variations in ear canal sizes and dimensions (Mueller & Hall, 1998, pp. 415–417). Intrasubject or patient differences are also possible for the right versus left ear. Standing waves can confound stimulus presentation with pure tone signals in any sound field, including the ear canal.

The standing wave problem is limited to DPOAE measurement, and only for higher stimulus frequencies (above 5000 Hz). The physical basis for standing waves in OAE measurement and guidelines for trouble-shooting standing wave problems in clinical measurement of DPOAEs are detailed in Chapter 5. The take-home message for clini-

Table 2–1. Summary of assorted external ear canal factors potentially influencing clinical OAE measurement.

Factor	Influence
NONPATHOLOGIC	
■ Probe tip placement or condition	✔ The soft (rubber or foam) probe tip on the rigid probe assembly extends medially beyond the stimulus or microphone ports and occludes either or all, *or*
	✔ Foam probe tip on the rigid probe assembly is compressed too much, narrowing or occluding one or more of the tiny tubular openings and preventing an adequate stimulus delivery to the ear canal or detection of the OAEs in the external ear canal
■ Probe insertion	✔ In a tortuous external ear canal with abrupt turns, the end of the probe tip on the rigid probe presses up against the canal wall
	✔ Blockage of stimulus energy delivery from the probe to the tympanic membrane
	✔ Blockage of OAE energy return from the tympanic membrane to the microphone probe
■ Standing waves	✔ Artifactual reduction or enhancement of DPOAE amplitude (for stimulus frequencies >5000 Hz)
	✔ Unreliable DPOAEs (for stimulus frequencies >5000 Hz)
	✔ Bogus or artifactually present DPOAEs (for stimulus frequencies >5000 Hz) when in fact DPOAE are absent
■ Cerumen or debris	✔ Occlusion of one or two stimulus ports (tubes) in the OAE probe, reducing stimulus amplitude
	✔ Occlusion of the tube leading to the microphone in the OAE probe
	✔ Blockage of stimulus energy delivery from the probe to the tympanic membrane
	✔ Blockage of OAE energy return from the tympanic membrane to the microphone probe
■ Vernix (neonates)	✔ Occlusion of one or two stimulus ports (tubes) in the OAE probe, reducing stimulus amplitude
	✔ Occlusion of the tube leading to the microphone in the OAE probe
	✔ Blockage of stimulus energy delivery from the probe to the tympanic membrane
	✔ Blockage of OAE energy return from the tympanic membrane to the microphone probe
PATHOLOGIC	
■ Stenosis	✔ Blockage of stimulus energy delivery from the probe to the tympanic membrane
	✔ Blockage of OAE energy return from the tympanic membrane to the microphone probe
■ External otitis or cyst	✔ Blockage of stimulus energy delivery from the probe to the tympanic membrane
	✔ Blockage of OAE energy return from the tympanic membrane to the microphone probe
	✔ Pain or discomfort preventing adequately deep probe fit within the external ear canal

DISTORTION PRODUCT OAEs

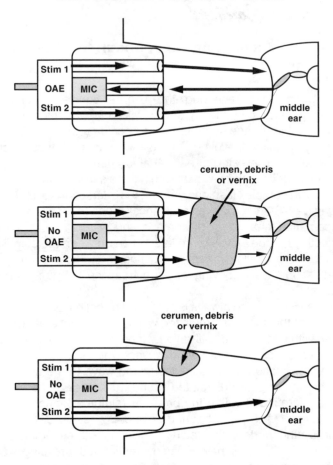

Figure 2–2. Illustration of inteference with OAE stimulus presentation and/or response detection due to external ear canal pathology, cerumen, or debris.

cians is that close otoscopic inspection of the external ear canal, and usually immittance measurement, is necessary whenever OAE findings are in any way abnormal. *Otoscopic inspection prior to all OAE measurements is an advisable clinical practice.* The exception to this general practice principle is OAE hearing screening.

MIDDLE EAR

Acoustic stimuli usually reach the ear as sound waves traveling through the air. These sound waves must be converted to mechanical vibrations before the energy reaches the inner ear. When mother

Clinical Concept

Standing Waves Can Be Found in the External Ear Canal

During OAE recording, the external ear canal contains sound generated by the patient (physiologic), the test environment (ambient), and sometimes the cochlea (e.g., SOAE without any stimulus or evoked OAE following appropriate acoustic stimulation). The external ear canal is, therefore, a very busy sound field. The sound waves within the external ear canal can interact in complex fashions. Among the interactions are *standing waves*. Standing waves are cancellations (nodes) and reinforcements (antinodes) of some sound waves due to either reflections of the waves or an interaction between the stimulus sound wave moving toward the tympanic membrane and the OAE sound wave moving outward from the tympanic membrane.

OAE recording always is preceded by calibration or equalization of the stimulus amplitude within the patient's ear canal. Even with appropriate calibration, standing wave problems can produce cancellation of sound waves, which reduce or eliminate propagation of the stimulus sound wave to the tympanic membrane or the OAE-related sound wave back to the equipment microphone within the probe or reinforce (enhance) the stimulus- or OAE-related sound waves. As a result, OAE amplitude is either underestimated (OAE is incorrectly assumed to be abnormal or not even present) or overestimated. Standing wave artifacts are most bothersome for high-frequency stimuli (>5000 Hz) used in DPOAE measurement. The only fail-proof solution to the problem of standing waves is placement of the microphone at the tympanic membrane which is, unfortunately, not clinically feasible at this time.

For more information, see Siegel (1994).

nature designed the middle ear, she no doubt was concentrating on optimizing this delivery of acoustic stimuli from the relatively low-impedance air medium to the relatively high-impedance fluid medium of the cochlea. The impedance matching provided by the middle ear effectively reduces the influence of this impedance mismatch, and thus enhances hearing sensitivity (Figure 2–3). The areal ratio difference between the tympanic membrane and stapes footplate, and the

IMPEDANCE MATCHING FUNCTION OF
THE MIDDLE EAR SYSTEM

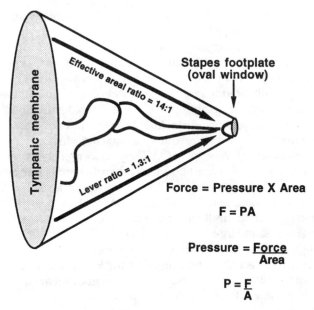

**Stapes footplate
(oval window)**

Effective areal ratio = 14:1

Tympanic membrane

Lever ratio = 1.3:1

Force = Pressure X Area

F = PA

Pressure = Force
          Area

$$P = \frac{F}{A}$$

Figure 2–3. Schematic diagram of middle ear anatomy and mechanical advantages that contribute to reduction of the impedance mismatch between the air in the ear canal and the fluid within the inner ear.

Assessment of middle ear status with immittance measures is essential whenever OAEs are not recordable. Meaningful interpretation of OAEs depends on documentation of normal middle ear function.

ossicular lever system, certainly offers an advantage for inward propagation of energy from the ear canal to the inner ear, including the stimuli used in OAE measurement. OAE measurement is, however, not limited to this inward propagation of energy. OAE measurement requires a round-trip ticket. Energy generated within the cochlea must find its way outward, and backward, through the middle ear system and into the ear canal. The air-to-fluid impedance mismatch mechanism does not enhance the fluid-to-air route taken by OAE energy. In fact, outward propagation is under the best of conditions (e.g., normal middle ear status) really an uphill journey against significant physical odds. No one has ever reported the actual strength or amplitude of OAEs in humans at the level of the cochlea, before the loss of energy due to the inefficient reverse passage through the middle ear system. It is likely, however, that up to 15 dB of OAE energy is lost from the cochlea to the external ear canal. Remarkably, using this estimate of energy dissipation and OAE amplitude values of 25 dB or more in some young and otologically normal subjects, one could infer actual OAE strength in the cochlea of over 40 dB, a value quite similar to enhancement of hearing sensitivity that is attributed to the cochlear amplification of outer hair cell motility.

The middle ear system is, therefore, a vital and unavoidable link in OAE measurement. The practical implication of this statement is clear and vital for clinical application of OAEs. Middle ear dysfunction, or even very subtle deviations from normal middle ear function, may have serious effects on OAE amplitude. Middle ear and/or tympanic membrane disorders or related aberrations are plentiful in a clinical setting, especially among pediatric populations, and include scarred, monomeric, or perforated tympanic membranes; ventilation tubes in the tympanic membranes; eustachian tube dysfunction and resulting negative middle ear pressure; otitis media; cholesteatoma; otosclerosis; and many others. Whenever OAEs are abnormal or not detectable, middle ear dysfunction must be effectively ruled out before any statement can be made regarding cochlear status. Put another way, one must always assume that OAE abnormality or absence is due to middle ear dysfunction until proven otherwise, even in persons with audiometric hearing thresholds within clinically normal limits. In general, slight middle ear disorders that may not entirely obscure OAE measurement affect OAE findings first for lower frequency stimuli. Clinically, immittance measurement to verify middle ear status is indicated whenever OAE results are abnormal.

Fortunately for clinicians, particularly those assessing auditory status of young or difficult-to-test children, there is a positive side to the dependence of OAE on middle ear status. If OAE findings are unequivocally normal, that is, OAE amplitude values are within an appropriate normal region for all test frequencies (e.g., 500 to 8000 Hz), then it is safe to conclude that middle ear function is reasonably normal. Thus, the clinician assessing the auditory function of a young child might begin with OAE measurement, rather than immittance measurement. If OAE findings are entirely and unequivocally normal, one can reasonably, and often quickly, conclude that middle ear and cochlear (outer hair cell) function is intact. This does not, of course, imply that "hearing" is normal. The interpretation of OAE findings in the context of the audiologic test battery is reviewed in detail in later chapters. If OAEs are abnormal or absent, however, further assessment with immittance, behavioral pure tone and/or speech audiometric, or auditory evoked response techniques is clearly in order.

COCHLEA

Overview

That OAEs are generated by cochlear structures is now a well-proven fact. A detailed review of cochlear, and specifically cochlear hair cell, anatomy and physiology is far beyond the scope of this book. However, because a clear and comprehensive understanding of this topic is essential for the clinician performing OAE procedures, the reader is directed to key references at the end of the chapter. Investment in a recent textbook devoted to a thorough review of cochlear structure, micromechanics, hair cell physiology (including motility), and the efferent auditory system would be money well spent. Slepecky (1996), in particular, provides an updated and detailed, yet readable, review of cochlear structure. The following information was drawn in part from her chapter in the book *The Cochlea.*

Located within the temporal bone, reportedly the hardest bone in the body, the human cochlea consists of a bony, coiled tube (bony labyrinth) that is subdivided into three compartments (Figure 2–4). The tube curls around a central core, the *modiolus.* Two of the compartments (the lower *scala tympani* and the upper *scala vestibuli*) are filled with perilymph (high in sodium), whereas the other compartment (*scala media*) is filled with endolymph (high in potassium). The stapes footplate is coupled to the scala vestibuli, so mechanical energy conveyed through the middle ear and reaching the stapes produces inward-outward pistonlike movements of the stapes footplate. Pressure vibrations are then transmitted from the base to the apex of the cochlea through the perilymph of the scala vestibuli. At the apex, perilymph of the scala vestibula continues into perilymph of the scala tympani via a small passageway, the *helicotrema.* The scala tympani ends, practically speaking, at the round window. Between the scalae vestibuli and tympani is the scala media, bounded on the lower side by a wall consisting, medially (from the modiolus) to laterally (toward the stria vascularis) of three continuous structures (the *spiral limbus*, the *basilar membrane*, and the *spiral ligament*) and on the upper side by Reissner's membrane (Figure 2–4). The stimulus-related vibrations in perilymph deform the flexible basilar membrane with a wavelike motion. Technically, these are the boundries for the cochlear duct, but not the fluid-filled cavity. Endolymph makes direct contact with the specialized cells (e.g., hair cells, Hensen's and Claudius' cells). Within the cochlea are dozens of anatomic structures, in addition to the major structures that are noted in Figure 2–4.

Research on how the cochlea works is progressing at a staggering pace. To confirm this statement, just check out the website for the Association for Research in Otolaryngology (www.aro.org). Most clinicians who've been out of graduate school for a few years will benefit from a thorough review of current information on cochlear anatomy and physiology. Some of the many recent books summarizing the results of basic hearing science are listed at the end of this chapter.

The traditional diagram of the scala media (shown in Figure 2–4) highlights most of the cochlear structures that play a role directly or indirectly in hearing, and generation of OAEs. In this figure, the central core of the cochlea (modiolus) is to the left and the lateral wall of the bony labyrinth is to the right. As the cochlea curls upward from base to apex, there are numerous modifications in the structures shown in this figure, and in their function. To appreciate the dynamic nature of the cochlear better, take a few moments to review some of the more prominant base-to-apex changes, as summarized in Table 2–2. The *basilar membrane* is suspended between two rigid structures that pro-

Clinical Concept

Nonlinearity Is Normal

Sources of nonlinearity in the peripheral auditory system. Nonlinearity in cochlear function is reviewed in detail elsewhere in this chapter.

■ *Linearity*: "The response to the sum of two stimulus signals is the sum of the responses to the stimuli separately. This property has the consequence that response magnitude is proportional to stimulus magnitude. From the same property it can be proven that the response to a sinusoidal stimulus is sinusoidal too."
(de Boer, 1996, p. 296)

■ In a nonlinear system, the amplitude of the response is not proportional to the amplitude of the stimulus. Nonlinearity is a feature of cochlear and eighth nerve function.

■ *Cochlear nonlinearity* is complex, mechanical, and usually compressive, i.e., response amplitude is less than stimulus amplitude. However, it is also characterized by components in the response that are not part of the stimulus, such as:
  ✔ *harmonics* (sinusoidal components at multiples of one or more stimulus frequencies),
  ✔ *intermodulation products* or *combination tones* (produced when the stimuli are two or more sine waves), which consist of not just the stimulus frequencies and harmonics, but also sounds that are integral combinations (e.g., $2f_1 - f_2$) of the primary frequencies (e.g., f_1 and f_2). Referred to as *distortion products*, their frequencies are mathematically predicted by the equation: $(n_1 f_1 \pm n_2 f_2)$, where f_1 and f_2 are integers.

■ *Neural nonlinearity* response measures include firing rates for auditory nerve fibers or neural components in the temporal response pattern. Some nonlinear effects due not to mechanical properties of the cochlea but, rather, neural synapses are:
  ✔ adaptation
  ✔ saturation
  ✔ refractory properties
  ✔ masking.

Source: de Boer (1996).

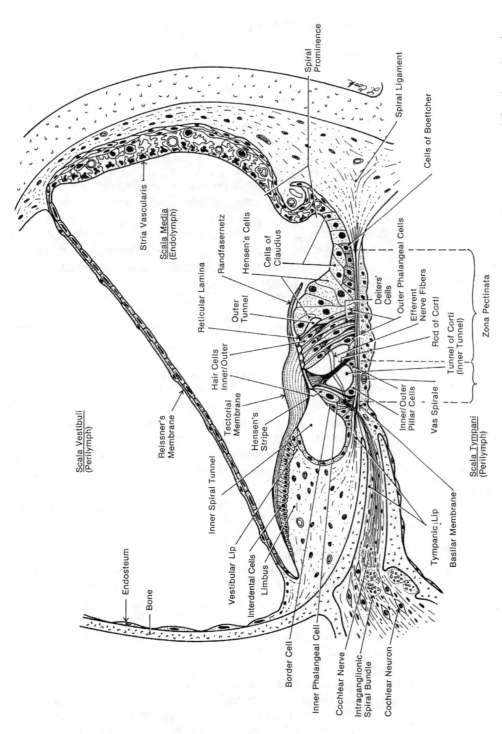

Figure 2–4. Traditional cross-sectional view of the cochlear showing the basilar membrane, organ of Corti, and major anatomic structures within the cochlea. The lateral cochlea (e.g., stria vascularis) is toward the right, with the medial extension to the modiolas on the left. Reprinted with permission from Schuknecht HR. *Pathology of the Ear* (2nd ed). Baltimore, MD: Williams & Wilkins, 1993, p. 50. Copyright 1993 Williams & Wilkins.

Clinical Concept

The Cochlea Is Where the Action Is

Active processes in the cochlea may occur without any stimulus, giving rise to spontaneous otoacoustic emissions. When a stimulus is presented to the ear, mechanical and electrical events together can greatly enhance vibrations of the basilar membrane. This is good for hearing, and coincidentally produces otoacoustic emissions.

Lots of activity requires lots of energy. Not surprisingly, metabolism of the cochlea is higher than most organs in the body (Johnstone & Sellick, 1972; Patuzzi, 1996). The clinical implication is also clear. Outer hair cell function is affected by almost anything that can go wrong with the cochlea, and otoacoustic emissions are an extremely sensitive measure of cochlear functioning. Much more on that topic can be found in Chapters 6, 8, and 9.

ject horizontally into the cochlea. The basilar membrane is connected medially to the spiral limbus (far left in Figure 2–4) and laterally to the spiral ligament, just below the spiral prominence, a bump in this ligament. Most of the cochlear structures, such as this ligament, are actually composed of numerous cells. Composition of the basilar membrane itself is quite complex, with several different layers and membranes, an extracellular matrix substance, along with several types of collagen and various proteins. As summarized in Table 2–2, there are base-to-apex alterations in basilar membrane size and mechanical properties. There are also two distinct zones or regions. One, the pars tecta (or arcuate zone) runs from the spiral limbus (medial end) to just under the outer pillar cells; whereas the pars pectinata (or pectinate zone) continues laterally to the spiral ligament. Completing the lateral wall of the cochlea, and forming the lateral boundary for endolymph, is the stria vascularis. The stria is a really important structure in the generation of OAEs and for interpreting OAE findings in certain patient populations (e.g., patients receiving ototoxic medications, such as furosemide).

Resting on the basilar membrane, directly or indirectly, are over a dozen specific types of cells and/or structures that have intimate and often complex interrelations. Toward the center of the basilar membrane is the *organ of Corti*, the most famous of these structures. The support for the organ of Corti is provided by the inner (medial, or left in

Table 2–2. Summary of changes in cochlear structures from the base to apex, and from the medial (inner toward modiolus) to more lateral (outer toward stria vascularis) portions.

Structure	Base	Apex	Inner	Outer
Diameter of bony labyrinth	wider	narrower		
Basilar membrane	narrower	wider		
	more stiff	less stiff		
Tectorial membrane	less mass	greater mass		
Inner hair cell stereocilia	shorter	longer	shorter	longer
	more stiff	less stiff		
Outer hair cell stereocilia	shorter	longer	shorter	longer
	more stiff	less stiff		
Deiters' cells	smaller	larger	smaller	larger
Boettcher's cells	present	absent		
Efferent innervation: inner hair cells	ipsilateral origin	contralateral origin		
Efferent innervation: outer hair cells	more terminals project over a limited region	less terminals branch to more distant outer hair cells	more terminals	less terminals
	more acetylcholine at synapses	more GABA at synapses		
Endolymph (scala media) DC resting potential	80 mV	slightly less		

Figure 2–4) and outer (lateral, or right in Figure 2–4) pillars. Between the pillars is the tunnel of Corti, which is filled with endolymph. Medial to the inner pillars is a single row of inner hair cells (see Tables 2–2 and 2–4) for specific information on these and other cochlear structures, and their relationships). Lateral to the outer pillars are three or four rows of outer hair cells. Below and to the lateral side of (but not closely adjacent to) the outer hair cells are other cells which provide either structural or metabolic support (e.g., Deiters' cells, Hensen's cells, Claudius' cells). The uppermost organ of Corti structure is the reticular lamina. Curious to know whose names are attached to these cochlear cells? Several are summarized in Table 2–3.

A prominent structure that contributes importantly to cochlear mechanics and sensory function is the *tectorial membrane* (Figure 2–4). The three-layered tectorial membrane is located just above and parallel to the recticular lamina. It is composed of gel-like substances arranged as a dense network of two different types of fibers (types A and B), with minimally three types of collagen and abundant glycoproteins. The presence of collagen contributes to the tectorial membrane's strength and resistance to stretching, that is, its capacity to withstand considerable mechanical stress associated with cochlear fluid vibrations, basilar membrane movement, and outer hair cell elongation and shortening. There is direct contact between the undersurface of the tectorial membrane and the tallest stereocilia of the outer

Table 2-3. Who were those people whose names are affixed to structures within the cochlea?

Claudius' cells: Friedrich Claudius (1822–1869) was an Austrian anatomist. A fossa in the posterior portion of the pelvis is also named for Friedrich.

Deiters' cells: Otto F. C. Deiters (1834–1863) was a German anatomist. He also gave his name to a nucleus and a process (within a neuron).

Hensen's cells: Victor Hensen (1835–1924) was a German anatomist and physiologist. He also had a disk (feature of striated muscle) and a stripe (a dark band on the under surface of the tectorial membrane) named after him.

organ of Corti: Alfonso Corti (1822–1888) was an Italian anatomist. A street in Milano is named after him, along with a tunnel (not in Milano, but within the organ of Corti).

Reissner's membrane: Ernest Reissner (1824–1878) was a German anatomist.

Nuel's space: Jean P. Nuel (1847–1920) was a Belgium oculist.

Cochlear Fluids and Cerebral Spinal Fluids Mingle, and the Cochlea Interacts With the Vestibular Portion of the Inner Ear

In the basal-most end of the cochlea, the scala tympani does not completely dead-end at the round window. The cochlear aqueduct, a narrow canal, provides a passageway for perilymph to blend with cerebrospinal fluid.

Also, the scala tympani and scala vestibuli connect at the apical end of the cochlea via the helicotrema (Gr. *helix* = coil + *trema* = a hole). The scala media continues on to the saccule via the ductus reunions.

---

hair cells (in a region known as Hardesty's membrane). Whether inner hair cell stereocilia normally attach to, or even contact, the tectorial membrane (if so, in the Hensen's stripe region) is debated. Further upward, *Reissner's membrane forms* the top border between the scala media and scala vestibuli. Avascular but metabolically active, Reissner's membrane consists of two layers of cells (epithelial and mesothelial), which make contact, respectively, with endolymph of the scala media and perilymph of the scala vestibuli.

Outer Hair Cells

The most important single contributor to OAE production is the unique motility of outer hair cells. Anatomy of the inner and outer hair cells is illustrated in Figures 2–5 and 2–6. Information in this section is adapted from Slepecky (1996), Patuzzi (1996), and other cited key references. Clearly, the two types of hair cells are distinguished by many features, as summarized in Table 2–4. Many of the distinctly different features of the outer hair cells contribute to their capacity for motility, whereas many inner hair cell features preclude their capacity for motility. In humans, outer hair cell length ranges between 30 and 70 μm (Oghalai et al., 1998). Beginning at the top, there are more than 100 delicate stereocilia sitting on the apical surface of the hair cells, arrayed in a "W" (for outer) or "U" (for inner) shape, which consist of microfilaments made of protein substances. Structural differences in stereocilia are found among the three rows and from base to apex (Table 2–2). Taller stereocilia are on the lateral side of the array, whereas shorter stereocilia face medially toward the modiolus. Stereocilia are tapered smaller toward the bottom.

For a "snap-shot" view of how outer hair cell motility contributes to cochlear function and hearing, skip forward to review the sequence of events illustrated in Figure 2–9 (found on page 52).

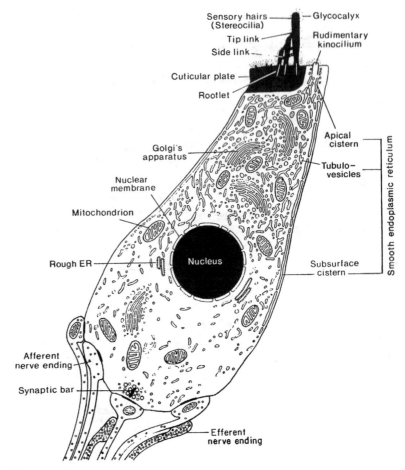

Figure 2–5. Inner hair cell anatomy. Reprinted with permission from Schuknecht HR. *Pathology of the Ear* (2nd ed). Baltimore, MD: Williams & Wilkins, 1993 p. 52. Copyright 1993 Williams & Wilkins.

A plasma membrane on the outside of each stereocilium has a negative electrical charge and helps to keep the stereocilia apart from each other. Rootlets, located within the central core of the stereocilia, are planted within the uppermost (apical) part of the hair cell, a region referred to as the cuticular plate. Tip links connect shorter and longer stereocilia within each row of a bundle, and cross-links connect stereocilia of different rows, again within each bundle, even down to the rootlets (see the highly schematic and simplified Figure 2–7).

These protein linkages among stereocilia are important, really critical, structures in the hair cell's response to stimulation, perhaps by triggering the opening of ion channels of the hair cell and initiating the biochemical processes that underlie motility. The cuticular plate is a specialized region of the hair cell, which also probably contributes to

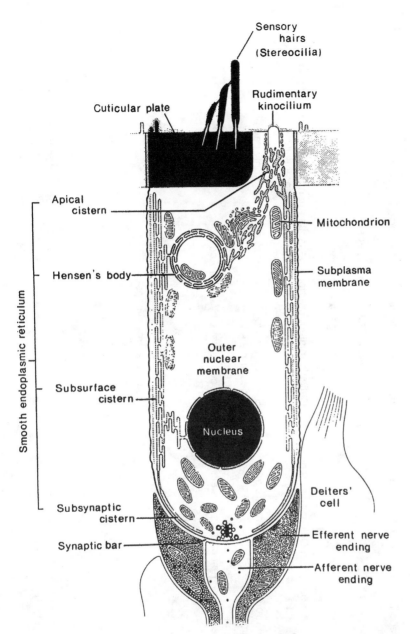

Figure 2–6. Outer hair cell anatomy. Reprinted with permission from Schuknecht HR. *Pathology of the Ear* (2nd ed). Baltimore, MD: Williams & Wilkins, 1993 p. 50. Copyright 1993 Williams & Wilkins.

structural and functional capacities of the hair cell. Most of the intracellular components (e.g., mitochondria, ribosomes, endoplasmic reticulum, nucleus, and many microfilaments and microtubules) are illustrated earlier in Figures 2–5 and 2–6.

Table 2-4. Summary of differences between inner and outer hair cells.

Inner Hair Cells	Outer Hair Cells
1 row	3 or 4 rows
$N = 3500$	$N = 12,000$ to $20,000$
On spiral lamina	On basilar membrane
No contact between stereocilia and reticular membrane	Tallest stereocilia firmly contact tectorial membrane
Stereocilia in flattened "U" shape	Stereocilia in flattened "W" shape
Stereocilia shorter and fatter	Stereocilia longer and thinner
Cuticular plate less homogeneous (than OHC), and made up of actin filaments and dense actin protein α-actinin	Cuticular plate more homogeneous (than for IHC), and made up of filaments arranged randomly and circumferentially
Stereocilia rootlets insert through the cuticular plate and even into apical cytoplasm of IHC	Stereocilia narrow toward base and project only partially into cuticular plate
Do not contact basilar membrane (rest on support cells)	Cupped at base by Deiters' cells
Support cells around IHCs do not have organized bundles of microtubules	
95% of afferents synapse	5% of afferents synapse
Purely sensory	Partly motor
Not motile	Motile
Single layer of discontinuous cisterns below plasma membrane, and connected to the membrane by cross-links	Parallel layers of membranous subsurface cisterns which are linked to mitochrondia and microtubules

Encompassed and touched by support cells	Supported on at top and bottom
IHCs are not separated from each other in the region near the nucleus	OHCs are separated in region near the nucleus (only contacting fluid)
Central nucleus	Nucleus at base of cell
Wine bottle, goblet, or flask shape	Test tube (cylinder) shape, and longer
Wider diameter	Smaller diameter
Single layer endoplasmic reticulum	Extensive subsurface cisternae in ER
Mitochondria are round and scattered	Mitochondria along perimeter of cell
Glycogen content low	Glycogen content high
No acetylcholine	Acetylcholine and γ-aminobutryic acid (GABA) (receptors at base)
Innervated by thick, myelinated type I ganglion cells	Innervated by thin, unmyelinated type II ganglion cells
Hair cell-to-neuron ratio = 1.8:1	Hair cell-to-neuron ratio = 5.7:1
Efferent fibers from lateral superior olive	Efferents from medial superior olive
Efferent fibers synapse on afferent dentrites	Efferent fibers synapse on base of hair cell

Source: Information contributed in part by Marleen T. Ochs, Ph.D., and adapted from Slepecky (1996).

A Few Points About Hair Cell Stereocilia Length and Activity

Stereocilia are arranged in a W- or U- shaped bundle, with the closed (bottom of the letter) portion pointing toward the stria vascularis (laterally). The longer stereocilia also are located on the lateral region of the array. Deflection of the stereocilia bundle toward the tallest produces an excitatory response in the hair cell, whereas a deflection the other direction (toward the modiolus) results in an inhibitory response.

Among the multiple differences between inner and outer hair cells, the most unique feature of outer hair cells is the complex and specialized architecture of the lateral walls. Outer hair cell walls consist of three different and distinct cylindrical components. From the outside-to-inside they are the plasma membrane, the intermediate cortical lattice, and the innermost, the subsurface cisternae (Figure 2–8). Critical mechanical properties of the outer hair cell walls are stiffness, resistence to bending, and elasticity. The walls consist of subsurface cisternae (SSC) that are, in turn, made up of densely arranged parallel lamellae and connected to mitochondria and some of the microtubules. The lateral cisternae, a special part of the endoplasmic membrane, provide structural support for the outer hair cell, but probably figure in high-frequency length changes. Because the cortical lattice on the outer portion of the lateral cisternae consists of chains of rigid segments, and of molecular substances with elastic properties, they are capable of length and shape changes. Finally, one must remember that, in addition to the inner and outer hair cells, a host of other structures are vital for cochlear function, as summarized in Table 2–5.

Outer Hair Cell Motility

Major steps in hair cell response to a sound stimulus, and resulting outer hair cell motility, inner hair cell functional changes, and otoacoustic emissions, are summarized in Figure 2–9.

Outer hair cells have active properties that increase mechanical energy within the cochlea, increasing stimulus-specific vibrations of the basilar membrane. The energy is transmitted to the inner hair cells and enhances hearing sensitivity and tuning (frequency selectivity). Briefly, stimulus-induced macromechanical vibrations of basilar membrane and organ of Corti produce micromechanical vibrations of hair cells. These can in turn exert a "feedback" influence on the macromechanics. Importantly, for outer hair cell activity, there is more basilar membrane vibration laterally, where it is more free to move and

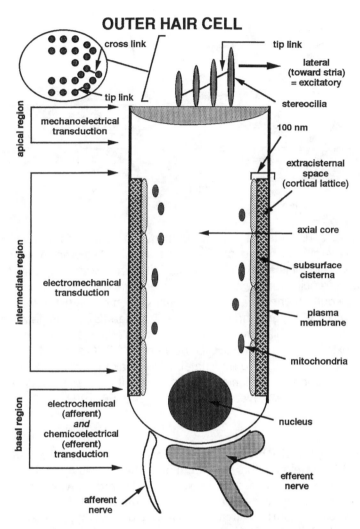

Figure 2–7. Schematic illustration of an outer hair cell with association of processes critical for motility with apical, middle, and lower portions.

where the outer hair cells are located. The initial mechanical events at the hair cell level are deflection of the stereocilia and tensions on the tip and cross-links. These events produce mechanoelectrical transduction (refer to the schematic illustration of an outer hair cell in Figure 2–7), involving current changes at the base of the stereocilia and the cuticular plate, and then the generation of a receptor potential within the hair cell. The changes in voltage across the plasma membrane, not the passage of ionic current, lead directly to outer hair cell length changes. This sequence of events also triggers an active process within the cochlea—stimulus-related oscillations of the outer hair cells. Deflec-

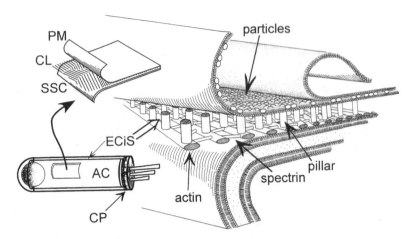

Figure 2–8. Detailed view of the unique structure of the outer hair cell lateral wall based on electron microcope studies. A simplied outer hair cell is shown in the lower left corner, with axial core (AC) and stereocilia roots within the cuticular plate (CP). The three layers of the outer hair cell wall are the plasma membrane (PM), the cortical lattice (CL), and the subsurface cisternae (SSC), as detailed in the upper left. Pillar molecules connect the PM to the CL. Fluid fills the extracisternal space (ECiS) between the SSC and PM. Reprinted with permission from Oshalai, Patel, Nakagawa, and Brownell. Fluorescence-imaged microdeformation of the outer hair cell lateral wall. *The Journal of Neuroscience 18*(1): 48–58, 1998, p. 49.

tion of stereocilia bundles toward the longest stereocilia (lateral), lengthening (elongation), and thinning of the hair cells (and decreased cell surface area) are associated with depolarization, whereas deflections in the opposite direction, shortening, and fattening (and increased cell surface area) are associated with hyperpolarization (Evans & Dallos, 1993). Outer hair cells are connected via Deiters' cells to the basilar membrane and, above, to the recticular lamina. Because the pillar cells of the organ of Corti are quite rigid and the tectorial membrane above is also somewhat stiff, oscillations of the outer hair cells are transmitted to the basilar membrane. The basilar membrane moves up and down, pivoting at the outer pillar, while the reticular lamina also pivots at the arch of Corti. Because the inner hair cells are located medially, partly over the highly rigid spiral lamina, and due to their structural features (review Table 2–4 again), they are incapable of as much movement. This energy normally increases lateral basilar membrane vibration dramatically and helps to overcome the loss of energy from the stimulus associated with the dampening and friction effects of cochlear fluids and mass. As noted by Patuzzi, *"It seems that the 'basilar membrane' should be named the 'basilar plate,' and it is more like a xylophone played under water than Helholtz's piano played in air"* (Patuzzi, 1996, p. 208).

Table 2-5. Cochlear hair cells that are neither inner nor outer (some with and some without filaments). See Figure 2-4 for the location of these cells.

Type	Description
With Filaments	The outer hair cells rest on the flexible basilar membrane. With acoustic stimulation, the basilar membrane is mechanically deformed and stressed. This group of cochlear cells provide a firm structural framework around the outer hair cells. Microfilaments and microtubules contribute to the rigidity of this structure. Flexibility, which is also essential, occurs because the cells are arranged in a criss-cross pattern comparable to a "children's folding gate" (Slepecky, 1996). That is, the apical surfaces (e.g., tops) of support cells are located a few outer hair cells away from their foot processes (e.g., bottoms). The wide base of each of these supporting cells rests on the basilar membrane, whereas the apical portions actually make direct contact with the reticular lamina.
Pillar cells: inner tunnel	The inner tunnel pillar cells separate the *inner hair cells* from the fluid within the tunnel of Corti. There is about one inner tunnel pillar cell for each inner hair cell. The footplates of the inner tunnel pillar cells rest on the basilar membrane. The middle parts of the cells consist of a series of straight microtubules and filaments running up to the reticular lamina. The inner tunnel pillar cells then flatten out along at their apical surface, where they make direct contact and tight junctions with the inner hair cells. However, nerve fibers wind through the inner tunnel pillar cells on the way to the outer hair cells.
Pillar cells: outer tunnel	Because there is one outer tunnel pillar cell for every *outer hair cell* in the first (inner) row, outer tunnel cells outnumber inner tunnel pillar cells. The tops of the outer tunnel pillar cells actually lie underneath the inner tunnel pillar cells and are snugly junctioned with the outer hair cells and Deiter's cells. Fluid surrounds the outer tunnel cells, and is continous with the fluid around the outer hair cells (in the space of Nuel). Importantly, these pillar cells (inner and outer) not only provide support to the cochlea, they also contribute to the transport of fluids from one cochlear compartment to another via pinocytosis.
Deiters' cells	Deiters' cells, which also contain microfilaments and microtubules, run from the basilar membrane to the reticular lamina. Along the way, they encompass the base of the outer hair cells. A unique portion of the Deiters' cells is a slender stalk running at an angle from the base of one outer hair cell at its lower portion to a slightly distant region of the reticular lamina at the upper portion. Similar to the inner and outer hair cells, the Deiters' cells contain mitochondria, cristae, and other organelles. Interestingly, Deiters' cells include a tubulovesicular system and lots of creatine kinase, suggesting considerable energy utilization and more than a simple structural role in the cochlea.
Without Filaments	
Hensen's cells	Column shaped and located outside of the third (last) row of Deiters' cells, Hensen's cells may run from the basilar membrane to the reticular lamina, or they may rest on Boettcher's cells (rather than the basilar membrane). Unlike the pillar cells, they do not contain microtubules or microfilaments. They do, however, contain lipid droplets. Hensen's cells are taller than Claudius cells.

(continued)

Table 2-5. *(continued)*

Type	Description
Claudius cells	Within the space between Deiters' cells and the lateral wall of the cochlea, Claudius cells sit on the basilar membrane and are cuboidal in shape. Technically, Claudius cells are not part of the organ of Corti. The shape of Claudius cells becomes shorter and flatter toward the lateral portion of the cochlea.
Boettcher cells	These cells are located mostly in the base and middle turns of the cochlea, but not in the apex. They lie between the basilar membrane and the Claudius cells.
External sulcus cells	The external sulcus cells form the junction of the basilar membrane with the lateral wall of the cochlea, with extensions from the cells projecting into the spiral ligament. Their uppermost portions come into contact with either endolymph or Claudius cells.

Source: Information adapted in part from Slepecky (1996).

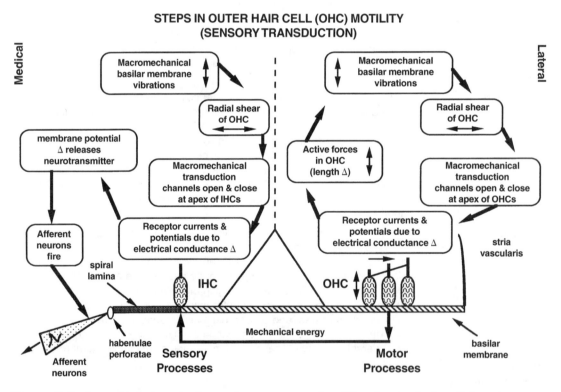

Figure 2–9. Important steps in the motor processes (motility of outer hair cells) and sensory processes (activation of inner hair cells and innervation of afferent fibers of the eighth cranial nerve). Energy from outer hair cell movement is transmitted from the more flexible lateral basilar membrane to the stiffer medial portion of the basilar membrane where the inner hair cells are located. Adapted from Patuzzi R. Cochlear micromechanics and macromechanics. In Dallos P, Popper AN, Fay RR (eds). *The Cochlea*. New York: Springer, 1996, p. 230.

Where's the Motor in the Cochlea?

The movement of the outer hair cells is known as a motor process, whereas the function of the inner hair cells is a sensory process. Where is the motor located? The answer may lie in the "tip theory of transduction."

One possibility is the actin cytoskeleton of the outer hair cell stereocilium. Parallel actin filaments are linked among stereocilia and for each stereocilium to the plasma membrane. The tip links connect to the stereocilium in this region. Evidence of substances such as calmodulin and myosin in the region suggest the presence of a molecular motor. A molecular myosin motor in this region may function in triggering opening or closing (depending on which direction the hair cell bundle is deflected) of the mechanoelectrical ionic transduction channels and in subsequent calcium entry into the stereocilia. These events, in turn, increase or decrease the outer hair cell receptor current (and potential), changes in outer hair cell length (recall that hyperpolarization means lengthening and depolarization means shortening), i.e., motility.

Sources: Patuzzi (1996), Slepecky (1996).

During outer hair cell high-frequency motility, the change in hair cell length is on the order of about 5% (at least in guinea pigs). Latency of these length changes to electrically-induced hyper- and depolarization is about 100 μs. Outer hair cells also can undergo relatively slow changes in length and shape, over the course of seconds or even minutes. It is possible that these slow motility mechanisms may contribute to temporary threshold shifts following extended noise exposure. Contributing to these complex cochlear processes are a variety of biochemical substances, as summarized in Table 2–6.

Blood Supply of the Cochlea

The blood supply to the cochlea originates from the vertebro-basilar system, and the posterior inferior cerebellar artery (PICA). The internal auditory artery from this system runs out to the cochlea through the internal auditory canal. Once in the cochlea, the internal auditory artery branches into the spiral modiolar artery. For the return blood flow, there is a corresponding spiral modiolar vein. Little arterioles radiate off of the spiral modiolar artery to supply blood to different regions and structures of the cochlea, from base to apex (Figure 2–10). Notably, membranes within the cochlea, such as the end portions of

Table 2-6. Summary of biochemical substances found in cochlear structures. Various proteins found in hair cells are shown in Figures 2-5 and 2-6.

Substance	Examples of Structures
■ Collagen	Tectorial membrane; basilar membrane
■ Polypeptides	Tectorial membrane
■ Proteoglycans	Tectorial membrane
■ Fibronectin	Basilar membrane
■ Cytoskeletal proteins	Basilar membrane
■ Actin protein fimbrin	Hair cell stereocilia
■ Spectrin protein	Hair cell walls
■ Profilin protein	Hair cells
■ Actin protein tropomysin	Hair cell stereocilia rootlet; Deiters' cells
■ Calmodulin	Hair cell stereocilia; inner hair cell bodies
■ Calbindin	Inner hair cells
■ Calsequestrin	Inner hair cells
■ Actin protein filaments	Hair cell stereocilia; cuticular plate; hair cell walls; pillar cells; Deiters' cells
■ α-actinin protein	Inner hair cell cuticular plate
■ Tubulin	Hair cells
■ Calcium (Na+)	Hair cells; stria vascularis marginal cells
■ Potassium (K+)	Hair cells; stria vascularis marginal cells
■ Enzymes	Hair cells
■ Cadherins (proteins)	Hair cells
■ Creatine kinase	Deiters' cells; stromal cells of spiral ligament and spiral prominance
■ Anhydrase	Spiral ligament
■ Acetylcholine	Efferent fibers
■ Acetylcholinesterase	Efferent fibers
■ GABA	Efferent fibers
■ Glutamic acid decarboxylase (GAD)	Efferent fibers
■ Dopamine	Efferent fibers
■ Tryosine hydroxylase	Efferent fibers
■ Vimentin	Stria vascularis (basal cells)
■ GLUTI (glucose transporter protein)	Stria vascularis

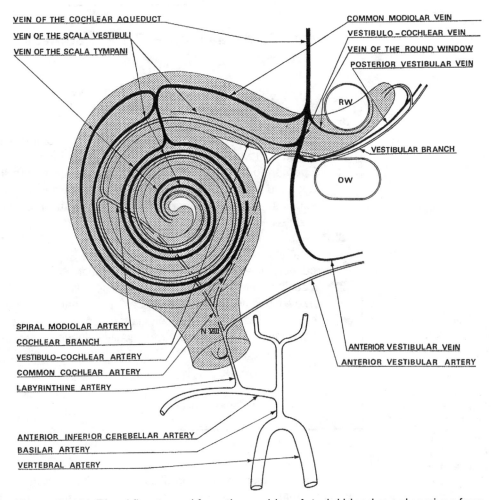

Figure 2–10. Blood flow to and from the cochlea. Arterial blood supply arrives from the vertebral-basal system. RW = round window; OW = oval window.

the basilar membrane, the tectorial membrane, and Reissner's membrane, are largely avascular and are not included among the destinations of the spiral modiolar artery. These in turn further branch off to form fine and complex capillary beds (capillaries are fenestrated), including those in the spiral ligament, the spiral prominence, and a branch to the most complex network in the *stria vascularis*. Located on the lateral wall of the cochlea and playing a critical role in maintenance of the endocochlear (endolymph) electrical potentials (via potassium secretion) that power the cochlea in general, and outer hair cell activity in particular, the stria vascularis is highly vascularized epithelial tissue. The stria consists of three cell types: tightly joined marginal cells making direct contact with endolymph, intermediate cells, and basal cells which are linked with the spiral ligament. Within the intrastrial

Thomas Gold Was Right—There Is an Active Process

A four-part convincing argument that outer hair cells do actively influence cochlear macromechanics (and therefore inner hair cell function and hearing).

■ Outer hair cells move (change length) when stimulated electrically and when their stereocilia bundles are deflected.

■ Spontaneous otoacoustic emissions, recorded in the absence of an external stimulus, reflect activity within the cochlea, a phenomenon incompatible with a passive cochlea.

■ Passive models fail to predict the degree of sensitivity and localization (frequency selectivity) that can be documented along the extent of the cochlea partition.

■ Cochlear sensitivity and frequency selectivity are impaired by even relatively subtle disruptions of cochlear metabolism, especially near the characteristic frequency; whereas passive vibrations are not as dramatically influenced by rather slight alterations of mechanical, biochemical, or electrical factors.

Source: Patuzzi (1996).

One readable account of cochlear structure and function, and a popular textbook in graduate courses, is "An Introduction to the Physiology of Hearing" by James Pickles (see Key References at the end of the Chapter). It is available from some of the booksellers found on the internet. Almost any book can, of course, be ordered by your local bookstore.

space, there is access to perilymph. This observation has suggested the possibility that endolymph is formed from perilymph, rather than from the blood supply to the cochlea. Closely related anatomically to the capillary beds are venules that collect the blood and lead to large veins coursing in a spiral and complementary fashion back into the modiolus.

Afferent and Efferent Cochlear Innervation

Afferent Innervation

Evidence continues to confirm that the descending, or efferent, auditory system plays a role in outer hair cell physiology and, therefore, influences OAE measures. It is difficult, however, to discuss the efferent innervation of the cochlea in isolation, without also mentioning the corresponding afferent innervation. Among a total of about 30,000 eighth cranial nerve fibers in the human, two clear types of afferent neurons can be identified, at least in the distal region near the cochlea.

The Place Relation Between Outer Hair Cell Movement (Motor Processes) and Inner Hair Cell Movement Enhancement (Sensory Processes)

Movement of the basilar membrane secondary to oscillations in outer hair cell length are transmitted radially (from the lateral to the medial portion of the basilar membrane). The result is an enhancement in inner hair cell function and improved hearing sensitivity and frequency selectivity.

Interestingly, however, the energy from the outer hair cells does not reach the inner hair cells directly medially, but rather inner hair cells that are located (away from the stapes footplate) in the direction of the traveling wave (from base to apex) along the cochlear partition.

Source: Patuzzi (1996).

Differences in the appearance of the two types of fibers are less striking more proximally in the eighth cranial nerve. There is actually some evidence that these two general types of eighth cranial nerve fibers can be subdivided, based on morphology and neurotransmitters, into as many as five subgroups. Type I (radial fibers) have bipolar cell bodies in the spiral ganglion and account for 90 to 95% of all of the neurons. Thick and myelinated, they directly innervate *inner hair cells* at the base (Figure 2–11). Each fiber innervates only one inner hair cell, although a single inner hair cell may be innervated by about 20 different fibers. For different species, the fiber-to-hair cell ratio is greatest in frequency regions along the cochlea where hearing is most sensitive (the mid-frequency region for humans). The presynaptic membrane between the type I nerve terminal and the inner hair cell is thin, whereas the post-synaptic membrane density is thick. Afferent fibers convey sensory information from the cochlea to auditory regions of the central nervous system. Individual nerve fibers leave the inner hair cells at the organ of Corti through little openings in the osseous spiral lamina known as habenulae perforatae. Upon reaching the spiral ganglion, they join fibers from other cochlear regions and form the afferent portion of the eighth cranial and continue on through the internal auditory canal as myelinated fibers to the cochlear nucleus in the pontine brainstem.

In contrast, type II (outer spiral) fibers are monopolar or pseudo-monopolar, and account for the remaining 5 to 10% of the neurons.

A Timely Quote About Outer Hair Cell Motility in Humans . . . Yes, People Like You and Me!

Sacrifice of the human inner ear is occasionally required during surgical removal of tumors of the temporal bone and posterior cranial fossa . . . We were able to harvest inner ear organs from this select patient population. (Oghalai et al., 1998, p. 2235)

From the cochlea, we isolated outer hair cells. In all six outer hair cells in which whole cell recording was attempted, we observed an electromotile response to voltage steps. Depolarization led to a decrease in length and an increase in width, whereas the reverse occurred with hyperpolarization. (Oghalai et al., 1998, p. 2238)

Our results indicate that outer hair cell electromotility in humans is qualitatively similar to that found in rodents. This suggests that, within humans, the high-frequency sensitivity and selectivity as well as the source of otoacoustic emissions derives from the outer hair cell. (Oghalai et al., 1998, p. 2238)

Source: Oghalai JS, Holt JR, Nakagawa T, Jung TM, Coker NJ, Jenkins HA, Eatock RA, Brownell WE. Ionic currents and electromotility in inner ear hair cells from humans. *Journal of Neurophysiology* 79:2235–2239, 1998.

Thin, unmyelinated (really enclosed by a single layer of Schwann cells), highly branched, and having small bouton endings, they innervate outer hair cells. Each single outer hair cell synapses with plenty of different type II fibers, yet due to the considerable branching each spiral fiber may be connected to up to 100 different outer hair cells, usually within the same row (Figure 2–12). In fact, most fibers of type II ganglion cells innervate outer hair cells within the first (more medial) row, with the extensively branched fibers reaching rows two and three. In contrast to inner hair cell afferent innervation, nerve fibers connect synaptically to an invagination in the outer hair cell. As they leave the cochlea, Type II fibers spiral together in groups toward the apex, often running through the tunnel of Corti for a distance of up to one quarter of a turn before departing medially past inner pillar cells to join the Type I (radial) fibers squeezing through the habenulae perforatae. Cytoplasm of the psuedomonopolar cell bodies of the Type II neurons is filled with an abundance of components, including mitochondria, endoplasmic reticulum, Golgi apparati, subsurface cisterns, ribosomes, and other assorted vesicles and intracellular bodies.

ORGAN OF CORTI

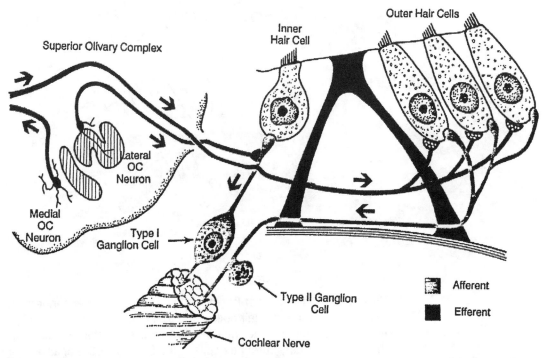

Figure 2–11. Afferent (*light lines*) and efferent (*dark lines*) innervation of the cochlea. Efferent fibers course to the cochlea from the olivary complex in the pons of the brainstem (the olivo-cochlear bundle). Note the indirect connection to the inner hair cells and direct synapse with the base of the outer hair cells (shown also in Figures 2–5 and 2–6). Inner hair cell afferent fibers involve Type I ganglion cells, whereas outer hair cell afferent fibers lead to Type II ganglion cells. Reprinted with permission from Schuknecht HR. *Pathology of the Ear* (2nd ed). Baltimore, MD: Williams & Wilkins, 1993, p. 67. Copyright 1993 Williams & Wilkins.

Efferent Innervation

Delineation of the efferent auditory pathways, and specifically the crossed and uncrossed olivocochlear bundles, dates back to the mid 1940s (Rasmussen, 1946, 1960). The inhibitory effects of the efferent auditory system on cochlear activity were clearly demonstrated by Galambos in 1956, and further described in 1962 by Desmedt and by Fex. Each of these investigators used auditory evoked response techniques to demonstrate the effects on cochlear and neural activity (e.g., for ECochG, increased amplitude for the cochlear microphonic and decreased amplitude of the action potential) associated with electrically induced efferent activity. Fex (1962) also showed that sound presented to the contralateral ear resulted in efferent system activation and affected cochlear function. The suppressive effects of efferent stim-

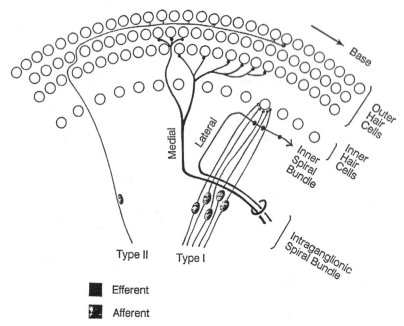

Figure 2–12. Relation of Type I and Type II afferent fiber connections to the inner and outer hair cells. Note that many afferent fibers (Type I) innervate a single inner hair cell, whereas one afferent fiber (Type II) innervates many outer hair cells. Actually, about 95% of all afferent fibers synapse with inner hair cells. Medial efferent fibers branch radially in a basal direction to innervate multiple outer hair cells. Lateral efferent fibers lead to inner hair cells. Reprinted with permission from Schuknecht HR. *Pathology of the Ear* (2nd ed). Baltimore, MD: Williams & Wilkins, 1993, p. 67. Copyright 1993 Williams & Wilkins.

Mother Nature Offers Protection From Overstimulation by Very Low Frequency Sounds

Imagine the problems a person would encounter in communicating if very high intensity, but very low frequency, pressure changes were always heard. In fact, it is likely that cochlear (especially outer hair cell) damage would result from such overstimulation. Sources of these low-frequency pressure fluctuations are commonplace and include swallowing, contraction of the stapedius and/or tensor tympani muscles, atmospheric pressure changes, hyrdostatic imbalances in cochlear fluids, and even postural changes.

The vibrations in cochlear fluids for most audible frequencies (>100 or 200 Hz) do not pass through the tiny opening at the apical end of the cochlea (the helicotrema). Rather, the energy of these vibrations is dissipated by moving the cochlear partition (basilar membrane, hair cells, supporting cells, etc.) at the stimulus frequency. Together, the mass and velocity of cochlear fluids at these frequencies exceed the capacity of the small cross-sectional area of the helicotrema, forming an "acoustic plug" (Patuzzi, 1996, p. 206).

Vibrations for very low frequencies, on the other hand, travel from the stapes footplate, up to and through the helicotrema, and then back to the round window membrane in the basal end of the cochlea. The energy of these very high-intensity, low-frequency vibrations is thus dissipated and is not expended directly on the cochlear partition. In addition to the helicotrema passageway, other mechanisms for reducing the impact of the low-frequency energy include the eustachian tube (mostly effective for atmospheric pressure changes), adjustments of the mechanoelectrical transduction process at the apical end of the hair cells, the nature of the viscous connection between the inner hair cells and tectorial membrane, and maybe even influences of the efferent system (Patuzzi, 1996).

Sources: Dallos (1970); Patuzzi (1996), pp. 206–207; Ruggero, Robles, & Rich (1986).

---

ulation by the presentation of ipsi- or contralateral sound on outer hair cell function and on spontaneous, transient, and distortion product otoacoustic emissions is reviewed in some detail in Chapters 3, 4, and 5. What follows here is an overview of general efferent system structure and function. For detailed reviews of efferent system anatomy and physiology, the reader is directed to Guinan (1996), as well as Warr, Guinan, and White (1986) and Warr (1992).

Inner hair cells are innervated by the efferent auditory system, although not as intimately as are the outer hair cells. Thin fibers originate from cell bodies within the ipsilateral or contralateral *lateral superior olive* in the auditory brainstem. These efferent fibers gain access to inner hair cells by spiraling through Rosenthal's canal toward the base and the apex of the cochlea from their entrance points in the basal and middle turns. They eventually turn in a lateral (radial) direction toward the organ of Corti through the obligatory openings in the osseous spiral lamina (habenulae perforatae) and reach the inner hair cells. Efferent synapses at the inner hair cells tend to be via the afferent fibers, rather than directly with the hair cell itself (see Figure 2–11). The lateral efferent system neurotransmitter is α-aminobutyric acid (GABA), and neurotransmitter-related substances include enkeph-

This modest section on the efferent auditory system is merely a superficial review. Consult some original articles or a book chapter devoted to the efferent pathways for a proper introduction to the topic. Remember,

"A little knowledge is a dangerous thing,
Drink deep, or taste not the pierian spring;
There shallow draughts intoxicate the brain, and drinking largely sobers us again."

Alexander Pope
(1688-1744)
[An Essay on Criticism]

Distinct Differences in the Efferent Innervation of Inner Versus Outer Hair Cells

■ *Inner hair cell* efferent innervation is characterized by:
   ✔ Origin in the lateral superior olive (LSO) nucleus in the pons.
   ✔ Unmyelinated axons forming the lateral olivocochlear bundle and traveling to the cochlea within the internal auditory canal.
   ✔ Efferent fibers terminating on the dentrites of the afferent radial fibers underneath the inner hair cells.
   ✔ Ipsi- and contralateral lateral contributions that are balanced toward the mid- and basal regions of the cochlea, with crossed lateral pathways more prominant toward the apex.
■ *Outer hair cell* efferent innervation is characterized by:
   ✔ Origin in large neurons found anterior, ventral, and medial to the medial superior olive (MSO) nucleus in the pons.
   ✔ Myelinated axons forming the medial olivocochlear bundle and traveling to the cochlea within the internal auditory canal. Myelination makes the medial efferent fibers more stimulable electrically; hence, more is known about the medial efferent pathways.
   ✔ Efferent fibers terminating directly on the outer hair cells.
   ✔ Medial efferent innervation, ipsi- and contralateral contributions that are balanced toward the mid- and apical regions of the cochlea, but crossed lateral pathways are more prominant toward the base.

Source: Guinan (1996).

alins and calcitonin gene-related peptide (CGRP). Latencies for medial efferent system effects on the cochlea may be fast or slow. The faster efferent effects have a latency on the order of 100 to several hundred milliseconds, with the delay largely related to accumulation of an adequate quantity of neurotransmitter at the presynaptic membrane, and also changes outer hair cell conductance related to Ca+ and K+ alterations. The slow component of efferent activity occurs over a time period of minutes, and produces similar effects on cochlear and neural responses.

Early Literature: Efferent Cochlear Innervation

Early investigations on the structure and function of the efferent auditory system's innervation of the cochlea. The topic of suppression of spontaneous, transient, and distortion product otoacoustic emissions by efferent stimulation is reviewed respectively in Chapter 6.

Desmedt JE. Auditory-evoked potentials from cochlea to cortex as influenced by activation of the efferent olivocochlear bundle. *JASA* 34: 1478–1496, 1962.

Fex J. Auditory activity in centrifugal and centripetal cochlear fibers in cat. A study of a feedback system. *Acta Physiologica Scandinavia* 55: 2–68, 1962.

Galambos R. Suppression of auditory activity by stimulation of efferent fibers to the cochlea. *Journal of Neurophysiology* 19: 424–437, 1956.

Geisler CD. Hypothesis on the function of the crossed olivocochlear bundle. *JASA* 56: 1908–1909, 1974.

Gifford ML, Guinan JJ Jr. Effects of electrical stimulation of medial olivocochlear neurons on ipsilateral and contralateral cochlear responses. *Hearing Research* 29: 179–194, 1987.

Kimura R, Wersall J. Termination of the olivocochlear bundle in relation to the outer hair cells of the organ of Corti in guinea pig. *Acta Otolaryngologica (Stockholm)* 55: 11–32, 1962.

Mountain DC. Changes in endolymphatric potential and crossed olivocochlear bundle stimulation after cochlear mechanics. *Science* 210: 71–72, 1980.

Rasmussen GL. The olvary peduncle and other fiber projections of the superior olivary complex. *Journal of Comparative Neurology* 84: 141–219, 1946.

Rasmussen GL. Efferent fibers of cochlear nerve and cochlear nucleus. In: Rasmussen GL, Windle WF (eds). *Neural Mechanisms of the Auditory and Vestibular Systems*. Springfield IL: Charles Thomas, 1960, pp. 105–115.

Smith CA. Innervation pattern of the cochlea. *Annals of Otology, Rhinology, and Laryngology* 70: 504–527, 1961.

Warr WB. Olivocochlear and vestibular efferent neurons of the feline brainstem: Their location, morphology, and number determined by retrograde axonal transport and acetylcholinesterase histochemistry. *Journal of Comparative Neurology* 161: 159–182, 1975.

Warr WB, Guinan JJ Jr. Efferent innervation of the organ of Corti: Two separate systems. *Brain Research* 173: 152–155, 1979.

> ### Where Is All This Basic OAE-Related Science Published?
>
> Don't expect the latest discoveries on outer hair cell physiology or cochlear anatomy to be published in your convenient clinical audiology journals. There are well over 1,000 published papers on topics related to OAE, including the anatomic and physiologic underpinnings, dating back over 20 years.
>
> Where are all of these articles hiding, you might ask? The findings are often initially presented at the Association for Research in Otolaryngology (ARO) Mid-Winter Meeting held in February in St. Petersburg Beach, Florida, and then published in major basic or general science journals, such as:
>
> ■ *Hearing Research*
> ■ *Journal of the Acoustical Society of America*
> ■ *Journal of Physiology*
> ■ *Journal of Neurophysiology*
> ■ *Journal of Neuroscience*
> ■ *Science*
> ■ *Nature.*

The final pathway for outer hair cell innervation by the efferent auditory system originates from cell bodies within structures near either the ipsilateral or contrateral (to the cochlea) *medial* (versus lateral) *superior olivary complex* in the auditory brainstem. As an aside, however, more rostral brainstem centers, such as the reticular formation and the inferior colliculus, and even perhaps cortical auditory regions mediating selective attention, exert some influence on medial efferents. After passing through the habenulae perforatae as myelinated fibers, the efferents lose their myelination and course underneath the inner hair cells. After traveling in a spiral fashion some distance through the tunnel of Corti, the efferent fibers turn laterally and then branch out toward the outer hair cells. As summarized in Table 2–2, there are differences in efferent outer hair cell innervation for the base versus apex of the cochlea, and for each of the three rows of outer hair cells. Efferent synapses with the outer hair cells are differentiated from those with inner hair cells by both the complexity of the pre- and postsynaptic membrane anatomy and the direct nature of the synapse with the outer hair cell. The primary neurotransmitter involved in outer hair cell medial efferent innervation is acetylcholine. Influences reported for the medial (not lateral) efferents when activated include control of the cochlear amplifier (and dynamic range of hearing) by raising hearing thresholds, improvement in attention to nonauditory signals, and protection from temporary threshold shift in excessive noise exposure.

Efferent Innervation of the Cochlea Is Not Always the Same, and There Is Also Autonomic Nervous System Innervation

■ There are more efferent terminals:
  ✔ on outer hair cells in the first (more medial) row than on outer hair cells in rows two or three.
  ✔ on each outer hair cell in the base of the cochlea than more apically.

■ Although most efferent fibers synapse on the base (bottom) of outer hair cells, to 25% of efferent fibers synapse on outer hair cells above the nucleus, at least in the apex of the cochlea.

■ Interestingly, single nerve fiber making a synapse with a single outer hair cell may involve both afferent and efferent types of innervation (in some species).

■ The sympathetic portion of the autonomic nervous system also extensively innervates the cochlea, and plays an important role in the regulation of cochlear vasculature. It is not yet clear whether sympathetic, and especially parasympathetic innervation, influence metabolism of cochlear structures (e.g., the hair cells, stria vascularis, or supporting cells). It is difficult to refrain from speculating on the potential part such innervation might play in certain patient populations, such as tinnitus or hyperacusis.

Sources: Slepecky (1996), pp. 88–89; Ross (1973); Spoendlin (1981); Laurikainen et al., (1993).

KEY REFERENCES

Cazals Y, Demany L, Horner K. (eds). *Auditory Physiology and Perception*. London: Pergamon Press, 1991.

Dallos P, Popper AN, Fay RR. (eds). *The Cochlea*. New York: Springer, 1996.

Flock A, Ottoson D, Ulfendahl M (eds). *Active Hearing*. Oxford: Elsevier, 1995.

Guinan, JJ, Jr. Physiology of olivocochlear efferents. In Dallos P, Popper AN, Fay RR (eds). *The Cochlea*. New York: Springer, 1996, pp. 435–502.

Pickles JO. *An Introduction to the Physiology of Hearing*. (3rd ed). New York: Academic Press, 1988.

Slepecky NB. Structure of the mammalian cochlea. In Dallos P, Popper AN, Fay RR (eds). *The Cochlea*. New York: Springer, 1996, pp. 44–129.

Yost WA. *Fundamentals of Hearing: An Introduction* (3rd ed). New York: Academic Press, 1994.

CHAPTER

3

Spontaneous Otoacoustic Emissions (SOAEs)

Why do some normal ears spontaneously produce sounds that can be measured in the external ear canal? What mechanism (s) is (are) responsible for generating SOAEs? Why are SOAEs more common in females than males? These are but a few of the fundamental questions that hold the interest of dozens of basic scientists who essentially devote their professional lives to the study of SOAEs.

SOAEs provide information on cochlear functioning and offer a useful tool for studying a number of cochlear mechanisms. SOAEs do not, and probably never will, however, be routinely applied clinically. The main disadvantage of SOAEs as a clinical tool is rather simple. The absence of SOAEs does not invariably imply abnormal cochlear function. That is, the prevalence of SOAEs in the general population is far less than 100%. Put another way, the absence of any detectable SOAEs is not a sign of auditory dysfunction or a reason for clinical concern. Early papers noted that less than 50% of normal-hearing persons showed evidence of SOAEs. With advances in instrumentation for measurement of SOAEs, specifically lower noise microphones, amplifiers, and algorithms, including spectral analysis factors for detecting acoustic signals within a noisy background, the apparent prevalence of SOAEs has steadily increased. This trend is evident in Table 3–1. Other factors have a marked influence on SOAEs prevalence, among them gender, laterality (right versus left ear), age from infancy to adulthood, and even very subtle and sometimes overlooked hearing loss. Another factor confounding the accurate determination of prevalence is the definition of SOAEs as reported in various studies. For example, prevalence is properly based on the presence of any SOAE activity in either ear of a subject rather than the presence in a proportion of ears within a group of subjects. At the least, the prevalence of SOAEs must be described separately for males and females, and as a function of age. These critical nonpathologic factors are reviewed in some detail in this chapter.

Although not destined to be a viable clinical procedure, SOAEs are an extremely valuable tool for investigations of basic hearing science. In fact, most of the hundreds of articles on SOAEs provide data on fundamental and extremely important cochlear mechanisms, such as the nature of active cochlear processes. In the review of cochlear anatomy and physiology in Chapter 2, there was discussion of the contribution of outer hair cell motility to the reduction energy loss due to damping effects within the cochlea. Research utilizing SOAEs is yielding vital details on this point and helping to resolve critical debates regarding cochlear function. For example, can the cochlea act as a power amplifier to produce gain exceeding unity? Do SOAEs reflect nonlinear oscillatory energy that underlies this amplifier? In answering these two questions, one must also take into account energy lost in the propagation of the SOAEs outward from the cochlea, through the middle ear to the external ear canal, and variations in the effect of the reverse transmission through the middle ear as a function of SOAEs frequency, and subject age. Or, on the other hand, is SOAE simply a form of output from a passive nonlinear system when stimulated or driven by a noise input? The background, and current status, of these issues are summarized in recent publications (e.g., Burns, Keefe, & Ling, 1998).

Table 3–1. Summary of estimates of SOAE prevalence among studies as a function of age and gender.

Study	Prevalence
Children	
Strickland et al. (1985) (SOAE = >5 dB above NF)	In infants: per ear, 26%; per subject, 38% In children aged 5 to 13 years: per ear, 31%
Bonfils et al. (1992)	In preterm and full-term neonates: per ear, 61%
Burns et al. (1992)	In preterm and full-term neonates, and infants: per subject, 64%
Kok et al. (1993)	In preterm and full-term neonates: per ear, 78%
Morlet et al. (1995)	In preterm and full-term neonates: per ear, 75% In preterm and full-term neonates: per ear, 84%
Khalfa et al. (1997)	In preterm, full-term neonates, and infants: per subject, 81%
Lamprecht-Dinnesen et al. (1998)	In neonates: per ear, >90% for females and 73% for males In children > 6 years old: per ear, 77% for females and 68% for males
Adults	
Schloth (1983)	Per ear: 34%; per subject: 45%
Bright and Glattke (1984)	Per ear: 37%; per subject: 43%
Weir et al. (1984)	Per ear: 27%; per subject: 38%
Dallmayr (1985)	44%
Lonsbury-Martin et al. (1990)	Per ear: 48%; per subject: 60%
Burns et al. (1992)	Per subject: 62%
Moulin et al. (1993)	Per ear: 32%; per subject: 41%

Given their somewhat relatively limited role in clinical audiology, SOAEs will not be reviewed comprehensively in this chapter. Rather, the emphasis will be on SOAE findings that impact most on our understanding and clinical measurement, analysis, and interpretation of DPOAEs and TEOAEs. The review also is biased toward more recent investigations.

GENERAL CHARACTERISTICS

SOAEs are very narrow bands (less than 30 Hz) of frequencies recorded in the external ear canal in the absence of an evoking acoustic signal (Figure 3–1). There are two general techniques for recording SOAEs. One is to average a number of samples (e.g., 20 to 40) of sound in the ear canal and to perform a spectral analysis of this averaged sound. This approach is probably more common clinically. With the other technique, referred to sometimes as synchronized SOAEs, a click is presented to the ear and SOAEs time-locked to the click are averaged.

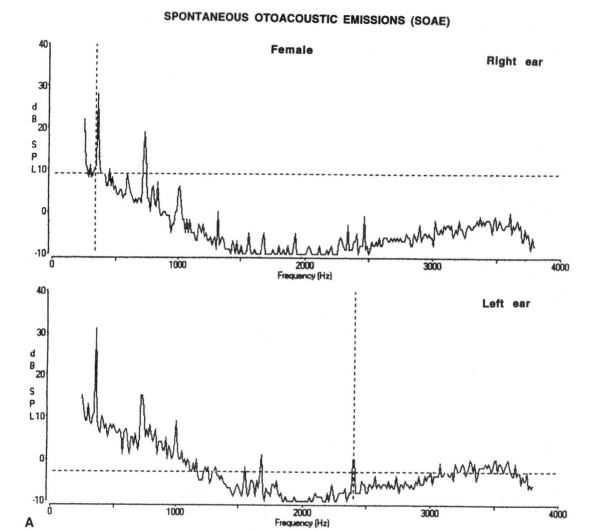

Figure 3–1. Spontaneous OAE (SOAE) recorded from a 26-year-old normal hearing female (**A**) and a 51-year-old male (**B**) with clinical instrumentation (GSI 60). The female has multiple SOAEs in each ear. *(continued)*

SOAEs are recorded using this technique with the ILO 88 device. The frequencies of SOAEs are usually between 500 Hz and 7000 Hz, although many studies did not measure lower frequencies due to excessive noise, nor higher frequencies due to equipment limitations. On the average, SOAEs in humans are most likely to be recorded within the most sensitive hearing region (1000 to 2000 Hz). SOAEs amplitude is most often in the range of −5dB to about 15 dB SPL. Deriving from active processes in the cochlea, SOAEs are detected with a sensitive and low-noise microphone housed within a probe assembly which, in turn, is fit snugly into the ear canal. As typically recorded, a

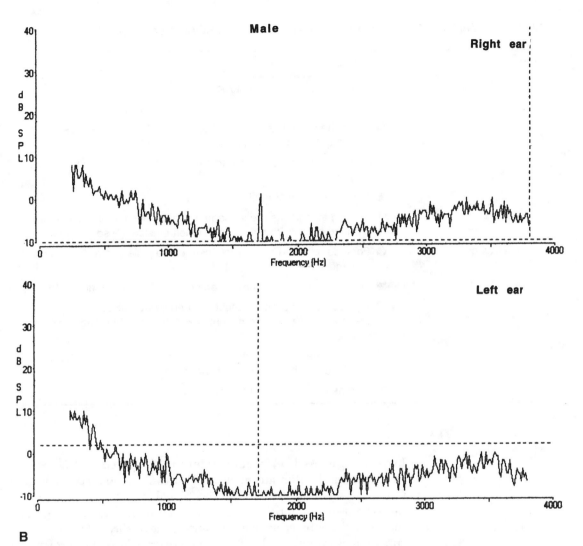

B

Figure 3–1. (B) *(continued)* For the male, SOAE activity was detected only in the right ear (at 1700 Hz). The subject has consistently documented an SOAE at that frequency for 7 years.

single SOAE appears almost as a spike at one frequency, arising sharply above the noise floor in the ear canal. Sound in the ear canal unrelated to SOAEs is unavoidable. In part, this sound consists of ambient environmental noise and patient movement noise, both of which can be reduced with appropriate modifications in the test protocol and often with patient instruction. Unwanted and inevitable sound during SOAE measurement, however, also is associated with obviously vital bodily functions, such as breathing and blood flow. Regardless of the source, most ear canal noise is greatest for the lower frequency region (less than 1000 Hz). Clinical strategies for reducing the noise floor in SOAEs measurement are summarized in Table 3–2.

Table 3–2. Techniques and strategies for noise reduction in SOAE measurement.

Source	To Reduce the Noise
Ambient environmental noise	■ Close the door to the test room.
	■ Seat probe tip deeply into the external ear canal.
	■ Move the patient as far away from the SOAE equipment as possible (the computer fan is the source of the noise).
	■ Turn the patient so that the test ear is facing away from the equipment.
	■ Increase the amount of signal averaging.
	■ If these techniques are inadequate, then relocate the patient inside a sound-booth with the equipment left outside the sound-booth.
Patient/physiologic noise	■ For older children and adults, instruct the patient to remain still and limit movement.
	■ For younger children, amuse and distract the patient during testing.
	■ For infants and difficult-to-test children, perform SOAE measurement while the patient is sedated for other diagnostic procedures.
	■ Stabilize the cord from the SOAE equipment to the probe tip to minimize rubbing with the patient or the chair.
	■ Increase the amount of signal averaging.

In recording evoked OAEs, amplitude can be increased to some extent by increasing the stimulus intensity. However, because spontaneous OAEs amplitude (the strength of the "signal" when a signal-to-noise ratio is considered) for a subject or patient cannot be manipulated by the tester, the only recourse for enhancing the quality of SOAEs measures, that is improving the signal-to-noise level, is to minimize measurement noise.

As summarized in Table 3–3, it is not uncommon for one ear to produce multiple SOAEs, or for multiple SOAEs to be produced by both ears. Examples of single and multiple SOAEs were shown in Figure 3–1. The frequency(ies) of SOAEs are not limited to any specific region in the spectrum, although likelihood of confident SOAEs detection increases for the mid- and high frequencies, as noise levels tend to decrease. As a rule, for an adult, SOAEs frequency remains constant (less than 1% variation) over periods of years, whereas amplitude may vary over time, even from hour to hour. Racial factors may also influence the absolute frequency(ies) of SOAEs, as noted below. Fluctuations in middle ear status, even subclinical changes, must be considered as a factor in the instability of SOAE amplitude. Indeed, any measurement of SOAEs is highly dependent on functional status of the

---

SOAEs Do Have Their Limits

The minimal frequency difference between SOAEs in ears with multiple SOAEs is about 50 Hz, or a distance along the basilar membrane of roughly 0.4 mm (Talmadge et al., 1993).

---

entire middle ear system (ossicular chain, tendons, muscles, and tympanic membrane), as well as the external ear canal cross-sectional area.

Although the possibility of SOAE was raised prior to 1970, David Kemp in 1979 described them clinically in normal-hearing persons. Since then, well over 100 papers have been published describing the complex effects on SOAE amplitude suppression and phase of characteristics of external signals (e.g., phase, frequency, intensity, duration), a variety of nonpathologic subject factors (e.g., ear side, gender, age), genetic influences, and findings in otologic pathologies and disorders, such as ototoxicity and noise-exposure, and the relation of SOAEs to certain otologic symptoms, among them tinnitus. This literature is

Table 3–3. Summary of features of spontaneous otoacoustic emissions (SOAE).

■ Recorded in the external canal without an acoustic stimulus.

■ Each SOAE consists of a very narrow frequency band, usually 1 Hz, which appears as a single frequency spike.

■ Present in approximately 70% of normal hearers (Penner, Glotzback, & Huang, 1993; Talmadge, Long, Murphy, & Tubis, 1993). The apparent prevalence of SOAE has increased over the years with technical advances for recording signals in the ear canal and reduction of the effects noise in the ear canal (e.g., very sensitive yet miniature microphones).

■ Frequencies of SOAEs for a person remain stable for long periods of time. That is, less than 1% change or, according to Dallmayr (1985) a change of less than 3 outer hair cells along the basilar membrane!), although high-frequency SOAEs may disappear and low-frequency SOAEs may emerge over the course of years among adults.

■ Amplitudes of SOAEs are characteristically rather modest (around 0 to 5 dB), or they may range from - 10 dB up to about 20 dB. For an adult, SOAE amplitude may fluctuate over time (less than 5 dB typically). With maturation from infancy to young childhood, SOAE amplitude values usually decrease.

■ For adults, SOAEs are most often present above 1000 Hz (especially in the 1000 to 2000 Hz region), whereas for infants and young children SOAEs are typically recorded at higher frequencies. However, with appropriate instrumentation SOAEs are recorded also for higher and lower frequencies.

■ Multiple SOAE frequencies are common in individuals.

■ If present in an individual, likely to be present in both ears.

---

reviewed now, again focusing on findings of practical interest to clinicians. A common theme in this review is the complexity of the interactions among most of these factors. There is no simple answer to the question: Could you describe the typical SOAEs? Thus, it is impossible to discuss any single factor, such as age, ear side, or gender, in isolation. Rather, one must also consider at least these three factors in combination, and control for two factors when assessing the effect of the third. For example, statements about gender effects on SOAEs should be made separately for the right and left ears (e.g., not for a mixture of right and left ears) and for a restricted age range (e.g., 6 to 8 years).

MEASUREMENT AND ANALYSIS

The main steps in SOAE measurement are summarized in Table 3–4. Technically, measurement of SOAEs differs little from measurement of evoked OAEs. The importance of minimizing noise is equivalent for all OAE measurements. Similarly, one must closely examine data in an attempt to differentiate a true SOAE from an artifact, particularly an equipment-generated electrical interference at a single frequency. One approach for ruling out the presence of an artifactual SOAE is to veri-

Table 3–4. Important steps in clinical measurement of SOAEs. The sequence of some steps may be varied.

- Enter demographic patient information into the SOAE device computer.
- Select the appropriate OAE program.
- Examine the patient's external ear canal otoscopically and defer testing pending medical or audiologic management if pathology or excessive cerumen in present.
- Select a clean and appropriately sized probe tip, place it on the probe assembly, and verify that all tubes and ports are open before inserting the probe tip into the external ear canal.
- Seat the probe tip deeply within the external ear canal.
- Instruct patient (for older children and adults).
- Take necessary steps to minimize measurement noise (*see* Table 3–2 on noise reduction steps).
- Begin signal averaging process.
- Extend signal averaging if noise levels are excessively high.
- Store SOAE data immediately after averaging process is stopped.
- At the conclusion of the averaging, inspect visually the spectrum of sound (usually ranging from 500 to 8000 Hz) for peaks (spikes) representing SOAEs.
- Using the equipment cursor, analyze amplitude and frequency of SOAE of interest.
- Record these data for later reporting, if desired.
- Repeat the measurement process for the other ear.

fy that a presumed SOAE is not present in a calibration cavity, or a dead ear if available. The suspicion of artifactual contamination of SOAE recordings, or even the erroneous identification of artifact as a SOAE, must be higher for low-frequency components, as certain types of electrical interference (e.g., 60-Hz line noise and harmonics) are more common, and SOAEs are less common, within this spectral region.

As stressed in Chapter 1 and noted above, the status of the middle ear system must always be considered in the measurement of SOAEs. For clinical SOAE recording, conventional tympanometry (i.e., impedance or admittance for a low [e.g., 226 Hz] probe tone, would be minimally required). Experimentally, if not clinically, data on aural input impedance (e.g., at the probe tip) and reflectance (Keefe et al., 1992; Keefe & Levi, 1996; Burns et al., 1998) should be incorporated into precise calculations of SOAE absolute amplitude values. More sophisticated documentation of the role of the ossicular chain, tympanic membrane, and ear canal in SOAE recordings, now essential for experimental investigations (Keef, Ling, & Bulen, 1992; Burns et al., 1994; Keefe & Levi, 1996; Tubis & Talmadge, 1998), might someday be incorporated at least partially into clinical applications. Certainly, thorough assessment of middle ear maturational stage and normal versus pathologic status with immittance measures is most important in the infant. Within the 1- to 6-month age range, it will be necessary in some cases to supplement conventional tympanometry (a 226-Hz probe frequency) with either multifrequency tympanometry (Holte, Margolis, & Cavanaugh, 1991; Hunter & Margolis, 1992; Hall & Mueller, 1997) or, at least, a higher frequency probe tone (e.g., 1000 Hz).

Several authors have described changes in SOAEs due merely to continuous measurement with a probe inserted in the external ear canal (Zurek, 1981; Rabinowitz & Widen, 1984; Whitehead, 1991; McFadden & Pasanen, 1994). Referred to as "initializing effects" (McFadden & Pasanen, 1994), and occuring after 20 to 30 minutes, the changes consist of slight increases in SOAE amplitude (2 or 3 dB) and frequency shifts of 6 to 10 Hz (higher or lower). Also, new previously unmeasured SOAEs sometimes emerge during this extended continuous measurement period. There may be interactions among these initializing effects and the effects of certain drugs, such as quinine, as described below. In addition to their theoretical interest, these effects have practical implications for extended clinical measurement of any type of OAE. Probe removal and reinsertion periodically should be considered to reduce the initializing effects. These manueveurs may, of course, introduce another source of variability into OAE measurement.

Finally, in contrast to the typically consistent presence or absence of SOAEs in an individual, and stability of SOAEs frequency(ies) and to a lesser extent amplitude, when present, there is one recent report of SOAEs appearing and then disappearing. After reviewing the charac-

Investigation of SOAEs is an international effort. Some of the more prolific authors in the United States of America are Ed Burns (University of Washington in Seattle), Glenys Long and Arnold Tubis (University of Purdue), Merilyn Penner (University of Maryland), and Dennis McFadden (University of Texas-Austin). European investigators include Antoinette Lamprecht-Dinnesen and colleagues (University of Munster in Germany), Pim van Dijk and Hero Wit (Groningen in the Netherlands), Patrick Brienesse and colleagues (Maastricht in the Netherlands).

The Principle of Conservation of Energy May Apply to SOAEs

First suggested by a rather obscure German physician, J. R. Mayer (1814–1878) and lent scientific evidence independently by English brewer James P. Joule (1818–1889), the principle of conservation of energy states that the total energy of any isolated system remains constant.

Under certain conditions, such as extended measurement with the probe continuously inserted in the external ear canal during administration of potentially ototoxic drugs (e.g., aspirin or quinine), "new short-lived" SOAEs may appear just as preexisting "long-lived" SOAEs at other frequencies disappear, at least temporarily. This phenomenon is referred as an "initializing effect" by Dennis McFadden and is similar to the "quasi-stable-state" behavior noted by Edward Burns and colleagues. In the words of Burns, "some frequency components are present in the SOAEs at one time, but not another, i.e., there appears to be more than one dynamical state, each of which is structurally stable. Transitions between a pair of structurally stable SOAEs are sometimes associated with intermittant tinnitus" (Burns, Keefe, & Ling, 1998, p. 473). Some time later, after the experiment is complete, the premeasurement SOAEs pattern for the ear returns. One interpretation for this rather interesting process is that there is a finite and constant pool of energy available within the normally functioning cochlea. When energy is lost at one place along the basilar membrane, it reappears at another place. SOAEs seem to jump spontaneously from one frequency to another in these conditions.

Sources: Burns, Strickland, Tubis, & Jones (1984); McFadden & Pasanen (1994).

teristic stability of SOAEs and carefully ruling out any possible technical, equipment, probe, or artifact problem, Merrilyn J. Penner of the University of Maryland, an experienced investigator of SOAEs, noted that, "it came as no small surprise therefore that a subject with no SOAEs on Monday or during the preceding month had as many as 10 of them on Wednesday and that all the SOAEs had vanished in a testing session occuring 85 days later" (Penner, 1996, p. 116). Even a potential circadian rhythm effect was minimized by scheduling the data collection within a 1-hour time slot (1 to 2 p.m.) each test day. Over an 85-day period (36 test sessions), a total of 51 SOAEs were recorded from the 18-year-old male college student. One day alone, the subject had 36 SOAE frequencies in his right ear. The author surmized that some of the apparent SOAEs were actually cubic difference tones (i.e., DPs produced by two closely and appropriately spaced primary SOAEs). Hearing sensitivity on days 1 and 98 was unchanged. Assessments continued on for 342 days without any reappearance of the SOAEs. Interestingly, the subject did demonstrate some typical features of SOAEs. For example, he had more SOAEs for the right than left ear, and the majority of the SOAEs were below 3000 Hz. Obviously, the main departure from normal for this subject was the highly unstable nature of the SOAEs and their disappearance despite apparently normal auditory function. This finding alone argues that not all SOAEs are inherited.

High-Level SOAEs

For over 30 years, and even before SOAEs were systematically described, reports have appeared documenting unusually high amplitude sounds, up to 30 dB SPL or higher, spontaneously recorded in the ear canal (e.g. Glanville et al., 1971; Huizing & Spoor, 1973; Yamamoto et al., 1987; Penner, 1988; Mathis et al., 1991). An example reported by Mathis, Probst, De Min, and Hauser (1991) is shown in Figure 3–2. Actually, this case is somewhat typical. The patient was a 6-month-old boy referred by his pediatrician for an audiologic assessment. The reason for the referral was an easily audible sound arising from the child's left ear. After an ABR (with click stimuli) was normal, the parents were assured that there was no reason for concern. Two years later the child was again evaluated audiologically. The sound was still present, and documented as shown in Figure 3–2. Six months after that visit, behavioral audiometry showed normal hearing in the 1000 and 2000 Hz region. Thresholds for other frequencies were not available. The presence of the SOAE in the left ear was confirmed. No SOAEs were detected in the right ear. Subsequent behavioral audiometry showed a moderate high-frequency sensorineural hearing loss bilaterally, greater for the left ear. Throughout all of this period, the child was never aware of the high-level SOAEs. Interestingly, and important for clinical documentation of SOAEs, this child's high-level SOAEs could not be synchronized by click stimuli.

High-level SOAEs are sometimes referred to inaccurately as "objective tinnitus." This term is misleading because the patient with the high-level SOAEs cannot hear it. High-level SOAEs are probably more common in children than adults and may coexist with sensory hearing loss. The author has, within the past 4 years, received personal communications from three different audiologists who encountered infants with high-level SOAEs that were extremely disconcerting to the child's parents and pediatrician. I have also had the opportunity to

No clinician will ever forget their first patient who presents with high level OAEs that can be easily detected with the naked ear (of the examiner). The patient is usually a young child whose parents probably have plenty of interesting, and amusing, tales to tell about the reaction of family doctors, and others, to their child's whistling ear. The "owners" don't perceive their spontanous otoacoustic emission, probably because they long ago habituated to the sound.

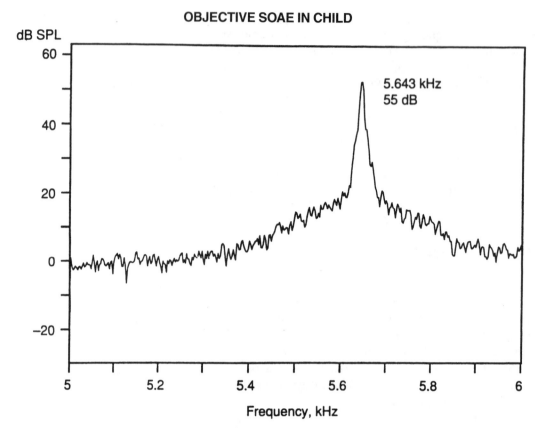

Figure 3–2. High level spontaneous otoacoustic emission recorded from the left ear of a 2.5-year-old boy with a sensitive microphone placed at the entrance of the ear canal (top portion). The child was never aware of the sound, although it was audible to examiners. From Mathis A, Probst R, DeMin N and Hauser R. A child with an unusually high level spontaneous otoacoustic emission. *Archives of Otolaryngology—Head and Neck Surgery* 117: 674–676, 1991.

evaluate a little girl with objective SOAEs, easily detectable as a high-pitched ringing sound by any normal hearing person within about 1 foot from her left ear. Given the relatively low incidence of high level SOAEs and the general correlation of SOAE with normal hearing, there is probably little cause for concern or alarm for patients with, or parents of children with, high-level SOAEs. There appears to be a hereditary component to the presence of some high-level SOAEs (Glanville et al., 1971; Wilson & Sutton, 1983).

Nonpathologic Factors

Ear Differences

For most audiologic measurements, interaural symmetry in normal-hearing persons is an underlying assumption. In fact, the experienced clinician will systematically troubleshoot the equipment (e.g., audiometer, immittance meter, evoked response system) setup, all connections between the equipment and the transducer, and right versus left earphones, and even patency of the tube within insert ear couplers, to rule out a technical explanation for the asymmetry. A common strategy during this process, to verify that a suspicious transducer or equipment channel isn't contributing to the asymmetry, is to perform the audiologic measurement, such as pure tone thresholds or ABR latency-intensity functions, using the one earphone and channel (right or left) in testing both ears. In essence this technique is always used for OAE recordings. That is, the same probe is routinely used for right and left ear measurements. Interaural symmetry in OAE measurements would, therefore, be expected. There is, however, considerable evidence to the contrary.

The prevalence of SOAEs is higher for the right versus the left ear, as is the actual number of SOAEs per ear. There is also a tendency for larger SOAE amplitude for the right ear. These conclusions regarding SOAE asymmetry must always be qualified by consideration of other nonpathologic factors. Most studies with adult subjects confirm the increased prevalence of SOAEs for the right ear (Burns et al., 1992; Penner et al., 1993; Whitehead et al., 1993; Khalfa et al., 1997), although there is some evidence to the contrary (Collet et al., 1993), and right versus left ear differences in SOAEs prevalence may vary for infants and young children versus older children and adults and for males versus females, particularly as a function of age. The complexity of these interactions is illustrated in Figures 3–3 through 3–5. Although the age effect in prevalence is consistently apparent, it differs as a function of age and for males versus females. The actual number of SOAEs is typically greater for the right than left ear in children and adults (Kok et al., 1993; Penner et al., 1993; Morlet et al., 1995; Khalfa et al., 1997; Lamprecht-Dinnesen et al., 1998), with numbers of multiple SOAEs per ear ranging from 2 to as many as 15 or 16. Whether gender is a factor in the asymmetry in number of SOAE is not clear.

Asymmetries in efferent system innervation and function may, at least in part, play a role in the side differences in SOAEs. Kalfa and Collet (1996) described more efferent system activity for the right side of the medial olivocochlear system in right-handed adults. An efferent-based explanation for the interaural asymmetry of SOAEs is supported by McFadden (1993). That is, if efferent inhibitory (medial olivocochlear system) effects are lower for right ears and in female subjects, than for left ears and males, then a greater number of SOAEs and larger SOAE amplitudes would be expected for right ears and females. It would be reasonable to theorize that immaturity of the efferent auditory system (medial olivocochlear system) in newborns and infants, especially brainstem pathways, might contribute to a developmental factor in the presence and size of SOAEs as well. That is, the immature efferent system would exert less inhibition of the cochlea, and specifically outer hair cells. This in turn would result in greater motility and

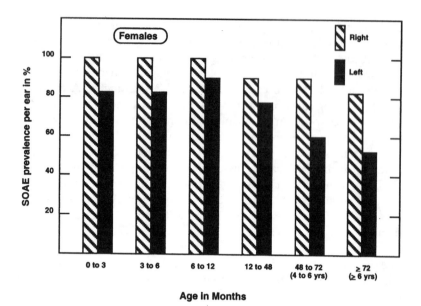

Figure 3–3. The prevalence of SOAE for right and left ears in female subjects as a function of age from neonates to school-age children (*N* = 267). Adapted from Lamprecht-Dinnesen et al. Effects of age, gender, and ear side on SOAE parameters in infancy and childhood. *Audiology & Neuro-Otology 3*: 386–401, 1998 (p. 390).

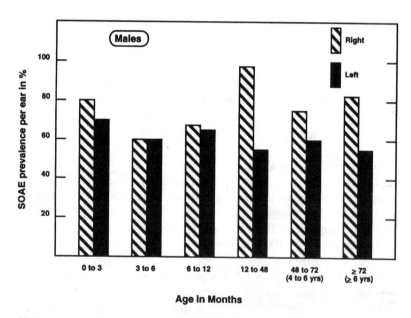

Figure 3–4. The prevalence of SOAE for right and left ears in male subjects as a function of age from neonates to school-age children (*N* = 267). Adapted from Lamprecht-Dinnesen et al. Effects of age, gender, and ear side on SOAE parameters in infancy and childhood. *Audiology & Neuro-Otology 3*: 386–401, 1998 (p. 390).

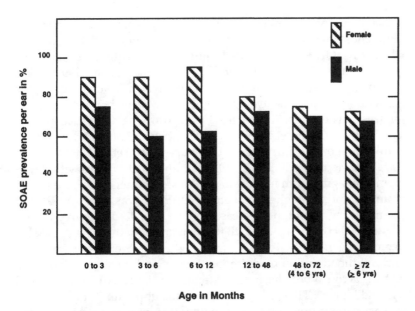

Figure 3–5. The prevalence of SOAE for male versus female subjects per ear (right and left) as a function of age from neonates to school-age children (N = 267). Note the lower prevalence for males versus females across the age range. Adapted from Lamprecht-Dinnesen et al. Effects of age, gender, and ear side on SOAE parameters in infancy and childhood. *Audiology & Neuro-Otology 3*: 386–401, 1998 (p. 390).

larger SOAE amplitudes. Increased prevalence of SOAEs for the right (79%) versus left ear (72%) is present beginning with preterm neonates (Morlet et al., 1995) and continuing for infants and young children (Burns et al., 1992; Kok et al., 1993; Lamprecht-Dinnesen et al., 1998), although once again the findings of Collet et al. (1993) support no side difference. Furthermore, whereas the right versus left ear asymmetry is mostly found for female infants and young children, other authors report that this asymmetry is more pronounced for male versus female adults (Talmadge et al., 1993; Whitehead et al., 1993). Despite the sizeable number of published studies on SOAEs, more information is needed to resolve some of the apparent contradictions in the relation among age, gender, and ear side.

Age

With development in children the prevalence, number/ear, and amplitude level, and perhaps the frequency, of the individual SOAEs all decrease from neonates to older children (e.g., Burns, Campbell, & Arehart, 1994; Lamprecht-Dinnesen et al., 1998). These trends, which have for the most part been confirmed by the numerous investigators of SOAEs, were illustrated in Figures 3–3 through 3–5. SOAEs can be detected in preterm neonates as early as 30 weeks (about 6 months)

There is much to learn about on the complex interactions among gender, genetics, and SOAEs. One way to keep updated on this fascinating topic is to follow the work of Dr. Dennis McFadden, an experimental psychologist at the University of Texas in Austin. Seek Dr. McFadden out on the internet or locate his publications via a Medline search.

conceptional age (Morlet et al., 1995). Although there are no significant differences in SOAEs for preterm versus term infants, the frequencies at which SOAEs are recorded shift upward with maturation for preterm infants followed longitudinally (Brienesse et al., 1997, 1998a, 1998b). Amplitude does not show an equivalent change during the same time period. The average number of SOAEs per ear may be as high as 6 in neonates (Morlet et al., 1995), dropping to about 3 in older children (Strickland et al., 1985), and to about 2.5 or slightly more for adults (Bargones & Burns, 1988; Lonsbury-Martin et al., 1990; Burns et al., 1992; Moulin et al., 1993). SOAE amplitude decreases with developmental aging from infancy to adulthood and tend to be most pronounced for the higher frequency SOAEs (Burns et al., 1992). For example, the amplitude decrease may be over 15 dB for frequencies about 3000 Hz and about 10 dB for frequencies in the 1000 to 2000 Hz region. In general, SOAEs shift from higher to lower frequencies during childhood and into adulthood. Infants and young children have SOAEs across a broader range of frequencies than adults (up to 5000 Hz and higher). Then, as age increases, the upper limits of SOAE frequencies move downward. Put another way, most SOAEs in children are in the 2500 to 5000 Hz region (Burns et al., 1992), whereas adult SOAEs are most common in the 1000 to 2000 Hz region (Weir et al., 1984; Strickland et al., 1985; Lonsbury-Martin et al., 1990; Martin et al., 1990; Whitehead et al., 1993; Martinez Ibarguen et al., 1995).

Measurement of SOAEs is, of course, dependent on transmission of energy from the cochlea outward through the middle ear system into the external ear canal. Explanations offered for the age effects on SOAEs amplitude and frequency, therefore, must include well-known developmental changes in external and middle ear resonance during infancy (Burns et al., 1994), although effects secondary to maturation of the efferent system must also be considered (McFadden, 1993; Burns et al., 1994). Ear canal resonance frequency decreases progressively from about 6000 Hz in neonates to about 4000 Hz in infancy and down to adult values of approximately 3000 Hz by age 2 to 3 years (Kruger & Ruben, 1987; Westwood & Bamford, 1992; Mueller & Hall, 1998). However, no study has systematically related actual measures of ear canal resonance to SOAEs findings.

The effect of advancing age on SOAEs in adults is less straightforward. Relatively early investigations (Bonfils, 1989; Lonsbury-Martin et al., 1991; Stover & Norton, 1993) appeared to demonstrate a clear decrease in the prevalence, number/ear, and amplitude level for older persons with normal hearing, as defined clinically as "with presbycusis but audiometric thresholds within normal limits relative to their age" (Bonfils, 1989, p. 752). Prieve and Falter (1995) found that sychronized SOAEs were recorded less often for subjects aged 40 to 60 years than for younger subjects (19 to 29 years). There were equal numbers of males and females in each group. However, there is some evidence that SOAEs recorded without an acoustic signal (free-averaged) from the ear do not show a negligible age effect when older subjects are matched rigorously with their younger counterparts for hearing thresholds and when subjects with age-related otologic dysfunction and even subtle hearing deficits are carefully excluded (Strouse & Hall, personal communication, 1996).

Gender

One of the most well-recognized and distinct characteristics of SOAEs is their prominence in females versus males (see Figure 3–3 through 3–5). The gender effect includes a higher prevalence, greater number per ear, and higher amplitude for SOAEs in females than males (Zurek, 1981; Strickland et al., 1985; Collet et al., 1993; Penner et al., 1993; Talmadge et al., 1993; Whitehead et al., 1993; Martinez Ibarguen et al., 1995; Morlet et al., 1995). Once again, however, the influence of age and ear differences must be taken into account. For example, although the gender difference is a consistent feature throughout childhood and adulthood, Lamprecht-Dinnesen and colleagues (1998) showed that the gender difference in SOAE prevalence was most obvious in the first year after birth. When SOAEs are present unilaterally in males, they are more likely to be emitted from the right ear.

Gender differences abound in studies of auditory function, as summarized in Table 3–5 and reviewed extensively by McFadden (1998). Explanations for the gender difference in SOAEs include an anatomical difference in the size of the cochlea, with females typically having a shorter cochlear length (Sato et al., 1991), more outer hair cells (Wright et al., 1987), slightly better hearing sensitivity (McFadden & Mishra, 1993), and possibly the smaller external ear canal volume (Martin et al., 1987). The gender difference in prevalence and amplitude of SOAEs may also play a role in the tendency toward robust TEOAEs in females versus males, as noted in the next chapter.

Genetic Factors

SOAE prevalence is, at least in part, genetically determined (Bilger et al., 1990; Whitehead et al., 1993; McFadden & Loehlin, 1995). SOAE characteristics, including the number and amplitude, are more similar for monozygotic cotwins than for dizygotic cotwins of the same gender (McFadden & Loehlin, 1995). According to McFadden and colleagues, about 75% of the variation in SOAEs among individuals can be accounted for by genetic factors (McFadden & Loehlin, 1995; McFadden et al., 1996; McFadden, 1998). Furthermore, although females in general are more likely to show SOAEs, more SOAEs per ear, and larger amplitude SOAEs than males, a female having a male cotwin characteristically has SOAEs more like her male counterpart. McFadden refers to this OAE tendency in opposite sex dizygotic twin females as the "prenatal masculinization."

Table 3–5. Summary of gender differences in auditory function.

Auditory Measure	Gender Effect
Physical differences	
■ Head size	Larger in males
■ Pinna size	Larger in males
■ External ear canal volume	Larger in males
■ Middle-ear volume	Larger in males
■ Cochlear length	Longer in males
Psychophysical	
■ Hearing sensitivity	Females more sensitive (at least above 2000 Hz)
■ Binaural tasks	
Sound localization	Males more sensitive to differences in interaural time and intensity
Binaural beats	Males detect them at higher frequencies
Right-ear advantage (REA)	Smaller REA (less asymmetry) in females
■ Noise-induced hearing loss	
Permanent	Greater in males
Temporary	Less in females below about 1500 Hz, but more above approximately 3000 Hz
■ Complex masking tasks	
Profile analysis	Males are more sensitive
Lateral suppression	Greater in males
Overshoot	Greater in females
■ Gap detection	More sensitive in females
Electrophysiologic	
■ Auditory brainstem response (ABR)	Wave V latency and interwave latencies shorter in females; Wave V amplitudes larger in females
■ Otoacoustic emissions (OAE)	More SOAEs in females
	Larger TEOAEs in females
■ Prenatal masculinization OAE	OAEs in females with a male cotwin are more similar to Male OAEs

Source: Reprinted with permission from McFadden D. Sex differences in the auditory system. *Developmental Neuropsychology 14*: 261–298, 1998, p. 263.

An apparent difference in SOAEs as a function of *race* may also be viewed as support for a genetic influence. According to Whitehead et al. (1993), and as illustrated in Figure 3–6, SOAEs are most common in African-Americans (mean number of 3.3), less common in Asians (mean number of 2.1), and least common in Caucasians with light eyes

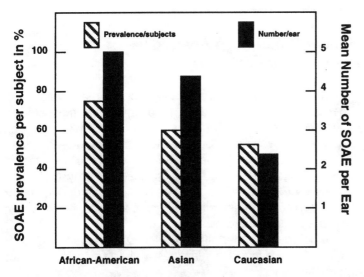

Figure 3–6. Prevalence of SOAE and mean number of SOAE per ear for three different racial groups (*N* = 10 males and 10 females in each group). Adapted from Whitehead et al. Spontaneous otoacoustic emissions in different racial groups. *Scandinavian Audiology 22*: 3–10, 1993.

(mean number of 1.2), a finding generally supported by Russell (1992). The differences in the number of SOAEs between the three groups of 20 subjects were highly significant (Whitehead et al., 1993). There was a tendency for more bilateral SOAE, and multiple (versus single) SOAEs among African-Americans. On the average, SOAEs in Asian ears tended to be higher in frequency (mean of 2794 Hz) than those from the African-American group (mean of 1950 Hz) or Caucasian group (2191 Hz). The expected higher number of SOAEs in females versus males was noted in this study.

Body Temperature

The effects of body temperature on some auditory measures, such as the ABR, are well-known and appreciated (e.g., Hall, 1992a). Increases in body temperature above normal (i.e., 98.6° Fahrenheit or 37° Centigrade) shorten latencies, particularly of later latency waves, whereas decreases in body temperature have the opposite effect on ABR latency. There are no reports addressing the possible effects of body temperature on SOAEs.

Diurnal and Monthly (Menstrual) Changes

The frequencies of SOAEs may change during the day (Wit, 1985; Wilson, 1986; Bell, 1992; Haggerty et al., 1993), with frequencies tending to be lower early in the morning or late at night. In interpreting the diurnal factor in auditory function, one must always rule out a body tem-

Gender Differences Abound in Auditory Function

There are relatively few investigations of the development of gender differences in auditory function. That is, most studies confirming differences in auditory functioning between females and males—psychoacoustic and electrophysiologic—are limited to adult subjects. However, gender differences for some auditory tasks and procedures, such as auditory brainstem response (ABR), appear to be more pronounced during and/or after puberty. This observation suggests a role for hormones in the explanation of the differences.

In contrast, gender differences in OAE, especially SOAE and TEOAE, are found in infants as well as adults, arguing for an origin at birth.

Source: McFadden D. Sex differences in the auditory system. *Developmental Neuropsychology 14:* 261–298, 1998, p. 263.

---

perature effect in assessing changes in sensory function during the day. From a review of the literature, it would appear that the possible influence of body temperature on diurnal rhythms in SOAEs has not been conclusively eliminated.

Some measures of auditory function, such as hearing sensitivity, vary during *the monthly (menstrual) cycle*. It appears that SOAEs are one of these measures, as on the average SOAE frequency is lowest immediately before menses and highest before ovulation (Wilson, 1986; Bell, 1992; Haggerty, Lusted, & Morton, 1993; Penner, Brauth, & Jastreboff, 1994; Penner & Glotzbach, 1994; Penner, 1995; McFadden, 1998). Hormonal influences on cochlear blood flow and/or metabolism of outer hair cell motility are offered as possible mechanisms. The maxima and minima in SOAE frequencies are reduced during natural or induced (birth control pill) anovulation (Penner, 1995). Monthly differences are, however, small (in a range of +0.6 to −0.6% of the frequency) and somewhat inconsistent. Furthermore, blood hormone levels were usually not documented to mark accurately the stage of ovulation, and the confounding effect of body temperature, which should be considered, has not always been accounted for.

Miscellaneous Factors

There is some evidence that SOAEs are influenced by *body position* (Bell, 1992), particularly hanging the head downward at a 30° angle.

This relationship would not be unexpected, as slight variations in middle ear status might be caused by changes in body position. As a small part of a study of SOAEs and tinnitus, Ciranic, Prasher, and Luxon (1998) recorded click-synchronized (versus purely spontaneous) SOAEs from 10 subjects (5 with and 5 without tinnitus) in the upright sitting position and then again with the subject's head downward 160° to 180°. Analysis of a total of 48 SOAE peaks showed no differences in SOAE variability between the two body positions. Given the discrepancy between these two papers and the lack of systematic study in general, further investigation of the effects of body position on SOAE (and importantly on middle ear functioning) is warranted.

Ipsilateral and Contralateral Acoustic Stimulation

When an acoustic signal is presented to an ear with SOAEs, and at a frequency or frequencies within the signal that match those of the SOAE(s), the phase of the SOAEs can be synchronized or locked into the phase of the external signal (e.g., Wilson, 1980; Wilson & Sutton, 1981; Wit et al., 1981; Long et al., 1991; Talmadge et al., 1991; Uppenkamp & Kollmeier, 1994). This relationship does not, of course, imply that stimulus-evoked OAEs (e.g., TEOAEs) are equivalent to SOAEs (Wable & Collet, 1994). Perhaps more valuable for study of the cochlea, SOAEs can be suppressed by either ipsilateral or contralateral sound signals. Just as tuning curves can be measured with psychoacoustical methods, suppression tuning curves can also be generated with SOAEs (e.g., Wilson, 1980; Ruggero et al., 1983; Dallmayr, 1985; Bargones & Burns, 1988; Zizz & Glattke, 1988). For *ipsilateral suppression*, the SOAEs are first recorded in quiet without an external signal. Then external signals of varying frequencies, some higher and some lower, are presented to the ear with SOAEs and SOAE amplitudes are systematically calculated. Reductions in the SOAE amplitude with presentation of the external signal are referred to as suppression. The more effective suppression occurs when external signals are close to, or actually at, the SOAE frequencies, whereas the effectiveness of the suppressing signal (suppressor) decreases for lower or higher frequency external signals, although not at the same rate. Factors that must be considered in SOAEs suppression include the amplitude of the SOAEs, whether the suppressor is higher or lower in frequency than the SOAEs, the intensity of the suppressor, the time elapsed after the suppressor is turned off, and the subject. The most effective ipsilateral suppression occurs when a tone is presented at a frequency slightly higher than the SOAEs' frequencies, although the growth of suppression is greater for tones presented at frequencies below the SOAEs' frequencies.

The suppressive effects of ipsilateral or contralateral noise on OAEs is a hot research topic. It seems likely that before long contralateral suppression techniques will be applied clinically in the assessment of the efferent auditory system, along with cochlear function. The topic is reviewed also toward the end of Chapter 5.

Contralateral acoustic stimulation may also influence SOAEs. That is, sounds presented to one ear at moderate intensity levels, insufficient to activate the acoustic reflex and less than interaural attenuation, can

> ## SOAEs Can Produce DPOAE
>
> SOAEs may occur as multiple peaks closely spaced together. Equally spaced triplets of SOAE peaks may reflect the presence of a pair of SOAEs ("primary SOAEs") and a distortion product (DP) generated by these two primary frequencies.
>
> *Sources*: Burns et al. (1984); Jones et al. (1986); van Dijk & Wit (1998).

alter amplitude of SOAEs recorded from the other ear (Mott et al., 1989). Contralateral SOAEs suppression is mediated by the efferent auditory pathways. The topic of OAE suppression (ipsilateral and contralateral) is addressed in more detail in Chapter 5. Factors influencing SOAE measurement are summarized in Table 3–6.

Table 3–6. Summary of factors influencing spontaneous otoacoustic emissions (SOAEs), with selected references. See Key References at the end of this chapter for more literature on SOAEs.

Ear

■ More common in the right ear than in the left ear (Bilger, Matthies, Hammel, & Demorest, 1990; Penner, Glotzback, & Huang, 1993; Lamprecht-Dinnesen et al., 1998; Strickland, Burns, & Tubis, 1985).

Gender

■ Up to twice as common in females versus males (Bilger, Matthies, Hammel, & Demorest, 1990; Lamprecht-Dinnesen et al., 1998; Martin, Probst & Lonsbury-Martin, 1990; Strickland, Burns, & Tubis, 1985).

■ Females are more likely to have SOAEs bilaterally and to have multiple SOAE frequencies in an ear (Bilger, Matthies, Hammel, & Demorest, 1990; Martin, Probst, & Lonsbury-Martin, 1990; Strickland, Burns, & Tubis, 1985).

Menstrual cycle

■ SOAE frequencies recorded from women fluctuate during the monthly cycle (Bell, 1992; Bilger, Matthies, Hammel, & Demorest, 1990; Haggerty, Lusted, & Morton, 1993; Martin, Probst, & Lonsbury-Martin, 1990; Penner, Brauth, & Jastreboff, 1994; Strickland, Burns, & Tubis, 1985).

Daily changes

■ During the course of a day, there are circadian changes in SOAE frequency (Bell, 1992; Haggerty, Lusted, & Morton, 1993).

Table 3–6. *(continued)*

Age

■ Comparable prevalence in infants, children, and young adults according to some studies (Bonfils, Francois, Avan, Londero, Trotoux, & Narcy, 1992; Burns, Arehart, & Campbell, 1992; Strickland, Burns, & Tubis, 1985), but others studies show distinct decrease in the prevalence and number of SOAE as age increases in infancy and childhood (Lamprecht-Dinnesen et al., 1998).

■ There are reports suggesting that SOAEs are less common, and fewer in number, in persons over age 50 years (Bonfils, 1989; Moulin, Collet, Delli, & Morgon, 1991). It is likely, however, that these findings are due largely to subtle age-related sensory deficits (presbycusis) rather than simply age. With careful control of hearing sensivity across the age range, SOAEs show no clear age-effect (Stover & Norton, 1993; Strouse, Ochs, Hall, & Bess, 1996).

Hereditary factors

■ There seems to be a genetic predisposition for having SOAE (Bilger, Matthies, Hammel, & Demorest, 1990). SOAE findings more similar for monozygotic cotwins than for same-sex dizygotic cotwins (e.g., McFadden & Loehlin, 1995).

Race

■ There is a tendency for African Americans to have more SOAEs than whites and Asians, and Asians to show more than whites (Whitehead, Kamal, Lonsbury-Martin, & Martin, 1993).

Measurement conditions

■ Whether or not SOAEs are recorded, the amplitude of SOAEs can be seriously affected by measurement noise (physiologic and environmental), and the noise-reduction processing strategy used during recording.

Hearing thresholds

■ Among persons with normal otologic function and normal hearing sensitivity, hearing thresholds of persons with SOAEs are approximately 3 dB better than those without SOAEs (McFadden & Mishra, 1993).

■ As a rule, SOAEs are not recorded in persons whose hearing thresholds exceed 30 dB HL (assuming normal middle ear function), although SOAEs may be absent in persons with hearing thresholds well within normal limits who experience tinnitus or report a history of noise exposure (Bonfils, 1989; Bright & Glattke, 1986; Moulin, Collet, Delli, & Morgon, 1991; Probst, Lonsbury-Martin, Martin, & Coats, 1987).

Middle ear status

■ When middle ear pressure is greater or less than 0 mmH$_2$O (or daPa), typically SOAE frequencies increase and amplitudes decrease. However, infrequently the reverse occurs (Hauser, Probst, & Harris, 1993; Schloth & Zwicker, 1983; Wilson & Sutton, 1981).

Tinnitus

■ There is no consistent association between SOAEs and tinnitus. Typically, SOAEs are not observed in the frequency region of subjective tinnitus (Penner, 1990; Penner & Burns, 1987; Rebillard, Abou, & Lenoir, 1987; Tyler & Conrad-Armes, 1982; Zurek, 1981). Penner (1988, 1992; Penner & Coles, 1992), however, have reported for a handful of female subjects SOAEs that appeared to be associated in frequency with tinnitus.

■ SOAEs are not consistent with "objective tinnitus," that is, sounds of up to 30 or 40 dB (at the pinna) that can be heard by an examiner or bystander. That is, unlike subjective tinnitus, persons whose ears emit relatively loud tones do not themselves hear the sounds.

SOAEs IN CLINICAL POPULATIONS

Ototoxicity

Drugs with known ototoxic effects on cochlear function alter SOAEs. Although not immediately considered ototoxic by many persons, *aspirin* was among the first ototoxic drugs to be investigated with SOAEs and is the drug most extensively investigated. SOAE amplitude is reduced, or SOAEs are not detected, with ingestion of aspirin at levels of about 4 grams per day (McFadden, Plattsmier, & Passanen, 1984; Long et al., 1986; Long & Tubis, 1988; Weir et al., 1988; Stypulkowski & Oriaku, 1991). As a rule, the smaller amplitude SOAEs in an ear are affected first (McFadden & Plattsmier, 1984), followed 20 to 50 hours later by the larger SOAEs.

Not that many years ago in tropical and subtropical cities (e.g., Houston, Texas), audiologists now in their 50s who were just getting started in their careers encountered occasional patients who reported taking large doses of *quinine* for treatment or prevention of malaria. Nowadays, although quinine is rarely required for malaria, at least in the United States, audiologists may still encounter patients taking quinine as a treatment for leg cramps and pains. Clinical experience confirms that quinine can induce tinnitus and, with sufficiently high doses, cause sensory hearing loss. Although the exact mechanism is not clear, quinine alters cochlear function by interfering with outer hair cell motility and, presumably, cochlear active processes (Karlsson & Flock, 1990; Karlsson et al., 1991). A specific alteration of K+ channel metabolism is also suspected (Karlsson & Flock, 1990; Puel et al., 1990). Not unexpectedly, therefore, quinine (sulfate) can also produce a usually temporary reduction or loss of SOAEs (McFadden & Pasanen, 1994). It is possible that quinine also exerts indirect, that is, vascular or perilymphatic hydropic and non-outer-hair cell, effects on cochlear function. The effect of quinine is not straightforward, though, as some enhancement of SOAEs amplitude may occur at times, but only for selected frequencies, within hours after the drug is administered (Stypulkowski & Oriaku, 1991; McFadden & Pasanen, 1994). In addition, SOAE frequencies tend to shift downward slightly during quinine intoxication. This process reverses as the effect of quinine diminishes. As with the effects of aspirin, SOAEs appear to be more susceptible to influence by quinine (at dosages of one 325 mg tablet every 4 hours) than are DPOAEs or TEOAEs (McFadden & Pasanen, 1994). In contrast to aspirin, however, quinine works more slowly. Remarkably, occasional subjects actually show new "short-lived" SOAEs during quinine drug ototoxicity (McFadden & Pasanen, 1994). This is similar to the emergence of new SOAEs during extended SOAE measurement with the probe continuously inserted, or the "intializing effect" (McFadden & Pasanen, 1994), mentioned above. Speculating on an explanation for this phenomenon, McFadden (1994) theorized that there is a "law of

SOAE energy conservation." That is, SOAE energy within the cochlea is drawn from a finite pool of energy. When SOAEs are diminished in one point within the cochlea, energy is essentially released. The product of this temporary "new source" of energy is the emergence of a new SOAEs at another frequency. It is as if the SOAEs are jumping from one frequency to another. A similar concept, has been referred to by Burns et al. (1984) as the "quasi-stable-state" behavior of the cochlea.

Sensory Hearing Loss

As a rule, SOAEs are inversely related to sensory hearing loss. That is, SOAEs are less common in persons with hearing loss of any degree, even quite mild. It has long been appreciated, however, that SOAEs can be recorded from persons with sensory hearing loss at frequencies removed from the SOAEs (Zurek, 1981; Tyler & Conrad-Ames, 1982; Penner & Burns, 1987; Probst et al., 1987). In fact, as noted above, there is evidence that hearing is actually more sensitive in the region of SOAEs (Ruggero et al., 1983; Schloth, 1983; Long et al., 1986).

Tinnitus

Just as SOAEs are typically not present in the frequency region of sensory hearing loss, SOAEs and tinnitus are generally considered mutually exclusive. SOAEs are usually not recorded in frequency regions of reported tinnitus (Penner & Burns, 1987). This is a logical relationship as tinnitus is a symptom associated with cochlear damage while SOAEs typically reflect normal cochlear function. As interest in tinnitus has increased among audiologists and hearing scientists, there has been a corresponding increase in clinical and basic investigation of tinnitus and OAEs, as summarized in the review paper by Ceranic, Prasher, and Luxon (1995). This group of investigators from London offered evidence suggesting that SOAEs can be recorded in at least some patients with the symptom of tinnitus.

Ceranic, Prasher, and Luxon (1998) measured SOAEs in a control group of 20 normal-hearing subjects (6 males and 14 females) who did not report tinnitus and 53 subjects complaining of tinnitus. The tinnitus population consisted of five groups: 20 subjects with normal hearing sensitivity and no otologic pathology (8 males and 12 females), 10 subjects with tinnitus and sensorineural hearing loss of unknown etiology (3 males and 7 females), 10 subjects with tinnitus secondary to head injury but with normal peripheral hearing status, 10 subjects (4 males and 6 females) with idiopathic endolymphatic hydrops and some hearing loss, and 3 male subjects with tinnitus and hearing loss secondary to noise exposure. Click-synchronized SOAEs were recorded with the ILO 88 device during two separate sessions within a 1 to 16 unit time period. Tympanometry was used as a measure of middle ear status at all SOAE sessions. The main finding of this study was a total SOAE prevalence of 53% in the tinnitus group (100% in head-injured subjects and 62% in those with endolympatic hydrops), which was equivalent to the 52% prevalence in the control group. In contrast, and more consistent with the expected relation of tinnitus and OAE, SOAEs were recorded from only 17.6% of the patients with sensorineural hearing loss due to noise exposure. Also notable was the significantly lower stability, or reproducibility, of SOAEs in the tinnitus subjects (23.8%) versus the control group (58.2%). The authors speculated on the importance of these findings to the mechanisms underlying tinnitus, including cochlear mechanics, the possibility of reduced central efferent auditory effects in some persons with tinnitus, and the possible neural basis for some forms of endolymphatic hydrops. It would of interest clinically for this study to be replicated using a conventional (nonsynchronized) SOAEs technique and with the inclusion of TEOAE and DPOAE measures.

Did this brief review pique your interest in spontanous otoacoustic emissions? Here are some of the hundreds of references on SOAEs. Most of these journals have a website which will assist you in tracking down specific references or the addresses and e-mail addresses of the authors.

KEY REFERENCES

Bell A. Circadian and menstrual rhythms in frequency variations of spontaneous otoacoustic emissions from human ears. *Hearing Research 58*: 91–100, 1992.

Bilger RC, Matthies JL, Hammel DR, Demorest ME. Genetic implications of gender differences in the prevalence of spontaneous otoacoustic emissions. *JSHR 33*: 418–432, 1990.

Bonfils P. Spontaneous otoacoustic emissions: Clinical interest. *Laryngoscope 99*: 752–756, 1989.

Bonfils P, Francois M, Avan P, Londero A, Trotoux J, Narcy P. Spontaneous and evoked otoacoustic emissions in preterm neonates. *Laryngoscope 102*: 182–186, 1992.

Burns EM, Arehart KH, Campbell SL. Prevalence of spontaneous otoacoustic emissions in neonates. *JASA 91*: 1571–1575, 1992.

Burns EM, Keefe DH, Ling R. Energy reflectance in the ear canal can exceed unity near spontaneous otoacoustic emission frequencies. *JASA 103*: 462–474, 1998.

Burns EM, Strickland EA, Tubis A, Jones K. Interaction among spontaneous acoustic emissions. I. Distortion products and linked emissions. *Hearing Research 16*: 271–278, 1984.

Haggerty HS, Lusted HS, Morton SC. Statistical quantification of 24-hour and monthly variabilities of spontaneous otoacoustic emission frequency in humans. *Hearing Research 70*: 31–49, 1993.

Hauser R, Probst R, Harris EP. Effects of atmospheric pressure variation on spontaneous, transiently evoked, and distortion product otoacoustic emissions in normal human ears. *Hearing Research 69*: 133–145, 1993.

Kohler W, Fritze W. A long-term observation of spontaneous otoacoustic emissions (SOAEs). *Scandinavian Audiology 21*: 55–58, 1992.

Kok MR, van Zanten GA, Brocaar MP. Aspects of spontaneous otoacoustic emissions in healthy newborns. *Hearing Research 69*: 115–123, 1993.

Lonsbury-Martin BL, Martin GK, Probst R, Coats AC. Spontaneous otoacoustic emissions in nonhuman primate: II. Cochlear anatomy. *Hearing Research 33*: 69–94, 1988.

Martin G, Probst R, Lonsbury-Martin BL. Otocoustic emissions in human ears: Normative findings. *Ear and Hearing 11*: 106–120, 1990.

Mathis A, Probst R, DeMin H, Hauser R. A child with an unusually high level spontaneous otoacoustic emission. *Archives of Otolaryngology 117*: 674–676, 1991.

Moulin A, Collet L, Delli D, Morgon A. Spontaneous otoacoustic emissions and sensorineural hearing loss. *Acta Otolaryngologica 111*: 835–841, 1991.

Penner MJ. Audible and annoying spontaneous otoacoustic emissions. *Archives of Otolaryngology 114*: 150–153, 1988.

Penner MJ. Linking spontaneous otoacoustic emissions and tinnitus. *British Journal of Audiology 26*: 115–123, 1992.

Penner MJ, Brauth SE, Jastreboff PJ. Covariation of binaural, concurrently-measured spontaneous otoacoustic emissions. *Hearing Research 73*: 190–194, 1994.

Penner MJ, Coles RRA. Indications for aspirin as a palliative for tinnitus caused by SOAEs: A case study. *British Journal of Audiology 26*: 91–96, 1992.

Penner MJ, Glotzbach L, Huang T. Spontaneous otoacoustic emissions: Measurement and data. *Hearing Research 68*: 229–237, 1993.

Rebillard G, Abou S, Lenoir M. Les oto-emissions acoustiques II. Les oto-emissions spontanees: Resultats chez des sujets normaux ou presentant des acouphenes. *Annals of Otolaryngology 104*: 363–368, 1987.

Ruggero MA, Rich NC, Freyman R. Spontaneous and impulsively evoked otoacoustic emissions: Indicators for cochlear pathology? *Hearing Research 10*: 283–300, 1983.

Stover L, Norton SJ. The effects of aging on otoacoustic emissions. *JASA 94*: 2670–2681, 1993.

Strickland AE, Burns EM, Tubis A. Incidence of spontaneous otoacoustic emissions in children and infants. *JASA 78*: 931–935, 1985.

Talmadge CL, Long GR, Murphy WJ, Tubis A. New off-line method for detecting spontaneous otoacoustic emissions in human subjects. *Hearing Research 71*: 170–182, 1993.

Tyler RS, Conrad-Armes D. Spontaneous acoustic cochlear emissions and sensorineural tinnitus. *British Journal of Audiology 16*: 193–194, 1982.

Whitehead ML, Baker RJ, Wilson JP. The bilateral symmetry and sex asymmetry of spontaneous otoacoustic emission (SOAE) incidence in human ears. *British Journal of Audiology 23*: 149, 1989.

Whitehead ML, Kamal N, Lonsbury-Martin BL, Martin GK. Spontaneous otoacoustic emissions in different racial groups. *Scandinavian Audiology 22*: 3–10, 1993.

Wilson JP. Evidence for a cochlear origin for acoustic re-emissions, threshold fine-structure and tonal tinnitus. *Hearing Research 2*: 233–252, 1980.

Zurek P. Spontaneous narrowband acoustic signals emitted by normal ears. *JASA 69*: 514–523, 1981.

CHAPTER

4

Distortion Product and Transient Evoked OAEs: Measurement and Analysis

PREPARATION AND SETUP
  Equipment Setup
  Selection of Stimulus and Acquisition
    Parameters
  Ear Canal Inspection
  Review of Prior Test Results
  Patient Instructions
  Probe Insertion
  After the Test

DPOAE MEASUREMENT AND ANALYSIS
  Verification of Probe Fit and Test
    Conditions
  Stimulus Factors and Parameters
  Response Factors and Parameters
                                        (continued)

This discussion of OAE measurement and analysis is as generic as possible, with an emphasis on principles of measurement and accepted clinical practices rather than simply a "cook-book, how-to" description of OAE recording with instrumentation marketed by a single manufacturer. What follows is an attempt, in part, to review the features common to all OAE devices. The reader is referred to the "Manufacturers Forum" (Chapter 7) for device-specific information on OAE stimulation, acquisition, and analyses. For a basic introduction to OAEs, and to put the following sometimes technical discussion into perspective, Chapters 1 and 2 should be read first.

From a technical standpoint, performing OAEs measurements from normal-hearing and cooperative adults and school-aged children, for instance, your friendly audiology co-workers or well-behaved offspring, is not very challenging. A manufacturer's representative or a colleague who has been using the technique for awhile can effortlessly demonstrate how easy it is to record good-looking TEOAEs or DPOAEs, usually in less than a minute. "There's really nothing to this test," they proclaim confidently. "Tell you what . . . sit in this chair, and I'll show you how it's done. Let's see . . . what color immittance probe tip fits your ear? The medium-sized pink one? Good. O.K. Now I'll just slip the probe tip into your right ear and we'll begin the test. You can watch the screen here during the test, but be sure to sit very still." About 45 seconds later, the rep proudly announces "Here's your TEOAEs (or DPOAEs). It sure looks normal to me. We've got an extra minute, let me explain to you how we interpret OAEs . . . listen up, you'll need to know something about analyzing OAEs if you're going to use them here in your clinic . . ."

Many audiologists have had an experience very similar to that little scenario. Actually, there's some truth to implication that OAEs can be recorded quickly and easily and that analysis and interpretation can be clearcut and straightforward. On the other hand, it is much more challenging clinically to perform OAE measurement in uncooperative patients or noisy settings, to determine what test protocol is feasible and will provide the information you need, to analyze OAE responses that are clearly not entirely normal, and to interpret OAE findings meaningfully in the context of the patient's medical and auditory status and other audiologic findings. At the very least, clinicians who intend to either incorporate OAEs into their practices or apply them in a specific program, such as newborn hearing screening, should make a sincere and substantial effort to: (1) acquire or update their understanding of basic science underlying OAEs, (e.g., anatomy and physiology); (2) read some of the germinal original literature on the topic (readings are noted throughout this book) and a book (like this one) on OAEs; (3) keep up with professional literature on OAE; (4) attend an OAEs workshop or seminar devoted to the topic; (5) strive to understand the rationale behind specific components of OAEs test protocols; (6) practice recording OAEs from as many people as possible in the clinical setting, analyzing and interpreting findings with knowlege of the patient's diagnosis and audiologic profile; and (7) maintain an innovative, inquisitive, and open-minded approach to continued education on OAEs and their clinical applications.

Who would consider entering a golf tournament without first developing a decent swing and putting in hours of practice? Why are drivers licenses not available to anyone through the mail for a fee? Why are there minor leagues for baseball players? OAE measurement is not as complex as neurosurgery, but it does involve technique which takes practice to develop. The wise clinician will log in plenty of OAE recordings with cooperative normal hearing adults before attempting to apply the technique clinically in the audiologic assessment of pediatric patients.

The remainder of this chapter is meant to provide a useful mix of practical, even common-sense, guidelines on OAEs measurement along with a review of both basic and clinical principles of OAE measurement and analysis. A primary goal is to provide answers to the "why" questions about the use of OAEs in clinical practice, as well as the "how to" questions.

PREPARATION AND SETUP

Preparation is very similar for measurement of SOAEs, TEOAEs, or DPOAEs. Guidelines for preparing to perform successful OAE recordings that are common to all types of OAEs will be presented first. In reviewing this information, it is relevant, and might be helpful, to consider the following paraphrase of a section on "Preparation and Precautions Before the Test" from a book on auditory evoked responses (Hall, 1992b, pp. 277–278).

An important ingredient in successful OAE assessment is adequate preparation before patient contact. Although the degree of preparation required and its impact on OAE assessment varies among applications, at least three main concerns should be addressed. First, it is extremely valuable to know what kind of patient is being scheduled for assessment and why. There are many questions to be asked. What is the patient's age? Is the patient a newborn (premature or full-term?), a young or an older child, a young or older adult? Is the primary objective of testing diagnostic or to screen hearing sensitivity? What is the tentative diagnosis, or what are the likely etiologies to be ruled out in the differential diagnosis? If a diagnosis is suspected, consult other portions of this text or additional reference sources, to determine what OAE findings might be anticipated, or what special recording problems might be expected. Has an OAE assessment been carried out before? What did it show, and are the results available? Does the referral source want an immediate report of the results? Will the patient be alert, lethargic, or asleep? Are there reasons why behavioral audiologic techniques cannot be use? If previous behavioral testing was done, what did it show? Does the patient have normal hearing audiometrically and, if not, what is the type and degree of hearing impairment?

Second, before the OAE testing is scheduled to begin, it is important to ensure that the necessary equipment, personnel, and supplies are in place. This determination is, in part, based on the answers to the preceding questions. Is there an adequate and varied supply of clean probe tips? Is the program for the planned OAE test protocol prepared and accessible? Is there enough disc space for storage of OAEs data? Special additional questions and steps, sometime appropriate for specific OAE applications, such as newborn hearing screening or diagnostic OAE assessment in difficult-to-test children, are addressed in Chapter 8.

Equipment Setup

Prior to the arrival of the patient to the test area, or on reaching the patient if the assessment will be conducted elsewhere, the equipment is powered on. The patient's name and other demographic and, perhaps, clinical information are entered. Verify that the computer shows the correct date and time. Most OAE software includes an option for indicating the name of the tester. Adequacy of hard or floppy disc space on the OAE system might be verified at this time, so time-consuming data deletions or disc reformatting is not required in the midst of a possibly hurried OAE assessment. Also, an adequate assortment of clean probe tips should be handy, especially in sizes that would be appropriate for the patient.

Selection of Stimulus and Acquisition Parameters

The next customary step is creation or selection of an appropriate test protocol. Actually, all of the many and varied factors to consider in developing OAE test protocols and choosing specific stimulus and acquisition parameters, along with the reasons for the selections, are the topic of a detailed discussion below. Test protocols designed for specific clinical applications in children and adults are also reviewed in Chapters 8 and 9. Most clinicians will rely on a handful of test protocols for commonly encountered patient populations and the typical clinical applications of OAEs. Development of these protocols, which are easily entered into the computer software soon after the OAE equipment is initially delivered to the clinic, should be based on experimental evidence as reported in the literature or acquired by the manufacturer. For many OAE test parameters, there is now growing consensus, due to systematic investigations, about which values are optimal or most appropriate. Often, it will become very apparent during an OAE assessment that the test protocol initially selected for use with a patient is inappropriate or simply not feasible for one or more reasons. As an example, measurement noise may obliterate the OAE response or prevent the acquisition of any OAE data. It is important for the clinician to know how to modify a protocol and how to quickly access another premade protocol. But, equally important, clinicians should clearly understand the rationale for why specific test parameters were selected initially and how changing any parameter might affect the OAE. As in behavioral audiology and auditory evoked response recording, clinical decisions regarding OAE strategies must often be made quickly and on-line during testing for the outcome of the assessment to be successful, or the data at least usable.

Ear Canal Inspection

It is good clinical practice to perform otoscopic inspection before inserting the probe tip and beginning OAE measurement. There are, of course, exceptions to this policy, including for example patients who have recently been evaluated with tympanometry or other audiometric procedures and whose ear canals were inspected at that time, patients seen by audiology after an ear examination by a physician, and newborn infants undergoing hearing screening. In addition to the conventional wisdom of verifying status of the ear canal before putting anything into it, there are four main reasons for the otoscopic inspection: First, the clinician can determine whether OAE assessment is contraindicated by an external ear canal disorder or disease. Second, the possibility of technical problems due to probe blockage or occlusion by cerumen or debris can be evaluated and perhaps avoided before testing begins. Third, the inspection might yield findings that contribute to the meaningful interpretation of the OAEs (e.g., observation of a ventilation tube in place or of a perforation of the tympanic membrane). Fourth, otoscopic verification of a healthy ear canal before *and* after OAE assessment, and proper written documentation of any unusual findings, will help in the defense against any later claims that the procedure posed undue risk, caused excessive discomfort, or was injurious to the patient (Table 4–1).

Even normal ear canal acoustics can influence OAE measurement. Pathology, cerumen, vernix, debris, and other assorted objects (e.g., small rocks, bugs, buttons, beads) in the ear canal can totally confound OAE measurement. Otoscopy goes hand-in-hand with recording OAEs. When in doubt, check it out.

Table 4–1. Summary of assorted external ear canal factors potentially influencing clinical measurement of OAEs.

Factor	Influence
Nonpathologic	
■ Probe tip placement or condition	✓ The soft (rubber or foam) probe tip on the rigid probe assembly extends medially beyond the stimulus or microphone ports and occludes either or all, or
	✓ The foam probe tip on the rigid probe assembly is compressed too much, narrowing or occluding one or more of the tiny tubular openings and preventing an adequate stimulus delivery to the ear canal, or detection of the OAEs in the external ear canal.
■ Probe insertion	✓ In a tortuous ear canal with abrupt turns, the end of the probe tip on the rigid probe presses against the canal wall.
	✓ Blockage of stimulus energy delivery from the probe to the tympanic membrane
	✓ Blockage of OAE energy returning from the tympanic membrane to the microphone in the probe assembly
■ Standing waves	✓ Artifactual reduction or enhancement of DPOAE amplitude for stimulus frequencies > 5000 Hz
	✓ Unreliable DPOAE (for frequencies >5000 Hz)
	✓ Bogus or artifactually present DPOAEs when in fact DPOAEs are absent (>5000 Hz)
■ Cerumen or debris	✓ Occlusion of one or two stimulus tubes in the OAE probe, reducing stimulus intensity
	✓ Occlusion of the tube leading to the microphone with the OAE probe
	✓ Blockage of stimulus energy delivery from the probe to the tympanic membrane
	✓ Blockage of OAE energy returning from the probe to the tympanic membrane to the probe
■ Vernix (neonates)	✓ Occlusion of one or two stimulus tubes in the OAE probe, reducing stimulus intensity
	✓ Occlusion of the tube leading to the microphone with the OAE probe
	✓ Blockage of stimulus energy delivery from the probe to the tympanic membrane
	✓ Blockage of OAE energy returning from the tympanic membrane to the probe
Pathologic	
■ Stenosis	✓ Blockage of stimulus energy delivery from the probe to the tympanic membrane
	✓ Blockage of OAE energy returning from the tympanic membrane to the probe
■ External otitis or cyst	✓ Blockage of stimulus energy delivery from the probe to the tympanic membrane
	✓ Blockage of OAE energy returning from the tympanic membrane to the probe
	✓ Pain or discomfort preventing adequately deep probe fit with the external ear canal

Review of Prior Test Results

Decisions about the strategy and approach to take in OAE assessment will often become quite apparent when the results of previous audiologic or medical studies are reviewed. For example, if previous behavioral audiometry of an overtly cooperative 14-year-old girl showed marked discrepancies between pure tone thresholds and speech thresholds and generally inconsistent responses, then it would be appropriate to perform a diagnostic OAE assessment covering a wide frequency range and, perhaps, both moderate and lower intensity stimuli. One goal would be to rule out peripheral (at least middle ear and outer hair cell) auditory dysfunction throughout the range of audiometric frequencies. For an infant who was untestable behaviorally, or for whom results were obtained for only one ear, it would be appropriate to start out with a screening OAE protocol encompassing the upper end of the speech frequency region (anticipating considerable measurement noise and precious little test time) and to begin for the untested ear. If previous test results are not available in advance of the OAE test session, the review might even be conducted during the assessment or immediately after, prior to interpretation of the findings. One of the most interesting and intellectually challenging aspects of OAE clinical application is the working through the diagnostic audiology process with the inclusion of OAE data. For some patients, putting together the diagnostic puzzle is entirely dependent on the piece of information provided by OAEs. Chapters 8 and 9 include detailed discussions on how OAEs can be integrated into the current clinical audiology test batteries used with children and adults.

Patient Instructions

Patient instructions are, of course, worthless for neonates and very young children. They are, however, an important part of the OAE technique for many preschool children and many more mature patients. You may perform OAE assessments day in and day out, but your patient is probably going through the testing for the first time. First of all, explain briefly the procedure by making a statement such as: *"For this test, I'm going to place this soft tip (show it to them . . . let young children feel it!) just barely into your ear canal. Once it's in place, you'll hear some sounds (clicking sounds or tones). They won't be loud. Pay no attention to these sounds. This is an automatic response from your ear. You don't need to tell me that you hear the sounds. This test should only take a minute or two for each ear. Please just sit still and relax during this time. I'll let you know as soon as the test is done."* Patients need to understand that they can assist you by sitting very still and remaining quiet throughout the procedure and that they do not need to tell you they hear the sounds. Discourage the patients from talking, chewing gum, reading (and moving their head vertically or horizontally), scratching their head, and so on. The suspected malingerer or pseudohypacusic patient is an exception to this instruction guideline. Keep them guessing about the nature of the test. It would certainly not be wise to give such patients tips on how they might confound or even invalidate the OAE assessment. Similar explanations should be given to parents of children to be tested, especially if the child will remain with and be held by a parent during the assessment. It is helpful to announce to the parents at the outset that you will explain the findings to them when the assessment is complete. During the testing, however, everyone will need to be as quiet as possible since very faint sounds produced by the ear are being recorded in the ear canal.

This is a good time to mention the importance of arranging for the patient, and the test ear, to be in a relatively quiet location. With few exceptions (e.g., there is an important clinical reason to evaluate cochlear functioning for frequencies below 1000 Hz), it is not necessary to conduct clinical OAE assessments in a sound-treated booth. OAE measurement in a sound booth, if it is convenient and will not disrupt the clinical routine (and perhaps reduce the likelihood of appropriate OAE utilization) is unquestionably a good policy. As described in some detail in Chapter 5, and also below in the discussion of Trouble-Shooting, noise is almost always a concern in OAE measurement as the overall objective is to detect faint sounds (the OAEs) in the presence of unwanted sound (noise) originating from the environment and the patient. Ambient (environmental) noise can be reduced substantially during OAE measurement if the patient is located in a sound booth and the equipment (potentially noisy computer) remains outside the booth. When OAEs are recorded in a nonsound-treated room, measurement noise can be minimized by closing the outside door to the room, moving the patient as far from the OAE computer as the probe cord will allow, turning the test ear away from the OAE equipment (a swivel chair for the patient is handy), and turning off any other noise-generating devices that are not being used (e.g., evoked response system, printer, radio, soap opera on TV).

Probe Insertion

In this author's clinical experience, optimal probe fit is by far the most critical single step in successful OAE measurement. The savy clinician will not take any short cuts when purchasing probe tips, selecting the best tip for the patient, or assuring a snug fit within the ear canal. During the otoscopic inspection, roughly estimate the size of the ear canal and note any atypical features. Then, select a probe tip size that seems appropriate. If you have just performed tympanometry with an adequate hermetic (airtight) seal, attempt the OAE recording with the same size, or even the same tip if it is compatible with the OAE device. Sometimes a probe tip the next size smaller than that used for immittance procedures will facilitate deep and firm insertion. Remember, an airtight seal is not necessary for OAE measurement. All manufacturers offer probe tips of varying sizes, ranging from probe tips for newborn infants to adult sizes, but some probe tip designs seem to fit ear canals better than others. Probe tips available from one manufacturer are sometimes compatible with probes for a competitor's OAE system. You might want to order a small supply of different brands of probe tips, or borrow a few from a colleague, and "experiment" with a diverse collection of normal subjects (even young siblings or offspring) and patients until you find the combination that seems to work best for you. Whether you use disposable or reusable probe tips, be sure to obtain a sizable number of all sizes. On busy clinical days, a fair number of probe tips of each size will either be discarded (disposable) or out-of-service during disinfection (reusable).

The next step is to couple the probe tip to the probe assembly. Take care to slide a new probe tip fully onto the probe. Several different probe designs are used with clinical OAE devices (see Chapter 7). With some OAE devices, the probe tip (usually made of soft rubber) forms a sleeve around the rigid tubular end of the probe assembly. For this design, the probe tip should be pushed onto the probe until the end is flush with the ear (lateral) end of the probe. Other equipment designs include probe tips of rubber, plastic, or foam formed around a straw-like stalk. The stalk, which may be a simple tube or may contain two or three small-diameter tubes, is slipped into or onto the proper receptacle on the probe. Consult with the manufacturers, their representative, and/or your equipment manual for specific guidelines on probe tip placement, probe assembly cleaning, probe maintenance, and so on.

If immittance measurement has just been completed successfully, and the probes for your immittance and OAE devices are compatible, use the same probe tip (or maybe one size smaller) in recording OAEs. A well-designed probe tip contributes immensely to successful OAE measurement — this is where the rubber meets the ear canal.

The technique used for inserting the probe depends, to a degree, on the style of the probe tip. Foam probe tips are usually compressed before insertion. For optimal insertion in adults, the tester grasps the upper part of the pinna of the ear with one hand and, while pulling gently upward and toward the back, inserts the probe with the other hand (as with the insertion of immittance tips). With neonates, infants, and young children, the tester grasps the ear lobe with one hand, while pulling downward and outward. Both of these maneuvers tend to straighten the ear canal and permit easier and deeper insertion of the probe tip. A slight twisting motion during the maneuver may facilitate insertion. In addition to selecting the proper size of the probe tip, it is important to reach an appropriate depth of insertion. As a rule, deeper is better because the probe tip will serve to attenuate more ambient noise and the stimuli will be delivered closer to the tympanic membrane. The angle of insertion is also important. The goal is to place the probe tip directly into the ear canal, whenever possible, so that the stimulus is delivered toward the center of canal, rather than diagonally toward the canal wall (another good reason for visual inpection of the ear canal before OAE measurement begins). Problems with probe fit will be addressed again in the discussion of Troubleshooting. If during the probe fit routine, or anytime during OAE recording, the stimulus is less than optimal, the first step that should be taken is inspection of the probe and then reinsertion.

After the Test

After removal of the probe tip from the ear canal, it is good practice to perform a cursory inspection of the ports and openings for cerumen or other debris, particularly if OAE findings were not entirely normal. If cerumen or debris is noted, it should be cleaned or the probe tip replaced. Then, OAE assessment should be repeated.

Immediately after it is disconnected from the probe assembly, the used probe tip (if not disposable) should be placed in either a container clearly marked for probe tips that need to be cleaned or directly into a container with hospital-approved disinfectant solution. Disposable probe tips should be properly discarded immediately after use. Infection precautions and control are more important now than anytime in the past. It is important to follow all hospital policies for prevention of the spread of bacterial and viral infection. For details on universal precautions and infectious diseases and their control, the reader is referred to Mueller and Hall (1998, pp. 797–808). Finally, colorful and cute probe tips may be attractive to young children. Kids might even find them appetizing. It's advisable to keep all probe tips out of reach of curious little hands.

DPOAE MEASUREMENT AND ANALYSIS

Verification of Probe Fit and Test Conditions

In this chapter, and elsewhere in the book, the abreviation "DP" will be used for distortion product, and will refer unless otherwise specified to the DP at $2f_1 - f_2$.

After visual inspection to assure that the probe tip is placed snugly within the external ear canal, probe fit is formally verified immediately before OAE data collection begins. The process is rather unique in hearing measurement, although not unlike probe microphone measurements in hearing selection, fitting, and verification. In conventional hearing measurement, such as pure tone or speech audiometry, instrumentation including transducers (e.g., earphones) meets national or international standards and is calibrated periodically during the year. The unspoken assumption is that the signal delivered to the patient has all of the desired characteristics, including precise intensity, frequency, and duration and is free from unwanted sound (noise, distortion, interference, artifact). In clinical audiology, during pure tone or speech audiometry, signal characteristics are not verified within the ear canal as they are in OAE measurement.

Verification of probe fit and stimulus characteristics are routinely completed before actual OAE measurement starts, critical properties of the stimulus or stimuli (intensity and sometimes frequency composition) are monitored either continously or periodically during measurement, and documentation is stored for later analysis. This is possible because the probe assembly, and sometimes attached transducers, functions not only in delivering the stimulus (stimuli) to the ear, but also in detecting acoustic signals (OAEs) within the ear canal. It is also necessary because differences in ear canal dimensions and acoustics among patients would create wide variations if stimulus intensity levels were fixed. The miniature microphone within the probe converts (transduces) sounds within the ear canal into electrical signals that are eventually sent in digital format to the computer software. The microphone built into the probe, therefore, permits continuous or periodic monitoring of stimulus intensity and frequency values to assure stimulus stability and balance between stimuli (f_1 and f_2). Recommendations and protocols for probe fit verification vary among manufacturers. Some probe fit routines are semi-automated, providing warnings to the equipment user when the fit is inadequate but otherwise leading directly to data collection. This approach is particularly useful with hearing screening OAE devices that are operated by technicians and other nonaudiologists. With other OAE devices, the operator manually starts and stops the probe fit routine and analyzes the quality of the stimulus before OAE measurement proceeds.

With any DPOAE device, the user should assume responsibility for verification of stimulus adequacy. Once the probe is inserted into the ear canal, stimulus presentation begins and the intensity levels, and of course frequency values, of the stimuli (f_1 and f_2) and the intensity level of noise in a narrow frequency region around the DP (usually $2f_1–f_2$) are displayed. Actual intensity values of the stimuli are compared to target (intended) values, and the intensity of the noise floor is determined and compared to expectations for that frequency. With most DPOAE devices, a message will be displayed if there is a critical problem with the probe, such as occlusion, or sometimes excessive noise levels. Interference of stimulus presentation, or OAE detection, by cerumen or other debris in the external ear canal is commonplace for both DPOAEs (Figure 4–1) and TEOAEs (Figure 4–2). Guidelines for evaluating stimulus properties during OAE measurement are reviewed below (Response Analysis), along with figures illustrating examples of the information displayed by several clinical devices.

Stimulus calibration recommendations also vary among DPOAE manufacturers. In general, the operator cannot actually calibrate the stimulus (stimuli). That is, the operator does not manually readjust stimulus intensity levels to meet some standard. Rather, the operator essentially verifies that stimuli are calibrated whenever DPOAEs are measured with a patient. Probe failure or damage is the most common

Don't expect the equipment distributor to calibrate your OAE system during the quarterly calibration of audiometers in the clinic. Read carefully the manual for your OAE device to learn as much as possible about how the accuracy of stimulus intensity and frequency is verified, and what to do if the system is out of calibration.

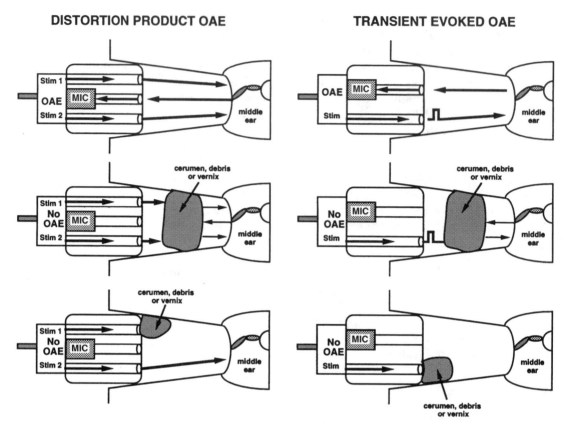

DISTORTION PRODUCT OAE

TRANSIENT EVOKED OAE

Figure 4–1. Illustration of interference with DPOAE stimulus presentation and/or response detection due to external ear canal pathology, cerumen, or debris. Occlusion of the external ear canal will reduce the effective stimulus intensity and block the outward propagation of the DPOAEs, whereas blockage of one or more ports will greatly reduce the intensity level of the primary stimuli (f_1 and/or f_2), or the DPOAE detected by the microphone. In either event, measurement is invalidated and a normal DPOAE will not be recorded.

Figure 4–2. Illustration of interference with TEOAE stimulus presentation and/or response detection due to external ear canal pathology, cerumen, or debris. Occlusion of the external ear canal will reduce the effective transient stimulus intensity delivered to the cochlea and will block the outward propagation of the TEOAEs. Blockage of either or both of the ports reduces the intensity level of transient stimuli and/or the TEOAEs detected by the microphone. In either event, measurement is invalidated and a normal TEOAEs will not be recorded.

cause for major deviation in stimulus intensity level that is not leveled, or adjusted, once the probe is fitted into a patient's ear. Reliability and durability of probe designs, and the probe cords/cables, naturally vary among manufacturers. With heavy use, including accidental physical abuse, probes may eventually malfunction. The solution is usually replacement of the probe by the manufacturer, and sometimes reloading a calibration software program for that specific probe.

Stimulus Factors and Parameters

As illustrated in Figure 4–3, the stimuli for DPOAE measurement are two pure tones, referred to as the "primary" tones, at frequencies f_1 and f_2. By convention, f_1 is always the lower frequency tone and f_2 is always the higher frequency tone, or $f_2 > f_1$. Although there is potentially an infinite array of intensity and frequency combinations and relationships for these two stimuli, basic and clinical investigations during the last decade have produced the rationale for certain stimulus values. The evidence from these studies will now be reviewed briefly for the DP and DP protocol stimulus parameters illustrated in Figure 4–4, and the DP protocols and DPgrams shown elsewhere in this chapter.

DPOAE Measurement

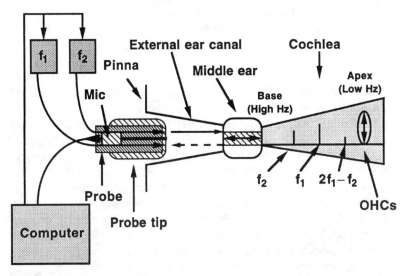

Figure 4–3. A schematic diagram of the general instrumentation used to record DPOAEs. In addition to a computer, the major components are two separate transducers (for f_1 and f_2). Stimuli are mixed when delivered to the enclosed ear canal. Within the probe assembly is a miniature, low-noise microphone for detecting the response (DPOAEs) produced apical to the stimulus place on the basilar membrane and propagated outward to the ear canal. The probe apparatus is coupled to a computer with software for generation of the signal(s), spectral analysis of sound within the ear canal, detecting and processing the response, and reducing noise, also detected in the ear canal.

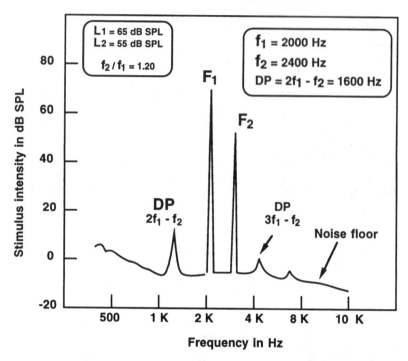

Figure 4–4. Major stimulus parameters in measurement of distortion product OAEs (DPOAEs). The stimuli, or primaries, are labeled f_1 (lower frequency) and f_2 (higher frequency). The intensity Level of these stimuli is indicated by the label L (i.e., L_1 and L_2). In this typical example, L_1 = 65 dB SPL and L_2 = 55 dB SPL. The relation or spacing between the two frequencies is described as the f_2/f_1 ratio (typically about 1.20). The distortion product (DP) recorded from the cochlea with presentation of these stimuli appears at other frequencies. The prominant DP in humans is at the frequency defined by the equation $2f_1 - f_2$, although DPs at other frequency regions are not uncommon. The noise levels or floors are always measured during OAE recording. Noise invariably is progressively greater for the lower frequency regions.

The Three Frequencies of DPOAEs

From a clinical point of view, it is important to know which of the three frequencies in DPOAE measurements (i.e., f_1, f_2, or $2f_1–f_2$) is most closely related to the cochlear place that effectively is being stimulated. In other words, when we analyze DP amplitudes for various stimulus frequencies in a DPgram, how do these findings relate to the audiogram frequencies? To answer this practical question, it is necessary to know whether the two primary stimuli have equal intensity ($L_1 = L_2$), or whether intensity for the higher frequency primary (f_2) is lower than that of the lower frequency primary (f_1), that is, $L_1 > L_2$. Discussion of frequency and intensity properties of the stimuli used in DPOAE measurement is somewhat cumbersome because neither of the two properties can be considered in isolation. The role played by each of the two primaries (f_1 and f_2) in activating outer hair cells along the basilar membrane is also dependent on their relative intensity levels. It might help to refer to the schematic illustrations of the three frequencies shown in Figure 4–5. DPOAEs are presumably generated in the frequency region where energy for the two primaries overlaps, illustrated as the shaded area in Figure 4–5 (Whitehead, Jiminez, et al., 1995; Whitehead, Stagner, McCoy, Lonsbury-Martin, & Martin, 1995). For both primary intensity conditions ($L_1 = L_2$ and $L_1 > L_2$), at low to moderate absolute stimulus intensity levels, the "tail" or "skirt" of the f_1 primary extends toward the base of the cochlea (Johnstone, Patuzzi, & Yates, 1986) and into the region of f_2 excitation. However, the ampli-

In clinical DPOAE measurement, it is handy to align some of f_2 and audiometric frequencies (e.g., 1000, 2000, 3000 Hz) to enhance the relation between the DPgram and audiogram. With a DPOAE stimulus intensity paradigm of L_1-L_2 = 10 dB, the cochlear place stimulated approximates the f_2 frequency. Of course, the same can be said for the stimulus frequency of a pure-tone signal.

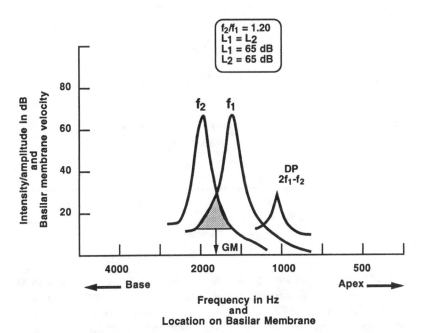

Figure 4–5. A schematic representation of the traveling waves associated with the two primary stimuli (f_1 and f_2) used to evoke DPOAEs. In this example, intensity level for each stimulus is 65 ($L_1 = L_2 = 65$ dB SPL). The shaded triangle approximately midway between the two stimuli (GM = geometric mean) is a region of the basilar membrane activated during stimulation, in addition to the f_1 and f_2 places. The DP measured in the ear canal is produced at the more apical place represented by the frequency defined by the equation $2f_1 - f_2$.

tude of basilar membrane vibration at the f_2 place (the basal spread) will be even greater as the f_1 intensity is increased. In fact, if L_1 is increased sufficiently, relative to L_2, the overlap is maximized and amplitude of the f_1 vibration approximates f_2 vibration at the f_2 place on the basilar membrane (Figure 4–6). In essence, at low to moderate stimulus intensity levels (up to about 70 dB), when $L_1 > L_2$ about 10 dB or more (i.e., $L_1 - L_2 \geq 10$ dB), cochlear stimulation is mostly at the f_2 place on the basilar membrane. At very high stimulus intensity levels (above 70 to 75 dB), the region of excitation for each primary is broad and, therefore, the f_1 vibration approximates f_2 vibration at the f_2 place on the basilar membrane for $L_1 = L_2$. Decreasing the f_2 primary level (L_1) may actually decrease the overlap, with a corresponding reduction in DPOAE amplitude (Whitehead, Jimenez, et al., 1995; White-

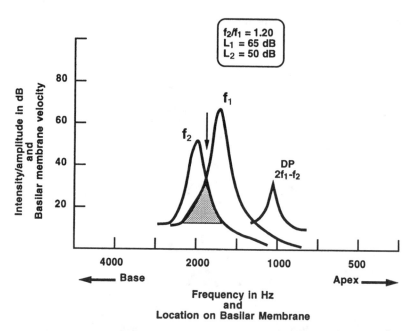

Figure 4–6. Another schematic representation of the traveling waves associated with the two primary stimuli (f_1 and f_2) used to evoke DPOAEs. In this example (in contrast to Figure 4–5), intensity level for the f_1 stimulus is 65, whereas intensity level for the f_2 stimulus is 50 dB SPL ($L_1 - L_2 = 15$ dB SPL). Because of this intensity difference, the region of overlap shifts toward the frequency place of the higher intensity stimulus (f_2). The peak of the shaded triangle, which is found close to the f_2 stimulus place, produces activation during stimulation, in addition to the f_1 and f_2 places. This additional energy is not part of either of the two stimuli, i.e., it is distortion. The DP measured in the ear canal is produced at the more apical place represented by the frequency defined by the equation $2f_1 - f_2$.

head, Stagner, et al., 1995). For equally intensity primaries (i.e., $L_1 = L_2$) at low-to-moderate absolute intensity levels, the site of maximum vibration on the basilar membrane is presumably closer to the geometric mean between the two frequencies (refer to Figure 4–5). So, the question posed earlier about relating DPOAE frequencies to the audiogram is best answered as follows. DPOAE amplitudes plotted as a function of f_2 would be expected to agree closest to the audiogram, assuming that $L_1 > L_2$ and the absolute intensity level is low to moderate (not over 70 dB). Clinically, it is useful to be sure that the effective DPOAE stimulus frequency corresponds to audiometric frequencies (e.g., 1000 Hz, 2000 Hz, 3000 Hz, etc.). Less attention needs to be given to the other two DPOAE frequencies—f_1 and $2f_1$–f_2—which are not directly related to the audiogram. The latter frequency ($2f_1$–f_2) reflects the place on the basilar membrane that the DPOAE is expressed, but it provides no information on the status of the cochlea in that region. Conceivably, a DPOAE could be recorded at the $2f_1$–f_2 frequency even if the outer hair cells at that place were nonfunctional. As noted later in this section of the chapter, DPs may also be present at frequencies other than $2f_1$–f_2. The numerous and interdependent effects of absolute and relative stimulus frequency and intensity variables are summarized in the next two sections of this chapter.

The f_2/f_1 Ratio

The frequency relationship or separation between the two primary tones is critical in DPOAE measurement (Wilson, 1980; Brown & Kemp, 1985; Harris et al., 1989). A DP will not be recorded if the two tones are spaced too far apart or if they are too close together. The distance between the two primary tones is described as the ratio of f_2: f_1, typically expressed as the f_2/f_1 ratio. DP amplitude drops off rather sharply as the frequency ratio is increased or decreased from a value of about 1.20. This effect is probably a reflection of filtering processes and tuning capabilities within the cochlea (e.g., Allen & Fahey, 1993; Brown, Williams, & Gaskill, 1993). Specifically, if one of the primaries is fixed while the other is varied systematically, and if this process is repeated for different absolute and/or relative f_1 and f_2 intensity levels for the primaries, and DPs are recorded at the different stimulus ratios and intensities, then the interactive effects among f_2/f_1 ratios and stimulus intensities on DP amplitude can be assessed. This has been done by a number of investigators during a 10-year period. In fact, as shown diagrammatically in Figure 4–7, the optimal ratio for generating maximum DP amplitude varies slightly as a function of the intensity level and frequencies of the primary tones between subjects and for humans versus other animal species (Harris et al., 1989; Gaskill & Brown, 1990; Bonfils et al., 1991; Nielsen, Popelka, Rasmussen, & Osterhammel, 1993). Within the 1000 to 3000 Hz frequency region, maximum DP amplitudes are recorded with an f_2/f_1 ratio of close to 1.30, whereas for higher or lower frequencies, a ratio of 1.20 produces the largest DP

With all DPOAE devices, the f_2/f_1 ratio can be manipulated easily. The effect of ratio on DP amplitude can be readily observed by recording a few DPgrams at ratios slightly above (e.g., 1.30 and 1.35) and below (e.g., 1.15 and 1.10) the generally optimally ratio of 1.20.

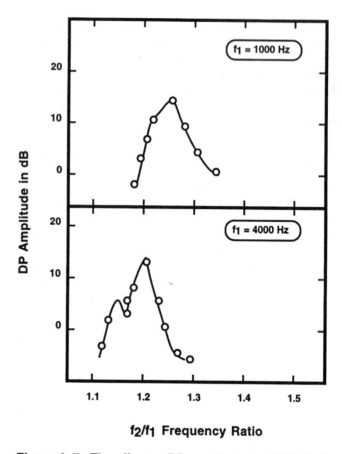

Figure 4–7. The effect on DP amplitude (in dB SPL) of manipulating the spacing or difference between the two primaries (f_1 and f_2) in DPOAE measurement. Maximum DP amplitude is associated with a narrow range of f_2/f_1 ratios, with sharp decreases in amplitude for higher or lower f_2/f_1 values. The optimal ratio, however, varies as a function of the absolute frequency of the primaries (e.g., 1000 versus 4000 Hz in the figure), the intensity levels of the stimuli, and individual differences between persons.

amplitude (Nielsen et al., 1993). According to these authors, if a ratio of 1.20 is used for primaries of any frequency, the DP amplitude will generally still be within 3 dB of what it was at the optimal ratio. DPOAEs are most often recorded clinically for frequencies of 1000 and higher. Therefore, the practical point is that, as stimulus frequency increases above 2000 Hz, the optimal ratio decreases from about 1.22 to 1.17. That is, if the ratio is kept at 1.22, then we would expect a progressive reduction in DP amplitude for higher frequency stimuli up to the limit for most clinical devices (8000 or 10,000 Hz). Also, generally speaking, as primary stimulus intensity increases, there is a corresponding increase in the optimal f_2/f_1 ratio.

The slope of the DP amplitude decrease (as the f_2/f_1 ratio is shifted above or below the optimal value) becomes steeper for higher frequencies, and when $L_1 > L_2$ versus $L_1 = L_2$ (Gaskill & Brown, 1990). Multiple peaks in this DP amplitude by f_2/f_1 ratio function are also sometimes observed. The effect of changes in the f_2/f_1 ratio on DP amplitudes is apparent in input/output functions (He & Schmiedt,1997), although the effect is dependent in a rather complex fashion on the intensity relation between L_1 and L_2 (He & Schmiedt, 1997). DPOAE fine structure (described below) also undergoes a frequency shift as a function of changes in the f_2/f_1 ratio, but once again these changes are the product of highly dependent interaction among absolute and relative primary intensity levels and the frequency ratio. The earlier f_2/f_1 ratio findings, cited above, for adult subjects, indicating that a frequency ratio of 1.20 produces robust DP amplitude under most combinations of primary frequency and intensity, have more recently been confirmed also for children, including neonates (Abdala, 1996). Age effects on OAEs will be reviewed in the next chapter. *The cumulative results of these studies confirm that, on average, an appropriate and clinically effective f_2/f_1 ratio for persons of all ages is somewhere within the range of 1.20 and 1.23.*

Intensity Level of f_1 and f_2 (L_1 and L_2)

The relative intensity level of the two primaries, as well as the absolute intensity levels, is another critical stimulus parameter in DPOAE measurement. The problem of selecting two stimulus intensity levels for one auditory signal is rare in clinical audiology. For most audiologic procedures, the signal is a single sound, a series of the single sounds, or a unit of sound. Examples of each would be a pure tone (pure tone audiometry), a series of hundreds or even thousands of clicks (ECochG or ABR), or a word (speech audiometry). One exception that comes to mind are a group of cortical electrophysiologic measures. Some long-latency auditory evoked responses, among them the P300 response and mismatch negativity (MMN) response, are elicited with two different signals, one presented frequently and predictably and another different signal presented only occasionally (the rare or deviant signal). In clinical audiology, most often in diagnostic or central auditory system test procedures, secondary sounds are presented ipsilaterally at the same time as the signal, but not as a stimulus. The secondary sound might be a masking noise (as in a masking level difference, or MLD, test), a babble or speech signal (as a competing message, for example, the synthetic sentence identification with ipsilateral competing message, or SSI-ICM test). Simultaneously presented contralateral signals are also employed in some procedures, such as dichotic speech tests. Unlike in DPOAE measurement, in none of these tests are both signals necessary components of the stimulus.

The intensity level of the primary stimuli is abbreviated "L". The three possible intensity relationships between the two primary signals are: $L_1 > L_2$, $L_1 < L_2$, or $L_1 = L_2$. Which of these should be used in DPOAE measurement, and why? One of the possibilities can be scratched off the list at the outset. DP amplitudes are invariably paltry and submaximal when recorded with intensity of the higher frequency primary exeeds that of the lower frequency primary, that is, with an intensity relation of $L_1 < L_2$. Consistently robust DPOAEs can be recorded with either of the other two intensity possibilities. Equal intensity primaries ($L_1 = L_2$) were in fact employed in many of the earlier experimental studies of DPOAEs and until about 1995 were also used in recording DPOAEs for clinical applications (e.g., Lonsbury-Martin et al., 1990; Spektor et al., 1991; Hall, 1993). Now, two major clinical advantages of utilizing an relatively lower intensity level for the f_2 primary, that is, $L_1 - L_2 = > 0$ dB or $L_1 > L_2$, are recognized, and this primary stimulus intensity relationship is an accepted and preferred feature of clinical DPOAE test protocols. The two advantages associated with the $L_1 > L_2$ intensity relation, at least absolute stimulus intensities up to about 75 dB SPL (low to moderate levels), actually provide a rare example, in clinical audiology, of "the best of both worlds," or "having your cake and eating it too." Namely, in comparison to the $L_1 = L_2$ relation, with $L_1 > L_2$ DPOAE amplitudes are larger usually by about 3 dB (Gaskill & Brown, 1990; Hauser & Probst, 1991; Whitehead, Lonsbury-Martin, & Martin, 1992; Rasmussen et al., 1993; Jiminez, et al., 1995; Whitehead, Stagner, et al., 1995) *and* there is enhanced DPOAE sensitivity to cochlear (outer hair cell) dysfunction secondary to a variety of clinically common etiologies, such as ototoxicity and excessive noise exposure (e.g., Mills et al., 1993; Mills & Rubel, 1994; Sutton et al., 1994; Jiminez, et al., 1995; Whitehead, Stagner, et al., 1995). A group of Danish investigators offered evidence to the contrary, however. Rasmussen et al. (1993) reported maxiumum DP amplitude when $L_1 = L_2$, a slight decrease in amplitude when $L_1 > L_2$ and, as expected, a very marked amplitude drop when $L_1 < L_2$. In their study, however, DPOAEs were evoked with stimuli at an intensity level of 75 dB SPL (from 7 normal hearers). Because a relatively high stimulus intensity level was used, the results may not be directly generalized and compared, to those using lower primary intensity levels. Virtually all published studies and accumulated clinical experiences have also confirmed that the sensitivity of DPOAEs to cochlear dysfunction increases as the absolute stimulus intensity levels decrease. Abnormal DP findings are, therefore, more likely for stimulus intensity levels of 55 dB (for either $L_1 = L_2$ or $L_1 > L_2$), for example, than at 75 dB (again for either $L_1 = L_2$ or $L_1 > L_2$).

If you enjoyed experimenting with the f_2/f_1 ratio, then you might want to also record DPOAEs with several intensity combinations. To demonstrate the importance of the relative intensity levels, run a DPgram with $L_1 - L_2 = 10$ db (e.g., $f_1 = 65$ dB and $f_2 = 55$ dB), then with $L_1 = L_2$ (e.g., $f_1 = 65$ dB and $f_2 = 65$ dB), and then with $L_2 - L_1 = 10$ db (e.g., $f_1 = 55$ dB and $f_2 = 65$ dB). Compare DP amplitudes as a function of stimulus frequency for these three Dpgrams.

Concluding Comments

Major stimulus parameters include the absolute frequencies of the primaries, the f_2/f_1 ratio, the absolute intensity of the primaries (from low levels of about 30 dB up to levels of 75 dB or higher) and the relative intensities of the primaries (e.g., fixing L_1 at 50 dB and increasing L_2 from 30 to 75 dB, or vice versa). It is beyond the scope of this discussion to review in detail the interesting and dynamic, yet somewhat complicated, effects on different DPOAE response parameters (amplitude, phase, and DP fine structure) brought about by the interactions among these DPOAE stimulus parameters. In addition, the potential effects of other stimulus factors, such as the rate at which the primaries are presented at each frequency were not mentioned, mainly because they apparently have not been formally studied. As noted in Chapter 10, with technical advances in instrumentation, clinical DPOAE measurement in the future may incorporate the findings of these studies into innovative, and probably more precise and efficient, test protocols. Meanwhile, the reader is referred to the following literature for a review of original data (Harris et al., 1989; Gaskill & Brown, 1990; Bonfils et al., 1991; Whitehead et al., 1992; Brown, 1993; He & Schmiedt, 1993; Nielsen et al., 1993; Whitehead, Jiminez, et al., 1995; Whitehead, Stagner, et al., 1995; Abdala, 1996; He & Schmiedt, 1997).

In summary, from the rather extensive experimental and clinical data now available, we can confidently make the final general statements regarding stimulus parameters:

■ decreasing L_2 below L_1 produces a modest amplitude augmentation of DPOAE amplitude (on the order of 3 dB for low to moderate absolute stimulus intensity levels).
■ decreasing L_2 below L_1 enhances the sensitivity of DP to cochlear deficits, that is, DP amplitude reductions associated with outer hair cell dysfunction are greater (for low to moderate absolute stimulus intensity levels).
■ decreasing absolute stimulus intensity enhances the vulnerability (sensitivity) of DPOAEs to cochlear dysfunction.
■ DPOAEs are fundamentally different for low to moderate stimulus intensity levels (dependent on active cochlear processes) than for high stimulus levels (dependent on passive cochlear processes).
■ the site of cochlear stimulation in DPOAE measurement is closest to the f_2 region along the basilar membrane (not the f_1 region or where the $2f_1–f_2$ is expressed). DPOAE amplitude is more dependent on the intensity of L_1 than the intensity of L_2.

Response Factors and Parameters

As just reviewed, the presentation of primary tones at an appropriate ratio and appropriate intensity levels to a normal cochlea generates combination tones or DPs within the cochlea that are propagated toward the stapes footplate and then outward through the middle ear system to the external ear canal (Table 4–2). DPs are not effectively generated with very low stimulus intensity levels. Spectral analysis of sound in the ear canal after the stimuli are presented will reveal stimulus-induced sounds at predictable frequencies (the DPOAEs). These combination tones can be found at frequencies defined by the equation: $/n\,f_1 - m\,f_2/$, where m and n are any pair of integers. In humans, with Fourier (spectral) analysis sound within the ear canal after presentation of the primary tones, the most robust DPs are found at $2f_1–f_2$ (Table 4–3). Some clinical DPOAE devices, however, offer an option for recording other frequencies. Features of specific DPOAE devices are reviewed by the manufacturers in Chapter 7.

DPgrams

The most common approach for reporting DP findings clinically is a graph of DP amplitude (in dB SPL) as a function of stimulus frequency. The term "DP audiogram," used occasionally in the late 1980s and

Table 4–2. Linearity/nonlinearity of the auditory system.

■ **Linearity**

When the input to the auditory system, such as an acoustic stimulus, is changed only in amplitude and/or phase of a signal before it emerges as the output of the system. There is a straight relation between input and output.

■ **Nonlinearity**

When sinusoids are found in the output of the auditory system that are not present in the input; that is, what comes out is more than what went in to the system. A simple waveform enters the nonlinear system and a complex waveform comes out the other end. The output may differ from the input in the *time domain*, as well as in the frequency domain.

■ **Harmonics**

Multiples of a single frequency put into a system in the output. For example, if the input frequency is f_1, e.g., 100 Hz, then higher harmonics might be $2f_1$, $3f_1$, etc. (or 200 Hz, 300 Hz, etc.).

■ **Combination tones (summation and difference tones)**

When two frequencies are put into a system at the same time, a nonlinear system has in its output the original two frequencies, the harmonics of each of the two frequencies, and also frequencies that are a combination of each of the two original frequencies, or *combination tones*.

Combination tones include *summation tones*, e.g., $f_1 + f_2$, $2f_1 + f_2$, and *difference tones*, e.g., $2f_1 - f_2$, $2f_2 - f_1$. Combination tones are mathematically predictable.

Table 4–3. Nonlinearities, combination tones, and harmonics. *Note:* the f_2/f_1 ratio is 1.20.

| Symbol | Harmonic Tones | Combination Tones | |
		Summation Tones	Difference Tones
f_1	830		
f_2	1000		
$2f_1$	1660		
$3f_1$	2490		
$2f_2$	2000		
$3f_2$	3000		
$f_1 + f_2$		1830	
$f_1 + 2f_2$		2830	
$f_1 + 3f_2$		3830	
$2f_1 + f_2$		2660	
$3f_1 + f_2$		3490	
$2f_1 + 2f_2$		3660	
$2f_1 + 3f_2$		4660	
$3f_1 + 2f_2$		4490	
$f_1 - f_2$			170
$f_1 - 2f_2$			1170
$f_1 - 3f_2$			2170
$2f_1 - f_2$			660
$3f_1 - f_2$			490
$2f_1 - 2f_2$			340
$2f_1 - 3f_2$			1340
$3f_1 - 2f_2$			90

Source: Adapted from Yost (1994), p. 55.

early 1990s, fell out of favor because it was inaccurate and misleading. In the early 1970s, the term "impedance audiometry" was discarded because tympanometry, static immittance, and acoustic reflexes are not measures of hearing. The term "DP audiogram" is inappropriate for the same reason. Several researchers from Denmark coined one of the more interesting terms for the DPgram—the "outer-hair-cellogram" (Rasmussen & Osterhammel, 1992). As noted in Chapter 1, with most clinical instrumentation DPOAE amplitudes can be plotted as a function of several different stimulus-related values, including f_2, f_1, the geometric mean between f_2 and f_1, or the DP frequency itself ($2f_1-f_2$). The rationale for plotting DP amplitudes as a function of f_2 was explained in the previous section of this chapter. Figure 4–8 shows an

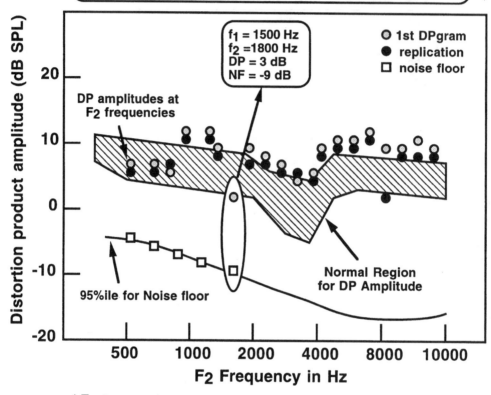

Patient Name: G.V.B
Test Date: July 29, 1999
Tester: Thomas Silver
DP Protocol*:: General diagnostic

Age: 98 years
Time: 6 a.m.
Clinic: Y2K Audiology Services

* Test parameters:
- ▢ F2 = 550 - 8800 Hz
- ▢ F2/F1 = 1.22
- ▢ L1 = 65 dB; L2 = 55 dB
- ▢ Frequencies/octave = 3

Figure 4–8. An example of a DPOAEgram or DPgram in which DP amplitude (vertical axis) is plotted as a function of stimulus frequency (for f_2 as illustrated) over a relatively wide range (from 500 to 8000 Hz). Test parameters are indicated in the lower portion of the figure. The hatched region encompasses a normal region (5%ile to 95%ile) for a group of adults with audiometric sensitivity thresholds of 15 dB HL or better at all test frequencies. The upper limit for acceptable (normal) noise floor (NF) at each frequency is indicated by the solid line, along with actual noise floors for test frequencies (open boxes). Notice the high degree of replicability (within ± 2 dB) between two separate DPgram runs for most stimulus frequencies. The highlighted region shows a DP-NF difference of 15 dB, much greater than the 3 dB minimum required to verify that any DP activity is present (versus simply noise). Test conditions were good (low noise and replicable responses). These diagnostic DP data are interpreted as normal, and consistent with cochlear outer hair cell integrity.

illustration of a DPgram. Amplitude of the DP for different frequencies, as measured by the microphone in the probe in dB SPL, is indicated on the vertical axis. The f_2 values are indicated on the horizontal axis. The number of stimulus frequencies presented per octave is entirely under user control. With most clinical DP devices, as few as one set of primaries per octave can be presented or up to 20 frequencies per octave can be presented. As a rule, the appropriate number of frequencies per octave varies depending on the objective of DPOAE measurement. This topic is discussed in more detail in the next section. Each DP symbol at a given frequency does not reflect the presentation of a single set of primaries (f_2 and f_1). The DP amplitude values are derived by averaging sound in the frequency region of the DP ($2f_1$–f_2) for multiple stimulus presentations. The number of stimuli presented (stimulus repetitions) is, with most clinical DP systems, determined separately for each frequency. Factors that enter into the determination include the size of the DP (the absolute amplitude), the amount of noise (noise floor) in the region of the DP, and, usually, the DP-to-noise floor (NF) difference. For each DP device, it is possible and rather easy to set the limits for acceptable values for each of these factors. Manufacturers offer protocols with combinations of these criteria—often referred to as stopping criteria—that differ depending on the intended clinical application of the protocol. The criteria are arranged logically as a series of "and/or" or "if/then" decisions. Preset stopping criteria essentially instruct the DP system when to continue averaging in search of the DP, how long the averaging should go on (the maximum time spent at each test frequency or number of stimuli that will be presented), and when to stop if a DP is present. These decisions are made based mainly on two types of data—the DP amplitude (if it's present) and the noise floor, both in dB SPL. Criteria may be rigorous in terms of the minimum amplitude signals accepted as a DP, how low the noise floor must be reduced by averaging, and the minimum difference between DP amplitude and the noise floor. Regardless of the DPOAE device or the analysis protocol (configuration) used, measurement time will be minimal whenever the DP amplitude is reasonably large (e.g., >5 dB) and noise is reasonable low (e.g., <10 dB). DPOAE measurement of a cooperative normal-hearing person, under ideal test conditions may require only 10 to 15 seconds, even for several frequencies/octave over a frequency region extending from 500 to over 8000 Hz. In contrast, if the patient has no detectable DP (e.g., in cochlear dysfunction or serious middle ear disorder), if there is considerable measurement noise (detected in the ear canal), and/or if stimuli are presented at many frequencies per octave over multiple octaves, then the time required to record a single DPgram can literally be infinite. Clinically, to get as much useful information as possible in a reasonable length of time, one must always select all DPOAE protocol parameters carefully. Examples of the various options available for modifying these criteria for different clinical DPOAE devices are provided by manufacturers in Chapter 7. Clinical DPOAE protocols and

Soon after purchasing a DPOAE system is a good time to create programs or test setups that will be used most often clinically. With the equipment manual (and maybe this book) handy, think about the types of patients who will be evaluated with DPOAEs, such as infants undergoing screening or persons being monitored for possible ototoxicity. Examples of clinical protocols are provided later in this chapter.

strategies for analyses including information derived from DPgrams, are discussed later (see DPOAE Test Protocols and Analysis).

DPOAE Fine Structure

For over 40 years, carefully conducted psychoacoustic studies have documented numerous peaks and valleys in auditory thresholds, referred to as auditory microstructure (Elliott, 1958; Thomas, 1975; Kemp & Martin, 1976). To some extent, attempts to explain this characteristic feature of cochlear function created the knowledge base and the research climate that led directly to the discovery of OAEs. Even casual inspection of the TEOAE spectral waveform will invariably reveal a jagged line, which is actually hundreds of little peaks and valleys in the response. These irregularities in the TEOAE spectrum are recorded from normal ears when the stimulus spectrum is perfectly flat, as described more fully in the following section on TEOAEs. When relatively few stimulus frequencies fall within an octave, DPgrams often appear flat, with relatively similar DP amplitude levels across a wide range of frequencies. The same statement applies to the audiogram for a person with normal hearing sensitivity. Thresholds for most or all octave frequencies may be at 0 dB, for example. However, the irregular pattern of OAE amplitudes viewed in a clinical TEOAE spectrum can be seen also in DPgrams when numerous stimulus frequencies are presented within an octave (Figure 4–9). The same pattern would be found in the audiogram if thresholds were measured for an adequate number of pure tone frequencies with rigorous psychoacoustic methods and small intensity increments (1 or 2 dB). In fact, the "audibility curve" is characterized by many peaks and valleys in auditory thresholds that cover an excursion of more than 10 dB. It is possible that the apparent peaks are "normal" threshold values and the valleys are really nulls, or momentary decreases in threshold values. This "ripple" phenomenon in the auditory threshold, first described over 40 years ago (Elliott, 1958) and then studied with psychoacoustic techniques in 1975 by David Kemp, provided one of the first clues that led to the discovery of otoacoustic emissions (Kemp, 1979a, 1979b, 1979c). The stability of the ripple pattern, when measured in a subject over time, is evidence that the peaks and valleys are not simply noise or the effects of noise on measurements of threshold (He & Schmiedt, 1993). The *fine structure* (or *microstructure*) of the DPOAE is characterized by peak-to-peak distances of approximately 3/32 octave (about 10 peaks/octave) and peak-to-valley excursions of up to 20 dB. The ripple effect in DPOAEs, which is less apparent for frequencies above 4000 Hz (He & Schmiedt, 1993), appears to reflect auditory threshold fine structure (Long, 1984; Zwicker & Schloth,1984; He & Schmiedt, 1993, 1997; Talmadge, Tubis, Long, & Piskorski, 1998).

The normal jagged "fine structure" or "microstructure" of hearing sensitivity is one logical explanation for why OAE findings do not always agree with an audiogram, even when signals for both measures are aligned in frequency. The curious reader will want to review one of the articles on fine structure cited herein to view this phenomenon firsthand.

DPOAE fine structure varies depending on the absolute and relative intensity levels of the primary stimuli (f_1 and f_2), and also the f_2/f_1 ratio. If L_1 is fixed (e.g., at 50 dB) and L_2 is increased (e.g., from 30 to 75

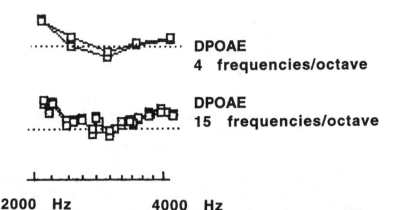

DPOAE
4 frequencies/octave

DPOAE
15 frequencies/octave

2000 Hz   4000 Hz

Figure 4-9. DPgrams for a normal adult ear recorded with 4 frequencies/octave (top) and 15 frequencies/octave (bottom). Stimulus intensity levels were $L_1 = 65$ dB and $L_2 = 55$ dB SPL. The peaks and valleys at adjacent stimulus frequencies characterizing fine structure of the DPgram are beginning to emerge as the frequency resolution is increased. At higher numbers of stimuli per octave, even greater irregularity in the DPgram structure is seen. This normal jagged pattern is observed when numerous stimuli frequencies are presented within an octave. The fine structure will not be apparent for DPOAEs evoked with relatively few stimuli per octave (e.g., 3 or 4).

dB), the fine structure shifts upward; whereas if L_2 is similarly fixed while L_1 is increased, fine structure shifts downward (He & Schmiedt, 1997). More shifts in DP fine structure were associated with closely spaced primary frequencies (i.e., small f_2/f_1 ratios of 1.11 versus primaries that were farther separated [ratios of 1.20 or 1.33]). This intensity-related change was interpreted as evidence that DP fine structure "largely reflects the place features within the overlapping area of the primary traveling waves," while the frequency effects "suggest that the frequency shift is a function of the amount of overlap of the primary traveling waves or the overall stimulation in the area of overlap" (He & Schmiedt, 1997, p. 3564). The fundamental relation of fine structure to cochlear function remains unknown, although theories have been offered and models developed to explain the cochlear mechanisms responsible for fine (micro) structure of both auditory thresholds and DPOAE. Independent of the exact mechanisms, however, consideration of fine structure may help to explain some of the apparent discrepancies between OAE measures and the conventional audiology measures.

Input-Output (I/O) Functions

The relation of stimulus intensity level to DP amplitude can be described by the input-output function. In recording I/O functions, absolute stimulus frequency and the frequency ratio are held constant while stimulus intensity is either increased from a low level or decreased from a high level. Recording DPOAE amplitudes at different intensity levels is comparable to the common practice in ABR measurement of recording wave V latencies at different stimulus intensity levels. Thus, the DP input/output function is equivalent to the ABR intensity/latency function. In clinical applications and published clinical studies, DPOAE findings are almost always displayed in the DPgram format. There is rather substantial literature on DPOAE data generated from input/output measurement techniques (Harris, 1990; Harris & Probst, 1990; Kimberley & Nelson, 1989; Lonsbury-Martin et al., 1990; Nelson & Kimberley, 1992; He & Schmiedt, 1993; Popelka et al., 1993; Stover & Norton, 1993; Kimberley, Kimberley, & Roth, 1994; Moulin, Bera & Collet, 1994; Popelka, Karzon, & Arjand, 1995; Nelson & Zhou, 1996; Stover et al., 1996). The results of the published studies of I/O measures in persons with normal and impaired hearing, noteworthy for their strong research design and thorough statistical treatment of the data, point to the following generalizations.

DP amplitude characteristically increases with primary intensity level, but the shape of the I/O function is highly variable among subjects and even for stimuli at different frequencies within subjects. I/O functions usually take on four or five characteristic shapes, as detailed below, but they typically are quite shallow for lower stimulus intensity levels. That is, amplitude growth begins slowly and increases more steeply for moderate to high stimulus intensity levels (see Figure 4–10). This is in contrast to nonphysiologic DPs, resulting from either artifactual sources or passively with very high intensity stimulation of the ear, which have an input/output slope of about 3 dB/dB (i.e., 3 dB of output for every dB of input). (As an aside, latency properties also differentiate physiologic [e.g., active processes within the cochlea] from nonphysiologic DPs, with the latter characterized by very fast changes in phase as the f_2 stimulus is varied. As DPOAE latency is not yet analyzed clinically, it is included in the discussion of Future Directions in Clinical OAE Measurement in Chapter 10.)

Software for recording DPOAE input-output functions is available upon request from manufacturers of selected clinical instruments. The clinician can always manually manipulate stimulus intensity and plot DP amplitudes and construct "home-made" I/O functions. As noted in Chapter 10, I/O functions will probably be incorporated into routine clinical practice with future generations of OAE equipment.

The intensity level at which the DP is initially detected, and the appearance of the low intensity "tail" of the DPOAE I/O function, is highly dependent on the noise floor. When I/O functions are recorded under suboptimal test conditions, the shape may appear linear because the tail is obscured by noise. In clinical settings, excessive noise more often affects DPOAE I/O functions for low-frequency stimuli. To define a DP "threshold" confidently and accurately, or a minimum detection level, and to plot the entire range of the I/O function properly, the noise floor must be as low as −20 to −30 dB SPL. Practical steps to accomplish this minimum noise requirement would include, in addition to patient instruction, performing the DP measurements in a sound booth (away from noise sources including the DPOAE instru-

DPOAE Input/Output Measurement

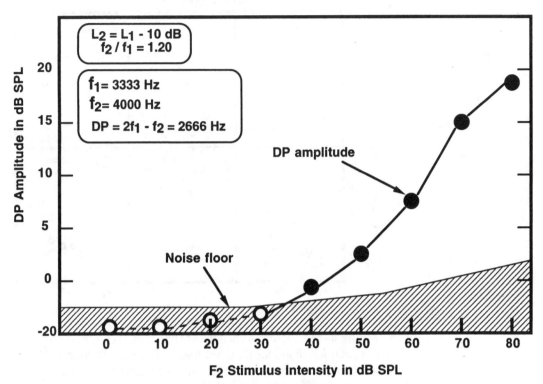

Figure 4–10. DPOAE input/output function. DP amplitude is recorded as stimulus intensity level is increased (or decreased) while stimulus frequency is held constant. DP input/output functions are greatly influenced by the level of noise during recording. In this figure, the filled circles (●) indicate the presence of DP activity, whereas data represented by the open circles (○) is indistinguishable from noise within the ear canal.

mentation), test protocol stopping criteria that mandate a very low noise level, and continuous signal averaging until the minimum noise level is reached. Although it is not impossible to perform such DPOAE measurements with clinical populations, including neonates (e.g., Popelka et al., 1995), the amount of time required currently precludes the routine clinical application of I/O functions for multiple stimulus frequencies (particularly for mid-to-lower stimulus frequencies). For example, according to Popelka et al. (1993), up to 45 minutes may be needed to achieve a noise floor of −40 dB and then to record a single I/O function, for an adult. These practical problems are prohibitive for potentially uncooperative patients in traditionally noisy test settings (e.g., intensive care unit).

There appear to be four or five normal variations in the shape of I/O functions (Figure 4–11), described as straight or linear, saturation,

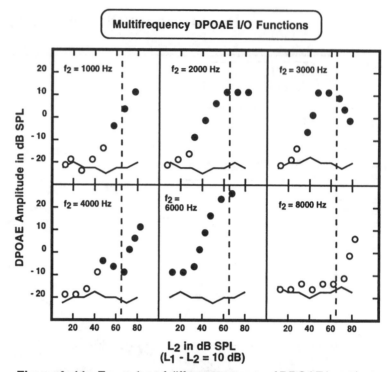

Figure 4–11. Examples of different patterns of DPOAE input/output (I/O) functions for different frequecies. Variations in DPOAE I/O functions may be observed among subjects for a single frequency or within subjects for different frequencies or for the right versus left ears. The level of noise during DP recording at the stimulus frequency is indicated by the solid line (—). In this figure, the filled circles (●) indicate the presence of DP activity, whereas data represented by the open circles (○) are indistinguishable from noise in the ear canal or below a minimum intensity level used as criterion for DP presence (−10 dB SPL). A vertical dashed line (┊) is drawn at a typical stimulus intensity level for DPOAE (65 dB SPL). Whether maximum DP amplitude is recorded at this stimulus intensity level depends on the DPOAE I/O pattern. Notice that, for the 8000 Hz stimulus (*lower right corner*), all symbols are open circles. It is possible that a DPOAE apparent only for very high stimulus intensity levels (above 70 dB) reflects passive energy from the cochlea, rather than activity of outer hair cells. Artifactual DPOAEs related to standing wave interference are especially likely for high stimulus frequencies.

plateau, and notched (Nelson & Kimberley, 1992; Popelka et al., 1993; Stover & Norton, 1993; Popelka et al., 1995; Stover et al., 1996). The expected proportion of different shapes has not yet been systematically defined in a large normal hearing population, although it would be convenient if a simple classification system was developed, much as tympanogram types were developed by Jerger in early 1970 as immittance measures gained clinical popularity (Jerger, 1970; Hall & Mueller, 1997). Preliminary findings suggest that the monotonic pattern may be recorded in over 50% of normal hearers, with the notched pattern (in the low-to-mid intensity region) recorded in about one-fourth (e.g., Popelka et al., 1993). Possible explanations for some of the shapes have been offered (Norton & Rubel, 1990; Whitehead et al., 1990; Nelson & Kimberley, 1992; Popelka et al., 1993; Stover & Norton, 1993). For example, He and Schmiedt (1997) have provided evidence suggesting that these discontinuities, or nonmonotonic notches, in the I/O function are related to frequency shifts in DP fine structure as stimulus intensity level is increased, whereas Moulin et al. (1992) and Stover et al. (1996) associated the notches with the presence of SOAE near the stimulus frequency. Steeper I/O slopes are often recorded from ears with mild-to-moderate hearing impairment, partly because passive cochlear mechanisms dominate as the generator of the high stimulus intensity DP response. Low level DPs are, in contrast, more dependent on outer hair cell motility (i.e., active cochlear processes). Even though there is clearly normal variation in I/O shapes, group data reported independently by a number of investigators confirm some rather consistent relations between stimulus intensity and DP amplitude. Reported rates of amplitude growth with intensity are in the neighborhood of 1 dB/dB (Popelka et al., 1993; Nelson & Zhou, 1996), although rate (slope of the function) varies as a function of both the intensity level (generally steeper slope for the linear low-level portion of the function, and decreasing rates for the often saturated high-intensity portion); the frequency of the stimulus, and, of course, whether the cochlea is functioning normally or not. The final word on I/O slopes is not in yet, as there are substantial discrepancies in the findings among studies (e.g., Gaskill & Brown, 1990; Lonsbury-Martin et al., 1990; Nelson & Kimberley, 1992; Popelka et al., 1993).

The concept behind input/output functions for DPOAE or TEOAE is very familiar to the clinical audiologist who regularly records ABR latency-intensity functions, probe microphone measures of hearing aid performance at multiple input, or performance-intensity functions for word recognition (PI-PB functions).

One take-home message of this discussion of I/O functions is reminiscent of early papers on speech audiometry. Then, Carhart and later others (e.g., Jerger & Jerger, 1971) cautioned against the use of a single intensity level for measuring word recognition, noting correctly that signal intensity level yielding maximum speech intelligibilty varied among normal hearing persons and, especially, persons with sensorineural hearing impairment. It was simply not appropriate to measure word recognition performance exclusively for a speech signal at a comfortable conversational level of 40 or 50 dB HL. This argument was the rationale, of course, for the clinical use of performance-intensity (PI) functions. The same point may be made for clinical DPOAE measurements. Reliance on a single stimulus intensity approach (e.g., L_1 = 65 dB; L_2 = 55 dB) in recording a DPgram may, in most cases, produce reasonably large DP amplitudes for some frequencies, but almost never the maximum possible DP amplitude for all frequencies. Indeed, reliance on DP amplitude data for a single intensity level is sure to contribute to incorrect interpretations of DPOAEs in some patients, including diagnostically both under- and overestimations of cochlear dysfunction and/or hearing impairment and, in screening applications, false-negative and false-positive errors. This point becomes readily apparent when DPgrams are reconstructed from I/O functions and when the maximum DP amplitude from the I/O function for each stimulus frequency is used to create the DPgram (e.g., Stover et al., 1996). Unfortunately, until there is some degree of standardization of instrumentation, absolute DP intensity levels obtained with clinical devices are somewhat artibrary. Because DP amplitude is reported in dB SPL (a known physical dimension of intensity) and stimulus calibration or leveling is performed for each test ear prior to data collection, one might assume that DP amplitude measures for well-defined test protocols would be consistent from study to study, clinic to clinic, or device to device. Review of the literature clearly shows that this is not the case. In fact, as noted in the following discussion of instrumentation for DPOAE recording and further on TEOAE recording, there are rather substantial differences in the OAEs recorded with instrumentation marketed by different manufacturers. Potential innovative clinical strategies for exploitating the DP information derived from I/O functions are discussed in Chapter 10.

It would be reasonable to wonder, at this point, whether the intensity at which the DP is first detected might be related to audiometric threshold and, extending this theme, whether audiometric thresholds in certain patient populations (e.g., infants or difficult-to-test children), might be predicted objectively with DPOAE I/O functions. There is almost universal agreement among the investigators cited above that hearing thresholds cannot be accurately predicted from DPOAE I/O data. Statistically, correlations between DP "thresholds" from I/O functions and audiometric thresholds are often very low (e.g., 0.40). The reasons for this conclusion are multiple and varied, including the confounding effects of noise on precise estimation of DP detection at low intensity levels, remarkable intersubject variability in DP amplitude data, even among normal hearers, differences in the place of cochlear activation for pure tone audiometric signals versus DPOAE stimulus frequencies, and the host of fundamental anatomic and procedural differences between pure tone audiometry and OAEs. The general lack of consistent correlation between OAEs and conventional audiometry was reviewed in Chapter 1.

Reliability

The sensitivity of OAEs to even subtle cochlear dysfunction involving outer hair cells is, in one sense, confirmation of their validity as an auditory measure. Clinically, however, reliability is also very important. Reliability may be defined as the "extent to which a test yields consistent scores on repeated measures" (Stach, 1997, p. 176). In deter-mining reliability of DPOAEs, consistency is appropriately assessed for quantifiable response parameters, such as absolute amplitude or an amplitude-noise measure. It might also be useful for some DPOAE applications, such as hearing screening, to define reliability according to the consistency with which one of two outcomes (pass versus fail) is obtained. There appear to be no studies formally addressing the relia-bility of DPOAEs, especially DPOAEs recorded from patient popula-tions (not normal adult subjects) in typical clinical test settings (not a sound booth) by clinical audiologists (not the principle investigator of the study) with commercially available devices. Limited knowledge of DPOAE reliability is more than an esoteric concern. There is consider-able potential value clinically to monitoring auditory function with DPOAEs. Two examples of this DPOAE application are monitoring ototoxicity and noise-induced damage. The success and clinical value of monitoring with DPOAEs is highly dependent on the reliability of the measure. Although it does not minimize the importance of prop-erly investigating DPOAE reliability, the same criticism can be direct-ed to most other widely used clinical procedures in audiology, among them tympanometry and all auditory evoked responses. Unfortunate-ly, it is common clinical practice to record single versus replicated DPgrams in one test session only, essentially yielding no means for even informally evaluating either test-retest consistency or reliability. As noted below, there are at least several published accounts of the reli-ability of TEOAEs, and with one device (ILO 88) the reproducibility parameter offers a convenient metric of internal consistency of the response, if not reliability from one test to the next.

Franklin, McCoy, Martin, and Lonsbury-Martin (1992) published one of the earliest, and only, papers describing test-retest reliability of DPOAEs (and also TEOAEs). The study appeared to be very carefully designed and conducted. Test reliability was defined as "the ratio of the variance or variability of the true scores over the variance of the observed scores" with good reliability viewed as a coefficient of 0.85 or higher (1.0 would be perfect). The authors concluded from a detailed and statistical analysis of their data that "the consistency of repeated measures of DPOAEs and TEOAEs was generally excellent" (Franklin et al., 1992, p. 428). Reliabilty for DPOAE improved for higher fre-quencies (above 1000 Hz), whereas for TEOAE reliability was best within the 1000 to 3000 Hz region and poorer at 4000 Hz. At least five features of the study, however, limit the clinical usefulness of the find-ings. First, there were only 12 subjects. Second, all subjects were coop-erative (i.e., quiet and instructable) adults (reliability might decrease with less agreeable subjects). Third, all subjects had normal auditory function (reliability might be lower with less robust or absent OAEs). Fourth, OAE measurement was conducted in a double-walled sound booth (with a very low noise floor). Fifth, DPOAEs were recorded with a specially designed device, because this study was conducted in the early 1990s before a variety of clinical FDA-approved instruments was on the market. The ILO 88 device was used for TEOAE measurement. In a more recent paper that included analyses of DPOAE reliability during a 24-hour period for 16 normal hearing adults, Cacace et al. (1996) reported average coefficients of 0.75 (range 0.64 to 0.90) for a stimulus intensity of $L_1 = L_2 = 55$ dB and an average reliability coefficient of 0.77 (range of 0.65 to 0.85) for a stimulus intensity of $L_1 = L_2 = 75$ dB.

Along with several colleagues (Sladen, Lamb, & Hall, 1996), this author conducted a study of DPOAE inter- versus intrasubject variability with a clinical device (Grason Stadler 60). Subjects were 10 young (20- to 30-year-olds) audiometrically normal subjects. All subjects had hearing thresholds of 15 dB or better at audiometric frequencies of 250 through 8000 Hz and normal tympanometry. None of the subjects reported a history of otologic pathology or recent exposure to high-intensity sounds. Subjects underwent DPOAE measurement 10 times. DPOAE data were collected in a quiet but not sound-treated room. There was at least an 8-hour interval between test sessions. At each session, replicated DPgrams were recorded from each subject with a total of 12 pairs of f_1 and f_2 stimuli over the frequency region of 500 through 8000 Hz using two stimulus protocols. For one protocol $L_1 = 65$ and $L_2 = 55$ dB SPL. For the other, $L_1 = 55$ and $L_2 = 45$ dB SPL. The f_2/f_1 ratio was fixed at 1.20.

OAEs are not real if they are not reliably recorded. Remember always "If OAEs do not replicate, you must investigate" and "If the OAEs do not repeat, then the test is not complete."

Intersubject DPOAE amplitude variability exceeded intrasubject variability under all test conditions by approximately a 2:1 ratio. DPgrams for the two stimulus intensity protocols for 5 representative frequencies from among the 12 frequencies assessed, averaged for the 10 subjects, are illustrated in Figure 4–12. Frequency is plotted for the f_2 primary stimulus. Predictably, DP amplitude varied as a function of stimulus frequency and was greater for the higher stimulus intensity level. Variability was significantly greater for the highest test frequencies and also tended to be greater, although not consistently, for the lower stimulus intensity protocol. As expected, absolute DP amplitude was consistently larger for a higher versus lower primary intensity level (Figure 4–13), and variability was greater for the lower set of primary intensities than for the higher set of intensities. The range of DPOAE amplitude values was clearly greater between subjects than within a single subject. For example, for the middle of the 5 frequencies the intersubject range was approximately 15 to 17 dB, whereas the intrasubject range was as low as 3 dB and typically 6 or 7 dB. Increased variability for the lower frequencies was in part due to differences in the noise floor in this frequency region among subjects, and among test sessions, whereas the increased variability for higher frequencies may have been related to previously described (Siegel, 1994) influences of ear-canal acoustics, especially standing waves, on DPOAE amplitude for test frequencies above 5000 Hz. As illustrated in Figure 4–14, inter-

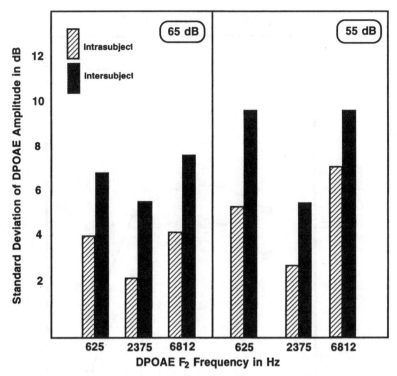

Figure 4–12. Intra- and intersubject variability in DPOAE amplitude values (represented by standard deviation of the mean on vertical axis) for two stimulus intensity paradigms ($L_1 = 65$ dB and $L_2 = 55$ dB, with $L_1 - L_2 = 10$ dB) and selected stimulus frequencies (horizontal axis). Subjects were 10 normal hearing adults tested on 10 separate days (with the GSI 60 device). Variability in DP amplitude was minimal for stimuli in the mid-frequency region (shown here by 2375 Hz) in comparison to low or high stimulus frequencies. More striking was the significantly greater DPOAE amplitude variability between subjects ($N = 10$) than among test sessions ($N = 10$) for individual subjects. Adapted from Sladen, Lamb, and Hall (1996).

subject variability in a representative session consistently exceeded variability for any of the 10 subjects over the course of the 10-test sessions. These results confirm the need for relatively large sample sizes in DPOAE measurement, even among cooperative normal hearing adult subjects. These findings cannot be generalized to DPOAE variability for other subject populations or test environments, nor to variability statistics for transient OAEs (TEOAEs).

In an even more clinically realistic investigation, Chase and Hall (1998) investigated test-retest reliability of DPOAE in infants using a clinical device (GSI 60). Subjects were 40 newborn infants (80 ears) screened in either a well-baby nursery ($N = 12$), a nursery treatment room ($N = 15$),

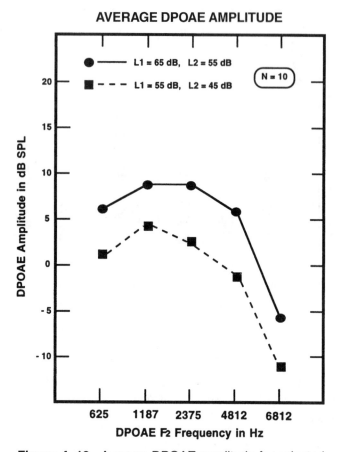

Figure 4–13. Average DPOAE amplitude for selected stimulus frequencies with two stimulus intensity paradigms ($L_1 = 65$ dB and $L_1 = 55$ dB, with $L_1 - L_2 = 10$ dB). Subjects were 10 normal hearing adults (thresholds of 15 dB or better for audiometric frequencies of 250 to 8000 Hz) tested with a GSI 60 device. DPOAE amplitude was significantly greater for the higher stimulus intensity levels and varied significantly as a function of stimulus frequency. Adapted from Sladen, Lamb, and Hall (1996).

or the mother's hospital room ($N = 13$). The average gestational age at birth was 40 weeks, and the average birth weight was 3,336 grams. Average time of testing after birth was 28 hours. Infant state varied from sleeping to awake and restless. All infants passed an automated ABR screening at the time of the DPOAE data collection. DPOAEs were recorded with three separate test protocols. One was the default protocol recommended by the manufacturer. Two were custom protocols with stimuli ($L_1 = 65$ dB and $L_2 = 50$ dB; $f_2/f_1 = 1.2$) presented 3/octave over a frequency range of 2000 to 5000 Hz either sequentially (one frequency at a time) or simultaneously (two sets of primaries

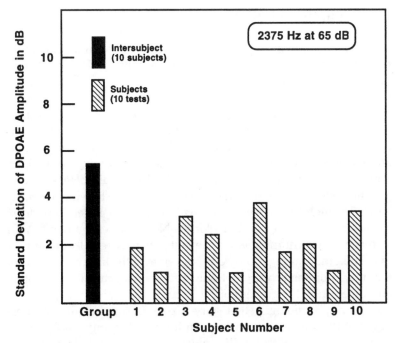

Figure 4–14. Intersubject variability in DPOAE amplitude values (black bar) and for 10 different normal hearing subjects (hatched bars, as represented by standard deviation of the mean on vertical axis for a stimulus intensity paradigm of $L_1 = 65$ dB and $L_2 = 55$ dB at a stimulus frequency of 2375 Hz. DPOAE amplitude variability between always exceeded the variability for individual subjects. Adapted from Sladen, Lamb, and Hall (1996).

separated by at least an octave presented at the same time). Otherwise, the custom protocols had the same test configuration. Two runs were completed for each protocol in random order. Importantly, the probe was removed from the ear canal after each tracing. DPOAEs recorded with the two custom protocols, using absolute DP values or DP-noise floor data showed moderate to strong correlation coefficients. The sequential protocol had the highest test-retest reliability.

In conclusion, intersubject variability in both DPOAE and TEOAE measurements is, as one would expect, considerably greater than intrasubject variability (Kemp et al., 1990; Lonsbury-Martin, Harris, Stagner, Hawkins, & Martin, 1990; Lonsbury-Martin, Whitehead, & Martin, 1991; Sladen, Hall, & Lamb, 1996). Even for DPOAE recordings with a clinical device from newborn infants in a hospital setting, test-retest reliability is acceptably high for appropriately designed protocols. Nonetheless, there is a need for additional carefully designed and clinically relevant studies of DPOAEs (and TEOAEs) reliability.

The Equipment Factor

Imagine the following nightmarish day in the clinic. You get in early, turn on each of the four audiometers in the clinic, and generally prepare for the arrival of the first patients. Being a good clinician, you ask your co-worker with "the golden ears" to help with the daily listening check of each audiometer. This morning's routine is uneventful for audiometer #1. But you become a little concerned when pure tone thresholds for audiometer #2 (acquired from another manufacturer) are hot (thresholds are better than they should be) by about 15 dB. You're truly alarmed after the listening check for audiometer #3 shows just the opposite pattern . . . the "golden ears" are showing a hearing loss in the high-frequency region. With dread, you patiently perform the listening check for audiometer #4. Now you're in a panic. Your stomach begins churning when the first patient cheerfully announces himself in the waiting room because results of the listening check for the final audiometer were not only at odds with the all of the other audiometers . . . the golden ear produced a 15-dB air-bone gap at 500 Hz! For any audiologist, that story is pure fiction and almost unbelievable. We rely on audiometric equipment standards and periodic calibration to verify that a dB is always a dB, not more and not less. Because standards do not yet exist for OAE equipment, this little saga is quite plausible, in fact probable, for DPOAE measures.

Are there really differences in the DPOAE amplitude data recorded among different clinical devices? This is a very important question clinically. As different DPOAE instruments are acquired for application in various patient populations, clinicians require normative DPOAE databases. Optimally, DPOAE databases would be collected systematically for all devices from a single sizable and well-defined subject sample. These comparative databases would permit cross-clinic comparison of DPOAEs and would facilitate meaningful clinical interpretation of DPOAE findings. Along with several colleagues, the author took a step in this direction by conducting a study aimed at generating normative adult databases, using a rather conventional test protocol, for the five commercially available DPOAE systems that were FDA-approved at the time (Hornsby, Kelly, & Hall, 1996).

We measured DPOAEs in a group of young adults aged 21 to 28 years. All subjects had hearing thresholds of 15 dB HL or better for audiometric test frequencies of 500 through 8000 Hz. In addition, all subjects had normal (type A) tympanograms. None of the subjects reported tinnitus or exposure to excessive levels of sound. The environment for DPOAE measurement was a quiet, but not sound-treated, room with an average ambient noise level of 56 dBC. Data collection was made by three graduate level audiology students who had received classroom lectures on OAE topics and clinical experience in OAE measurement.

The cubic distortion product ($2f_1-f_2$) was analyzed following simultaneous stimulation with two primary tonal stimuli (f_1 and f_2). This measure was defined as DPOAE amplitude. The two stimuli were presented with a f_2/f_1 ratio of 1.22. Stimuli were presented across a frequency region of 500 to 6000 Hz. Two different stimulus intensity protocols were used. For one protocol, the two stimuli were at an intensity level of 65 dB SPL ($L_1 = L_2 = 65$ dB SPL). For the other protocol, $L_1 = 65$ dB SPL and $L_2 = 55$ dB SPL. For four of the five devices, we recorded DPOAE amplitude and the noise floor in the adjacent frequency region of the distortion product ($2f_1-f_2$) for a total of six frequency pairs per octave. One of the devices permitted the presentation of only two frequency pairs per octave. The actual measurement parameters used for each device were carefully documented and held constant across devices (parameters are summarized in the tables of normative data displayed at the end of this chapter). We followed manufacturer recommendations for settings specific to their devices for efficiently recording optimal DPOAE amplitudes while also minimizing noise floor levels. Thus, the configurations or test set-ups which usually incorporated criteria for acceptance of a DP data point and for definition of an acceptable noise floor level (i.e., stopping criteria) necessarily varied among devices according to manufacturer recommendations. Algorithms for processing DP amplitudes and noise floors also varied among manufacturers. We also plotted the DPOAE amplitude as a function of either the geometric mean of the two stimulus frequencies, or as a function of the f_2 frequency, as recommended by the manufacturer. In either case, this plot is referred to as a DPgram. Finally, we always performed replicated DPgrams to ensure that the DPOAE data were repeatable.

Standardization does not yet exist for the manufacture of OAE equipment. Design of devices, including probes, software, calibration strategies and measurement algorithms vary considerably, as detailed by manufacturers in Chapter 7.

For each device, normative databases were established for each of the two stimulus intensity protocols described above. The recommended protocol, however, was for intensity of the f_2 frequency to be lower by 10 dB than the intensity level of the f_1 frequency, specifically, $L_1 = 65$ dB SPL and $L_2 = 55$ dB SPL, a decision based on published evidence summarized earlier in this chapter that DPOAE measures are more sensitive to cochlear dysfunction when there is this relationship in f_2 and f_1 intensity levels (L_2 lower than L_1 by 10 to 15 dB). Recall that, with this relative intensity difference, the cochlea is maximally stimulated very close to the frequency region represented by f_2. DPOAE data for each device are displayed as tables in Appendix A.

The importance of utilizing normative data collected specifically with the DPOAE device that is used in a clinical setting is highlighted in the Figure 4–15. There were distinct, and statistically significant differences among devices in DP amplitude. The differences were especially evident in certain frequency regions. Disparity among the devices was greatest for the highest test frequencies. This finding may be related to variable effects of ear canal acoustics. For stimulus frequencies

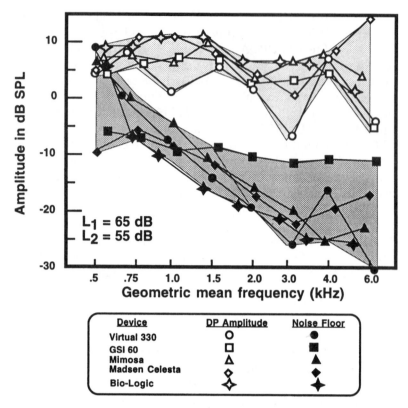

Figure 4–15. DPOAE amplitude for selected stimulus frequencies with a stimulus intensity paradigm of $L_1 = 65$ dB and $L_2 = 55$ dB. Subjects were 30 normal hearing adults (thresholds of 15 dB or better for audiometric frequencies of 250 to 8000 Hz) tested with five different FDA-approved devices. DPOAE amplitude varied significantly among devices, and as a function of stimulus frequency. Adapted from Hornsby, Kelly, and Hall (1996).

above 5000 Hz, DPOAE measurement may be confounded by interference from standing waves (Siegel, 1994), a point discussed further in Chapter 5 (section on ear canal acoustics). Standing wave influences are likely to vary among commercially available devices as they are related, in part, to the distance of the microphone from the tympanic membrane. The effects of "internal coupling (cross-talk) between the sound source and probe microphone" (Siegel, 1995); that is, leakage of stimulus energy from within the silicone tubing in the probe assembly to the microphone used to detect the DPOAE may contribute to measurement artifacts and may have a negative influence on the accuracy of DPOAE recordings. Differences in the extent of this problem among devices is likely to have contributed to the disparity in DP amplitude values. Two practical implications are apparent from this simple study. First, normative data collected with the particular brand of DPOAE device used in a clinic must also be used in the analysis and interpretation of DPOAE data for patients. Also, there is a clear need for guidelines and perhaps even standards for the design and manufacture of clinical DPOAE devices and related components (e.g., probes). Differences in probes probably account for much of the variation in DPOAE findings among devices and from one study to the next. Some OAE devices are coupled to probes designed and contructed by the manufacturer (see Chapter 7). With other devices, marketed by various manufacturers, the probes or components are supplied by a common vendor, such as Etymotic Research or Knowles Electronics. Examples of Etymotic Research probe system types include the the ER-10, ER-10B, or the ER-10C microphones, typically used in combination with ER-2 or ER-3A insert earphones. A Knowles Electronics microphone used in OAE measurement is model EA 1843, and this critical clinical issue will be addressed again for TEOAE devices later in this chapter.

DPOAE Test Protocols and Analysis Strategies

Protocols

The specific protocol used to record DPOAEs depends largely on the clinical objective of the assessment. To increase the likelihood of a successful DPOAE assessment, and to minimize test time without eliminating critical data, the test protocol needs to take into account the patient population, the test setting, and exactly what clinical audiologic information is required. For example, a very different test protocol would be used for screening the hearing of a newborn infant versus monitoring the hearing of a preschool child receiving cis-platin for an inoperable brain tumor for ototoxicity. Examples of DPOAE test protocols are summarized in Table 4–4. The rationale for selection of the values used for parameters in this table is explained throughout this chapter. Other DPOAE protocols would also be appropriate clinically for a variety of applications in children and adults. It is important to remember that not all the parameters or settings affecting the DPOAE measurement are shown in the table. Behind these protocols, there are several other settings specific to devices designed by different manufacturers which may have a profound influence on test accuracy and test time (see Chapter 7). To cite a few examples, settings for sampling rate, the time period allotted for collecting data at each stimulus frequency (set of primaries), the number of averages or sweeps completed at each frequency, and noise conditions must be selected. As with the parameters shown in Table 4–4, most of these other settings will be altered, depending again on the patient population, the test setting, and exactly what clinical audiologic information is required. Note that the exact terms used to refer to each of these settings may differ among manufacturers.

There are an infinite number of possible OAE test protocols. Rather than relying on the sample protocols supplied by a manufacturer, the clinician is advised to develop "customized" protocols which are best-suited for specific test settings, patient populations, and clinical objectives.

As more clinical DPOAE systems are introduced, and as available systems evolve and undergo software updates with technologic advances or as a result of clinical data, we can expect to see changes in design and size, with more flexibility and more options. We will also witness more user sophistication, and experiment, in "fine-tuning" protocols for

Table 4–4. Summary of main features of selected DPOAE test protocols

Test Parameters	General	Diagnostic[a]		Screening[b]
		High Frequency	Low Frequency	
Stimuli				
Intensity level[a]	→	$L_1 - L_2$ = 10 dB e.g., L_1 = 65 dB L_2 = 55 dB	→	L_1 = 65 dB L_2 = 65 dB
Ratio	f_2/f_1 = 1.20	f_2/f_1 = 1.20	f_2/f_1 = 1.20	f_2/f_1 = 1.20
Frequency range	500 to 8 kHz	2 to 10 kHz	500 to 1000 Hz	2 to 5 kHz
Frequencies/octave	3	≥ 6	4	4 or 5
Acquisition				
Repetitions (averaging)	Conventional	Fewer	More	More
Noise algorithm	Conventional	Low noise	High noise	High noise
Examples of applications	General[c] diagnostic assessments	Ototoxicity Noise-induced SNHL	Ménière's disease	Newborn screening

[a]Decreasing stimulus intensity level will increase sensitivity (i.e., the chance that any cochlear dysfunction will be detected), whereas increasing stimulus intensity (up to about 70 dB) will increase specificity (i.e., an abnormality is more likely to be associated with communicatively important hearing loss, 30 dB or greater).

[b]*General* = routine diagnostic assessment of a cooperative adult with suspected otologic etiology, a suspected malingerer, suspected retrocochlear dysfunction (including auditory neuropathy), initial testing of tinnitus, or a school-aged child for central auditory processing disorders (CAPD).

[c]Examples of clinical applications for screening protocol include neonates and infants, children who are difficult-to-test with behavioral audiometry, and uncooperative patients of any age.

various clinical applications (Musiek & Baran, 1996; Kim et al., 1997; Zapala, 1998). The paper by Frank Musiek (of Dartmouth Medical School) and Jane Baran (1996) provides an excellent example of this trend. Using a GSI 60 clinical DPOAE device, they developed an abbreviated screening DPOAE test protocol, requiring fewer stimulus averages and a limited frequency range that shortened test time from over 2 minutes for a standard diagnostic protocol to about 12 seconds for the "Dartfast" protocol. Then, Musiek and Baran (1996) applied these protocols in a series of adults with normal hearing or sensorineural hearing loss. The study demonstrated statistically that the shortened protocol yielded results that were in agreement with the longer protocol without sacrificing test accuracy. The authors pointed out advantages of the new protocol for hearing screening.

A recent study by Kim et al. (1997) provided another example of innovation in the design of DPOAE protocols. With the objective of increasing test speed, these authors applied a "multiple-tone-pair" option available with a clinical DPOAE device. This software (available on the GSI 60 device) permits simultaneous presentation of several sets of primaries (f_1 and f_2). Data were obtained from 98 normal-hearing ears and 94 ears with sensorineural hearing loss using three sets of primaries. The results of this custom test protocol were in good agreement with those obtained from the same subjects using a conventional one primary pair protocol, but test time was two to three times faster. Again, the advantages of this strategy for screening were noted. As an aside, we (Chase & Hall, 1998) have demonstrated that the simultaneous stimulus presentation technique, even though it saves test time, has comparable reliability to the conventional DPOAE protocols, even in newborn infants tested in a hospital setting. Results of the study are summarized below in the section on Reliability.

Measurement and Analysis

Some basic steps in DPOAE measurement are listed in Table 4–5. The overall objective is to record high quality and reliable DPOAE data. There are a host of potential pitfalls in measurement that can invalidate DPOAE measurement, usually resulting in smaller amplitude responses or even no detectable response when, in fact, normal DPOAEs should be recorded. As with any audiologic activity, one should proceed deliberately step-by-step, always inspecting findings and troubleshooting when they are inconsistent with expectations. This process is summarized graphically in Figure 4–16.

Once valid and reliable DPOAE data are collected for an ear, or a patient, analysis is performed. Guidelines for DPOAE analyses are displayed in Table 4–6. At this stage in the clinical development of OAEs, however, there is no "preferred method" for measurement or analysis of TEOAE or DPOAE. The intial analysis will lead to one of three gen-

Table 4–5. Steps in distortion product otoacoustic emissions (DPOAE) measurement.

■ Prior to OAE data collection

■ Verify that the actual stimulus intensity level is within ± 1.5 to 3 dB of target intensity level.

■ Verify that noise levels (noise floor or NF) are not excessive in the ear canal. Compare to normal expectations. See DPOAE normative tables in the Appendix.

■ Data collection

■ Monitor each of these parameters visually on computer screen as the DPgram is performed.

■ Replicate (at least twice) the DPgram for each protocol in each ear. Superimpose the two DPgrams for rapid evaluation of replicability.

■ Verify that you have stored the DPOAE data for each run on the computer hard or floppy disc.

■ Analyze OAE data for amplitude and noise floor as a function of stimulus frequency.

■ Interpret OAE data versus normative data as a function of stimulus frequency. See DPOAE normative Tables in Appendix.

Source: Hall JW III, Mueller HG III. *Audiologists' Desk Reference. Volume 1.* San Diego, CA: Singular Publishing Group, 1997.

eral outcomes. The DPOAE may be entirely normal—replicated DPOAE amplitudes for all frequencies are well within an appropriate normal region and noise floors at these frequencies are sufficiently low. A second possible outcome is that no replicable DPOAEs are detectable at any stimulus frequency. That is, DPOAE data are within the noise floor (again presuming that measurement noise is below maximum permissible levels). The third analysis alternative, and a very common one, is really a combination of the first two. DPOAEs are abnormal, or not detectable, at some frequencies, but within normal limits for other stimulus frequencies. With clinical experience, DPOAE patterns become more recognizable and easily interpreted. Certain characteristic features of DPgrams, and differences in DP findings among different devices, also become appreciated. To cite just one example of a typical variation in DPgram appearance, DPOAE amplitude is normally consistent across most stimulus frequencies with two exceptions. A slight dip in amplitude is often apparent in the 3000 Hz region (Lonsbury-Martin et al., 1991; Gorga et al., 1993; Strouse, Ochs, & Hall, 1996; Dorn et al., 1998). Also, as seen in the DPgrams displayed throughout the book, and normative data in Appendix A, amplitude also tends to diminish for the highest frequencies. The former may be

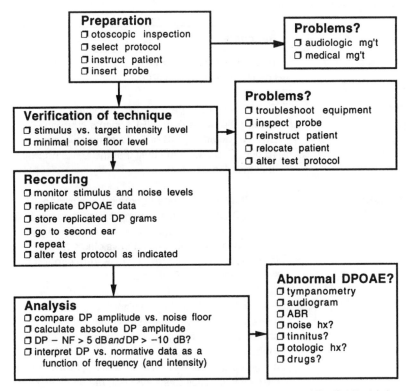

CLINICAL MEASUREMENT OF DPOAEs

Preparation
☐ otoscopic inspection
☐ select protocol
☐ instruct patient
☐ insert probe

Problems?
☐ audiologic mg't
☐ medical mg't

Verification of technique
☐ stimulus vs. target intensity level
☐ minimal noise floor level

Problems?
☐ troubleshoot equipment
☐ inspect probe
☐ reinstruct patient
☐ relocate patient
☐ alter test protocol

Recording
☐ monitor stimulus and noise levels
☐ replicate DPOAE data
☐ store replicated DP grams
☐ go to second ear
☐ repeat
☐ alter test protocol as indicated

Analysis
☐ compare DP amplitude vs. noise floor
☐ calculate absolute DP amplitude
☐ DP − NF > 5 dB and DP > −10 dB?
☐ interpret DP vs. normative data as a
   function of frequency (and intensity)

Abnormal DPOAE?
☐ tympanometry
☐ audiogram
☐ ABR
☐ noise hx?
☐ tinnitus?
☐ otologic hx?
☐ drugs?

Figure 4–16. A clinical approach for measurement of DPOAEs highlighting important steps in preparation, data collection and analysis, and troubleshooting.

related to the influence of middle ear function (and resonance) on the outward propagation of OAE energy, whereas the latter is probably in part a reflection of subtle cochlear deficits among subjects that are normal hearing audiometrically, at least for pure tone signals up to 8000 Hz. Whenever normal OAEs are not recorded or technical problems arise during measurement, the clinician must immediately begin troubleshooting in an attempt to determine the source of the problem, and likely solutions (see Table 4–7).

TEOAE MEASUREMENT AND ANALYSIS

Verification of Probe Fit and Test Conditions

The important steps in ensuring adequacy of the coupling between the OAE probe and the ear canal, reviewed earlier in this chapter for OAEs

Table 4–6. Distortion product otoacoustic emissions (DPOAE) analysis strategy. See also flow-chart showing DPOAE test sequence (see Figure 4–16).

Step	Rationale
■ Analyze each test frequency separately.	Take advantage of the incredible frequency specificity offered by DPOAE.
■ Does DP amplitude exceed noise floor?	To be considered present, DP amplitude must exceed the noise floor (NF). Minimal criterion is a DP - NF difference >3 or 5 dB (some might require 10 dB). This does not imply that the DP is normal, only that it is detectable.
■ Calculate absolute DP amplitude.	Does the DP amplitude (ignoring the NF for a moment) exceed some minimum limit, such as ≥10 dB or ≥15 dB. The assumption is the very small DP amplitudes are probably not physiologic activity from the cochlea, but rather noise from either the environment or OAE device.
■ Are DPOAE data replicable?	Remember, "if it doesn't replicate, you must investigate!" The absolute DP amplitude values should be reasonably similar from one DPgram run to the next (e.g., ± 2, 3, or 5 dB). There are no accepted guidelines for DP reliability. However, it is wise clincal policy to always require two similar sets of DP data before proceeding with analysis and interpretation.
■ Is DP amplitude within the normative region?	DPOAE interpretation must be done with reference to an appropriate normative database. The database should be derived from an adequate number of carefully selected normal subjects (e.g., normal middle ear status and hearing thresholds of ≤ 15 dB across the audiometric region). And, DPOAE for a patient should be recorded with a protocol equivalent to that used in normative data collection. Whether the DPOAE is normal or abnormal (or absent) is determined for most (although not necessary all) of the stimulus frequencies per octave that you use in your criteria for DP presence (e.g., 4 or 5 out of 6 frequencies). Due to fine structure, some DP data points may fall below the normal region even though cochlear function is intact.

Table 4–7. Troubleshooting problems during OAE recording.

Problem	Possible Solutions
No stimulus?	✔ Verify that power for the stimulus external box is on.
	✔ Verify that all tubes and cords leading to/from the computer to the probe are completely plugged in.
Very low stimulus intensity level (as detected by device)?	✔ Verify that you selected the appropriate stimulus intensity.
	✔ Verify by ear check that a stimulus is present at the level of the probe.
	✔ Make sure that the probe is fitted properly in the ear canal.
	✔ Inspect probe ports and tubes for debris (e.g., cerumen).
	✔ Inspect the external ear canal for excessive cerumen.
Stimulus intensity outside tolerance limits?	✔ Is the probe size appropriate for patient (i.e., newborn versus child versus adult)?
	✔ Inspect probe ports and tubes for slight blockage or compression.
	✔ Inspect the external ear canal for excessive cerumen.
	✔ Make sure that the probe is fitted properly in the ear canal.
Excessive noise levels?	✔ Is the patient quiet and not moving or chewing, etc?
	✔ Is the outside door to the test room closed?
	✔ What is the typical ambient noise level in the test room?
	✔ Is the test ear away from the OAE device and other sources of sound in the test room (e.g., ABR computer, door, air-conditioning vent)?
	✔ Is the probe fit well and deeply into the external ear canal? Try inserting deeper to reduce noise levels.
	✔ Are you averaging an adequate number of times per frequency? Maybe more processing is needed to reach a suitable noise level.
	✔ If all else fails, you should consider averaging OAE only for test frequencies above 1000 Hz to avoid the frequency region where noise is greatest.

Source: Adapted from Hall JW III, Mueller HG III. *Audiologists' Desk Reference. Volume I.* San Diego, CA: Singular Publishing Group, 1997.

in general, are directly applicable to TEOAEs. As noted by the discoverer of TEOAEs,

> Fitting the probe is the single most important part of making an acoustic emission measurement . . . outside of the laboratory it is often difficult to achieve an ideal fit, due to the wide variety of meatal configurations, and limited time for testing. Fitting criteria are vital and are quite different to those for tympanometry. There is less emphasis on an air tight seal. Instead, the primary factors are the inserted frequency response and the level of noise exclusion obtained (Kemp, 1990, pp. 97 and 98).

The four overall objectives in fitting the probe for TEOAE measurements are to obtain: (1) a well-formed and a clean temporal waveform, with little or no ringing; (2) a flat stimulus spectrum (a smooth frequency response); (3) the desired stimulus intensity level for the age of the patient (e.g., infant, child or adult). Keep in mind that the target will vary among TEOAE devices, and (4) an adequately low noise level in the enclosed ear canal, as documented by the device. The lower the noise level the better, but it should definitely fall below the manufacturer's recommended upper limit (usually less than 53 dB SPL). Noise is not a trivial factor in OAE measurement. In fact, for any patient and any test setting, it is one of the most important determinants of the success or failure of the procedure. In view of the critical role noise plays in the detection and analysis of OAEs, noise is addressed separately in the next chapter on nonpathologic factors influencing OAE measurement. There literature is reviewed, and practical guidelines for dealing with noise are offered.

Recording OAEs is technically quite straightforward. Analysis of OAEs, i.e., inspection of the findings and describing whether they are normal or how they are abnormal, is more complicated. Most challenging is the interpretation of OAE outcome in the context of other audiologic test results, and taking into account multiple nonpathologic and pathologic subject factors.

The first clue that there is a problem with the probe fit should be apparent from visual inspection of the stimulus temporal and/or spectral waveforms. Most manufacturers of OAE equipment provide guidelines for obtaining an adequate probe fit in the manual for their devices (see Chapter 7). Furthermore, the TEOAE devices on the market require that the operator follow a routine for verifying the quality of the probe fit before actual data collection begins. While the TEOAE measurement is underway, the device displays either numerical or graphic signals on stimulus intensity, which allow the operator to monitor the integrity of the probe fit. Finally, after TEOAE measurement is complete, the device displays documentation of stimulus intensity level, and stability or consistency of stimulus intensity from the beginning to the end of the recording. Widespread application of TEOAEs in newborn hearing screening since 1988 has resulted in a vast clinical experience in probe fitting under very demanding test conditions, (i.e., tiny external ear canals of sometimes wiggly infants in noisy test settings). This experience, which has led to a number of practical guidelines for improving probe fit and verifying of the adequacy of the probe fit and test conditions, among them changing the tip size, increasing the number of stimulus repetitions (the amount of averaging), and performing an otoscopic inspection. Specific guidelines are reviewed in a detailed discussion of newborn hearing screening with OAEs (Chapter 8). For a thorough review of issues important in click stimulus calibration, the reader is referred also to a recent paper by Chertoff and Guruprasad (1997).

Stimulus Factors and Parameters

The foregoing discussion of DPOAE stimulus factors and parameters, admittedly not an exhaustive review, referenced dozens of experimental and clinical studies of virtually every property of the stimuli used to evoke DPOAEs and the interactions among these properties. Among these studies, DPOAE data were recorded with a varied array of laboratory and clinical instruments. With the exception of the papers published by a few research centers, such as the Miami group (Brenda Lonsbury-Martin and colleagues), clinical DPOAE papers were infrequent. The corresponding literature on experimental investigation of TEOAE stimulus parameters is remarkably sparse. Most of the comprehensive investigations of TEOAEs, utilizing strong research-design and high-powered statistical analyses (e.g., Gorga et al., 1993; Prieve et al., 1993) reported data collected with one device (the ILO 88) using the default settings. Yet, ironically, from 1988 until the last year or two, the majority of publications describing clinical applications of OAEs and OAE findings with various patient populations (reviewed in Chapters 8 and 9) focus on TEOAEs, not DPOAEs.

Since 1988, the majority of TEOAE research has been conducted, and clinical experience acquired, with the ILO 88 device. Most researchers and clinicians have consistently recorded TEOAEs with the default settings of this device. This is a curious turn of events for at least three reasons. First, during the same time period, rather innovative and diverse measurement approaches were taken with DPOAEs. Second, prominent researchers and clinicians have, over the years, repeatedly advised more experimentation with TEOAE stimulus parameters and analysis strategies. Susan Norton and Judy Widen, in a 1990 article (Norton et al.) on TEOAEs in children, pointed out that,

> It is uncertain, even in adults, which parameters of otocoustic emissions are most appropriate for clinical applications. Questions include which evoking stimulus (tone pips or clicks) would be most useful clinically; which parameters of a given emission (threshold, latency, spectrum, or input-output function) will provide the most information; and how much analysis is needed and/or reasonable in order to judge an emission present and normal? (p. 121)

These words ring true even today. Four years after this Norton and Widen paper was published in a 1990 *Ear and Hearing* Supplement devoted to OAE, along with some colleagues I observed that,

The majority of the clinical studies of TEOAE were conducted with [the ILO 88 device] and used default stimulus and response parameters established by the manufacturer" and that "the use of default parameters may well have hindered study of the effect of measurement parameters on TEOAE outcome in clinical populations . . . documentation that the default parameters are optimal in varied clinical populations, such as infants or patients with sensory impairment, is not available—at least not based on the results of comprehensive published studies" (Hall et al., 1994, p. 29)

and, finally, that "widely accepted criteria, or at least guidelines for interpreting TEOAE data clinically are lacking." (Hall et al., 1994, p. 31)

Finally, repeatedly in the literature authors have cited analogies between OAEs and auditory evoked responses, especially the ABR. For example, each technique is electrophysiologic, both OAEs and ABR require signal averaging for detection, amplitude for both types of responses increases with stimulus intensity, and, clearly, OAEs and ABR are valuable components of the complete audiologic test battery. Yet, quoting again from Hall and colleagues (1994, p. 25), "the influence of stimulus and acquisition parameters on ABR findings have been extensively investigated in normal subjects and varied clinical populations . . . there are now test protocols for major clinical applications of ABR." To put this divergence in the clinical strategies taken for TEOAEs versus ABR into perspective, at least for readers who regularly apply ABR clinically, consider the inadequacy of a diagnostic ABR protocol for children that consisted exclusively of a single recording always for alternating polarity click stimuli presented at an intensity level of 90 dB HL and at a rate of 11/s for the same electrode array with analysis of latency only for wave V. Such an oversimplistic and rigid test protocol is inconceivable for the ABR, but its equivalent is often used in clinical application of TEOAEs. What is known about the effect of stimulus parameters on TEOAEs is summarized next.

It is probably safe to say that stimuli used to evoke TEOAEs are simpler than those used to evoke DPOAEs. The effects of some of the stimulus characteristics on DPOAEs that have been studied extensively, such as the frequency ratio and the relative intensity levels of the primaries, are not an issue with TEOAE measurement. The term transient evoked OAEs (TEOAEs) refers to a category of OAEs that are evoked with abrupt and very brief-duration stimuli. The two main types of transient stimuli are clicks (click-evoked OAEs are sometimes abbreviated CEOAEs) and tone bursts, or tone pips, although other stimuli have been used (e.g., Gaussian shaped or filtered clicks, single or half sinusoids, and chirps). In evoked response vernacular, a tone burst can be used in reference to any brief duration tonal signal that has a rapid rise time and might include one or several cycles of the frequency, whereas a tone pip technically has only a single cycle of the frequency at maximum amplitude. The first topic reviewed here is the effect of these types of stimuli on TEOAE response parameters.

Types of Stimuli

Clicks. The click stimulus contains a broad band of frequencies limited, usually, by the properties of the earphone (transducer) and the quality of the probe fit to the ear canal. It is desirable to present a stimulus characterized by a flat frequency response. That is, all possible frequencies within the stimulus are represented at approximately the same intensity level across the spectrum. In essence, the frequency response of the TEOAEs emitted from the cochlea is only as flat as the frequency response of the stimulus presented to the ear. The relationship between click stimulus spectrum and recorded TEOAEs has been clearly demonstrated experimentally (e.g., Norton & Neely, 1987) and by accumulated clinical experience. The typical TEOAEs for a click producing a flat frequency response consist of energy throughout the region of 500 to 6000 Hz, although peaks and valleys are typically present idiosyncratically for each subject/ear (Zwicker & Schloth, 1984; Elberling et al., 1985; Kemp et al., 1986; Probst et al., 1986; Abdo et al., 1992). It is certainly possible to record an abnormal TEOAE even when the stimulus frequency response is optimal. This pattern is, of course, quite common and entirely expected for patients with cochlear dysfunction. However, it is not possible to record an entirely normal TEOAE from even an entirely normal cochlea if the stimulus lacks energy in certain frequency regions. Put another way, an abnormal TEOAE can be interpreted as consistent with an abnormal cochlea if, and only if, the stimulus reaches and stays at the target intensity level, and is flat from one end of the spectrum to the other. Keep in mind the well-worn computer science adage "garbage in, garbage out."

Tonal signals. Clicks, clearly the most widely used stimuli in TEOAE measurement, contain relatively less energy than more frequency-concentrated stimuli, such as tone bursts. When the intensity level for clicks is increased to very high levels in an attempt to maximize stimulus effectiveness in evoking robust TEOAEs, the limit of the electro-acoustic transducer is exceeded and excessive distortion is produced. The distortion, in turn, contaminates the TEOAE response. Tonal stimuli offer a clinically feasible approach for maximizing stimulus acoustic energy, while minimizing distortion.

Beginning with the classic paper first describing OAEs published in 1978 by David Kemp, papers describing TEOAEs evoked with tone-burst stimuli have occasionally appeared in the literature (e.g., Elberling, 1985; Probst et al., 1986; Grandori, 1987; Norton & Neely, 1987; Harris & Probst, 1990; Stover & Norton, 1991; Xu et al., 1994). TEOAEs have more high-frequency energy, and shorter latency values, when elicited by high-frequency stimuli (Kemp et al., 1990). The relation between tone-burst frequency and TEOAE latency is, approximately, as follows: 4000 Hz at 5 ms; 3000 Hz at 7 ms; 2000 Hz at 9 ms; 1000 Hz at 12 ms; and 500 Hz at 15 ms. Also, importantly, with tone-burst stimuli, the OAE spectrum is limited to energy that matches the restricted frequency limits of the stimulus.

A relatively recent systematic study of TEOAEs elicited by tonal stimuli was reported by Lichtenstein and Stapells (1996). There were 72 subjects (31 males and 41 females). As an aside, many authors fail to specify the gender distribution of their subjects, even though gender is an important factor for TEOAE recordings. Among these subjects were 35 normal-hearing (less than or equal to 20 dB HL) and 51 sensorineurally impaired (hearing threshold greater than 20 dB HL) subjects. Stimuli were clicks (120 μs), and brief tones at 500 Hz and 2000 Hz linearly shaped with rise/fall times of 2 cycles and a plateau of 1cycle, presented at an intensity level of 80 dB peak equivalent SPL. A total of 520 sweeps was made for each response.

TEOAE analysis was performed with manufacturer's ILO 88 software for octave bands, and also half-octave bands, centered at 500 Hz, 1000 Hz, 2000 Hz, and 4000 Hz. The investigators also analyzed TEOAE data with an independent custom-written program. The major emphasis in data analysis was test performance for TEOAE findings relative to hearing status. Data were analyzed statistically using a signal detection theory approach, including hits, misses, false alarms, correct rejections, and relative operating characteristic (ROC) curves. Test performance for this, and other selected studies, is described in detail in Chapter 6 (TEOAEs and DPOAEs: Effect of Auditory Dysfunction). Relevant to this discussion, the authors concluded that "the use of the 500 Hz tones improved the identification of normal and impaired ears at 500 Hz for both the broadband TEOAEs (i.e., the whole reproducibility) and the 500 Hz octave-wide and half-octave-wide filtered TEOAEs. Results obtained for the 2000 Hz tones were similar to those obtained for clicks for the audiometric frequency of 2000 Hz" (Lichtenstein & Stapells, 1996, p. 133). In other words, for higher frequencies there was no clear advantage in using a tonal stimulus rather than a click stimulus with a frequency-specific analysis approach (octave band filtered TEOAE analysis). Use of the 500-Hz tone stimulus (in combination with a 30 ms sweep time), however, did improve frequency specificity of the TEOAE recording.

Chirps are another form of tonal stimulus that has been used to evoke OAEs. A chirp signal is "a sinusoidal signal with an instantaneous frequency that changes monotonically" (Neumann et al., 1994, p. 18). The objective in using chirp stimuli is to assess basilar membrane function in a highly selective frequency region. Neumann et al. (1994) delivered the chirp stimuli to 25 adult subjects (aged 24 to 71 years) with an Etymotic ER-2 insert earphone, and recorded the OAE with a Knowles EA 1843 microphone. Three types of chirp stimuli were utilized: a wide band "bark" chirp (500 to 6000 Hz), a low-frequency chirp (500 to 1000 Hz), and a high-frequency chirp (3000 to 6000 Hz). The authors concluded from this study that, at maximum amplitude settings, chirp-evoked OAEs had a higher acoustic level and better signal-to-noise ratio than click stimuli. Additional innovative approaches to TEOAE stimulation and analysis, most not quite ready for clinical application, are summarized in Chapter 10.

Bone-conduction. Virtually all reports of TEOAE measurement utilize stimuli presented by air conduction. In hearing assessment with pure tone audiometry, auditory brainstem response, and sometimes even speech audiometry, bone-conducted signals are often used to assess sensory function when middle ear dysfunction is associated with a conductive hearing loss. Clinically, it would be desirable if an equivalent technique could be developed for measurement of OAEs, that is, a technique not dependent on status of the middle ear system. Such a technique might permit the application of OAEs as a sensitive measure of cochlear function, even in persons with middle ear disease. There is at least one paper describing bone-conduction OAEs. Collet and colleagues, a prolific OAE research group in Lyon France, recorded TEOAEs with bone-conducted click stimuli utilizing specially designed instrumentation. OAEs were recorded from both ears of 10 otologically and audiometrically normal subjects. However, as the authors' pointed out: "The technique seems as yet to be of purely experimental interest . . . application in clinical exploration is more questionable, as in middle ear effusion OAEs are not present" (Collet et al., 1989, p. 45). This point is very important. OAEs are highly dependent on the middle ear system not only for transmission of the stimulus to the cochlea but also, of course, for propagation of the OAEs from the cochlea to the ear canal. Presumably, bone-conduction stimulation would not offer a feasible or effective approach for circumventing the deleterious influence middle ear dysfunction has on OAE measurement.

The majority of authors of publications, and clinical audiologists, have recorded TEOAEs with default test parameters. Research and clinical experience with various stimulus and acquisition settings is lacking.

Stimulus Polarity

As noted above, the use of a special version of alternating click stimuli (three signals of one polarity and a fourth more intense signal of opposite polarity) is a common strategy to minimize the linear components in the averaged TEOAE so that the nonlinear response of the cochlea can be detected (Figure 4–17). The effects of manipulations of stimulus polarity, other than this sequence, have, to my knowledge, not been assessed clinically. Lina-Granada and Collet (1995), in a study of inter-stimulus interval on TEOAEs mentioned below, did comment on the complete reversal of TEOAE polarity when stimulus was reversed, as had been reported in several early papers on TEOAEs (Kemp, 1978; Anderson, 1980).

Stimulus intensity level. Stimulus intensity level is a critical determinant for the presence or absence of TEOAEs and, when TEOAEs are

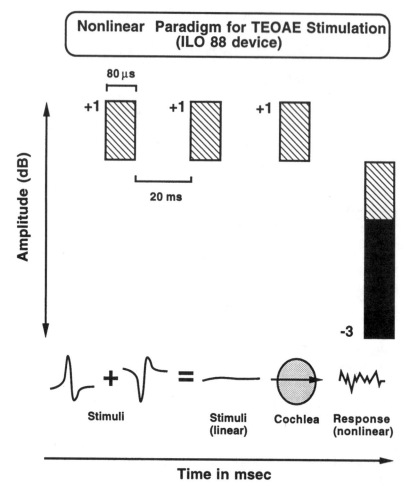

Figure 4–17. Schematic illustration of the nonlinear stimulus paradigm utilized for TEOAE recording with the ILO 88 device (Otodynamics, Ltd.) to minimize undesirable influence of residual stimulus energy in the measured response. Details on Otodynamics products, including the ILO 88 device, are provided in Chapter 7.

present, the correlation between waveforms and the amplitude at all frequency regions. Of course several other factors also affect these TEOAE characteristics as well, principally the status of the cochlea and middle ear. In the very first paper on OAEs in humans published by Kemp in 1978, TEOAEs were recorded from 15 subjects using either click or tone burst stimuli presented at different intensity levels. He noted linear growth of TEOAE amplitude for low stimulus intensity levels. Soon after, other authors confirmed that the I/O function for TEOAEs is linear for low-intensity levels and then shows a distinct saturation for moderate-to-high intensity levels (Wit & Ritsma, 1979; Kemp & Chum, 1980; Wilson, 1980b; Zwicker, 1983). The specific descriptions of the I/O reported in these papers, however, are not entirely consistent, and intersubject variability in I/O functions was a common finding. Furthermore, all of the studies predated the intro-duction of clinical instrumentation for TEOAE measurement. The combined results, therefore, shed little light on the potential clinical value of I/O functions.

As clinical devices became available around the world, the prevailing opinion on TEOAE I/O functions was concisely summed up by Dr. Kemp:

> The use of strong stimulation (90 dB SPL peak) for initial screening is recommended because the wider range of OAE frequencies are obtained . . . With low stimulus levels, not only are smaller OAEs collected but the response becomes dominated by any frequency components which are near to the self sustaining-spontaneous oscillation condition. (Kemp, 1990, p. 100)

But he immediately added that,

> The growth of OAEs with stimulus intensity is of interest. This can be very small in some ears with strong emissions (down to 0.1 dB/dB). The average is around 0.4 dB/dB, and can approach near to linearity. This has been found in some neonates. The growth rate is highly frequency dependent. (Kemp, 1990, p. 100)

Since the early 1990s, consistent with Dr. Kemp's initial recommen-dation, a single (default) intensity level of approximately 80 to 85 dB SPL has been almost always used in clinical applications of TEOAEs.

In one of the few reports describing TEOAE I/O functions from a clin-ical perspective, and relative to DPOAE data, Norton (1993) included several figures illustrating growth in the amplitude of TEOAE tem-poral waveforms from an intensity level of 21 dB up to about 45 dB, and then apparently similar waveform amplitude for higher intensity levels. Another figure showed a pronounced flattening of I/O func-tions, beginning in the intensity region of 45 to 50 dB SPL, for TEOAEs evoked with click and with tone-burst stimuli. Data were recorded on several young normal-hearing adult subjects. That year, Norton, and a colleague also recorded TEOAE I/O functions for click and tone-burst stimuli in a study of the effects of aging (Stover & Norton, 1993). Their results almost invariably confirmed saturation of TEOAE amplitude as intensity approached 50 dB peSPL for clicks and for 5 tone-burst stimuli (from 1000 Hz to 3000 Hz). No significant age effect was ob-served for the I/O functions.

In a study of TEOAE reliability (described below), Marshall and Heller (1996) collected data for stimulus intensity levels of 80, 74, 68, and 62 dB SPL. I/O data were described for 25 ears of 15 subjects. Reliability was high for all intensity levels. Slopes for TEOAE amplitude as a function of stimulus intensity, reported for three octave bands, were

0.70 for 625–1250 Hz, 0.57 for 1250–2500 Hz, and 0.40 for 2500–5000 Hz. Slope was affected by analysis bandwidth, with shallower slopes found for higher center frequencies. In addition, slope increased as hearing level increased (only subjects with normal hearing or a mild sensory hearing loss were included in this study). Marshall and Heller (1996) suggested that, "changes in the slope of the I/O function may be a viable way to determine whether an ear has been affected by oto-toxic factors. Additional data are needed in this area" (p. 245). Indeed, systematic clinical investigation of TEOAE amplitude as a function of intensity is long overdue. Among the factors that might be included, minimally, as variables in such studies are: (1) age (especially a look at possible developmental effects), (2) gender, (3) type of stimulus (click and tone burst), (4) cochlear status, (5) middle ear status, (6) contralateral suppression, and (7) DPOAE measurements.

Stimulus Rate/Interstimulus Interval

A theme developed earlier in this chapter was the distinct contrast between the pathways taken in research of TEOAEs versus ABR. There has been extensive clinical investigation of stimulus and acquisition parameters for ABR, yet relatively little study of these parameters for TEOAEs. This point is clearly evident in the size of the literature describing the effects of stimulus rate on ABR versus TEOAEs. Within 15 years after the classic initial publication on the ABR in 1971, dozens of clinical papers appeared describing the effects of stimulus rate in adults, children, and neonates and in patients with a wide variety of pathologies (Hall, 1992a). Until recently, papers on stimulus rate and TEOAEs were few and far between, limited to normal adult populations, and mostly limited to relatively slow to moderate rates of under 60 stimuli/s (Kemp, 1978; Anderson, 1980; Grandori, 1985). An exception is the recent interest in applying maximum length sequences (MLS) techniques to TEOAE measurement (e.g., Thornton, 1993). This topic is included in "Future Directions in Clinical Research" (Chapter 10).

In a study of the effect of interstimulus interval on TEOAEs, Lina-Granade and Collet (1995, 1997) found a significant reduction in amplitude as the stimulus rate increased from 50/s up to over 1000/s, and interstimulus intervals correspondingly decreased from 20 ms to below 1 ms, respectively. Subjects in these two studies were normal-hearing adults. Other previous investigations (Kemp & Chum, 1980; Thornton, 1993b; Thornton, 1994; Picton et al., 1993), utilizing various strategies for rapid presentation of clicks, such as pairs of click stimuli, pseudorandom pulse trains (PPT), and maximum length sequence (MLS), also showed diminished TEOAE amplitude at very high stimulus rates and as interstimulus intervals were shortened. Because OAEs are preneural, and therefore not subject to the neural adaptation associated with auditory evoked responses (e.g., ECochG, N1, and ABR), cochlear mechanisms are presumably accountable for these effects. Two possible explanations for these changes at high stimulus rates and short interstimulus intervals include incomplete recovery of adaptation of outer hair cell physiologic processes and ipsilateral efferent auditory system activation (see the discussion of OAE suppression Chapter 6). In any event, further clinical investigation of the effect of rate on TEOAEs would seem warranted.

Response Factors and Parameters

In the first 5 or 6 years after the introduction of the ILO 88 device (the ILO refers to the Institute for Laryngology and Otology and the 88 to 1988, the year the device became commercially available), many dozens of papers appeared describing TEOAE findings in normal subjects and various patient populations. As noted above, with very rare exceptions, TEOAE data for these studies were collected with the default test parameters. This rather strict adherence to manufacturer recommendations for stimulus and acquisition settings may have stifled innovation, and perhaps delayed the discovery of more efficient or effective test strategies for specific test conditions or clinical applications. Nonetheless, the consistency in technique facilitated the comparison of findings among studies. During the same time frame (1988 until about 1994), ILO 88 software underwent many upgrades and developments. Although the technologic progress was certainly positive, it quickly diminished the relevance of the findings of many earlier studies. For example, in the early years, analysis was almost limited to a description of overall reproducibility (in %) and/or overall amplitude level (in dB SPL). Unfortunately, these general response measures do not take advantage of the exquisite frequency-specific information available in TEOAE recordings. The dominant TEOAE frequencies are within the region of 500 to 4000 Hz, as recorded with available transducers. This frequency range is, of course, only a small portion of the normal human cochlear frequency response of 20 to 20,000 Hz. The restriction in spectral analysis is not a feature of all OAE measurements. For instance, with an appropriate probe system (transducers and microphone), it is possible to record DPOAEs for stimuli up to 20,000 Hz.

Is there any clinical value in recording both TEOAE and DPOAE together in audiologic assessment? Clinical data is insufficient to answer this question.

Therefore, neither overall or "whole reproducibility" (correlation) nor "echo level" (TEOAE amplitude) are an accurate reflection of the status of cochlear functioning across a wide range of audiometric frequencies. A high reproducibility value, interpreted as "normal," might be recorded in a patient with a serious sensory deficit for some audiometric frequencies, as long as there was normal cochlear function for a portion of the frequency range. Exactly the opposite interpretation was, of course, also possible. That is, a reproducibility value below the normal cut-off did not necessary rule out normal hearing within the audiometric region. The same limitation held true for reliance on overall "echo level." This concept is by no means original. Similar statements have been made for over a decade by various authors (Kemp et al., 1986; Probst et al., 1987; Hurley & Musiek, 1994; Lichtenstein & Stapells, 1996). As a consequence of this limitation in the sophistication of analysis software, the findings and, to some extent conclusions, of many otherwise thorough and systematic studies of TEOAEs in normal subjects (e.g., Vedantam & Musiek, 1991), in large populations of hearing impaired patients (e.g., Bonfils et al., 1989), and in series of neonates undergoing hearing screening are in retrospect quite limited. To be sure, most of these investigations are the product of an extensive, collaborative, research effort. Many made important, often innovative, contributions to our understanding of OAEs, and significantly advanced the clinical application of OAE. Yet, even generic discussions from these investigations regarding, for example, the most appropriate criteria for definition of normal versus abnormal TEOAE responses, such as an overall ("whole") reproducibility or correlation of 50% (e.g., Kemp, Bray, Alexander, & Brown, 1986; Kok et al., 1993) versus 60% (Prieve et al., 1993) versus 70% (e.g., Vedantam & Musiek, 1991) are now outdated.

Given the technologic constraints of the earlier investigations (prior to about 1994), the following discussion focuses mostly on one general and four frequency-specific response parameters that can be analyzed with clinical TEOAE devices. The one general response parameter is the temporal waveform. The four frequency-specific parameters, each assessed within octave bands or more restricted spectral regions, are: (1) reproducibility, (2) absolute amplitude, (3) the amplitude-to-noise difference or ratio, and (4) estimation of TEOAE "threshold" or minimum detection intensity level.

Temporal Waveform

A common initial approach for analyzing TEOAEs is to inspect the response temporal waveform visually. Actually, the display usually includes two waveforms recorded concomitantly during the averaging process from, respectively, odd and even stimulus presentations. The temporal waveforms of TEOAEs reflect the actual sound waves emitted from the cochlea, plus any noise present in the ear canal during the measurement. Even if recorded from the same ear of a subject, the appearance of the waveform, however, will vary to some degree from one device to another as it is altered by characteristics of the microphone within the probe and by the data processing strategy utilized. (Instrumentation is discussed more later.) As with an ABR, the TEOAE waveform provides immediate confirmation of the presence or absence of a response, and a rough overview of the amount of noise (components not common to both waveforms) in the recording. Estimations of the amplitude of waves within different time segments of the waveform (e.g., the first 5 ms versus later segments) also yield an overall impression of the relative frequency composition of the response. Because the temporal waveform, by definition, reflects the appearance of the TEOAE in the external ear canal over time, there is a general relationship between the latency of portions of the waveform and the place along the cochlea where the TEOAE was generated. TEOAE activity generated at the base of the cochlea reaches the external ear canal first, whereas TEOAE activity from more apical regions of the cochlea requires more time for the outward propagation basalward along the basilar membrane, outward through the middle ear, and in a lateral direction into the external ear canal to the microphone in the probe.

Also similar to ABR analysis, it is not possible to extract precise information on specific TEOAE response parameters, such as the correlation between two simultaneously averaged waveforms or specific amplitude or latency data from this visual inspection. Amplitude, or the response-to-noise difference, can be calculated in dB for the entire waveform or for designated frequency regions, as can correlation values for the two simultaneously recorded waveforms. These amplitude and correlation values typically are utilized in clinical applications of TEOAEs. In one respect, ABR and TEOAE analysis differs markedly. Latency calculations are the mainstay of ABR analysis and interpretation. Precise measurement of TEOAE latency is not possible clinically, as discussed below. For each of these parameters, a patient's TEOAE findings may be evaluated according to clinical criteria for response presence or absence (e.g., a response is present if overall correlation is 50% or greater), or any or all patient findings can be compared to an established normative data base. Specific strategies for clinical TEOAE analysis are discussed below and for patients in Chapters 8 and 9.

Analysis Time and Windowing

The duration of the analysis period after stimulus presentation is a measurement parameter that can be manipulated by the equipment operator. The default analysis time is typically in the range of 20 ms (see Chapter 10). However, there are clinical indications for recording TEOAE with shorter or longer analysis times. For example, one common modification of test parameters when TEOAEs are used in newborn hearing screening is to shorten the analysis time from 20 ms to 10 ms. This alteration in analysis time serves two valuable purposes: First, test time is reduced because the end point for analysis of the response for each stimulus is cut in half and also because there is less temporal information to process once the data reach the device. Second, the second half of the 20-ms analysis time window (from 10 to 20 ms) contains lower frequency TEOAE energy. By eliminating this time period from the analysis, much of the unwanted noise, which tends to be concentrated in the lower frequency region, is eliminated as well. The topic of measurement noise, always pertinent to OAE recording clinically, is discussed in detail in the next chapter.

Electrophysiologic information in the time domain (the temporal waveform) can be converted to information in the frequency domain (the spectral waveform), typically with a technique called fast Fourier transformation (FFT). Any complex waveform can be analyzed in terms of its frequency composition. Continuing the ABR analogy, FFT is used to obtain a display of the spectral composition of the ABR temporal waveform. So, instead of viewing waves I, III, and V, and calculating their latencies and amplitudes, analysis is performed for a series of energy peaks at different frequencies from about 100 Hz up to 1000 Hz. The FFT technique is used regularly in the analysis of TEOAE data in the form of the overall response spectrum, and the calculations of TEOAE correlation and amplitude (or amplitude-noise) values for specific frequency regions (e.g., octave bands centered around 1000 Hz, 2000 Hz, etc.). FFT involves a windowing process. A detailed explanation of this process is beyond the limits of this review (see Hall, 1986; Norcia, Sato, Shinn, & Mertus, 1986; Hall, 1992). However, it is important clinically to appreciate that the analysis time used to capture the response can substantially influence the outcome of the windowing process. If a response—an ABR, TEOAE, or any other electrophysiologic waveform—falls well within the center of the analysis time frame, windowing will usually have very little effect on the data. But, when the response undergoing FFT extends to the limit of the analysis time, then the window process may distort data. That is, the spectral display of the response, in this case the TEOAE, may lack some of the energy present in the temporal waveform. This problem was identified in clinical TEOAE measurements by Lichtenstein and Stapells (1996), as mentioned in the earlier section on tone-burst TEOAE.

With appropriate manipulations of important test parameters, such as stimulus intensity, TEOAE and DPOAE appear to be comparably sensitive to cochlear dysfunction within the frequency region of 1000 to 4000 Hz.

Latency

Latency of TEOAEs varies predictably as a function of the frequency composition, as noted above. Precise definition of TEOAE latency is problematic for several reasons. The shortest latency components, generated in the basal region of the cochlea, are obscured by leftover stimulus energy in the ear canal. The nonlinear technique typically used to record TEOAEs also can influence the accuracy of latency measures. The wide range of latency values for TEOAEs reported over the years lends further empirical evidence of the difficulty in precisely defining the temporal aspects of TEOAEs. Because latency is not a clinically analyzed parameter of TEOAEs, it will not be discussed further here. A review of the literature on OAE latency measures in general is found in Chapter 10.

Reliability

According to early studies (Johnsen & Elberling, 1982; Antonelli & Grandori, 1986; Kemp, Bray, Alexander, & Brown, 1986) and subsequently many others with the ILO 88 device (Harris, Probst, & Wenger,

1991; Vedantam & Musiek, 1991; Franklin et al., 1992; Prieve et al., 1993), TEOAE stimuli and response parameters are highly reliable. As an example, correlations for stimulus level, absolute TEOAE amplitude, the TEOAE amplitude-noise floor difference, and the reproducibility measure higher than 0.90 for normal subjects and sensory impaired patients in the age range of 4 to 81 years, even with probe replacement between trials (Prieve et al., 1993). Test-retest reliability for TEOAEs was similarly high as reported in a paper by Franklin et al. (1992). For the most part, the authors of these studies relied on default stimulus settings (e.g., as a single high-intensity level, 80 dB SPL). Perhaps the most comprehensive investigation to date was conducted by Marshall and Heller (1996). These investigators examined several important factors not addressed in most earlier studies, including the influence of stimulus intensity, bandwidth of the TEOAE, spectral shape of the stimulus, and hearing loss. It is important to note that the subjects were 13 adults and that all TEOAE data were collected in a double-walled, sound-treated room. In summary, this study showed that: (1). TEOAE amplitudes were reasonably reliable independent of stimulus intensity level across the range of 62 to 80 dB SPL, (2) slight-to-mild sensory hearing loss was associated with a slight, but not statistically significant, reduction in reliability, (3) reliability was equivalent among the frequencies for which the TEOAE could be measured (625 Hz to 5000 Hz, although data from hearing impaired subjects were limited for narrowband analyses for lower stimulus intensity levels), and (4) reliability was progressively poorer as the bandwidth analyzed (broadband, octave, ½ octave, ⅓ octave, and ⅙ octave) decreased. The broadband analysis was clearly most reliable but, of course, not frequency specific. This paper is recommended for a thorough review of TEOAE reliability and as a source of clinically useful information on the topic.

TEOAE Test Protocols and Analysis Strategies

Test Protocols

Protocols recommended by manufacturers of clinical TEOAE devices are summarized in Chapter 7. A TEOAE protocol for newborn hearing screening is described, along with guidelines for measurement, troubleshooting, and analysis, is presented in the section on newborn hearing screening in Chapter 8.

Bandwidth for Analysis

Current software for TEOAE devices permits frequency-specific analysis of the response. Earlier researchers and clinicians were limited, essentially by the stimulus spectrum transduced by the probe, to a description of either TEOAE amplitude or reproducibility for a broadband of frequencies. Now TEOAE analysis can be performed for narrower frequency regions, such as octaves, in addition to the entire broadband response. The narrower analysis bands offer the important clinical advantage of frequency specificity. As noted by Marshall and Heller (1996), a ⅓ octave bandwidth actually approximates psychophysical critical bandwidths, and a ⅙ bandwidth begins to approach, at least in theory, the frequency-specificity of the pure tone signals used to evoke DPOAEs. Unfortunately, poor reliability for these restricted bandwidths probably limits their value in TEOAE measurement.

Instrumentation

A study documenting significant variation in amplitude data recorded with DPOAE devices marketed by five different manufacturers was described earlier in this chapter. Presumably, DPOAE amplitude differences also would be found among the four or five devices introduced since the study was conducted. For TEOAE measurement, the picture does not appear to be quite as complicated because few devices are on the market. For the past 10 years only one device (the ILO 88 by Otodynamics) has been readily available and licensed for clinical use in the United States. A review of the "Manufacturers Forum" (Chapter 7) indicates that this picture will soon change, as additional manufacturers will be permitted to introduce TEOAE devices into the clinical marketplace. The rather heavy reliance on one TEOAE device to date and the relative consistency in data reported among studies should not be taken as evidence that TEOAE response parameters are uniquely consistent and dependable. There is, in fact, some evidence to the contrary.

As noted by British investigator Roger Thornton and colleagues in a paper comparing neonatal TEOAEs recorded with two types of devices: "Recording for the same stimulus, from the same ear should give the same TEOAE if the two instruments have similar characteristics" (Thornton et al., 1994, p. 99). This group studied TEOAE data recorded on three separate test days from over 100 neonates with the ILO 88 device and another TEOAE device (the Programmable Otoacoustic Measurement System, or POEMS, device). One example of the differences found between the two devices, a difference in power spectra, is illustrated in Figure 4–18. For higher frequency regions of the TEOAE response, differences of over 6 dB were reported. The results of this study were in agreement with previous findings from adult populations of device-specific differences in TEOAE data (e.g., Lutman et al., 1994). As shown in Figure 4–18, Lutman et al. (1994) confirmed substantial differences in the TEOAE temporal waveform that could be attributed to differences in the design and construction of the probes used with the two devices. These authors concluded their arti-

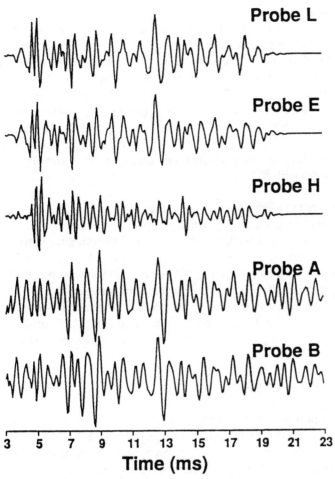

Figure 4–18. Influence of probe design on TEOAE waveforms. The top three waveforms were recorded with the ILO 88 probe, but each with a different probe. The lower two waveforms were recorded with the POEMS device with two different probes. Note the distinctly different temporal waveform characteristics depending on the probe used for the TEOAE recording. From Lutman et al. Coloration of click-evoked otoacoustic emissions by characteristics of the recording apparatus. In Grandori F (ed). *Advances in Otoacoustic Emissions Volume I.* Milan, 1996 (p. 43).

cle with the statement: " standardization of probe design and construction is required before TEOAE waveforms can be combined meaningfully across instruments" (p. 47). The same statement applies also to DPOAEs.

Lichtenstein and Stapells (1996) compared TEOAE reproducibility as calculated with the ILO 88 system versus a custom software program. In the study described above in the section on tone-burst stimuli, TEOAE data were recorded from 86 ears of 72 normal hearing or hearing-impaired subjects. With the custom program, a 30-ms analysis sweep was employed (versus 20 ms for the ILO 88), and reproducibility was assessed using a different windowing strategy in which "zeroed (windowed)" points were not included in the calculation (they are included with the ILO 88). The custom program appeared to improve TEOAE test performance (identification of hearing loss), as quantified with ROC curves.

ANSI and ISO standards are not yet available for TEOAE and DPOAE equipment.

Clinicians are likely to concur with the conclusion of Dr. Thornton and colleagues that major equipment-dependent differences in TEOAE findings for this neonatal population are disturbing. Industry should heed Dr. Thornton's eloquent and data-based plea for more consistency among OAE instruments: "With the increasing sophistication of equipment and the increasing use of more complex and quantitative measures, the time has come to grasp the nettle and consider detailed design factors and some form of standardization" (Thornton et al., 1994, p. 109). This statement rings true as well as for DPOAEs.

TEOAEs Analyses

Stimulation and acquisition parameters important in the measurement of TEOAEs are illustrated in Figure 4–19. This discussion will be limited to the review of generic characteristics of TEOAEs, rather than measurement and analysis with a specific brand and model of equipment. The first step in TEOAE measurement is the delivery of an optimal stimulus. Typically, the clinician completes a stimulus verification or "probe fit" routine or sequence before TEOAE data are collected. For an alternating polarity click stimulus (the most common type), the optimal *temporal waveform* should be characterized by two distinct deflections, one positive and one negative in polarity, with little or no subsequent activity. Undesirable features of a click temporal waveform include very small (low intensity) deflections, ongoing deflections of gradually smaller intensity (stimulus ringing), or, of course, no apparent stimulus.

Another important stimulus parameter that must be evaluated prior to TEOAE measurement is the *spectral waveform* . Optimally, for a click stimulus, the spectrum should be wide and flat, with approximately equal energy across the frequency region of 0 to 6000 Hz. The old computer adage "garbage in, garbage out" takes on very clear meaning for TEOAE. To record a normal TEOAE, reflecting outer hair cell activity from basal to apical regions of the basilar membrane, there must be

TRANSIENT EVOKED OTOACOUSTIC EMISSION

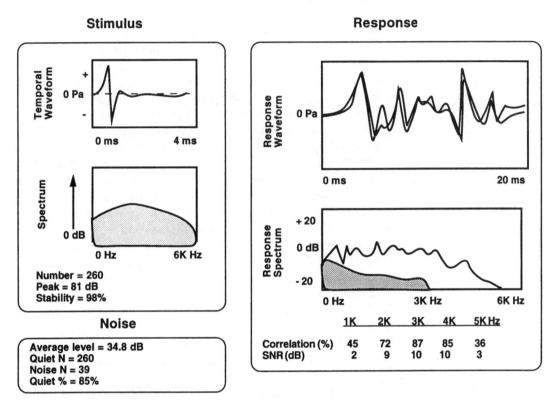

Figure 4–19. Stimulus and response parameters in the clinical measurement of transient OAEs (TEOAEs). Parameters were described in detail in Chapter 1 (see Figure 1–8). In this example, the temporal waveform is optimal for the click stimuli of alternating polarity (full amplitude without excessive ringing artifact) and the spectral waveform (frequency response) of the stimuli is flat across the range of 0 to 5000 Hz. Stimulus intensity level (peak = 81 dB) is close to the target of 80 dB SPL, and the stability of 98% confirms that the stimuli were consistently near the target for 260. Average noise level in the external ear canal during OAE measurement was relatively low (34.8 dB) and 85% of the 260 stimuli presented when noise was lower than the rejection level. Inspection of the temporal waveform of the TEOAEs measured in the external ear canal shows a clear and reliable response (*top portion*) with energy (*solid line*) well above the noise floor (*shaded area*) across the frequency region of 0 to 5000 Hz (*lower portion*). Correlation (reproducibility) values were highest for the 2000 to 4000 Hz octave bands, as were the signal-to-noise ratio (SNR) for the TEOAE versus noise floor. For accurate analysis, and interpretation of the TEOAE data as normal or abnormal, one would compare these response parameters to a normal adult database. Clearly, however, a TEOAE is present in the mid-frequency region.

energy in the stimulus from low-to high-frequency regions. The TEOAE recorded from an ear may not be normal due to cochlear dysfunction, but TEOAE findings will be normal in ears without cochlear dysfunction only if the stimulus spectrum includes all frequencies. In addition, the intensity of the stimulus must reach the desired criteria, often about 80 dB SPL. The clinician must, at the outset of TEOAE measurement, verify that stimulus temporal waveform is appropriately brief, the intensity level is within a decibel or two of target (the desired level), and the spectrum is broad and flat. Then, periodically during and again at the end of data collection (for a single run of stimuli), the stability of constancy of the stimulus should be verified. Clinically, it is not uncommon for the probe to shift, or even slip out of the ear canal, during the course of TEOAE or DPOAE stimulus presentation. With a quiet and cooperative subject, TEOAE measurement for a series of 200 to 300 stimuli may require only 1 minute or less. Some patients, however, are not quite so compliant and cooperative. How many stimuli should be presented in averaging a TEOAE? There is no single correct answer to that practical clinical question. The question is really: When is the desired signal-to-noise (TEOAE-to-noise) ratio reached? Although a default number of stimuli (e.g., 260) is almost always employed with some TEOAE devices, this number may be excessive under ideal test conditions, yet insufficient under adverse conditions when there is much noise and/or an abnormally small amplitude TEOAEs. Once the TEOAEs have reached maximum amplitude and remains stable, further stimulus presentation simply wastes test time. This parameter is under the control of the tester and stimulus presentation can be terminated or lengthened, as appropriate, during testing.

Clinically, two response properties of TEOAEs are quantified and described. One is a display of the response in the time domain. This temporal display of the response is invariably shown as one or two waveforms beginning about 2 to 3 ms after the stimulus and continuing out to about 20 ms. The temporal waveform for TEOAEs is, therefore, much like the ABR waveform. For TEOAEs the amplitude of the waveform (often reported with a unit of pressure such as the Pascal, Pa, rather than μV for the ABR) varies over the course of the analysis time. The earliest portions of the temporal waveform reflect TEOAE activity produced by the basal regions of the basilar membrane, whereas later portions of the waveform arise from more apical regions. When two separate waveforms are overlayed, it is possible to judge visually, albeit not precisely, the agreement, correlation, or reproducibility of the response. Of course, the more similar the multiple waveforms are, the more likely the response reflects cochlear activity rather than noise. In early clinical reports of TEOAEs, temporal waveforms were shown at progressively decreasing intensity levels, until no response was detected. Again, this follows a clinical convention used with the ABR.

Visual inspection of TEOAE temporal waveform fails to capture much clinically valuable information, especially regarding the status of the TEOAE at various audiometric frequencies. Thus, spectral analysis of the TEOAE waveforms provides additional frequency information. TEOAE findings are often displayed in the frequency domain. A TEOAE response spectrum clearly reveals the presence of TEOAE activity across the frequency region of 0 to 5000 Hz. For meaningful analysis of the TEOAE response spectrum, it is important to view the noise floor simultaneously during the measurement, also as a function of frequency. These visual displays are typically quantified for more precise analysis. TEOAE absolute amplitude, or the TEOAE amplitude-noise difference, is calculated at individual frequencies or summarized for bands of frequencies (e.g., octaves or some fraction of an octave). The agreement of two waveforms, recorded simultaneously (each the response to alternative click stimuli) is also shown as a percentage (correlation in %) for the different frequency bands. Assuming normal middle ear status and that stimulus intensity was at or close to the target level and the spectrum was flat, then any reduction in the TEOAEs signal-to-noise ratio or correlation in any frequency region would reflect cochlear (outer hair cell) dysfunction. Normative data can be derived for interpretation of these quantified TEOAE data. Finally, TEOAE measurement is summarized graphically in Figure 4–20.

CONCLUDING COMMENTS

Well, there may be more to OAE measurement and analysis than you thought at the beginning of this chapter. It is important to understand the principles underlying each and every step in measurement, including the selection of an appropriate test protocol, the quality of the probe fit, what can go wrong during measurement and how to fix it, and, last but certainly not least, the analysis of the response. This final step has not yet been fully addressed. A variety of nonpathologic factors, and OAE patterns in pathologies, will be discussed next (Chapters 5, 6, 8, and 9). But, above all, practice makes perfect. You now have more than enough knowledge to find a subject and begin recording OAEs. There is no other way to develop clinical technique and really learn OAE measurement and analysis.

CLINICAL MEASUREMENT OF TEOAE

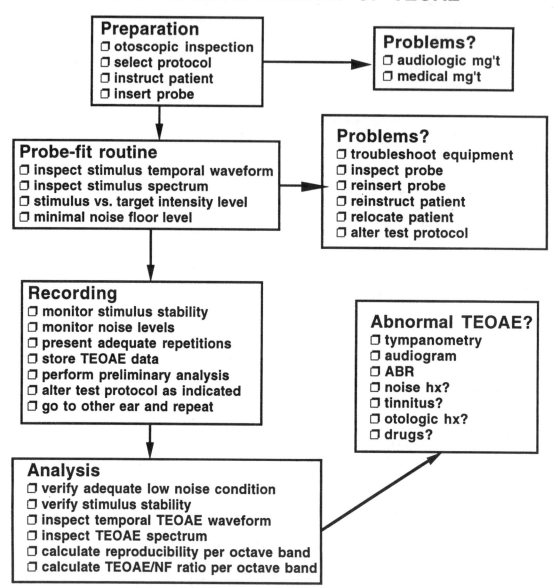

Preparation
- ☐ otoscopic inspection
- ☐ select protocol
- ☐ instruct patient
- ☐ insert probe

Problems?
- ☐ audiologic mg't
- ☐ medical mg't

Probe-fit routine
- ☐ inspect stimulus temporal waveform
- ☐ inspect stimulus spectrum
- ☐ stimulus vs. target intensity level
- ☐ minimal noise floor level

Problems?
- ☐ troubleshoot equipment
- ☐ inspect probe
- ☐ reinsert probe
- ☐ reinstruct patient
- ☐ relocate patient
- ☐ alter test protocol

Recording
- ☐ monitor stimulus stability
- ☐ monitor noise levels
- ☐ present adequate repetitions
- ☐ store TEOAE data
- ☐ perform preliminary analysis
- ☐ alter test protocol as indicated
- ☐ go to other ear and repeat

Abnormal TEOAE?
- ☐ tympanometry
- ☐ audiogram
- ☐ ABR
- ☐ noise hx?
- ☐ tinnitus?
- ☐ otologic hx?
- ☐ drugs?

Analysis
- ☐ verify adequate low noise condition
- ☐ verify stimulus stability
- ☐ inspect temporal TEOAE waveform
- ☐ inspect TEOAE spectrum
- ☐ calculate reproducibility per octave band
- ☐ calculate TEOAE/NF ratio per octave band

Figure 4–20. A clinical approach for measurement of TEOAEs highlighting important steps in preparation, probe fit routine (to verify adequate stimulation), troubleshooting, data collection, and TEOAE analysis.

CHAPTER

5

Distortion Product and Transient Evoked OAEs: Nonpathologic Factors Influencing Measurement

DIURNAL (TIME OF DAY) EFFECTS

GENETICS

RACE

BODY POSITION

STATE OF AROUSAL AND ATTENTION

EAR CANAL ACOUSTICS

OAE PREVALENCE IN NORMAL EARS IS
LESS THAN 100%

CONTRALATERAL AND IPSILATERAL
ACOUSTIC SUPPRESSION

FINAL COMMENTS

Every measure of auditory function, behavioral or electrophysiologic, is influenced by normally-occurring subject characteristics. OAEs are no different. The first steps in successful clinical measurement and analyses of TEOAEs and DPOAEs were detailed in Chapter 4. Meaningful, and accurate, interpretation of OAE data is highly dependent on an appreciation of the influences of a variety of nonpathologic factors. Some of these factors are summarized in Table 5–1. Not every factor must be taken into account for each patient. Some factors, such as gender, which invariably exist for each patient may be of little concern for some responses (e.g., DPOAEs) and very important for others (e.g., SOAEs and TEOAEs). Our understanding of which factors can influence OAEs, and the extent of their effect, is still evolving. What follows is a review of the characteristics that can or might influence clinical measurement of DPOAEs and TEOAEs and that should be considered in the interpretation of OAE findings.

AGE

Developmental Factors

In discussing the possible effects of age on evoked OAEs, one must distinguish between developmental changes in newborn infants, older children, and adolescents versus changes associated with advanced aging in older adults. A distinction should also be made between TEOAEs and DPOAEs. Although not yet taken into account in developmental investigations, it may be important also to consider which

Table 5–1. Nonpathologic factors to consider in interpreting otoacoustic emissions (OAEs) data.

Type of Factor	Description	Explanation of/for Factor
Anatomic		
External ear status	cerumen, vernix caseous, cockroaches, debris in the ear canal	occlusion of probe; small or absent OAEs
Middle ear status	age-related changes in transfer function; subclinical abnormalities of aural Impedance and/or reflectance	decreased amplitude with age in childhood; alteration of spectral composition; decreased OAE energy with abnormality
Cochlear status	subclinical outer hair cell dysfunction (see Chapter 6 for review)	abnormal OAE findings in normal hearing
Age		
children	larger amplitudes, wider spectrum in infants and young children than adults	possible age-related anatomic factors (ear canal resonance, middle ear transmission, cochlear function)
adults	advancing age alone does not appear to have major influence on OAE amplitudes (with normal hearing sensitivity)	reduced amplitude in aging only for high stimulus frequencies
Gender		
TEOAEs	larger amplitudes and higher correlation in females	possible anatomic factors, e.g., cochlear size; poor auditory sensitivity in males
DPOAEs	not a major factor for DPOAE amplitude; effect on latency unknown	
SOAEs	Can influence TEOAEs and, to lesser extent, DPOAEs	TEOAE amplitude is increased for frequency regions in which SOAEs are present
Ear canal acoustics	not a factor for TEOAEs influences DPOAEs > 4000 Hz	standing waves can interfere with stimulus calibration and seriously affect DPOAE measurement for stimulus frequencies in the 5000 to 7000 Hz region
Noise	a major factor in OAE measurement	affects both TEOAE and DPOAE identification and analysis especially below 2000 Hz
Body temperature	not a factor for clinical OAE recording	within the range of patient body temperatures encountered clinically, OAEs are unaffected
Body position	OAEs may be reduced In horizontal position	there is little clinical data on this factor
Anesthetic agents	do not reduce OAE amplitude	nitrous oxide may be associated with changes in middle ear pressure which may have a secondary effect on OAEs.

specific device was used for recording OAEs, that is, to conduct studies of age-related changes in OAEs with more than one brand of OAE system to rule out the possibility of device-specific factor in the age effects. Some early clinical papers on pediatric applications of OAEs reported that amplitude was unusually robust, and reproducibility higher, in infants than older children and, especially, adults (Norton & Widen, 1990; Kemp, Ryan, & Bray, 1990). As recorded with the ILO 88 device, TEOAE measurement in infants often yields an overall amplitude value of over 30 dB SPL, in contrast to a typical adult amplitude of 8 to 12 dB SPL (e.g., Kok et al., 1993). Within a few years, a variety of investigators confirmed with different measurement devices the robust nature of neonatal and infant TEOAEs, with some also showing a similar trend for DPOAEs (Uziel and Piron, 1991; Collet et al., 1993; Kok et al., 1993; Smurzynski et al., 1993; Zorowka et al., 1993; Smurzynski, 1994; Thornton et al., 1994). Amplitude diminishes significantly throughout childhood, but the most noticeable decrease is from birth to months after the neonatal period. Other TEOAE parameters also show age effects, including the response spectra, with a flat spectral response in neonates and progressively less high frequency energy (constriction of the response bandwidth) and the development of multiple notches of reduced amplitude through childhood and into adulthood (Johnsen et al., 1989; Kemp, Ryan & Bray, 1990; Norton & Widen, 1990). Whether or not TEOAE latency also varies with age in children is not clear. As noted in Chapter 4, precise calculation of TEOAE latency values is difficult. Several earlier reports noted larger DPOAE amplitudes for children versus adults (Bonfils et al., 1992; Lasky et al., 1992; Brown et al., 1995). Lately, development of DPOAEs has also been systematically investigated (e.g., Abdala et al., 1996a, b; Prieve et al., 1997; Lasky, 1998a, b;). As with TEOAEs, amplitude values for DPOAEs are greater for term than preterm infants. Then, DPOAEs are highest for infants less than 1 year, with amplitude decreasing during the 1 to 3 year age range, and decreasing even further for older children and teenagers, until adult values are reached. Information on developmental changes in OAEs for infants and children is particularly important clinically as the application of OAEs is most useful in these patient age groups.

Despite the well-recognized developmental effects on OAEs, age-corrected normative OAE data for infants and young children are generally lacking. There is a serious clinical need for pediatric normative OAE databases.

Explanations of Developmental Age Effects

What factors should be considered in any explanation of these developmental age effects? Without doubt, one is the combination of intensity level of the stimulus and anatomy of the ear canal, including volume, length, resonance properties, and compliance of the walls. Ear canal volume increases as a function of age from infancy to childhood. Sound intensity is inversely related to the volume of a cavity. Therefore, unless stimulus intensity (and stimuli spectra) were carefully calibrated for individual ear canals prior to OAE measurement, stimulus intensity levels would decrease with age through childhood due to progressive changes in anatomic dimensions. Of course, as stimulus intensity decreased, so would OAE amplitude. The possible effect of smaller ear canal volume on measurement of the OAEs has not been addressed. During outward propagation of the OAEs from the cochlea, acoustic energy is generated in the ear canal by tympanic membrane vibration. The amplitude of the OAEs would be unaffected by ear canal volume if a microphone detected the energy at the tympanic membrane. However, with clinical OAE devices the microphone is located laterally within the probe assembly. Thus, ear canal volume may influence, specifically enhance, OAE amplitude measurements.

There are at least three other potential factors related to anatomic/acoustic variables that may contribute to the developmental trends in OAE amplitude and spectral parameters. Ear canal acoustics definitely change as a function of age in young children. The resonance frequency for an adult ear canal is the region of 2500 to 3000 Hz, whereas ear canal resonance values are about 4000 to 4500 for children in the age range of 10 days to 6 months, and over 6000 Hz for neonates (Kruger, 1987; Upfold & Byrne, 1988; Dempster & Mackenzie, 1990; Westbrook & Bamford, 1992). An everyday confirmation of the importance of these ear canal acoustic characteristics is the reliance on real ear correction differences (RECDs) in pediatric hearing aid selection, fitting, and verification. Again, the enhancement of the higher frequency energy in the youngest children may influence the spectrum of OAEs emitted into the ear canal as well as the stimulus spectrum. In both cases, the result would be augmentation of high frequency composition of the OAEs. In addition, during TEOAE measurement of infants, resonance characteristics, and in some cases also a less-than-optimal probe coupling to the tiny ear canal, can produce marked "ringing" of the stimulus temporal waveform, which may affect the overall effectiveness of the stimulus in evoking the TEOAEs. Ear canal volume and resonance play a role in TEOAE and DPOAE outcome (Gvelesiani, Gunenkov, & Tavartkiladze, 1998).

External ear, middle ear, and cochlear anatomy and physiology involved in OAE generation and measurement are reviewed in Chapter 2.

The second anatomic factor that must invariably be kept in mind in any discussion of OAEs is middle ear function. This topic was reviewed already in the section of Chapter 2 on the effect of early age on SOAE frequencies and amplitudes. In theory, at least, age-related changes in middle ear status could be a factor in OAEs for young children or older adults. There is clear evidence that aural input impedance (e.g., at the probe tip), reflectance, phase, and the transfer function of the middle ear change as a function of age in children reflectance (Holte, Margolis, & Kavanagh, 1991; Keefe et al., 1992; Naeve, Margolis, Levine, & Fournier, 1992; Keefe & Levi, 1996; Burns et al., 1998). Age effects on middle ear function should be factored into analysis of OAE amplitude and spectra, although this has not been systematically accomplished in developmental investigations. Developmental maturation of efferent function is a final anatomic factor that may contribute to changes in OAEs during infancy. There is evidence, obtained with contralateral suppression OAE measurement techniques, that the efferent auditory system may not be fully mature until well after 1 year of age (Goforth, Hood, & Berlin, 1998). This would be consistent with the well-known immaturity of afferent auditory brainstem pathways until about 18 months, as evidenced by latency values for ABR waves III and V in infants versus older children and adults (e.g., Hall, 1992). Since the efferent auditory system exerts an inhibitory or suppression effect on cochlea activity (via the outer hair cells), it is reasonable to expect that reduction of efferent function due to immaturity would be reflected by increased OAE amplitudes. Indeed, this is the general pattern observed in term infants.

Other stimulus properties, such as overall intensity level (e.g., 50 versus 80 dB SPL), the type of stimulus (e.g., click, half-sinusoids, tone bursts), and rate should also be considered as relevant in developmental investigations. That these properties of the evoking stimulus, and perhaps recording equipment (including probe design), are factors in the apparent age-effect is supported by discrepancies among studies, with some investigators reporting marked differences in TEOAEs between infants and adults (Norton & Widen, 1990; Prieve, 1992) and others reporting little or no differences (Johnsen et al. 1983; Bray & Kemp, 1987). As noted in Chapter 4, input/output functions are rarely recorded in studies of TEOAEs. Rather, TEOAEs are recorded for a single high-intensity level. In 1990, Kemp, Ryan, and Bray mentioned that "our initial examination of growth rate with stimulus level showed that neonatal (nonlinear differential) emissions grow more rapidly with stimulus level than adult emissions" (Kemp, Ryan, & Bray, 1990, p. 101). Preliminary data reported by Johnsen et al. (1983), and later by Norton and Widen (1990), also suggested that I/O functions appeared steeper for infants than for older children or adults. To some extent, differences in OAEs for children versus adults also vary as a function of the stimulus intensity level (Prieve, 1992). This would certainly not be an unexpected finding, and argues for the inclusion of stimulus intensity manipulations, e.g., I/O functions, in further study of developmental and advanced age effects on OAEs. The topic of development age influences on OAEs, especially the possiblity of immature cochlear development in preterm infants, is addressed further in the discussion of newborn hearing screening found in Chapter 8.

SPONTANEOUS OTOACOUSTIC EMISSIONS (SOAEs)

Background Information

There is long-standing suspicion that OAE energy within the ear canal at all times (SOAE) might contribute to, or enhance, OAEs in the ear canal following the presentation of an appropriate stimulus (TEOAEs or DPOAEs). The SOAE contribution to DPOAEs is, to some extent, a "hit-or-miss" proposition. That is, the frequency of the SOAEs needs to fall within the narrow band of frequencies near the $2f_1$–f_2 region that is spectrally analyzed in DP measurements. An SOAE occurring precisely at the frequency of one primary (f_1 or f_2) could either enhance or minimize DP measurements, but the odds of these coinciding frequencies for a single subject are presumably low. SOAE effects on TEOAE measurements are more likely. If a person produced SOAEs at several frequencies within the 1000 to 2000 Hz region, for example, it is not hard to imagine that this acoustic energy in the ear canal could augment TEOAE energy, detected in the ear canal, for octave bands centered around 1000 Hz and 2000 Hz. The possible influence of SOAEs on TEOAEs was noted earlier in the review of explanations offered for the relatively larger TEOAE amplitudes found in females versus males, for the right versus left ears, for the progressive decrease in TEOAE amplitude with age from neonatal to childhood years, and even for genetically-related TEOAE characteristics (e.g., Kok et al., 1993; Osterhammel et al., 1996; Kulawiec & Orlando, 1995).

For a number of years, authors have suggested that DPOAE amplitudes are enhanced in the frequency region of SOAE (Kemp, 1979; Burns et al., 1984; Furst et al., 1988; Wier et al., 1988; Cianfrone et al., 1990; Lonsbury-Martin et al., 1990; Moulin et al., 1993; Prieve et al., 1997). Generally, the effect of SOAE decreases when the DPOAE frequency is more than 50 Hz away from the SOAE frequency (Furst et al., 1988). The most common methodologic approach in studies reporting group (versus single subject) findings was to divide a subject population into two groups, one with SOAEs and the other without. Then, DPOAE amplitude data were analyzed and compared between groups. Recognizing the possibility that with this experimental design extraneous variables might influence DPOAEs in addition to the presence or absence of SOAEs, Turkish investigators Ozturan and Oysu (1999) examined DPOAE findings for a group of 43 young (19 to 31 years) adult subjects who showed SOAEs in only one ear. DPOAE input/output functions were recorded with the Madsen Celesta 503 device. Amplitudes for DPOAEs evoked by stimuli within the intensity range of 40 to 65 dB SPL were significantly higher ($p < 0.05$) for ears with SOAEs than for ears without SOAE. The difference in DPOAE amplitude between groups was from 6 to 7 dB at lower intensity levels and decreased to 2 to 3 dB for higher intensity levels, reaching an insignificant difference at 70 dB SPL. This finding highlights the principle that DPOAE sensitivity to cochlear influences increases as stimulus intensity decreases (e.g., Brown, 1987; Norton & Rubel, 1990; Norrix & Glattke, 1996). In the Ozturan and Oysu (1999) study, gender was not assessed as a factor in the findings due to the unequal proportion of males versus females.

SOAEs, and factors influencing their measurement, are reviewed in detail in Chapter 3.

Clinical Conclusions

The presence and number of SOAEs produced by an ear may augment TEOAE amplitude, at least within the corresponding frequency regions. The contribution of age-related differences in the prevalence and number of SOAEs must be considered in this review of TEOAEs. There is little doubt, as pointed out below, that ears producing SOAEs are, in general, likely to be characterized by larger amplitude TEOAEs. The question of SOAEs playing a role in the progressive decrease of TEOAE amplitude during infancy was raised by Bonfils at al (1992) and by Kok (1994). SOAEs and TEOAEs do interact in adult subjects. Osterhammel and Danish colleagues (1996) studied this relationship in a group of 25 normal-hearing subjects. OAEs were recorded with custom-made instrumentation. One half of the subjects (12) produced no SOAEs; the other 12 subjects had at total of 31 SOAEs (about 2.6 per ear). The two groups were matched for age and gender. A sample of their findings (Figure 5–1) clearly reveals larger TEOAE amplitudes in the group of subjects with SOAEs. The authors noted that stimuli for TEOAE measurement will at typically high intensity levels synchronize the SOAEs, as shown by others (Gobsch & Tietze. 1993). The findings of the Danish study were in close agreement with those reported earlier by a group of French investigators (Moulin at al., 1993).

Advancing Age

Discrepancies also characterize studies on advancing age and OAEs. Initial studies consistently found evidence of significantly decreased TEOAE amplitude and reproducibility, and lower likelihood of recording a TEOAE, with advancing age, especially beyond about 60 years (Bonfils et al., 1988; Collet at al., 1990; Robinette, 1992). Although these investigators took care to exclude subjects with obvious peripheral hearing loss, criteria for inclusion of subjects may have been too lax. In most cases, older subjects had hearing thresholds that were viewed as normal for their age (e.g., 25 dB or better), rather than equivalent to those of younger subjects. Stover and Norton (1993) raised the logical and important question of age-related changes in hearing sensitivity as a potential factor in these OAE findings. More recent investigations which have taken great efforts to match younger and older subjects for hearing sensitivity have failed to demonstrate major differences in TEOAE amplitude as a function of advancing age. For example, criteria for subjects enrolled in the study conducted by Prieve and Falter (1995) included auditory thresholds of 15 dB HL or better at all audiometric frequencies from 250 to 8000 Hz, normal tympanometry, and even no history of middle ear disease, and no excessive cerumen. In fact an attempt was made to equate subjects in younger and older groups for hearing threshold levels, and compos-

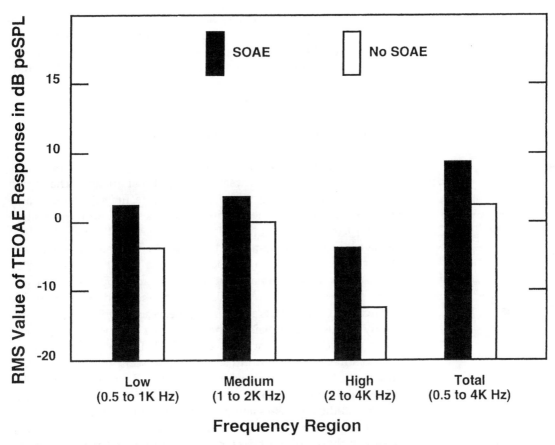

Figure 5–1. Mean TEOAE amplitude values for a group of 12 young adults with SOAEs and an age- and gender-matched group of 12 young adults with no detectable SOAEs. TEOAEs were measured with a custom-designed device using a nonlinear stimulus technique at an intensity level of 80 dB peSPL (Adapted from Osterhammel et al., 1996).

ite audiograms for both groups (shown in a figure in the paper) were clearly equivalent. TEOAE to click stimuli (COAE) were recorded with the ILO88 device from 20 subjects in the 19 to 29 year range and 20 subjects aged 40 to 61 years. This author heartily agrees with the comment of Prieve and Falter that "the mean age of subjects in our older group was 49, far from what would be considered 'old ears'" (Prieve & Falter, 1995, p. 527). Older subjects were not included due to the difficulty of finding any meeting their rigorous criteria for normal hearing. In addition to the close attention to hearing sensitivity, the design of this study was noteworthy for four other reasons. First, the authors generated I/O functions for stimulus intensity levels of 40 to 80 dB SPL, rather than simply analyzing TEOAE for a single high intensity level. Second, TEOAE "threshold" or minimal detection level was analyzed. Third, for each stimulus intensity level, noise values were reported in addition to TEOAE amplitudes. Finally, having demonstrated that SOAEs were less prevalent and fewer in number for the older group (see Chapter 3 for discussion), TEOAE analysis was performed for subgroups of subjects differentiated on the basis of SOAE findings. The authors concluded that TEOAE findings (amplitude and threshold values) were not significantly different for the younger versus older subject groups.

The findings of the Prieve and Falter (1995) study argue against an age effect, at least up to 60 years, and suggest that apparent changes in TEOAEs with aging reported previously were, in fact, related to age-related alterations in other pertinent variables (e.g., hearing sensitivity or SOAEs). These findings do lend support to the results of some earlier studies, which similarly had failed to document age alone as a factor in OAE measurement. Bertoli and Probst (1997) also studied TEOAEs in elderly patients, but with a different approach. Click and tone burst stimulus-evoked OAEs were recorded with an ILO88 device from 201 subjects aged 60 to 97 years who "volunteered for the study because of complaints concerning their hearing" (p. 286). Those with middle ear dysfunction were excluded. In other words, these authors made no attempt to screen out subjects with sensorineural hearing loss. Quite the contrary, they purposely included unselected older persons to evaluate the value of including TEOAEs as part of routine audiologic assessment in a typical older clinical population. Bertoli and Probst (1997) found that 39% of the subjects showed evidence of click-evoked OAEs (amplitude of at least 3 dB) for the better hearing ear (by PTA). OAEs were present only when the PTA was 30 dB HL or better, and 40% of the subjects with a PTA ≤ 30 dB HL did not have OAEs (or a prevalence of 60%). Although OAE amplitude tended to decrease with hearing level in the −5 to 30 dB HL range, there was poor correlation between OAEs and hearing, and considerable intersubject variability. Relevant to this discussion, age was not a significant factor in the presence or absence of click-evoked OAEs. The likelihood of recording tone burst OAEs decreased for higher frequencies. Among subjects with detectable click-evoked OAEs, 70% had an OAE for a 1000 Hz tone burst, 49% for 2000 Hz, and 25% for 3000 Hz tone burst stimuli. The authors concluded "that evaluation of TEOAEs is of little clinical value in the routine evaluation of elderly persons with mild to moderate hearing loss" (Bertoli & Probst, 1997, p. 292).

In the absence of age-related changes in hearing sensitivity (i.e., in perfectly normal hearing older adults), the effects of aging on OAEs are minimal. Decreased OAE amplitude in older clinical patients is usually secondary to age-related cochlear dysfunction (presbycusis), along with other pathologies.

The preceding discussion was largely limited to TEOAEs. Others have reported possible age effects on DPOAEs (Lonsbury-Martin et al., 1991; Kimberly et al., 1994), although hearing status was not entirely equivalent for young versus old subjects. An investigation reported by Strouse, Ochs, and Hall (1996) will be noted as one example of the independence of DPOAEs from the influence of aging. DPOAE data were presented in DPgrams and I/O functions for subjects in four age groups: 20 to 29 years; 50 to 59 years; 60 to 69 years; and 70 to 79 years. With hearing assessment of many potential subjects over age 60 years, it was possible to find a small, but audiometrically-elite, number with hearing thresholds of 15 dB or better for octave and half-octave frequencies from 250 to 8000 Hz, word recognition scores better than 90%, normal tympanometry, and normal otologic history. All but two subjects were female. Replicated DPgrams were recorded with primaries (f_2/f_1 ratio = 1.21 and $L_1 = L_2$) from 500 to 8000 Hz for 12 frequencies per octave. I/O functions were generated in 2 dB steps for stimulus intensity levels of 30 to 76 dB SPL at frequencies of 1, 2, 3, 4, 6, and 8 KHz. DPgrams or I/O functions were equivalent among groups and well within a normal range for younger subjects. The authors conclude that advancing age-corrected normative data are not needed for clinical interpretation of DPOAE findings or, put another way, if DPOAE amplitudes are abnormal for an older patient, then this finding is probably related to peripheral auditory dysfunction, rather than simply the patient's age.

After reviewing this literature thoroughly and critically, Dorn, Piskorski, Keefe, Neely, and Gorga (1998) concluded that "the findings from these reports do not provide a clear picture as to whether age alone, or age in conjunction with threshold shifts, significantly affects otoacoustic emissions" (p. 965). These prolific authors and other colleagues from Boys Town National Research Hospital have accumulated an impressively large OAE database, as described in other papers (e.g., Gorga et al., 1997). They expressed concerns about the small number of subjects enrolled in the studies of Stover and Norton (1993) and Strouse, Ochs, and Hall (1996), which had found no age effect on DPOAEs. Subjects in the Dorn et al. (1998) study were divided into two groups on the basis of hearing thresholds. For one group (ages 5.0 to 69.9 years), stringent hearing criteria permitted only persons with thresholds of 20 dB or better for all octave and half-octave audiometric frequencies. With the other larger group, formed by less stringent criteria and consisting of persons aged 5.0 to 79.9 years, DPOAE data were analyzed so long as hearing thresholds at the stimulus frequency were 20 dB or better, without regard to hearing at other regions of the audiogram. For both groups, age was subdivided into decades and there were usually at least 12 subjects for each decade (as many as 133 for the 40 to 49 year group). The more stringent "normal-across-frequency" group, however, had only 6 to 10 subjects in the 60 to 69 age category. Too few subjects over that age limit met normal hearing criteria to permit analysis of DPOAE data. Using a clinical device (Bio-logic Scout), DPOAEs were recorded with f_2 values ranging from 750 to 8000 Hz, with $L_1 = 65$ dB and $L_2 = 55$ dB, and with a f_2/f_1 ratio of 1.22.

Findings of the study by Dorn et al. (1998) may be summarized as follows. As one might expect, the group of subjects meeting more stringent criteria for normal hearing had larger DPOAE amplitudes than the other group, highlighting the importance of careful documentation of auditory status, although an age effect was evident, even for the group selected with more stringent criteria, but limited mostly to the highest frequencies (6000 and 8000 Hz). As the authors noted "in the normal-across-frequency group there were no main effects," (p. 969) for age, threshold and frequency. A statistical explanation is offered for this negative finding. Finally, over the clinically normal range of hearing thresholds from −5 dB to 20 dB DPOAE amplitude decreased, on the average, from about 5.5 dB down to −2 dB SPL. This extremely important observation is stressed further when the effect of cochlear dysfunction is discussed in Chapter 6. Given the clear inverse relation between hearing thresholds (within the 20 dB and under range) and DPOAE amplitude for the normal-across-frequency group in the Dorn et al. (1998) study, it would be interesting to view a display of hearing thresholds as a function of age for this group, even though statistically age and threshold did not significantly interact. One might expect a bias toward younger subjects having better thresholds and older subjects poorer thresholds. Also, is it possible that slight age-related changes in middle ear function, as detected by sophisticated measures of immittance and reflectometry (Keefe et al., 1992; Keefe & Levi, 1996) might contribute to the findings of the study? Although normal middle ear status for the subjects was confirmed "by tympanometry and/or otologic examination," details on the type of tympanometry employed were not provided. The authors of this study concluded that "we do not feel that corrections to DPOAE measures for these variables are warranted at this time" (p. 970), although age effects should taken into account for stimulus frequencies of 6000 Hz and higher.

OAE fine-structure or microstructure is discussed in the DPOAE section of Chapter 4.

He and Schmiedt (1996) conducted a detailed investigation of DPOAEs, which emphasized fine structure of the response. There were four groups of subjects. One consisted of 12 normal hearers aged 23 to 36 years (a young group). A second group was made up of 12 older subjects with normal or "near-normal" hearing (average age of 72 years, and ranging from 65 to 81 years). Then, there was a young and an older group with sensorineural hearing loss. DPOAEs were measured with custom laboratory instrumentation for 32 frequencies/octave over four one-third octave regions centered around frequencies of 2000, 3000, 4000, and 6000 Hz. Conclusions of this study were that DPOAE fine structure is consistent within subjects, and not affected by age or hearing loss. Age does not affect DPOAE amplitude when hearing loss is accounted for. In fact, DPOAEs are recorded in the presence of greater hearing loss for older subjects in comparison to hearing-impaired younger subjects. In explanation of this latter conclusion, the authors suggested that noise-induced hearing loss (common in the younger subjects) is associated with more outer hair cell dysfunction than presbycusis, which may also involve age-related neural or stria vascularis dysfunction. The possible fundamental difference in the nature of the sensory hearing loss for young and old subjects should be considered in large-scale investigations of OAEs and hearing. We will return to this point in the discussion of cochlear dysfunction in Chapter 6.

Clinical Conclusions

Age itself does not exert a major influence on either TEOAEs or DPOAEs, especially for stimulus frequencies up to about 6000 Hz. A modest decrease in OAE amplitude can be attributed to aging, although the precise site of the effect (middle ear or cochlea) would not necessarily be known. When OAE findings for an older patient are abnormal, however, a cause other than simply aging must be considered. Clinically, there are multiple possible explanations for abnormal OAE findings in older patients, although be age-related hearing loss is probably at the top of the list.

GENDER

Background Information

Gender differences are found for almost all measures of peripheral and central auditory function, as summarized in Table 5–2. Invariably, males as a group show less sensitive, smaller, lower, and slower responses to acoustic signals than age-matched females. Clinically, differences are apparent for pure tone audiometry, speech audiometry, immittance measures, and auditory evoked responses. Reasons for all of these gender effects are not yet known. There are clearly differences in anatomic dimensions (i.e., length and size) of auditory pathways and structures from the cochlea to the cortex. In addition, there are functional distinctions between males and females among some anatomic regions. A variety of explanations for the physiologic gender effects have been offered over the years. The most common are endocrinologic (hormonal) factors, perhaps affecting neurotransmission. The confounding influence of gender-related differences in body temperature on auditory function must always be considered. For example, for the ABR females characteristically demonstrate shorter latencies and larger amplitudes than males (see Hall, 1992, for review). Yet, females also tend to be slightly warmer than males, especially at certain times of the day and month. And, there is longstanding evidence that increases in body temperature are associated with decreased ABR latency (Hall, Bull, & Cronau, 1988). Therefore, unless ruled out by careful documentation and meticulous research design, gender differences in body temperature might explain at least some of the apparent gender differences in the ABR.

Gender (sex) differences in OAE amplitude measures are most prominent for SOAEs and TEOAEs, and minimal for DPOAEs. There are few studies of the possible influence of gender on OAE latency measures.

Table 5–2. Summary of gender differences in auditory function.

Auditory Measure	Gender Effect
Physical differences	
head size	larger in males
pinna size	larger in males
external ear canal volume	larger In males
middle-ear volume	larger in males
cochlear length	longer in males
Psychophysical	
hearing sensitivity	females more sensitive (at least above 2000 Hz)
binaural tasks	
sound localization	males more sensitive to differences in interaural time and Intensity
binaural beats	males detect them at higher frequencies
right-ear advantage (REA)	smaller REA (less asymmetry) in females
noise-induced hearing loss	
permanent	greater in males
temporary	less in females below about 1500 Hz, but more above approximately 3000 Hz
complex masking tasks	
profile analysis	males are more sensitive
lateral suppression	greater in males
overshoot	greater In females
gap detection	more sensitive in females
Electrophysiologic	
auditory brainstem response (ABR)	wave V latency and interwave latencies shorter in females; wave V amplitudes larger in females
otoacoustic emissions (OAEs)	more SOAEs In females larger TEOAEs in females
prenatal masculinization OAE	OAEs in females with a male cotwin are more similar to male OAEs

Source: McFadden D. Sex differences In the auditory system. *Developmental Neuropsychology 14*: 261-298, 1998, p. 263.

Gender is a factor in some OAE measures, but apparently not others. Several groups of investigators have independently found that TEOAE amplitudes and reproducibility values are significantly higher in females than males (Robinette, 1992; Baer & Hall, 1994; McFadden, 1998). This pattern is illustrated in Figure 5–2 and further detailed in normative data displayed in Table 1-A in Appendix A. At least five

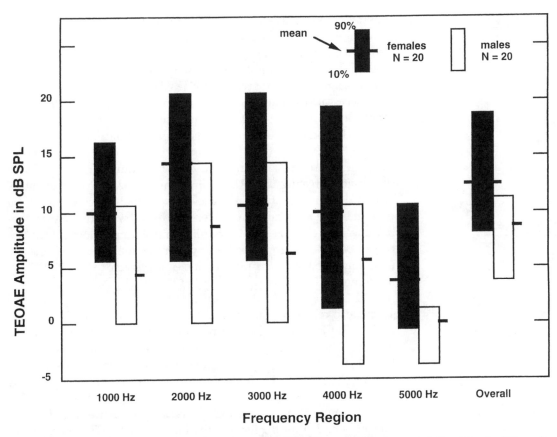

Figure 5–2. TEOAE amplitudes for 40 audiometrically normal young adult subjects (20 male and 20 female). The bars represent the range of values, whereas the thick horizontal lines bisecting the bars indicate mean values. Normative TEOAE data are displayed numerically in Appendix A. (Adapted from unpublished paper by Jane Baer, Ph.D., 1994.)

possible factors are considered in attempts to explain the differences in TEOAEs for reported for males and females. One factor that may be related to the gender effect in TEOAEs, and least click-evoked OAEs, is the apparent difference in the cochlear length for males versus females (Sato, Sando, & Takahashi, 1991). In addition to this anatomic evidence, is evidence of male versus female differences at the cochlear level of the auditory system (Don, Ponton, Eggermont, & Masuda, 1993) . Numerous investigators have, of course, confirmed statistically and clinically significant differences in electrophysiologic responses arising from neural auditory regions from the eighth nerve through the brainstem (see Hall, 1992, for review).

Second, slight and, clinically insignificant differences in hearing sensitivity could account for part of the gender differences in TEOAEs reported by some investigators. As noted above, gender differences in hearing sensitivity have been recognized for many years (see McFadden, 1993, for review), with females tending to have more sensitive hearing than males. Simply ruling out hearing loss by history or pure tone screening for an otherwise unselected group of males and females does necessarily equate the groups. Even if males show subtle decrements in hearing threshold levels in comparison to females, e.g., less than 10 dB and with all thresholds still within clinically-normal limits ($\leq$ 20 dB HL), then TEOAEs with smaller amplitude and lower reproducibility would be anticipated. Some of the differences in auditory sensitivity affecting TEOAE findings might occur for frequencies within the traditional audiometric octave signals, and might not be detected even with careful pure tone audiometry. Studies of the gender effect on TEOAEs must carefully control for auditory sensitivity, preferably by using small intensity increments (e.g., 2 dB) and by including signals at as many frequencies as possible (e.g., with Békésy audiometry).

Third, also related to the possibility of subtle "subclinical" cochlear deficits in males, all subjects reporting tinnitus and history of noise exposure should be excluded from study. There is abundant evidence that OAE abnormalities are possible in such persons despite normal hearing threshold levels, and might be more commonly encountered in males. Fourth, gender differences are pronounced in SOAEs. With a typical group of normal hearing adults, the prevalence would be significantly higher for the females than for the males. The energy from the SOAEs will augment TEOAE amplitude, at least for some frequency regions (Zwicker, 1983; Probst et al., 1986; Kulawiec & Orlando, 1995; Osterhammel et al., 1996). To parcel out this factor, it would be best to study groups of males and females matched for SOAE status. The relatively minimal gender effect for DPOAEs versus TEOAEs argues for the contribution of SOAEs. That is, SOAEs are less likely to influence DP measurements because two extremely narrow bands of frequencies (the SOAE and the DPOAE frequency at $2f_1-f_2$) would need to be aligned closely. This must be a rare occurrence indeed. In contrast, SOAEs would be expected to very often fall somewhere within the broad TEOAE spectrum (600 to 5000 Hz). Fourth, to minimize the possible influence of diurnal factors and body temperature, data should be collected for the two groups (males and females) at the same time of day, and temperature documented at the time of the testing.

Gender differences exist also for DPOAE response measures. Citing agreement with the study on cochlear differences by Sato et al. (1991), Kimberly, Brown, and Eggermont (1993) reported longer DPOAE latency (phase) values for males than females for selected frequency regions. Larger amplitudes have also been reported for females in comparison to males, again for some but not all frequencies (Gaskill & Brown, 1990; Lonsbury-Martin, Cutler, & Martin, 1991; Moulin et al., 1993; Cacace et al., 1996). Pure-tone thresholds were closely examined in two of these studies (Lonsbury-Martin et al., 1991, and Cacace et al., 1996), and the larger DPOAE amplitudes for females were concomitant with slightly better pure-tone thresholds versus males for the same frequency regions.

Finally, definition of the gender factor as simply "male versus female" may be inadequate. One of the more fascinating discoveries in recent years has been the demonstration of significant differences in click-evoked OAEs for heterosexuals versus homosexuals (McFadden & Pasanen, 1998) and in opposite-sex dizygotic twins versus monozygotic twins, same-sex dizygotic twins, or non-twins (McFadden & Loehlin, 1995). Differences for click-evoked OAE amplitude among males and females of varying sexual orientations are illustrated in Figure 5–3. A total of 237 subjects were studied by McFadden and Pasanen (1998). Both sex and ear differences can be observed. OAE amplitudes are significantly larger for heterosexual females than heterosexual males and for the right versus left ear. In addition, homosexual and bisexual females yielded smaller OAE amplitude values than heterosexual females. A different pattern of findings emerged for males. OAE amplitudes were equivalent for hetero- and homosexual males. The authors of this innovative study note that "the present CEOAE data can be interpreted as evidence that prenatal exposure to higher-than-normal levels of androgens in homosexual and bisexual females produced a partial masculinization of both their peripheral auditory systems and some brain structures involved with sexual orientation" (McFadden and Pasanen, 1998, p. 2712). They further caution that "the individual variability in CEOAE amplitude is considerable, meaning that CEOAEs presently could not be used as an indicator of sexual orientation in individual people" (p. 2713). In another related paper, McFadden and colleagues (1998) at the University of Texas-Austin described the appearance of SOAEs in a human male who was receiving estrogen treatment before a sex-reversal operation. The authors speculated that a treatment-related decrease in androgen levels diminished suppression of cochlear mechanisms that produce SOAEs, permitting their release. Further study of OAEs in transsexuals are planned.

It would be valuable to know whether the gender differences in TEOAEs are limited to click-evoked OAEs, or if they are apparent also for tone-burst evoked OAEs. And, for tone-burst evoked OAEs, whether the gender differentially affects some frequencies (e.g., lower frequencies). Although gender differences seem to be found mostly for TEOAEs, the absence of apparent DPOAE amplitude differences between males and females does not necessarily rule out the possibli-

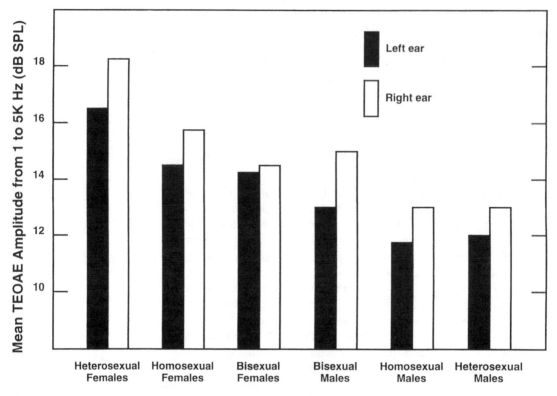

Figure 5–3. Mean TEOAE amplitude for a 75 dB click stimulus intensity level in males and females differentiated on the basis of sexual orientation (Adapted from McFadden and Pasanen, 1998).

ty of a gender influence on other parameters. The gender differences in ABR, for example, are far more striking for wave component latency than amplitude. The TEOAE gender differences are attributed, at least in part, to anatomic diffferences (i.e., shorter cochleas in females than males). One area warranting research is the search for gender differences in DPOAE phase and latency parameters. It seems reasonable to suspect that any DPOAE gender differences would affect latency of the response, with females more likely to show shorter latencies due to the reduced cochlear length.

Clinical Implications

Gender should be taken into account in the clinical application of TEOAEs. Given the magnitude and consistency of the differences in major response parameters (i.e., amplitude and reproducibility) maintenance of separate normative databases for males and females is a wise clinical policy.

EAR DIFFERENCES

Background Information

Hearing surveys of large numbers of apparently normal hearing persons have repeatedly showed slightly poorer hearing for the left versus right ear, especially for higher frequencies (e.g., Ward, 1957; Axelsson et al., 1981). The results of most early studies of TEOAEs showed comparable responses (amplitude, spectrum, and threshold of detection) for right and left ears (Probst et al., 1986; Bonfils et al., 1988; Johnsen et al., 1988). Some more recent reports have noted a tendency for some features of TEOAEs, such as amplitude, to be slightly more prominent for right versus left ears in adults (Robinette, 1992; Baer & Hall, 1994) and children (Glattke et al., 1995). This tendency is clearly apparent in Figure 5–4 and was evident also in the illustration of gender differences (Figure 5–2).

Toward the top of the list of explanations for ear differences in TEOAE amplitude is the contribution of SOAEs. As reviewed in Chapter 3, SOAEs are more prevalent and are found in greater numbers for the right versus left ear. In a study of 81 normal-hearing adult subjects (38 male and 43 female), Kulawiec and Orlando (1995) presenting convincing evidence that SOAEs, synchronized by the click stimuli, do contribute to TEOAE measurement. The SOAE frequencies corresponded to the frequency regions showing the largest amplitude within the TEOAE spectrum. And, TEOAE amplitude increased directly with the number of SOAEs produced by an ear. The authors concluded the substantial normal variability found in TEOAE amplitude (see Table 1 in Appendix A) is a product of the presence or absence, and varying number, of SOAEs in normal ears. Specific to this discussion, SOAEs were clearly a factor in the ear differences for TEOAE amplitude (Figure 5–5 from this paper). On the average, TEOAE amplitude was larger for the right ear when SOAEs were present in that ear, and vice versa for the left ear. Related to thisdiscussion is the remote possibility of a difference for some OAE parameter between right- and left-handed persons. In a study of over 5000 persons, using pure-tone audiometry and conventional clinical methodology, Pirila et al. (1991) were unable to demonstrate an effect of handedness in hearing asymmetry. Whether or not handedness is a factor in OAE measures has not been addressed, to my knowledge. Finally, in speculating on mechanisms for ear differences, and also gender differences, McFadden (1993) proposed that "these lateral asymmetries and sex differences may all result from differences in the 'strength' of the efferent inhibition delivered to individual cochleas. Specifically . . . the amount of efferent inhibition is relatively less in right ears and in females than in left ears and males" (p. 143).

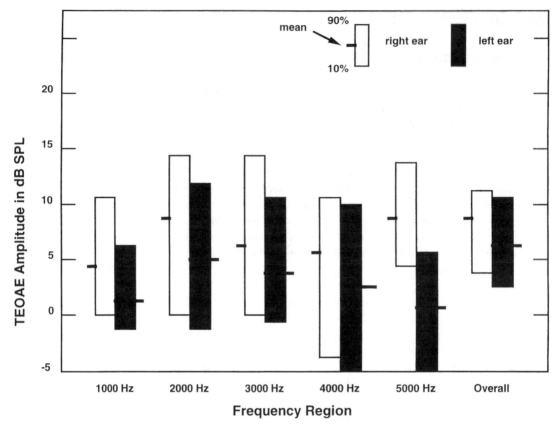

Figure 5–4. TEOAE amplitudes for right and left ears of 20 audiometrically normal young male subjects. The bars represent the range of values, whereas the thick horizontal lines bisecting the bars indicate mean values. Normative TEOAE data are displayed numerically in Appendix A. (Adapted from unpublished paper by Jane Baer, Ph.D., 1994.)

DIURNAL (TIME OF DAY) EFFECTS

Background Information

As noted in Chapter 3, biologically controlled rhythms throughout the course of a day may influence SOAEs (Bell, 1992; Haggerty, Lusted, & Morton, 1993). These diurnal factors may interact with other non-pathologic subject factors, such as body temperature and gender. Several studies failed to demonstrate that the time of day of OAE measurement influenced the response, at least during normal waking hours (Froehlich et al., 1988; Endahl et al., 1994), although the later investigators did observe larger TEOAE amplitudes during normal sleeping hours at night. In the only comprehensive report utilizing DPOAEs, Cacace and colleagues (1996) found a very modest (less than

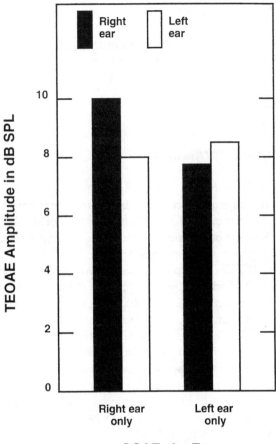

SOAEs by Ear

Figure 5–5. Mean TEOAE amplitude values for a group of 11 normal hearing adults with one of more SOAE only in the right ear and a group of 7 normal hearing adults with one or more SOAE only in the left ear. TEOAEs were measured with the ILO 88 device using default parameters. (Adapted from Kulawiec and Orlando, 1995).

1 dB) influence of time of day on DPOAE amplitude when rather copious amounts of data (for 12 stimulus pair frequencies) were collapsed (combined) and "converted to the frequency domain by computing the power spectrum of the time series with the discrete Fourier transform (DFT) before submitting the data to ANOVA" (p. 1141). The authors understandably concluded that the circadian effect was not large.

Clinical Conclusions

The time of day at which OAEs are recorded is not of clinical concern, especially during normal waking hours.

The literature on genetic factors in SOAEs (e.g., inherited and familial trends and patterns) is cited in Chapter 3.

GENETICS

Background Information

A theme already mentioned, and noted again below, enters also into the discussion of genetic factors in TEOAE measurement. The apparent genetic patterns in the prevalence and number of SOAEs, reviewed in Chapter 3, might be passed on directly to TEOAEs. It would be reasonable to suspect that some families with more SOAEs would tend to show larger TEOAEs. The data and arguments presented for heritability of SOAEs (McFadden, 1993; McFadden & Loehlin, 1995; McFadden, 1998) can, to some extent, be applied also to other types of OAEs. For example, the female in a set of opposite-sex dizygotic twins typically have TEOAE responses that resemble those of males, rather than females (McFadden, Loehlin, & Pasanen, 1996). The explanation was mentioned above in the discussion of sexual orientation and gender effects in OAEs, namely, that fetal exposure to androgens reduces OAE activity. Male fetuses produce androgens which have this effect, and the female fetus in the pair of opposite-sex twins is exposed to the male twin's androgens via amniotic fluids.

Clinical Conclusions

Genetic factors in OAEs must be considered. There is the possibility for inherited OAE characteristics among normal hearers. Also, OAE response patterns will be more seriously affected in selected genetically based cochlear pathologies, as noted in Chapter 6.

RACE

Background Information

Whitehead, Kamal, Lonsbury-Martin, and Martin (1993) reported racial distinctions for SOAEs (see Chapter 3). Given the relation noted above between SOAEs and TEOAEs, race could be a factor but I am not aware of any published studies.

BODY TEMPERATURE

Background Information

General neurophysiologic effects of body temperature on metabolism include reduced membrane resting potentials, decreased nerve conduction velocity, and extended duration of action potentials (e.g., Kochs, 1995). Body temperature is clearly a factor clinically in the measurement of auditory evoked responses, such as the ABR (see Hall, 1992, for review). Specific to the cochlea, experimental investigations in animal models have demonstrated the influence of temperature directly on the endocochlear potential, mechano-electric transduction properties, outer hair cell length, shape, and mechanics, and hair cell afferent synapses (Gitter, 1992; Ohlemiller & Siegel, 1994; LeCates, Kuo, & Brownell, 1995; Chen & Brownell, 1999). Using a guinea pig experimental model, these investigators found that an increase from room temperature (22° Centigrade) to body temperature (39° Centigrade) produced only a slight (10%) and no statistically significant decrease in stiffness of the outer hair cell lateral wall. However, strength of the attachment of the cortical lattice to the lateral wall was clearly reduced with increased temperature, and "increased temperature leads to more rapid deterioration of the integrity of the OHC" (Chen & Brownell, 1999, p. 49). Length of the outer hair cell increases directly with temperature (Gitter, 1992) and electromotility is also temperature- dependent (Ashmore & Holley, 1988).

Note: equations used for converting temperature back-and-forth from Centigrade to Fahrenheit are as follows:

$$F = 9/5 \, (C) + 32 \qquad\qquad C = 5/9 \, (F - 32)$$

where $9/5 = 1.8$ and $5/9 = .55$

Not unexpectedly, given these findings, OAEs and related cochlea-dependent properties of hearing (e.g., frequency selectivity) may be influenced by changes in temperature (Eatock & Manley, 1981; van Dijk & Wit, 1987; Manley & Koppel, 1994). Temperature may also be a factor in susceptibility to noise- induced outer hair cell dysfunction (Berndt & Wagner, 1981; Henry & Chole, 1984). However, because most of the data on these relationships are derived from animal models, sometimes cold-blooded (poikilothermic) animals such as frogs and lizards, and often at temperature extremes not encountered clinically, the conclusions can not be confidently generalized to mammals including humans. In fact, there is some agreement that frequency selectivity, or tuning, within the cochlea is not affected by temperature fluctuations (Wilson, 1985; Whitehead, Wilson, & Baker, 1986).

Studying human subjects, Ferber-Viart et al. (1995) reported a TEOAE amplitude decrease on the order of about 1 dB SPL with every 1 degree increase in body temperature above normal (i.e., in hyperthermia). However, no signficant alterations in SOAEs were found in humans (O'Brien, 1994). Similarly, even with very rigorous statistical data analysis Cacace et al. (1996) failed to demonstrate a relation among oral temperature, resting pulse, and DPOAE amplitude. Since temperature (hypo- and hyperthermia) definitely is a factor in the clinical interpretation of some other auditory measures, such as the auditory brainstem response (e.g., Hall, Bull, & Cronau, 1988), it is reasonable to question whether temperature might be a factor also in clinical OAE measurement. Since most published reports on temperature and OAEs describe findings for nonhuman animals, that literature will be reviewed briefly along with the few clinical studies. One study in rabbits showed no significant temperature effect on DPOAE amplitude or threshold of detection (Noyes et al., 1996). Khvoles, Freeman, and Sohmer (1998) investigated the effect of temperature on TEOAEs and DPOAEs in 8 rats using clinical instrumentation (Madsen Cochlear Emissions Analyzer). Within the temperature range of 33° to 39° Centigrade [note: 37 degrees is normal for humans] TEOAEs and DPOAEs amplitudes remained constant. Above and below these limits, amplitudes for both types of OAEs were markedly reduced, especially for lower intensity stimuli. Likely mechanisms for this finding were mentioned by the authors. The endocochlear potential, which presumably powers outer hair cells, decreases by about 10% as body temperature is lowered by 8° to 10° Centigrade (Konishi et al., 1981; Ohlemiller & Siegel, 1992). Hypothermia also diminishes cochlear microphonic amplitude (Konishi et al., 1991), although these temperature extremes are not encountered in most clinical populations. Probably secondary to the changes in outer hair cell function, cooling of about 3° to 6° Centigrade is associated with a blunting of the tip of tuning curves (Brown et al., 1983).

The influence of extreme induced hypothermia on TEOAEs, for 30 patients undergoing open heart surgery, was investigated by Seifert and colleagues (1998). TEOAEs were recorded with the ILO88 device during cooling to temperatures as low as 26.07° Centigrade or Celsius (corresponding to 78° Fahrenheit), as measured vesically, and 24.86 degrees Centigrade (76.7° Fahrenheit), as measured nasopharyngeally. Then, the patients were rewarmed to normal body temperature. TEOAE amplitude and reproducibility values decreased with temperature, and TEOAEs were no longer measurable (i.e., reproducibility < 60% and 0 dB amplitude) at temperatures lower than 33.41° vesical and 30.16° nasopharyngeal. The relationship of both TEOAE amplitude and reproducibility values with temperature was different during cooling than it was during warming. For example, during rewarming mid-frequency TEOAE bands reappeared at a lower temperature than they had disappeared (an average difference of 4.66° Centigrade), although TEOAEs in the high-frequency band did not reappear until temperature had increased another 2°. Importantly, these authors ruled out experimentally the influence of general anesthesia. Changes in middle ear pressure associated with the anesthesia are most often related to the use of nitrous oxide, which was specifically avoided in this study. Negative pressure, associated with hypothermia (Doyle & Fria, 1985), tended to increase as temperature decreased. The authors concluded, however, that the changes in TEOAEs with hypothermia exceeded what would be expected from middle ear effects alone. Similarly, the authors in their experimental design and data analysis minimized the potential confounding influences of age and gender, as well as blood and brain pressure. Among the intriguing mechanisms cited as possibly playing a role in the temperature effects were alterations in the energy supply to the outer hair cells (endocochlear potential), and in efferent innervation of the outer hair cells (e.g., Inamura et al., 1987). The authors logically concluded that temperature must be recognized as a factor in measurement of TEOAEs.

Three different clinical studies showed no changes in TEOAEs or DPOAEs as a function of the normal temperature fluctuations (less than 1°) occurring across a 24-hour day, or longer time periods (Froehlich et al., 1993; Cacace et al., 1996). This negative finding is consistent with earlier assertions that cochlear-based frequency tuning mechanisms are not altered by relatively minor temperature variations (Wilson, 1985; Whitehead et al., 1986).

Clinical Conclusions

There is limited information from humans on whether OAEs are influenced by substantial changes in body temperature. Further investigations would be welcome. Based on data from several animal studies, however, it is unlikely that the relatively modest temperature variations encountered in clinical populations will have any important effect on OAEs. This is in contrast to the quite distinct relationship between temperature and the ABR. That temperature affects ABR latencies but not OAE amplitudes, however, is consistent with our understanding of the anatomy of these two general electrophysiologic responses and the mechanism for temperature effects. Fluctuations from normal body temperature either slow down (hypothermic change) or speed up (hyperthermic change) neurotransmission events at synapses in the nervous system. ABR interwave latency values, therefore, shorten or lengthen, respectively, with increases or decreases from normal temperature. Since OAEs reflect preneural activity in the auditory system, before even the first synapse, they are relatively unaffected by even pathologic alterations from normothermia.

BODY POSITION

Background Information

For many years, the effect of body position has been demonstrated for middle ear immittance and hearing thresholds (e.g., Corso, 1962; Miltich, 1968; Macrae, 1972; Daniel et al., 1985; Phillips & Marchbanks, 1989). Hearing thresholds decrease (worsen) on the order of 4 to 5 dB, and acoustic immittance (impedance) increases while the tympanogram peak shifts in a positive pressure direction. One suspected mechanism for these changes is increased intracranial pressure, which is reflected in the cochlea as increased static perilymph pressure and, in turn, in the middle ear system via outward motion of the stapes footplate and middle ear pressure via outward motion of the round window membrane. There may also be increased cochlear venous blood pressure, and middle ear mucosal volume in the reclining (supine or prone) position. The combined findings of these studies imply that auditory function is optimal in the upright position.

The possible effects of body position on OAEs were evaluated in some of the earliest studies. For example, within a year of Kemp's classic paper in 1970, another Englishman, J.P. Wilson, showed that the auditory threshold fine structure was less pronounced as the body was tilted backward from an upright position, almost disappearing in the horizontal position (Wilson, 1980). Then, with the subject inverted, the peaks and valleys in the microstructure "approximately interchanged." Average hearing threshold during these maneuvers was unaffected. The author presumed that changes in body position altered oval window pressure. He then demonstrated a reversal of the direction of auditory microstructure (peaks and valleys) during positive and negative manipulations of middle ear pressure with the Valsalva maneuver. Wilson (1980) explained that at high negative and positive middle ear pressures the middle ear is stiffened (stiffness-controlled), whereas in the upright position the middle ear is mass-controlled. When the normal impedance matching of the middle ear to the cochlea is disturbed, energy produced by the cochlea may be reflected back into the cochlea where it can interfere with and alter ongoing active processes there.

In view of these findings, and suspected mechanisms, it is not surprising that several investigators have more recently examined the effect of body position on OAEs, but only for TEOAEs and in small numbers of normal-hearing subjects (Antonelli & Grandori, 1991; Phillips & Farrell, 1992). Data from these studies suggest that TEOAE latency decreases from the upright (+90 degree) position to a supine (0 degrees) or head-hanging (e.g., −10 to 20 degree) positions. However, Froehlich et al. (1988) found no change in TEOAE response for different body positions (sitting versus supine).

Clinical Conclusions

If body position influences OAEs, the effect is not likely to be dramatic. Nonetheless, more research is warranted with subjects of different ages as otoacoustic emission measurements are often performed clinically with patients in recumbent positions (supine, prone, or on one side or the other), especially in infants and children. Future studies might include TEOAEs and DPOAEs, with attention to fine structure of responses, as well as sophisticated documentation of middle ear status with multifrequency tympanometry and/or reflectometry.

STATE OF AROUSAL AND ATTENTION

Background Information

Outer hair cells receive efferent innervation from the olivocochlear bundle, which arises in the superior olivary complex within the pontine brainstem (see Chapter 2). Results of psychophysical studies in humans have raised the question of a possible "attentional filter" phenomenon in which efferent modulation of cochlear (outer hair cell) active processing is influenced by subject attention to stimuli (Scharf et al., 1987). This line of thinking has led, logically, to investigations of attentional effects on OAEs. Froehlich et al. (1988) reported that TEOAEs were independent of alertness level. Theorizing that the olivocochlear bundle efferent system innervating the outer hair cells might be involved in selective attention, Michie et al. (1996) enrolled 70 normal-hearing adult subjects in an investigation with click and tone-burst evoked OAEs. Subjects were told to pay attention to specific frequencies during the OAE measurement in a series of six related experiments. The results of this very detailed study failed to demonstrate an attention effect for TEOAEs. These conclusions for OAEs are in agreement with the trend of findings for a number of studies attempting to show evidence of a selective attention influence on the ABR (see Hall, 1992, for review). Michie et al. (1996) also present a reasonable explanation, based on methodologic differences, for the discrepancy between the negative outcome of their study versus the suggestion of possible attention effects in some earlier papers published exclusively by French researchers (Puel et al., 1988; Froehlich et al., 1990; Avan & Bonfils, 1991; Froehlich et al., 1993; Meric & Collet, 1992, 1993). In one other study (Giard et al., 1994), an extremely small reduction in OAE amplitude (usually less than 1 dB) when the stimulus was ignored, but the effect was not consistently observed for the same frequencies in each ear.

Some of the same investigators have described a consistent increase in TEOAE amplitude (up to 4 dB) with sleep during night time hours

As with ABR, the independence of OAEs to state-of-arousal and drugs that influence subject state, such as sedatives, is a major clinical advantage, especially in children.

(Froehlich et al., 1993). Subjects in this study were 9 young normal-hearing adults. The frequency region of the amplitude change, which was greatest between 2200 and 0200 hours (10 PM to 2 AM), sometimes varied among subjects. Then, other French investigators similarly found very modest increases in TEOAEs recorded from 6-week-old full-term infants during sleep. No change in TEOAE amplitude, however, was associated with sleep stage (as documented with polygraphic EEG techniques). The authors concluded that "sleep seems not to impair the use of TEOAE recordings, according to these preliminary results, as an auditory screening test in infants" (Morlet et al., 1994, p. 119).

Being an electrophysiologic measure of cochlear functioning, OAEs may be applied intraoperatively in the objective assessment of auditory function for diagnostic purposes or in monitoring status of an at-risk cochlea during surgical procedures (see Chapter 9). For meaningful interpretation of OAE data in this test venue, it is important to know how anesthesia affects the response. As with possible attentional effects on OAEs, one presumed mechanism for the influence of anesthetics is the efferent auditory system. There is some evidence from ECochG type measurements of cochlear function, for example, that activity of the olivocochlear bundle fibers diminishes as a function of depth of anesthesia (Liberman, 1989). In a study of anesthesia effects on OAEs recorded from avians (chickens and starlings), no consistently clear pattern of findings was demonstrated (Kettembeil, Manley, & Siegl, 1995). Harel et al. (1997) studied the effects of anesthesia (ketamine or barbiturates) on TEOAEs and DPOAEs recorded from chinchilla. TEOAEs were measured with the usual default test protocol, whereas DPOAEs were evoked with stimulus intensities of $L_1 = L_2 = 50$ dB SPL over the range of 1000 to 6000 Hz (the f_2/f_1 ratio was 1.22). With sodium pentobarbital anesthesia, TEOAE amplitude increased significantly (usually between 8 and 18%) for a 1000 Hz frequency region, but not significantly for other frequencies. In contrast, DPOAE amplitudes showed no change with this clinically encountered drug. Ketamine anesthesia was associated with TEOAE amplitude increases (up to 31%) for frequencies across the 2000 to 3000 Hz region. Changes were insignificant for other frequency bands. For DPOAEs, significant amplitude increases (of up to 34%) were observed at all frequencies with ketamine anesthesia. In this study, other factors that might have influenced OAE findings, such as changes in middle ear impedance, probe fit, and prolonged stimulation, were carefully ruled out. The authors cautiously speculated that "one possible interpretation of this results of our study is that anesthesia depresses the activity of cochlear efferents either directly, or via pathways (ascending or descending) that synapse onto olivocochlear neurons. Such as change might disinhibit the mechanisms responsible for OAEs" (Harel et al., 1997, p. 32). A group of investigators from Japan also assessed the effects of pentobarbital and ketamine on

DPOAEs, but in a gerbil animal model (Zheng et al., 1997). The prima-ry finding in this study was barbiturate anesthesia-induced negative middle ear pressure which, in turn, significantly reduced DPOAEs. DPOAEs were apparently unaffected by ketamine.

In a clinical study, Hauser et al. (1992) found no clear or significant change in TEOAE amplitude during anesthesia with a combination of other drugs (a muscle relaxant plus methohexital, fentanyl, and propo-fol or midazolam). Amplitude tended to decrease with nitrous oxide, perhaps due to an increase in middle ear pressure, but the effect was not statistically significant. Finally, inner ear blood flow may be altered by some anesthetics when blood pressure is controlled. Preckel et al. (1998) reported changes in inner ear blood flow which were associat-ed with TEOAE amplitude reduction during propofol anesthesia, whereas no correlation was found for isoflurane anesthesia.

Clinical Conclusions

Neither attention to stimuli, nor sleep in infants, are clinically impor-tant factors in the interpretation of TEOAE findings. Clinical anesthet-ic or sedative agents (e.g., pentobarbituates) may have a slight effect on TEOAEs but not, apparently, DPOAEs. Nitrous oxide is likely to influ-ence OAE detection by altering middle ear function. There are no com-prehensive human investigations of the effects of anesthetic agents. This is a clinically feasible topic for further study.

EAR CANAL ACOUSTICS

Background Information

As experimental and clinical experience with OAEs accumulated, anecdotal accounts of apparent OAE activity recorded from nonhear-ing (dead) ears or inanimate cavities (e.g., hard-walled cavities, rubber ears, and cadaver ears) began to circulate among the audiology com-munity. These observations naturally caused concern among clini-cians who were already applying OAEs in various patient popula-tions. Rumors ran rampant about which brands of equipment were most likely to produce "bogus" or "artifactual" OAEs, to the manu-facturer's chagrin. Those professionals who had prematurely con-cluded that OAEs were simply research tools, or were being reckless-ly and irresponsibly applied in certain populations (e.g., newborn infants) vigorously used the anectotal accounts as evidence in support of their positions. Adding to the confusion was a naivity about OAE measurement. Many clinicians routinely used test protocols and strategies that were, in retrospect, very inappropriate. There were sim-ply no accepted or evidence-based guidelines for OAE analysis. For example, DPOAE measurements at high stimulus intensities (e.g., greater than 70 dB SPL were commonplace because they invariably produced the most robust response. Normative data were nonexistent, so DPOAEs were often declared present whenever activity was detected above the noise floor. This finding was incorrectly viewed by some as consistent with normal cochlear function. The concept of cochlear and OAE fine structure or microstructure (see Chapter 4) was not widely appreciated clinically, so an isolated robust DP amongst mostly noise or, conversely, an single frequency island of noise only within an otherwise normal DPgram was overly interpreted. And fundamental principles of clinical OAE measurement, for example mandatory replication of data, were ignored. The issue seemed to go public in 1994.

Guidelines for recognizing, and minimizing, deleterious influences of ear canal acoustics, especially standing-wave interference, are offered in the DPOAE section of Chapter 4.

An example of the problem is illustrated in Figure 5–6. DPOAEs were recorded in July 1994 from a 1.0 cavity (syringe) with a then-just-

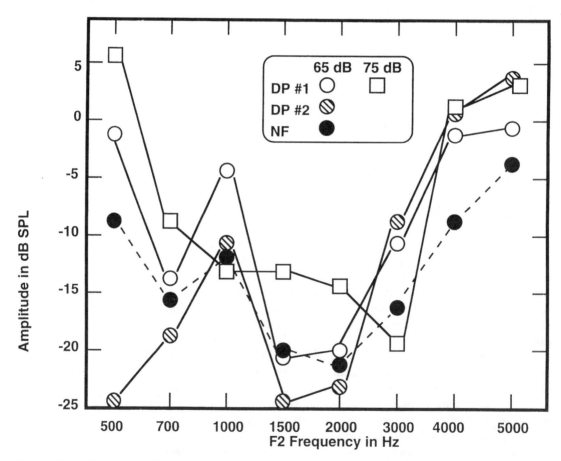

Figure 5–6. DP amplitudes recorded from a 1 cc syringe with a clinical DPOAE device. Two sets of DP data are shown for an primary intensity levels of $L_1 = L_2 = 65$ dB SPL (with noise floor values for the first run), and one set of data are shown for $L_1 = L_2 = 75$ dB SPL.

released, commercially available DPOAE device. At least five observations can be made from this figure that are pertinent to this discussion. Keep in mind that all references to "DPs" are really artifactual, that is, they are not DPOAEs and do not reflect active processes within the cochlea. First, apparent DP-noise floor (NF) differences exceeding 3 or even 5 dB (accepted criterion for the presence of a true DPOAE) can be recorded even when the probe is fit into a cavity (with no outer hair cells anywhere nearby!). Second, absolute "DP" amplitude values may be consistent with actual DPOAE amplitudes recorded from clinically normal hearing ears (e.g., greater than 0 dB at some frequencies). Third, artifactual DPs tend to be more pronounced for a higher stimulus intensity level. Fourth, the appearance of bogus DPs varies as a function of frequency, being more obvious for low and high frequencies and minimal within the 2000 to 4000 Hz region. Finally, repeatability is generally poor for these pseudo-DPs. A major qualifying statement is immediately in order. A hard-walled cavity is not an appropriate correlate to a human ear canal. The points just made are to highlight some of the facets of the problem with artifactual DPOAEs, not an illustration of what might happen clinically with real patients.

In the early 1990s, several authors presented or published papers noting the possibility of instrument-related "otoacoustic nonemissions" versus biologic OAEs (Probst & Hauser, 1990; Hotaling, Blank, Park, Matz, and Raffin, 1994; Gorga, 1994). One of the most extensive was the study reported by Hotaling and colleagues at Loyola University Medical Center near Chicago. Using several brands of clinical OAE devices, this group searched diligently for, and found, artifactual DPs in live patients, fixed hard-walled cavities, variable hard-walled cavities, rubber ears, and cadaver ears. The conclusions of the study, and a follow up investigation (Raffin, Blank, & Hotaling, 1995) were in agreement with most of the points made upon inspection of Figure 5–6.

During this time frame, the specific problem of ear canal standing waves in OAE measurement, and related weaknesses in OAE instrument probe design, was addressed by Jonathan Siegel at Northwestern University (Siegel, 1994; Siegel & Hirohata, 1994; Siegel, 1995). Siegel (1994) noted that, "Standing waves arise from sound reflected by the eardrum due to incomplete absorption. Regardless of the source impedance of the sound delivery system, the microphone will measure a null relative to the eardrum pressure when roughly one-quarter wavelength at the stimulus frequency corresponds to the distance of the entrance of the probe tube from the drum. Depending on the degree of the mismatch the sound pressure at the eardrum can be as much as 15–20 dB greater than that measured by the microphone" (p. 2589). Complicating the problem of standing wave interference, and preventing the use of correction factors, are: (1) the variability in

DISTORTION PRODUCT OAE

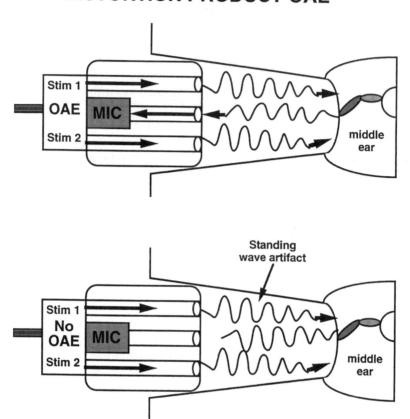

Figure 5–7. Schematic illustration of the problem of standing wave interference in DPOAE measurement for frequencies in the 4000 to 7000 Hz region. Placement of the microphone within 5 mm of the tympanic membrane would essentially eliminate the problem, but is not clinically feasible.

external physical dimensions, such as ear canal length and width; (2) intersubject, plus age- and gender-related, differences in acoustical properties of the ear canal; 3. differences in the depth of probe insertion; (4) inconsistencies among devices in the location of the microphone within the probe; and (5) cross-talk between the sound source and the microphone within probes of clinical devices (Siegel, 1994, 1995). Thus, the extent of the inaccuracy in OAE measurement, and the frequency or frequencies where it occurs, varies markedly among subjects. The problem would be eliminated by locating the microphone (not just a tube extending from the microphone) at the eardrum, but this is not feasible clinically. Underestimation of sound pressure at the eardrum (in stimulus calibration) is most serious (up to 20 dB) for frequencies in the 5000 to 7000 Hz region, although standing wave interference in DPOAE measurement is negligible only below about 3000 Hz (Siegel, 1994). Unfortunately, there is considerable potential value in measuring DPOAEs for the higher frequency region in certain clinical applications, such as ototoxicity monitoring (see Chapter 8). As an aside, the work of Siegel (1994) and others (e.g., Hotaling et al., 1994) prompted some modifications of probe design for several clinical DPOAE devices. It should be emphasized that standing waves are not a concern in recording SOAEs or TEOAEs.

Clinical Implications

When DPOAEs are recorded for stimulus frequencies above 4000 Hz, the possibility of the ear canal standing wave factor must always be considered. Inspection of normative data often shows greater variability for these higher stimulus frequencies. Manufacturers should provide users with information on probe design and stimulus/microphone calibration techniques, along with some documentation of device performance in the frequency region of concern. In addition, it is good clinical practice to replace the probe after each DPgram or I/O function for the higher stimulus frequencies, and then closely inspect data for reliability. Deviations of DPOAE amplitude values between repeated runs must be viewed as a warning sign of possible standing wave interference. These data should not be included in clinical interpretations. Exclusive reliance on DPOAEs for frequencies above 4000 Hz in, for example, newborn hearing screening or ototoxicity monitoring is ill-advised, even though it is tempting due to the characteristically low noise floor in this frequency region and the theoretical advantage of early detection of high frequency sensory hearing loss. Ultimately, the influence of standing waves in DPOAE measurement may be minimized by probe designs permitting deep insertion plus a probe mic arrangement, as calibration artifacts will be insignificant when the probe is within 5 mm of the eardrum. These problems with in-the-ear calibration for frequencies above 2000 Hz are not only pertinent to DPOAE recordings. Reflection of sound waves at the tympanic membrane may also affect SPLs measured within the ear canal during behavioral audiometric threshold measurements with insert earphones (Neely & Gorga, 1998).

Noise: Acoustic and Physiologic

Background Information

For most auditory measurements, with the exception of procedures using bone-conduction signals, an acoustic signal is delivered to the ear canal and then a change in status or a response from the auditory system is detected electrophysiologically or behaviorally. The change in status refers to alterations in middle ear immittance, whereas the responses refer to signal-induced activity in auditory regions from the cochlea to the cortex. The OAE response is detected as sound in the ear canal. Naturally, detection of OAEs is very much affected by any other sound present in the ear canal during the measurement. Clinically, there is always some sound in the ear canal when OAEs are recorded. The three general sources of the noise are equipment-related, environmental (ambient), and physiologic (from the patient). Equipment noise (electrical and thermal) must be assumed, although it cannot be easily quantified by the user. Given the differences in equipment and probe design, variation in the noise produced among OAE devices, and in the ability of OAE devices to effectively reduce other sources of measurement noise, would be expected. The amount of environmental sound in the ear canal during OAE recording can be markedly reduced by following rather common-sense guidelines, as summarized in Table 5–3. Unless information on low-frequency OAE energy (e.g., below 1000 Hz in the OAE spectrum) is important for a specific

Table 5–3. Strategies and techniques for reducing noise in OAE measurement (and improving OAE detection).

Source of Noise		To reduce the Noise
Ambient environmental	✔	close the outside door to the test room
	✔	move the patient as far from the OAE equipment as possible (the computer fan is the noise source)
	✔	turn off other equipment that generates noise
	✔	locate the patient in a sound-booth while keeping OAE equipment outside the sound-booth; turn the patient so that the test ear is facing away from the OAE equipment
	✔	reseal the OAE probe-tip deeper within the ear canal
	✔	locate the patient in a sound-booth while keeping OAE equipment outside the sound-booth
	✔	increase the amount of signal averaging during OAE recording
Patient/physiologic	✔	for older children and adults, instruct the patient to remain very still, including elimination of chewing and jaw movements
	✔	for younger children, amuse and distract the patient during testing
	✔	for infants, consider performing OAE while the patient is sleeping or sedated for some other diagnostic procedure
	✔	stabilize the cord to the OAE probe to prevent rubbing against clothing or body
	✔	increase the amount of signal averaging during OAE recording

clinical application, it is typically not necessary to record OAEs in a sound-treated booth. An appropriate test setting is a quiet room, with carpeting and acoustic ceiling tile, that is isolated from traffic in major hallways. Ambient noise in this setting can usually be reduced rather simply. Obvious sources of noise should be eliminated in the room. For example, printers, fax machines, telephones, ABR equipment, radios, and televisions should be shut off or turned down. The patient should be located as far from the OAE computer and other sound sources as the probe cord will permit, with the test ear turned away from these devices (a swivel chair for the patient comes in handy). If there are other people in the room, they should be politely told to refrain from talking and moving about during the test. This comment may seem self-evident, but the average person may not immediately perceive that quiet is important for a "hearing test". A sign on the door stating something to the effect of **"QUIET . . . hearing test in progress"** helps to consistently lower noise levels.

It is somewhat reassuring to observe some physiologic noise in an OAE recording. Only cadavers lack any body sounds. Excessive sounds generated by the patient, however, can totally obscure any evidence of OAEs, even for normal hearers with robust responses. For cooperative older preschool and also school-aged children, and of course adult patients, the most effective first step in noise reduction is to explain simply what the test is all about, and what you expect and don't expect from them. Your standard litany might go like this: "I'm going to be measuring some tiny sounds in your ear canal that are produced by your ears. You'll be hearing some [clicks or beeping sounds], but you don't need to listen for them or tell me when you hear them. All you need to do is sit very still. Try to remain quiet during the test, without moving or talking. The test only takes a few minutes." Young preschool children often remain relatively still for a quick OAE record-ing when amused by an tester assistant who plays puppet games or furiously blows bubbles. Young children generally find OAE record-ing more tolerable than tympanometry and certainly less demanding and quicker than behavioral audiometry. Therefore, even though in your clinical judgment a child is untestable using these two tech-niques, OAE measurement might still be a feasible procedure for pro-viding some information on auditory status. The best test conditions for OAE recordings from neonates and older infants are when they are sleeping. Timing OAE recordings for immediately after a feeding is a wise policy. This is an appropriate juncture to mention a rather unex-pected advantage of recording OAEs in the young and the restless. Clinicians with experience in pediatric ABR applications are acutely aware of the excessive measurement artifact associated with sucking. Even though a hungry child is usually physically calmed by nursing or taking a bottle, the myogenic artifact caused by the sucking activity and detected with the recording electrodes precludes valid waveform analysis and accurate estimation of auditory threshold levels. This author has, in contrast, had very positive experiences in recording OAEs while children are nursing or taking a bottle, particularly with test protocols that exclude low frequency stimuli and processing algorithms designed for high noise conditions. An example of this OAE dividend is presented the section on ototoxicity monitoring in Chapter 8.

Infants sedated already for ABR estimation of auditory status are in an excellent state of arousal for OAE recording as well. Similarly, if a characteristically uncooperative child requires general anesthesia for a surgical procedure that does not involve the tympanic membrane or middle ear, the operating room offers another choice option for recording OAEs with minimal physiologic noise. Although operating rooms can be noisy settings for neurotologic surgery, they tend to be much quieter for when the operation is a relatively minor procedure performed in a day surgery suite. Keep in mind that certain anesthetics, such as nitrous oxide, may alter middle ear pressure which, in turn, can influence OAE recordings. Also, OAEs are not regularly recorded from children undergoing tonsillectomies, adenoidectomies, or, of course, insertion of ventilation tubes or grommets, due to the adverse effects of middle ear dysfunction. In Chapter 8, cases illustrating OAE recordings from children in each of these settings are presented in a discussion of various clinical applications of TEOAEs and DPOAEs. Examples of the inverse relationship between DPOAE noise floor and frequency are found throughout the book. Noise floors almost always diminish steadily from low frequencies up to about 1500 to 2000 Hz. Remember, however, that for DPOAEs plotted as a function of f_2 stimuli the frequency region critical for noise floor effects on measurement is centered around the lower $2f_1-f_2$ frequency.

General steps for dealing with the ever present problem of noise in OAE measurement are discussed in Chapter 4, whereas strategies for noise reduction in newborn hearing screening are detailed in Chapter 8.

In addition to reducing environmental noise in the test setting, as outlined above and in the Table 5–3, and helping or coercing the patient to minimize bodily sounds, the tester can always take several technical steps in an attempt to record OAEs with acceptably low noise levels. Reviewed in Chapter 4, these steps include, minimally: (1) a deep and secure probe fit in the external ear canal; (2) an adequate number of stimulus repetitions (i.e., signal averages); (3) appropriate stopping criteria that require low noise and a clear signal-to-noise (OAE-to-noise floor) ratio; (4) emphasis on or exclusive presentation of signals at frequencies higher than 1000 Hz, and (5) protocol (for DPOAE) that presents signals from higher to lower frequencies. Other test protocol manipulations, such as increasing stimulus intensity levels to enhance OAE amplitude, must be exploited only as a last resort and with an appreciation for the resulting reduction in sensitivity of the measurement to cochlear deficits and increase in the likelihood of measurement artifact.

Although the importance of noise is recognized by clinicians experienced in recording OAEs, it would appear from the clinical literature that reliance on default test protocols continues to be a common practice, that is, protocols that are not varied on the basis of measurement noise. In fact, there are relatively few formal investigations of the effects of noise on OAEs. In most clinical papers, the methodology section includes an assurance that OAEs were recorded in a sound-treated room. For many clinical applications, however, OAEs are infrequently recorded in such an ideal environment. Newborn hearing screening with OAEs in a nursery setting is an excellent example of this point. Some published accounts of TEOAE-based newborn hearing screening have stressed the high noise levels encountered in that population and test environment (e.g., Hall & Chase, 1993; Jacobson & Jacobson, 1994; Hall & Mueller, 1997). The potential problem of high noise levels within the ear canals of infants during TEOAE and DPOAE measurement in intensive care unit and the well baby nursery settings is addressed, and illustrated with several cases, in the section of Chapter 8 on newborn hearing screening.

Rhoades et al. (1998) systematically assessed the effect of background noise on TEOAEs for 40 young and cooperative (i.e., still) adult subjects (all females). TEOAE measurement was conducted with the ILO88 device using both default settings and QuickScreen option in a sound-treated booth. Importantly, the maximum number of stimulus presentations (i.e., averages) was 260 and the default setting for noise rejection was 47.3 dB. If after 200 stimulus presentations, the quiet-to-noisy ratio was less than or equal to 5%, then the noise reject cutoff was raised to 51 dB. If more than 95% of the stimuli continued to be presented in excessive noise, the test was aborted. Initially, recordings were made in a quiet condition (noise less than 35 dBA). Then, during TEOAE measurement, calibrated white noise was presented via a loudspeaker at intensity levels of 50 dB, 55 dB, and 60 dBA. These noise levels were chosen because they are representative of infant screening environments. Among the TEOAE parameters evaluated, for the default and QuickScreen techniques, were overall amplitude, an index of noise in the recording (the difference between the two simultaneously recorded waveforms, the A-B difference), the whole (overall) reproducibility, reproducibility by frequency bands, the percentage of quiet versus noisy responses (those exceeding the noise rejection limit of 47 or 51 dB), and test time. Selected findings reported by Rhoades et al. (1998) are summarized in Table 5–4. Because the results of this study are highly relevant for clinical application of TEOAEs, the reader is urged to examine the trends evident from this summary. Clearly, for the default settings (e.g., a fixed number of stimulus presentation and a fixed intensity level), there are no invariable and absolute values for any of the TEOAE response parameters, nor test time. Rather, even the most fundamental response indices can vary dramatically depending on noise level. As the authors noted: "The study indicated a significant reduction

Table 5–4. Summary of selected effects of noise on TEOAE parameters. Click-evoked OAEs were recorded from 40 cooperative, normal-hearing female adults with the ILO 88 device in the default and QuickScreen modes of operation.

Parameter	Default Mode Noise Level				QuickScreen Mode Noise Level			
	Quiet	50 dBA	55 dBA	60 dB A	Quiet	50 dBA	55 dBA	60 dBA
Changed default noise rejection limit required (% of subjects)	0%	8%	22%	100%	0%	5%	30%	100%
Mean overall amplitude (in dB)	11.1	10.7	9.5	3.9	9.7	9.5	8.7	5.3
Mean whole reproducibility (in %)	89.2	75.45	56.5	23.5	91.7	81.2	68.9	33.6
Whole reproducibility ≥ 50% (in %)* (<50% is a criterion for screening failure)	100	88	64	20	100	94	82	40
Proportion of quiet responses (in %)	95.5	88.8	63.1	37.6	96.7	87.9	71.3	45.1
Mean reproducibility by octave band for default/QuickScreen (in %)*								
1000/800 Hz	86	64	40	8	80	63	41	22
2000/1600 Hz	90	75	53	25	96	77	62	25
3000/2400 Hz	90	84	73	40	94	86	76	37
4000/3200 Hz	77	74	68	40	98	89	89	52
5000/4000 Hz	30	30	28	16	88	78	74	47
Test time (in seconds)*	47	50	120	130	58	70	80	122

* Approximated from data displayed In figures from Rhoades et al., 1998.

in 9 of the 11 selected variables across 50 to 55 dB A of noise for default and QuickScreen modes of the ILO 88 operation" (Rhoades et al., 1998, p. 461). For example, from the quiet to the noisiest condition, average overall TEOAE amplitude went from over 11 dB down to less than 4 dB (and the range extended from 21 to 0 dB), while average overall reproducibility went from over 89% to less than 24% (and the range from 99 to 0%). Test duration was three times longer for the noisiest versus the quiet condition. The results of this clinic study are highly relevant for clinical application of TEOAEs. Without doubt, the deleterious influences of noise on each of these response parameters would be at least as serious in some typical clinical populations, as the authors excluded excessive physiologic (body) noise by limiting their subjects to cooperative adults. In some patient groups (e.g., young children), the negative effects of environmental noise would be compounded by noise secondary to physical movement (mouth, jaw, head, crying, etc.), although for normal hearing young children the response might be more robust. Quoting Rhoades et al. (1998) once again: "Hospital wards, school rooms, and physician's offices have ambient noise levels that may exceed 50 to 55 dBA and, hence, when using CEOAEs in these environments, noise reduction strategies must be implemented and alternatives to the default program should be employed" (p. 461).

An alternative approach to considering the effect of noise on TEOAEs is to manipulate one test parameter which directly influences the signal-to-noise ratio. Signal averaging is a technique employed successfully in the clinical measurement of auditory evoked responses and otoacoustic emissions. For a given OAE (i.e., signal) level and a given noise level, the ratio will improve with increased signal averaging. Amplitude of the OAEs, which is time-locked to the stimulus, is maintained with repeated presentations of the stimulus, whereas background noise (ambient and physiologic) which is, for the most part, random and unrelated to the stimulus will be progressively cancelled (or averaged) out with repeated stimulus presentations. Thus, extraction of the response from background noise is enhanced with averaging, as illustrated in Figure 5–8. With a larger response and/or less noise, fewer averaging are needed. However, when the response is not robust and/or noise levels are higher, more averaging is needed. An alternate approach for recording OAEs, used typically in AER measurement, is to determine in advance criteria for the optimal response, or response presence versus absence, and then to continue presenting stimuli (averaging) until these criteria are met, or some maximum limit for test time or stimulus presentations is reached. This strategy is sometimes employed in newborn hearing screening with OAEs, as noted in Chapter 8, but it can be exploited also in any OAE application. Noise affects lower frequency octave bands more than those above 2000 Hz. In addition to minimizing obvious sources of noise, and obtaining a snug probe fit with sound-attenuating probe tips, the tester can improve TEOAE response quality by simply adapting the amount of averaging to the test conditions.

Manufacturers of DPOAE equipment employ different algorithms and techniques for noise reduction, as detailed in the "Manufacturers' Forum" found in Chapter 7.

In displays of DPOAE data, in either DPgram or I/O formats, noise floor levels are invariably plotted for each stimulus frequency (set of primaries). Noise calculations are limited to a very constricted region of frequencies centered around the DPOAE frequency (usually $2f_1-f_2$), e.g., 30 Hz above and below that frequency. Noise potentially interfering with DPOAE measurement covers a rather broad band of frequencies. The narrower the bandwidth of frequencies subjected to fast Fourier transformation (spectral analysis), the more effective the detection of the DP, the larger the DP-to- noise ratio, the quicker the criteria for DP presence are met, and the shorter the test time. In contrast, the spectrum of noise potentially influencing TEOAE measurement is often limited only by the frequency response of the microphone used to detect the response, unless a low-frequency filtering option or shortened analysis time is utilized (analysis of the earlier post-stimulus times and higher frequencies of the response). Noise affecting any type of OAE—SOAE, TEOAE or DPOAE—will always be most prominent and troublesome in the low frequency region. Casual inspection of many figures of TEOAE plots and DPgrams scattered throughout this book repeatedly confirms that noise floors decrease from the lower frequency limit of measurement (about 500 Hz) up to about 1500 to 2000 Hz. That is not to say that excessive noise is never present for higher frequencies. Excessive physiologic (body) noise may traverse the entire OAE spectrum analyzed by clinical devices. As a rule, however, ambient environmental noise does not preclude DPOAE detection or confound accurate calculation of amplitude for higher frequencies. Algorithms and protocols employed in DPOAE measurement typically include data for absolute noise levels and the DP-to-noise difference in stopping criteria. That is, processing is more extensive, and takes more time, when there is more noise and vice versa. This adaptive measurement approach, varying as a function of noise, is in contrast to the practice of presenting a fixed number of stimuli in the averaging process without consideration of noise conditions.

Noise can affect any DP measurement (Whitehead, Lonsbury-Martin, & Martin, 1993). The influence is greatest when the noise floor is high and approaches the amplitude of the DP (small DP-to-noise ratio), whereas it is negligible, or even nil, when the noise floor is below the lowest stimulus intensity level producing DP activity (below the level of DP detection). In clinical terms, when noise levels are less than −15 dB SPL the noise is not an important factor in DP analysis. For DPgrams recorded at moderate-to-high intensity levels the signal (DP) is larger, and so is the signal-to-noise ratio in most cases. Consequently, noise levels exceeding −15 dB SPL may still not have any practical effect on DP measurements. With higher levels of noise, however, there is a possibility that DP amplitude will be overestimated (Whitehead et al., 1993). DP values sometimes appear to ride above high noise floors, dropping and rising along with the noise. Absolute DP amplitude varies, even though the DP-noise floor difference remains constant. Noise reduction is more crucial for estimation of DP threshold at low stimulus intensity levels when the signal-to-noise ratio is almost always smaller. The lower the noise floor, the more accurate the analysis of the low intensity tail of the DP I/O function. Also, the amount of noise during DPOAE measurement directly influences the slope of the I/O function. As noise levels increase, I/O slope is underestimated (the slope appears less steep than it really is).

Clinical Conclusions

Among all of the nonpathologic factors in OAE measurement reviewed in this chapter, noise is by far the most important one under the most control by the tester. Noise has a pronounced influence on the quality of OAE recordings. In fact, the success of OAE measurement and the accuracy of OAE interpretation is highly dependent on noise. By regularly following some common-sense guidelines (summarized earlier in Table 5–3), the clinician can usually minimize ambient and, to a lesser extent, physiologic noise at its source. Then, if needed, OAE measurement can proceed with modification of the test protocol with, perhaps, increased test time and/or loss of data for selected frequency regions. In the real clinical world, however, there will be times when excessive noise will obscure a response or preclude valid OAE measurement. If noise levels exceed maximum acceptable limits, then the wisest policy is to attempt OAE assessment at a later time, another location, and/or with the patient in a quieter state of arousal. No audiologic procedure is always successful performed with all patients.

OAE PREVALENCE IN NORMAL EARS IS LESS THAN 100%

Background

According to the conventional wisdom during the initial period of OAE research and clinical application, prevalence of TEOAEs was 100% (Kemp, 1978; Kemp et al., 1986; Bonfils et al., 1988; Vedantam & Musiek, 1991; Reshef et al., 1993), or nearly 100% (Grandori, 1983; Probst et al., 1986; Stevens, 1988; Probst et al., 1986; Stevens, 1988; Dolhen et al., 1991; Probst, Lonsbury-Martin, & Martin, 1991; Lutman & Saunders, 1992). Failure to detect normal OAEs in presumably normal ears was often attributed to either equipment malfunction, poor technique, an inadequate test environment (e.g., excessive noise), analysis criteria, or unidentified otologic pathology. As clinical experience accumulated, it became clear that on rare occasions OAEs appeared abnormal, or simply were undetectable, even from normal-hearing subjects with no obvious otologic dysfunction by history, clinical examination, or basic audiometry (e.g., Hall et al., 1994). In a formal investigation of this clinically important issue, at least for the presence of TEOAEs as determined by a cross-correlation (reproducibility) response parameter, Kapadia and Lutman (1997) found among a group of 397 ears a prevalence of 99.2%. However, close inspection of the ears without apparent TEOAEs failed to "unequivocally show absence of TEOAE characteristics in any ear with normal hearing threshold levels" (Kapadia & Lutman, 1997, p. 3566). There is to date no equivalent investigation with DPOAEs.

The occasionally inexplicable absence of OAEs is illustrated in Figure 5–8. The subject was a 30-year-old female audiologist with hearing threshold levels of 15 dB or better at all audiometric frequencies from 250 to 8000 Hz, including 3000 and 6000 Hz, and normal aural immittance findings. She had a normal otologic history, including no exposure to excessive noise. When pressed to reveal everything about her hearing, she admitted to occasional, brief periods of ringing. This phenomenon, known as spontaneous transient tinnitus, is normal. TEOAEs were not detected from either ear during repeated recordings over a 2-year period. DPOAEs (not shown) were abnormal but present bilaterally.

Clinical Conclusions

The absence of any recordable OAE activity does not invariably confirm cochlear pathology and certainly does not imply the presence of a pure-tone hearing loss. The prevalence of OAEs even in a random and adequately large normal-hearing population is not quite 100%. With extensive clinical experience in recording OAEs, every audiologist will eventually encounter a person who meets all criteria for audiologic and otologic normality save one . . . OAEs will be undetectable.

CONTRALATERAL AND IPSILATERAL ACOUSTIC SUPPRESSION

Introduction

Presentation of a sound ipsilateral or contralateral to a normal ear from which OAEs are being recorded reduces, or suppresses, the amplitude of the OAEs. Sound-induced suppression of OAEs is a normal phenomenon mediated by the efferent, or descending, auditory system.

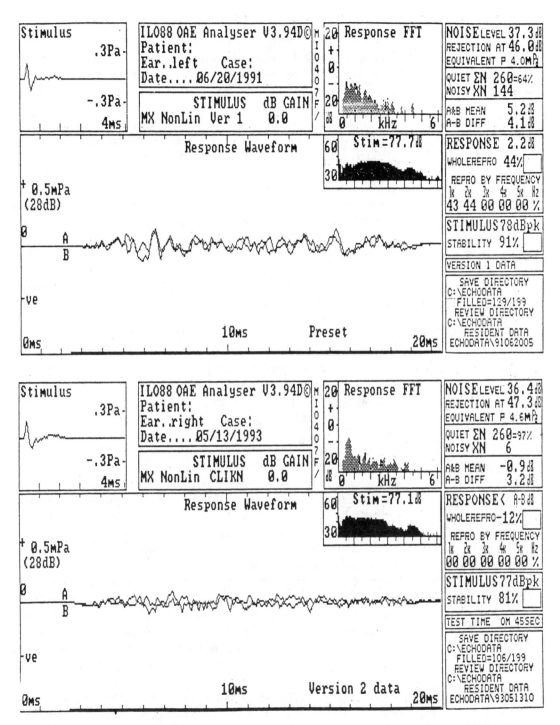

Figure 5–8. TEOAEs recorded from young female with hearing thresholds of 15 dB or better at all audiometric and inter-octave frequencies, normal middle ear function, and unremarkable otologic examination and history. No TEOAEs were detected for either ear in multiple recordings over a 3-year period.

Efferent system anatomy is reviewed briefly in Chapter 2, with reference to in depth readings on the topic.

Indeed, lack of suppression is a pathologic finding implicating dysfunction of the efferent auditory system. To review simply, the cochlea and, specifically, the organ of Corti is innervated by the olivocochlear bundle of the efferent system (efferent system anatomy is reviewed in Chapter 2). An ipsilateral lateral olivocochlear bundle runs from one side of the pons to the cochlea on the same side, and makes a synapse with afferent neuron dentrites close to the inner hair cells, with subsequent release of cholinergic and opioid neurotransmittors (Musiek, 1992). Keep in mind that, in contrast to innervation of outer hair cells, efferent fibers do not make direct contact with the base of the inner hair cells. A second and anatomically distinct efferent system pathway is of greater relevance to OAEs. It involves the medial olivocochlear bundle which arises, as the name implies, from cell bodies within the medial nuclei of the superior olivary complex on one side of the pontine brainstem (Robertson, 1985). The medial olivocochlear system (MOCS) fibers then cross the midline of the brainstem near the floor of the fourth ventricle and run distally through the internal auditory canal to synapse directly at the base of the outer hair cells in the contralateral cochlea, perhaps mediated at least partly by acetylcholine neurotransmittors (Kujawa, Glattke, Fallon, & Bobbin, 1993). Our understanding of the anatomy of the efferent system is the product of careful investigations beginning with those of Rasmussen in the 1940s (Rasmussen, 1946; Smith & Rasmussen, 1963) and perpetuated by Warr and Guinan, among others (Warr, 1975; Warr et al., 1986; Warr & Guinan, 1979; Guinan et al., 1983, 1984).

The functional effect of efferent auditory system activation is inhibition of cochlear activity, mostly via the outer hair cells. This conclusion is based on long-standing electrophysiologic investigation beginning in the 1950s (e.g., Galambos, 1956; Fex, 1959), and continuing on to the present. Initially, cochlear activity was measured with ECochG techniques or with direct recordings from the auditory nerve. Galambos (1956), and subsequently others showed clearly in animal experimentation that electrical stimulation of the efferent system at the brainstem level, in the region of the fourth ventricle investigators (Fex, 1959; Desmedt & Monaco, 1961; Wiederhold & Kiang, 1970; Guinan & Gifford, 1988), or contralateral acoustic stimulation (Fex, 1962; Rajan & Johnstone, 1988; Buno, 1978; Murata et al., 1980; Liberman, 1989; Warren & Liberman, 1989; Kawase & Liberman, 1993; Nieder & Nieder, 1970 a,b) produced several related effects, among them reduction of the amplitude of the ECochG action potential as recorded at the round window, lowering of the discharge rate of the auditory nerves and of the endocochlear potential, and an increase in cochlear microphonic activity. Later investigators confirmed some of these findings in humans (Folsom & Owsley, 1987). Conversely, when these efferent pathways are disenabled chemically or by surgical sectioning, the inhibitory effects are eliminated (e.g., Rajan, 1988; Liberman, 1989).

One of the latest lines of basic research on the role of the efferent auditory system on cochlear function utilizes electrical stimulation of brainstem structures with descending projections to the olivocochlear bundle region (Scates, Woods, & Azeredo, 1999). Although the focus of most research and clinical interest is the olivocochlear bundle (pons to cochlear connections), efferent system pathways and functions extend rostrally in the central auditory nervous system to the midbrain and even the temporal lobe. Stimulation of the external and central subnuclei of the inferior colliculus in rats suppressed DPOAE amplitude from 7 to 25 dB initially. This suppression persisted for 25 to 30 ms, and was followed by a later phase of suppression on the order of 3 to 15 dB. External subnuclei electrical stimulation produced equivalent DPOAE suppression as measured on ipsilateral and contralateral ears, whereas stimulation of the central subnuclei resulted in mostly contralateral suppression, which was of smaller magnitude. And, stimulation of the dorsal subnuclei of the inferior colliculus was associated with little or no suppression of DPOAEs. When middle ear muscles were severed, these findings were unchanged, effectively ruling out the acoustic reflex as a factor.

With the discovery of OAEs in the late 1970s, the next logical step was to assess the effect of efferent auditory system stimulation and inactivity on the outer hair cell responses as determined by evoked OAEs, first in animals (Mountain, 1980; Mountain, Geisler, & Hubbard, 1980; Siegel & Kim, 1982; Puel & Rebillard, 1990) and more recently in humans. Decreased amplitude of SOAEs, and an upward shift of SOAE frequency, with contralateral stimulation was also demonstrated (Grose, 1983; Mott et al., 1989; 1993). To a large extent, our initial knowledge of the influences of the efferent system on OAEs in humans was the result of pioneering work by a group of French investigators from Lyon (Collet et al., 1990, 1992; Morlet, Collet, Salle, & Morgon, 1993; Veuillet et al., 1991, 1992; Maison et al., 1997) and Chuck Berlin and colleagues at LSU and Kresge Hearing Research Laboratory in the United States (Berlin et al., 1993, 1994, 1995, Huang et al., 1994) with, not unexpectedly, contributions from David Kemp and several of his British co-investigators (Ryan et al., 1991). Other investigators , however, also made valuable contributions with early reports of contralateral acoustic suppression of OAEs (e.g. Brown & Norton, 1990). The characteristic effect of efferent system stimulation with contralateral sound is suppression of outer hair cell function, with subsequent reduction of OAEs amplitude.

This is an appropriate juncture to make a few comments about the terminology used to describe this phenomenon and the concepts underlying it. First, it would be reasonable to ask, "What's so interesting about the alteration of a cochlear response by a masking-type sound? Clinical audiologists use masking techniques daily to eliminate the nontest ear from contributing to, and confounding, assessment of a variety of auditory measures (e.g., pure-tone and speech audiometry.) With conventional masking in clinical audiology a masker that includes maximal energy in the region of the signal is presented to the nontest ear at the same time that the signal is presented to the test ear. The goal is to eliminate the possibility of a response, at high signal intensity levels, to signal energy that has crossed over from the test to nontest ear. The goal in suppression of OAEs is quite different. The contralateral signal (noise is most effective) is presented at a relatively low intensity level, certainly below the level which could cross over to the test ear (from which OAEs are being recorded), and also below an intensity level that might elicit an acoustic stapedial reflex. The contralateral sound (noise) activates the contralateral cochlea and, in turn, afferent eighth (auditory) cranial nerve fibers. In the lower brainstem (pons), specifically within the olivary complex, there are neural connections (synapses) among *afferent* auditory nuclei and efferent auditory nuclei. The contralateral sound-induced activation of efferent regions results in the transmission of efferent signals through two sets of olivocochlear bundles back to each cochlea. Ipsilateral pathways in the lateral system permit efferent innervation of outer hair cells in the cochlea to which the noise was presented, whereas contralateral pathways in the medial system run a course to contralateral (to the noise) cochlear outer hair cells. Clinical audiologists will recognize the similarity of the anatomic bases of acoustic suppression of OAEs and the traditional acoustic stapedius reflex. There are certainly some commonalites in the overall anatomic components for each auditory phenomenon. The final descending pathways and destinations are, of course, different. The acoustic reflex utilizes the seventh (facial) cranial nerve and innervation of the stapedius muscle, rather than efferent fibers within the OCB and innervation of the outer hair cells. Secondly, the term "suppression" suggests that OAEs are totally abolished by contralateral acoustic signals. To be precise, the effect of contralateral noise on OAEs is a minor alteration in the response, limited to a rather modest reduction (several dB) in amplitude.

The Contralateral Suppression Literature

Clinicians, particularly American audiologists, may be surprised to learn that the literature describing investigations of OAE suppression by acoustic stimulation is quite extensive. For readers who wish to study this topic further, a representative sampling of references on suppression and OAEs is listed in Table 5–5. Many of the studies were conducted with various animal models, and the majority were published in either basic science journals (e.g., *Hearing Research* or *Journal*

Table 5–5. Studies of auditory suppression of otoacoustic emissions arranged chronologically. References to clinical subjects or patients with pathology are italicized. Full citations for each study are provided in the bibliography at the end of the book.

Study (Year)	Type of OAE	Number of Subjects	Type of Subjects
Contralateral Suppression			
Veuillet, Collet, & Morgon (1992)	TEOAE	11	normal human adults
Collet, Veuillet, Bene, & Morgon (1992)	TEOAE	40	normal human adults
		77	*adult humans with SNHL*
Berlin et al. (1993)	TEOAE	3	normal human adults
		2	*adolescent and adult with unspecified auditory dysfunction*
Norman & Thornton (1993)	TEOAE	20	normal human adults
Morlet et al. (1993)			
Froelich et al. (1993)			
Chery-Cloze et al. (1993)			
Moulin, Collet, & Duclaux (1993)	DPOAE	40	normal human adults
		7	*unilateral SNHL due to mumps*
Morlet, Collet, Salle, & Morgon (1993)	TEOAE	20	normal human adults
		42	*preterm neonates*
Berlin, Hood, Hurley, & Wen (1994)	review article		
	TEOAE	5	*adults and children with various pathologies*
Pujol (1994)	review article		
Collet et al. (1994)	review article		
Lind (1994)	TEOAE	? ?	normal human adults
Thornton (1994)	TEOAE	10	normal human adults
Thornton (1994)	TEOAE	8	normal human adults
Graham & Hazell (1994)	TEOAE	6	normal human adults
		6	*humans with unilateral tinnitus*
Prasher, Ryan, & Luxon (1994)	TEOAE	24	normal human adults
		18	*adults with CPA lesions*
		11	*adults with brainstem lesions*

(continued)

Table 5–5. *(continued)*

Study (Year)	Type of OAE	Number of Subjects	Type of Subjects
Contralateral Suppression *(continued)*			
Chery-Croze, Truy, & Morgon (1994)	TEOAE	3	*adults with tinnitus*
Aran, Erre, & Avan (1994)	TEOAE	??	guinea pigs
Castor, Vueillet, Morgon, & Collet (1994)	TEOAE DPOAE	60	*young versus old adults*
Thornton & Slaven (1995)	TEOAE	8	normal human adults
Souter (1995)	SFOAE	4	normal human adults
Veuillet, Duverdy-Bertholon, & Collet (1996)	TEOAE	64	normal human adults
Attias, Bresloff, & Furman (1996)	TEOAE		*human adults with tinnitus*
Maison, Micheyl, Chays, & Collet (1997)	TEOAE	31 11	normal human adults *adults post vestibular neuronectomy*
Maison, Micheyl, & Collet (1997)	TEOAE	86 3	normal human adults unilateral SNHL due to mumps
Maison et al. (1997)	TEOAE	20 8	normal human adults *adults post vestibular neuronectomy*
Lina-Granade, Liogier, & Collet (1997)	TEOAE	22	normal human adults
Pratt, Shi, & Polyakov (1998)	TEOAE	10	normal human adults
Hood et al. (1999)	TEOAE	61	*young versus old adults*
Ipsilateral Suppression			
Kemp (1979)	TEOAE		
Wit & Ritsma (1980)	TEOAE		
Wilson (1980)	SOAE		
Zurek (1981)	SOAE		
Brown & Kemp (1984)			
Bargones & Burns (1988)	SOAE	40	normal full-term newborn infants
Harris et al. (1992)			
Kevanishvili et al. (1992)	TEOAE		normal human adults (forward masking)
Gobsch et al. (1992)	TEOAE	8	normal human adults (forward masking)
Long et al. (1993)			
Tavartkiladze et al. (1994)	TEOAE	7	normal human adults

Table 5–5. *(continued)*

Study (Year)	Type of OAE	Number of Subjects	Type of Subjects
Ipsilateral Suppression *(continued)*			
Cianfrone et al. (1994)	DPOAE	6	normal human adults
Thornton (1994)	TEOAE	10	normal human adults
Thorton (1994)	TEOAE	8	normal human adults
Kummer et al. (1995)			
Abdala, Sininger, Ekelld, & Zeng (1996)	DPOAE	15	normal human adults
		16	normal term newborn infants
Neumann (1997)	TEOAE	9	normal human adults
Neumann, Uppenkamp, & Kollmeier (1997)	TEOAE	4	normal human adults
Heitmann, Waldmann, & Schnitzler (1998)	DPOAE	??	normal human adults

of the Acoustical Society of America) or European otolaryngology/audiology journals.

Collectively, the results of these studies lead to the following general conclusions. Contralateral acoustic stimulation (CAS) reduces amplitude of both TEOAEs and DPOAEs, but usually at the most by only 1 to 3 dB. This effect is illustrated for DPOAEs in Figure 5–10. Latency of OAE suppression after the suppressor signal is presented is typically on the order of 8 to 15 ms, and depends in part on the type of suppressor (e.g., clicks vs. noise). These values include the time taken by OAEs in traveling along the cochlear membrane, through the middle, and into the external ear canal, estimated to be 4 ms (Kemp et al., 1990). In a departure from the rather brief suppressor durations employed in most studies, however, Moulin and Carrier (1998) demonstrated that with contralateral broad band noise stimulation ranging from 30 seconds to 20 minutes, the duration of the suppressive effect was as short as 2.6 seconds or was sustained for the full 20 minutes. When the noise was presented for over 2 minutes, some residual suppressive effect persisted for more than a minute after the noise offset. Greater suppression occurs for ipsilateral and binaural signals, respectively. The strength of the suppression, that is, the reduction of amplitude, is highly variable among normal subjects. Suppression is relatively greater for OAE responses, particularly TEOAEs, within the mid-frequency

(1000 to 2000 Hz) region. Suppression effects are more pronounced for OAEs evoked with low stimulus intensity levels (versus high intensities), as illustrated in Figure 5–9. OAE phase or latency parameters may also be affected (decreased or advanced). Broad band noise is a more effective suppressor than narrow band signals, and especially pure tones. When narrow band suppressor signals are employed, the effect on OAE amplitude is frequency-specific and greatest when the suppressor frequency band is centered on the frequency, or major frequency region, of the OAEs. Subject age appears to influence CAS. Preterm infants show less suppression than term infants, and both groups show less suppression than adults. There is also some evidence that the magnitude of CAS decreases as a function of advancing age over the range of 10 to 80 years. Even subject factors such as handedness, eyedness, footedness, as well as gender, in medial olivocochlear efferent system function have been investigated (Khalfa, Veuillet,& Collet, 1998). There is some evidence that this efferent system is more effective for the right ear among right handers, while functioning symmetrically for lefties. The effects of suppression are most evident for moderate (versus near threshold) suppressor intensities (refer again to Figure 5–9), but high suppressor intensities are not recommended because of the potential contamination of acoustic reflexes and acoustic cross-over. In any attempt to measure CAS clinically care must be taken to avoid activation of the acoustic reflex and/or acoustic crossover the contralateral signal to the ear from which the OAEs are being recorded. Suppressor intensities should be less than the levels of acoustic reflex thresholds and intra-aural attenuation. The foregoing factors or variables that can influence contralateral acoustic suppression of OAEs are summarized in Table 5–6.

The inhibitory, or suppressive, influence of the efferent auditory system on the cochlea can be eliminated surgically, and by selected clinical pathologies and lesions. There is a close anatomic proximity between the olivocochlear bundle and the vestibular portion of the eighth cranial nerve as both sets of fibers run via the internal auditory canal between the brainstem and the peripheral auditory-vestibular apparatus. Sectioning of the vestibular nerve surgically, a therapeutic option for patients with unilateral Ménière's disease, usually also serves the efferent pathways. Several investigators have confirmed that contralateral suppression disappears in humans following vestibular neuronectomy (Scharf et al., 1994; Williams et al., 1993, 1994; Giraud et al., 1995; Maison et al., 1997). Patients with vestibular nerve section have also been studied to differentiate possible ipsilateral efferent effects versus intracochlear processes in TEOAEs recorded with very high stimulus rates (Hine, Thornton, & Brookes, 1997). A similar loss of the suppression effect was previously shown with experimental midline sagittal sectioning of efferent pathways near the floor of the fourth ventricle within the brainstem (Puel & Rebillard, 1990). Although neuropathology is less site-specific than surgical sectioning techniques,

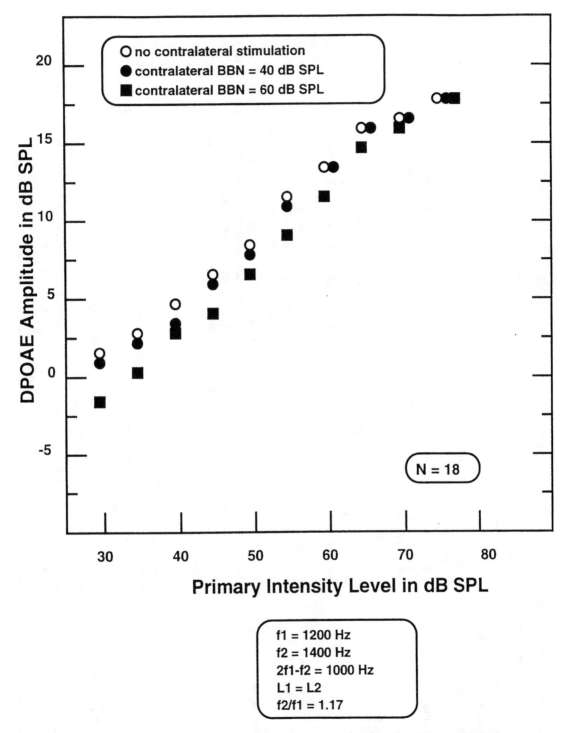

Figure 5–9. Example of the effect of contralateral acoustic stimulation (CAS) with two different suppressor intensity levels (40 and 60 dB) on DPOAE amplitudes, as a function of DPOAE stimulus intensity. Note the greater suppression (reduced DPOAE amplitude) for higher intensity suppressor, and lower stimulus intensity levels. (Adapted from Moulin, Collet & Duclaux, 1993.)

Table 5–6. Factors influencing contralateral acoustic suppression (CAS) of otoacoustic emissions (OAEs).

Factors	Description of Effect
Nonpathologic subject factors	
Intersubject variability	Some normal subjects show little or no effects, whereas others show a clear and robust suppression of OAE amplitude
Developmental age	Suppression is minimal or not demonstrable for preterm newborn infants, perhaps due to immaturity of either the efferent auditory brainstem pathways, olivocochlear bundle, and/or synapse at the outer hair cells. Term infants may show slight suppression effects.
Advancing age	There is some evidence of reduced suppression with aging.
Acoustic reflex	CAS will be contaminated and the effect on OAEs invalidated by contraction of the stapedius muscle and the resulting alteration of middle ear transmission. Acoustic reflex induced changes in middle ear transmission will greatly affect the inward/outward propagation of energy in OAE measurement and totally obscure the relatively slight true efferent effects. Use of adequately low suppressor intensity level will rule out acoustic reflex involvement. In early studies, the possible contribution of acoustic reflex activity in CAS was ruled out by measurements made in persons with facial nerve disorders due to Bell's palsy and other causes for absence of middle ear muscle reflexes (Collet et al., 1990; Berlin et al., 1993).
Acoustic crossover	Similar to the potential acoustic reflex problem in CAS, excessive suppressor intensity levels raise the possibility of crossover of the suppressor signal from the contralateral to ipsilateral (OAE) ear. The result is ipsilateral masking of either the OAE stimulus and/or response which invalidates documentation of CAS. Low level suppressor intensities, and the use of insert (versus supra-aural) earphones eliminates this problem.
Suppressor factors	
Intensity level	Suppressor intensity must be just audible to produce an effect, but the effect increases as intensity level is increased to moderate levels. The intensity level, however, must be less than the acoustic reflex threshold and less than the subject's intra-aural attenuation to eliminate possibility of crossover to OAE ear and ipsilateral masking.
Amplitude modulation	Greater modulation depth of an amplitude-moduluated tone produced more suppression (Maison et al., 1997). This suppressor type was frequency specific.
Frequency	Broad band noise is most effective. Narrow band noise signals will produce suppression of the OAE response within the suppressor frequency band. Clicks are less effective than narrow bands of noise, and pure tone suppressors are least effective.

Suppressor factors

Duration	For activation of the OCB, rather long stimulus durations of 50 ms or longer (up to 500 ms) are required (e.g., Liberman & Brown, 1986; Berlin et at., 1995).
Laterality	Suppression is greatest for noise signals presented binaurally, less for ipsilateral presentation of noise, and least for contralateral acoustic stimulation. Medial olivocochlear fibers innervating the outer hair cells are activated by both contralateral sounds (about one-third of the fibers) and ipsilateral sounds (about two-thirds of the fibers). Therefore, binaural suppressor signals (activating ipsi- and contralateral fibers) are maximally effective (Berlin et al., 1994).

OAE stimulus factors

intensity	CAS is most robust for OAEs recorded with relatively low versus higher stimulus intensity levels (e.g., click stimuli less than 65 dB SPL). CAS effects diminish as the input-output function for OAEs begins to saturate.

OAE response factors

amplitude	Suppression Is typically on the order of 2 to 3 dB, but characterized by considerable intersubject variability. TEOAE amplitude Is typically reduced by contralateral suppression but, under selected conditions, DPOAE amplitude may increase.
frequency	Suppression tends to be greatest within the 1000 to 2000 Hz region, with a broad band noise suppressor or when narrow band suppressors are compared.
latency	Phase of all OAEs may shift with contralateral acoustic stimulation. Onset latency of suppression, i.e., the time lag between presentation of the suppressor signal and the initial evidence of reduced OAE amplitude, may range from less than 40 ms to more than 140 ms (for TEOAEs). Offset latency of suppression, i.e., the time after suppressor presentation needed for the OAEs to return to baseline values, may be as long as 100 ms. That is, some evidence of suppression persists for up to 100 msec after the suppressor signal ends. Latency limits the rate at which stimuli can be presented to produce maximum suppression.
TEOAEs	Under equivalent conditions, greater suppression is typically observed for TEOAEs than for DPOAE.
SOAEs	Amplitude is reduced and SOAE frequency is shifted upward (not observed for TEOAEs or DPOAEs).

Papers on high rate stimulation of OAEs with the maximum length sequence (MLS) technique by Dr. Thornton and others are summarized in Chapter 10.

acoustic tumors within the internal auditory canal may compress the nerve fibers leading to the ear and compromise efferent system function. Thornton (1994) produced what was viewed as an ipsilateral suppression effect on TEOAEs by presenting click stimuli at extremely high rates (up to 2000 clicks/sc). His premise that suppression effects were produced by rapid stimulus presentation was based on his evidence (Thornton & Slaven, 1995) that contralateral acoustic suppression (the "Collet effect") disappeared at such high stimulus rates. He reported a patient with an acoustic neuroma who showed no decrease in TEOAE amplitude on the ear ipsilateral to the tumor, whereas the normal contralateral ear showed a substantial decrease in TEOAE amplitude at high stimulus rates. In a later paper, however, Thornton and colleagues (Hine, Thornton & Brookes, 1997) provided evidence of reduction in amplitude when TEOAEs were recorded at high stimulus rates from vestibular neurectomy patients. This finding led to the rejection of hypothesis that high stimulus rates induced efferent effects. The authors speculated that the explanation might instead be related to intracochlear processes.

The Ipsilateral Suppression Literature

There are essentially two approaches for assessing the effect of ipsilateral suppressors on OAEs. With one approach, a suppressor signal (ranging from a click to a relatively extended duration noise band) is presented to an ear prior to the presentation of an OAE-evoking stimulus. Suppressive changes in the OAE response secondary to the noise signal, and presumably to efferent system activation, are documented. This is sometimes called an "ipsilateral forward masking paradigm." Among the test variables examined in ipsilateral suppression studies, and their general effects, are; (1) The intensity level of the stimulus used to evoke the OAEs: less suppression of OAE for higher stimulus intensity levels; (2) The intensity level of the suppressor signal (masker): more suppression for higher masker intensity levels; (3) The nature of the suppressor signal (broad band or narrow band noise, clicks, pure tones): greater suppression with noise; (4) The duration of the suppressor signal (e.g., ranging from maximum suppression for longer duration (continuous) noise signals to minimal or no efferent-based suppression with transient click signals); (5) The time difference or delay between the suppressor signal and the OAE-evoking stimulus; Suppression effects are greatest within the first 5 ms after a transient (e.g., click) masker. They then diminish over the next few milliseconds; (6) The presentation rate for the suppressor signal and for the OAE stimulus: greater suppression for slower suppressor signal rates (to permit a complete response of the olivocochlear system) but for higher stimulus rates (probably enhances ipsilateral efferent system activation); (7) Intracochlear (versus efferent) processes secondary to forward masking; and (8) The type of OAEs recorded (i.e., SOAEs, TEOAEs, or DPOAEs): there are significant differences in magnitude and nature of suppression between the types of OAEs as a function of the above variables. As one would expect, suppression is dependent on rather complex interactions among these variables, as well as subject factors such as age, peripheral auditory status, central auditory status, and anesthesia (with animal experimentation). Detailed discussions of the interactions among these variables in investigations of ipsilateral suppression can be found in the original papers listed in Table 5–6. The reader is especially referred for more information on ipsilateral suppression of TEOAEs to the clinical work of George Tavartkiladze and his Russian colleagues (Tavartkiladze et al., 1994, 1996) and Chuck Berlin and associates (Berlin et al., 1995).

With the other approach, the suppressor is one or more tones presented simultaneously with an OAE- evoking stimulus, at nearby frequencies. Tonal suppression techniques, especially two-tone suppression (2TS) in which the response of the cochlea to one tone is diminished by the simultaneous presentation of a second tone, have been used in experimental animal studies of cochlear mechanics (e.g., Rhode & Robles, 1974; Rhode, 1977; Ruggero et al., 1992; Nuttall & Dolan, 1993; Cooper, 1996; Cooper & Rhode, 1996), outer and inner hair cell electrical activity (e.g., Sellick & Russell, 1979; Cheatham and Dallos, 1989, 1990, 1992; Nuttall & Dolan, 1993), and auditory nerve responses (e.g., Sachs & Kiang, 1968; Abbas & Sachs, 1976; Arthur, Pfeiffer, & Suga, 1971; DeIgutte, 1990). Tonal suppression methodology has also been applied clinically with SOAEs (Wilson, 1980; Zurek, 1981; Bargones & Burns, 1988; Long et al., 1993), DPOAEs (Brown & Kemp, 1984; Harris et al., 1992; Kummer et al., 1995; Abdala et al., 1996; Heitmann, Waldmann & Schnitzler, 1998), and TEOAEs (Kemp, 1979; Wit & Ritsma, 1980; Folsom et al., 1995; Neumann, 1994; Nuemann, Uppenkamp, & Kollmeier, 1997). Other authors have described similar findings for OAE suppression studies conducted with a menagerie of animal models (e.g., bats, rodents, gerbils, rabbits, lizards). With the technique, it is possible to produce OAE "suppression tuning curves" or STCs. STCs described with OAEs are one example of physiologic measures of cochlear frequency resolution, others approaches including ECochG and ABR (e.g., Teas et al., 1982; Klein, 1984; Folsom, 1985; Folsom & Wynne, 1987).

Tuning curves derived from selective tonal suppression of OAE responses have similar characteristics (width, slope, and Q_{10} values) to the traditional psychoacoustic tuning curves, although the latter tend to be narrower and have steeper slopes (Abdala et al., 1996). (*Note:* recall that the Q_{10} measure is a measure of tuning curve width calculated by determining the bandwith 10 dB above the tip of the tuning

Ipsilateral tonal suppression techniques are being used in studies of DPOAE properties and generators, as noted in Chapter 10. They are also being incorporated into at least one clinical DPOAE device (see the Hortmann contribution in Chapter 7 and the Heitmann et al., 1998).

curve, and dividing this bandwidth into the tip frequency.) These clinical investigations, conducted with infants (Bargones & Burns, 1988; Abdala et al., 1996), as well adults, have produced much basic information on frequency resolution of the cochlea and, in particular, the processes underlying OAEs. For example, early on Kemp and Brown, and others (Kemp & Brown, 1983; Brown & Kemp, 1984; Martin et al., 1987) reported that introduction of a suppressor tone between the f_1 and f_2 primary frequencies, and closest to the f_2, substantially reduced DPOAE amplitude, thus confirming that this region of overlap between the two traveling waves generated by the primaries was essential for the generation of DPOAEs. The tip of the STC, the frequency at which the suppressor is most effective (i.e., the lowest suppressor intensity level is needed to produce the predetermined criterion for suppression) corresponds mostly closely with the f_2 frequency. In contrast, even high suppressor intensity levels have less effect on the DPOAEs when presented at the actual DP place, or $2f_1-f_2$ (Brown & Kemp, 1984; Harris et al., 1992; Kummer et al., 1995). The contribution of both the f_2 region of the cochlea and the so-called DP place ($2f_1-2f_2$) to DPOAE responses has been, and continues to be, the topic of considerable research efforts (e.g., Kemp & Brown, 1983; Martin et al., 1987; Heitmann et al., 1998; Martin et al., 1999). There is some agreement that the DPOAEs we record in the ear canal, although mostly generated by cochlear activation in the f_2 region, can include energy reflected from the DP place under certain conditions when phase of the two components is aligned. In effect there is sometimes a primary, and a secondary, generator for DPOAEs. The energy arising from the DPs place is essentially a stimulus frequency OAE (SFOAE). Interactions (additive and subtractive) between these two generators may be responsible for the fine structure (peaks and valleys) in the DP gram (Shera & Zweig, 1991; Zweig & Shera, 1995; Heitmann et al., 1998). This explanation for DPOAE generation is supported by application of suppression techniques involving the presentation of a third tone in addition to f_1 and f_2 in the region of $2f_1-f_2$, which may either augment or diminish DPOAE amplitude, depending on the intensity levels of the tones and underlying DP fine structure (Heitmann et al., 1998). The reader is referred back to Chapters 2 and 4 for a detailed discussion of DPOAE generation and the underlying anatomic and physiologic concepts.

A recent paper by Carolina Abdala and colleagues (Abdala et al., 1996) at the House Ear Institute describing DPOAE suppression tuning curve findings for normal hearing healthy infants ($N = 16$) and adults ($N = 15$) will be highlighted in the explanation of this phenomenon. First, the authors recorded DPOAEs in the typical fashion, without a suppressor signal. Selected test parameters, such as the absolute and relative intensity levels of the primaries and the f_2/f_1 ratio, are summarized in Figure 5–10. Note that somewhat low primary intensities were used to enhance the likelihood of a suppression effect, as described

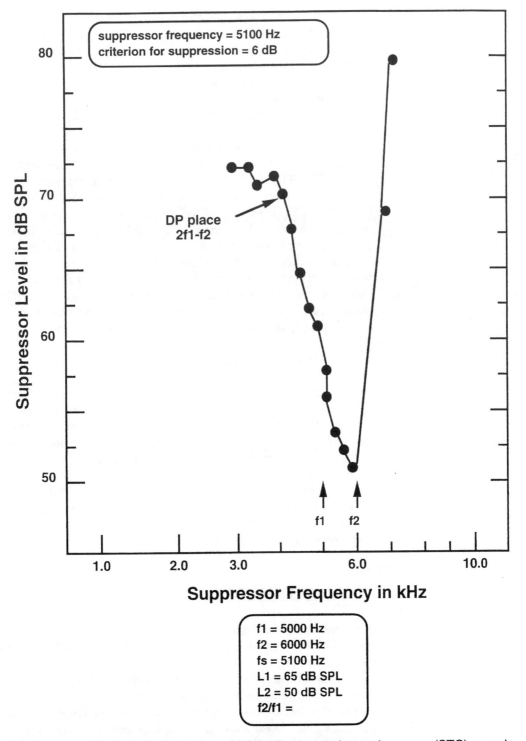

Figure 5–10. Schematic illustration of DPOAE suppression tuning curve (STC) record-ed from a normal hearing adult. (Adapted from Abdala et al, 1996.)

above. STCs were measured primaries representing low- (1500 Hz), mid- (3000 Hz), and high- (6000 Hz) frequency regions. Suppressor tones of different frequencies, some below and some above the f_2 frequency, were then presented during DPOAE measurement. Suppressor tone intensity was increased in 2 dB steps until the DPOAE amplitude for a given set of primaries was decreased by 6 dB. This was the criterion for suppression used in generating the STCs, following recommendations of Brown and Kemp (1984), which were based on minimizing the effects of measurement noise and increasing the speed of data acquisition. That is, the data points plotted in the example of a DPOAE STC illustrated schematically in the figure represent the suppressor intensity levels (verticle axis) that produced a 6 dB reduction in DPOAE amplitude for each of the suppressor frequencies (horizontal axis). In addition to developing DPOAE STCs, the authors collected psychoacoustic tuning curve (PTC) data from the adult subjects for the three above-mentioned frequencies. Among the authors' conclusions was the important observation that neonatal cochlear frequency resolution, at term birth, is similar to adults within the mid- and high-frequency region. As Abdala et al. (1996) suggest, "subsequent investigations applying the DPOAE suppression paradigm to other subject populations, such as premature infants, the elderly or mild to moderately hearing impaired individuals are warranted." (p. 48).

Even after a thorough review of the effects of the efferent system on OAEs, and the literature on contralateral and ipsilateral acoustic suppression, the clinician is justified in asking: "How does the efferent auditory system influence hearing?" With extended durations of noise (> 200 ms), which might be found in everyday listening environments, alterations in outer hair cell (and subsequently inner hair cell) function secondary to efferent effects reduce the responsiveness of the auditory system to the noise. Speech perception performance in noisy listening environments might then be improved (Humes et al., 1986; Kawase and Liberman, 1993 a,b; Licklider, 1948).

FINAL COMMENTS

Although OAEs are electrophysiologic responses, and OAE measurement is objective, analysis and interpretation of the findings is clinically challenging and very much influenced by a host of non-pathologic factors, as summarized at the beginning of this chapter (in Table 5–1). Many of these factors, such as subject age and gender or measurement noise, are ever present and unavoidable. Others, for example, ear canal acoustics and genetics, only need to be accounted for with certain test protocols and patients. And some factors, such as anesthetic agents, body temperature, or state of arousal, probably exert little or no influence on clinical measurement of OAEs for almost all patients.

CHAPTER

6

Distortion Product and Transient Evoked OAEs: Effect of Peripheral Auditory Dysfunction and Hearing Loss

THE EXTERNAL EAR
  Cerumen
  Vernix Caseosa in Newborn Infants

MIDDLE EAR DYSFUNCTION AND
CONDUCTIVE HEARING LOSS
  Experimental Variations in External Ear
    Canal Pressure
  Middle Ear Function and Dysfunction
  Comments

COCHLEAR DYSFUNCTION AND
SENSORY HEARING LOSS
   TEOAEs
   DPOAEs
   Summary

CLINICAL RELATION BETWEEN OAEs
AND SENSORY HEARING LOSS
   General Relation Among OAEs and
      Hearing Loss
   Cases Illustrating the Relation Among
      DPOAEs and Audiograms

The general relation between auditory dysfunction and OAEs is reviewed in this chapter. The discussion is limited to the two types of clinically evoked OAEs—transient and distortion product OAEs. A comparable review was presented for SOAEs in Chapter 3. Clinical applications of evoked OAEs in specific patient populations with various pathologic entities for auditory dysfunction are described in Chapters 8 (children) and 9 (adults).

THE EXTERNAL EAR

Cerumen

As stressed in Chapter 4, the external ear canal is a vital anatomic link in OAE measurement. Whenever OAS cannot be detected, or stimulus intensity is below the target level, the clinician is obligated to rule out occlusion by cerumen (earwax) of the ear canal or probe assembly port(s). Cerumen problems may interfere with OAE measurement in adult and pediatric populations. For adults and older children, otoscopic inspection of the ear canal is advisable before OAEs are recorded. Cerumen is never found in the ear canals of neonates and is not likely to be excessive in infancy and early childhood. Some patients in this age range often reject attempts at otoscopic inspection only if technical problems are encountered. Whether or not cerumen interferes with OAE measurement depends, to some extent, on the probe design and the consistency of the cerumen. There are, not unexpectedly, no formal published investigations of OAEs and cerumen.

Vernix Caseosa in Newborn Infants

Vernix caseosa—typically referred to simply as vernix—is a fatty (neutral lipid) residue of amniotic fluid found on a baby's skin immediately after delivery. The fetus was covered with vernix for the final few months of pregnancy. The chemical composition of vernix differs somewhat for preterm versus term infants (Wysocki, Graunaug, O'Neill, & Hahnel, 1981). Although vernix does not appear to have antibacterial properties, it may offer a mechanical barrier to passage of bacteria from the external environment through the skin (Joglekar, 1980). Vernix is generally washed off within hours after birth during baby's first bath. For a day or two, however, it may remain as a white or grayish-white, creamy, lotionlike substance within cracks and crevices in babies' skin and also in the external ear canal. When an OAE probe is inserted into the ear canal of a newborn infant within this time frame, vernix may become lodged in the ports (tubes) carrying the stimulus to the ear canal or directing the OAEs from the ear canal back to the microphone. Either possibility can interfere with OAE measurement. It is also possible, although less likely, for vernix to totally occlude the ear canal lumen (opening), thus attenuating stimulus delivery to the cochlea and outward transmission of the OAEs to the probe. The problem of vernix and related debris in the external ear canal of neonates is not inconsequential. Eavey (1993) noted that ear canal debris precluded examination of the tympanic membrane in over 25% of a series of infants in an NICU. In a healthy series of 81 full-term babies, Cavanaugh (1987) reported that vernix obscured the eardrum in 19%, even 72 hours after birth. In an earlier study, McClellan and Webb (1961) encountered his problem in 47% of a series of healthy infants.

Papers published in 1993 by two groups with expertise in newborn hearing screening are most relevant to this discussion (Chang, Vohr, Norton, & Lekas, 1993; Thornton, Kimm, Kennedy, & Cafarelli-Dies, 1993). In a series of healthy term neonates reported by Chang et al (1993), 10% had total obstruction by vernix of the external ear canal, and there was partial obstruction for another 33% of the infants. The TEOAE failure rate was very high (34%) prior to ear examination. Clearing of the external ear canal with a pediatric swab moistened by an alcohol wipe failed to remove all debris for 30%. Nonetheless, the failure rate dropped to only 9% after ear examination and cleaning. TEOAE amplitude also increased from the initial recording to the OAE recording after the ear examination and cleaning. Citing clinical experiences, these authors along with several colleagues in a related publication noted that collapsing ear canals were a factor in the obstruction of some infants, in addition to or in combination with, vernix and debris (Chang et al., 1993; Vohr et al., 1993). Chang and colleagues concluded that, "an examination of the ear canal is warranted whenever an ear fails to pass the OAE test" (p. 281). The feasibility of including ear examinations into protocols for newborn hearing screening is discussed in Chapter 8.

The results of a British group of investigators (Thornton et al., 1993) confirm the important negative effects of vernix and collapsing ear canals on OAE outcome, also noting that, "it would appear that neonatal screening, carried out within the first 3 days postpartum, could be improved by cleaning the ear canal and removing any debris" (p. 324). However, according to these authors, hearing screening pass rates for a TEOAE technique were still rather low on day 1 (after birth), even after ear canal cleaning.

Pass rates and TEOAE amplitude, especially in the 1000 to 3000 Hz region, continued to increase within the next few days. Analysis of TEOAE changes as a function of frequency, in combination with tympanometric data on middle ear function, suggested to Thornton et al. (1993) that factors in addition to vernix and middle ear transmission were affecting the OAE findings in the days after birth.

Vernix, which is not soluble in water and cannot be removed by simple irrigation of the external ear canal, clearly must be reckoned with if OAEs are to be recorded from neonates. The negative impact of vernix on OAE screening outcome, and suggestions for circumventing this practical problem, are described in the section on newborn hearing screening in Chapter 8.

MIDDLE EAR DYSFUNCTION AND CONDUCTIVE HEARING LOSS

The middle ear is, as stressed already in Chapters 1 and 2, an unavoidable and critical anatomic link in the measurement of any type of OAE (Table 6–1). Most procedures for assessing auditory function require transmission of the stimulus inward to the cochlea with measurement of either a behavioral or electrophysiologic response from more central (proximal) regions of the auditory system. OAE measurement, in contrast, requires a "round-trip ticket" through the middle ear. The middle ear, therefore, influences inward propagation of the stimulus and outward propagation of the response (the OAE). Furthermore, the well-recognized amplification of the stimulus strength provided by the middle ear system during inward transmission of energy presumably does not contribute appreciably, or perhaps at all, in the other direction. Indeed, in comparison to inward or forward transmission, OAE energy is lost, rather than gained, during the return trip from the cochlea to the ear canal by up to about 15 dB, as estimated by Kemp (1980). The critical and dual role of the middle ear in OAE measurement, even in otologically normal subjects, is often cited in the OAE literature (e.g., Kemp, Ryan, & Bray, 1990; Probst, Lonsbury-Martin, &

Table 6–1. Factors influencing the effect of middle ear status and dysfunction on otoacoustic emissions (OAEs) and contributing the wide range of variability in OAE findings clinically.

✔ Effect of middle ear status on forward (inward) propagation of stimulus energy to the cochlea

✔ Effect of middle ear status on backward (outward) propagation of OAE energy to the external ear canal

✔ Frequency region of the stimulus (e.g., low frequencies are more affected by the common stiffness abnormalities in middle ear functioning)

✔ Intensity level of the stimulus used to evoke the OAEs

✔ Type of middle ear dysfunction/disorder (e.g., perforation of the tympanic membrane, negative middle ear pressure, otitis media, osscicular chain fixation, disarticulation of the ossicular chain)

✔ Influence of the middle ear dysfunction on aural immittance/impedance and/or reflectance (i.e., the greater the effect on these measures of middle ear function, the greater the predicted effect on OAEs)

✔ Combined influence on middle ear function of pathology and the effect of anesthetic agents and/or sedation

✔ Whether OAEs are measured at ambient pressure or compensation for middle ear pressure

✔ Magnitude of the conductive hearing loss component (i.e., the air-bone gap)

Martin, 1991; Naeve, Margolis, Levine, & Fournier, 1992; Owens, McCoy, Lonsbury-Martin, & Martin, 1992; Osterhammel, Nielson, & Rasmussen, 1993; Thornton et al., 1993; Wada, Ohyama, Kobayashi, Sunaga, & Koike, 1993; Engdahl, Arneson, & Mair, 1994; Richter, Hauser, & Lohle, 1994). The importance of considering middle ear status is even greater in clinical applications of OAEs, particularly among patients in whom the prevalence of middle ear disorders is high, namely, infants and young babies. Beginning with the earliest clinical papers on OAEs, the impact of various common middle ear diseases, such as otitis media and otosclerosis, on OAE measurement has been repeatedly cited (e.g., Bonfils, Bertrand, & Uziel, 1988; Bonfils & Trotoux, 1989; Bonfils et al., 1990; Margolis & Trine, 1997). Further complicating the interpretation of clinical OAE findings is the dependence on frequency of inward and outward transmission of energy through the middle ear, and the possibility that one type of middle ear anomaly or pathology might exert a greater influence on inward propagation of the stimulus, whereas another might have more impact on the outward propagation of the OAEs (e.g., Margolis & Trine, 1997). The clinician would, no doubt, prefer a straightforward and rather simple answer to the practical question: How does middle ear dysfunction influence OAEs? In reality, however, there is no single or simple answer to this question. Rather, as summarized in Table 6–2, the answer for any given patient can vary widely due to complex and usually unpredictable interactions among many diverse factors producing different effects on OAEs. Even in the otologically pristine normal ear, there is a clear relationship between middle ear transmission properties, or "dynamic characteristics" (Wada et al., 1985), such as the resonance frequency and the OAE response parameters (e.g., amplitude).

Table 6–2. Effects of middle ear disorders on otoacoustic emissions, summarized from the literature and clinical experience.

Type of Disorder	Description of the Effect
Negative middle ear pressure	✔ OAEs are recorded except In extreme negative pressure when the air-bone gap exceeds about 15 dB.
	✔ OAE amplitude is usually below normal limits.
	✔ Low frequency OAE components (<2000 Hz) are affected first, and more seriously, than high-frequency OAEs.
Tympanic membrane perforation	✔ OAEs are recorded if there Is only a small perforation which is not associated with active middle ear pathology (e.g., otitis media with effusion, cholesteatoma).
	✔ OAE amplitude may be within normal limits across the frequency region of 500 to 8000 Hz, or within normal limits only for higher frequencles.
Ventilation tube	✔ OAEs may be recorded If there Is a patent (open) tube, and no active middle ear pathology, and hearing sensitivity is normal, but the likelihood of OAE presence under these conditions is less than 50%.
	✔ OAE amplitude may be withIn normal limits across the frequency region of 500 to 8000 Hz or within normal limits only for higher frequencles.
	✔ For TEOAEs with click stimuli, the temporal waveform may show an unusual triphasic pattern (expected intensity level Initially, followed by smaller intensity level, and then back to the expected level).
Otitis media	✔ OAEs are rarely recorded unless the air-bone gap is small (less than 15 dB).
	✔ OAE amplitude invariably below normal limits for all frequencies.
Otosclerosis	✔ OAEs typically not detected at any frequency for any degree of hearing loss.

Sources: Owens et al., 1992; Prieve, 1992; Kemp, Ryan, & Bray, 1990; Cullington, Kumar, & Flood, 1998.

Careful documentation of middle ear status by otoscopy and even more so, aural immittance (impedance) or reflectance measurements certainly will provide at least a partial answer to the question in many cases (Holte, Margolis, & Cavanaugh, 1991; Hunter & Margolis, 1992; Ling, & Bulen, 1992; Wada, Ohyama, Kobayashi, Koike, & Noguchi, 1993; Burns, Campbell, & Arehart, 1994; Wada et al., 1995; Keefe, Keefe & Levi, 1996; Tubis & Talmadge, 1998). And understanding what is known about the effect of middle ear dysfunction on OAEs is important for exploiting the application of OAEs in most clinical populations. Literature on the relationship between OAE findings and middle ear status will now be reviewed.

Experimental Variations in External Ear Canal Pressure

Several investigators have described the effects on the three major OAE types of manipulation in external ear canal pressure among otologically and audiometrically normal subjects (Naeve et al., 1992; Trine, Hirsch, & Margolis, 1993). Although not necessarily equivalent to actual middle ear pressure dysfunction (see below), OAE findings with experimentally induced pressure differences do isolate the immediate effects of pressure (versus indeterminable residual influences of prior middle ear pathology plus pressure changes) and provide some clinically useful information. The basic premise with this methodology is that the introduction of positive pressure into the external ear canal essentially simulates naturally occurring negative middle ear pressure. That is, the eardrum is pushed inward, producing a mechanical effect on middle ear function similar to a retracted tympanic membrane. These studies also shed some light on the effects of ear canal pressure changes on the spectra of both the stimulus and the OAEs. As noted in Chapter 3, ear canal pressure clearly is a factor in SOAE measurement (e.g., Schloth & Zwicker, 1983). This discussion will focus exclusively on literature reported for TEOAEs and DPOAEs.

When external ear canal pressure is altered from normal atmospheric pressure (0 daPa) by 100 daPa or 100 mm H_2O, amplitude is reduced by approximately 2 to 3 dB for TEOAEs and up to 8 dB for DPOAE (Bray, 1989; Robinson & Haughton, 1991; Naeve et al., 1992; Veuillet, Collet, & Morgon, 1992; Osterhammel, Nielsen, & Rasmussen, 1993). The decrease in amplitude (and for TEOAEs a corresponding reduction in reproducibility) occurs for both positive and negative pressure directions, is additive for each unit of 100 daPa, and is greatest for the lowest frequencies within the OAE spectrum (500 to 1000 Hz) and progressively less for higher frequency bands. Therefore, even modest negative ear canal pressure may reduce OAE response values (amplitude and/or reproducibility) to below normal limits. It is likely that equivalent amounts of negative middle ear (versus ear canal) pressure change produce even more pronounced reductions in OAEs (Owens et al., 1992). According to Margolis and Trine (1997), these changes are mostly due to the effect of increased middle ear stiffness on outward (backward) transmission of OAE energy from the cochlea to the ear canal.

There are also several investigations of external ear canal pressure manipulations with DPOAEs (Lonsbury-Martin et al., 1990; Hauser et al., 1991; Osterhammel, Nielsen, & Rasmussen, 1993). In a study of 16 ears of 8 adult subjects with normal haring and normal middle ear function, Osterhammel and colleagues (1993) found a sizeable decrease (about 8 dB) in DPOAE amplitude for primary frequencies in the 1000 Hz region as pressure was deviated 100 daPa in the positive or negative direction from 0 daPa (the reduction was approximately 3 to 4 dB for a change of 50 daPa), and amplitude decreased a total of 15 dB by +200 or −400 daPa. The effect of pressure changes was much less obvious for higher stimulus frequencies consistent with earlier findings (e.g., Bray, 1989; Hauser et al., 1993). In fact, positive pressure changes in the ear canal actually were associated with an increase in DPOAE amplitude for stimulus frequencies of 6000 and 8000 Hz. In general, negative pressure changes in the ear canal had a greater effect on DPOAE amplitude than positive changes, which is also consistent with earlier findings (e.g., Robinson & Haughton, 1991). There was considerable individual variability in the pressure effects, which has implications for clinical interpretation of DPOAEs in middle ear dysfunction. Osterhammel et al. (1993) reminded the reader that positive pressure in the ear canal is analogous to negative middle ear pressure, as the tympanic membrane is moved inward (medially), and both conditions increase stiffness of the middle ear system. However, with actual negative pressure in the middle ear space, the stapes footplate is displaced outward relative to the cochlea, whereas the opposite relative displacement occurs with positive external ear canal pressure.

Hauser, Probst, and Harris (1993) published the only description of the effect of pressure manipulations on SOAEs, TEOAEs, and DPOAEs. A total of 61 normal-hearing adult subjects were subjected to atmospheric pressure changes, in a chamber, from positive 9000 Pa down to −2500 Pa. The mechanism was somewhat like the pressure changes associated with flying. There were SOAE data for 21 subjects, TEOAE data for 20 subjects, and DPOAE data for 20 subjects, all seated in the pressure chamber. The authors concluded that pressure-related reductions in amplitude for each of the three types of OAEs were greater, on the average, for lower (e.g., up to about 1000 Hz) versus mid-frequencies (especially for DPOAEs). As an example, the average reduction in amplitude for a 1000 Pa pressure change for TEOAEs was 1.08 dB SPL at 500 Hz and 0.23 dB SPL at 4000 Hz, whereas for DPOAEs the reduction was 5.96 dB SPL at a primary geometric mean (GM) of 1000 Hz (DP at 614 Hz) and actually +0.13 dB SP at a GM of 6000 Hz. Among the three types, pressure changes in the high-frequency region were relatively greater for SOAEs, less for TEOAEs, and least for DPOAEs. Importantly, for clinical applications, there were substantial intersubject differences in the effects of pressure changes on OAEs.

Finally, among papers describing the effect of ear canal manipulations on OAEs, one of the most unique was published by Stephen and Badham (1996). TEOAEs were measured as usual with air in the external ear canal, and immediately after, leaving the probe position unchanged, with infusion of first helium and then with the external ear canal filled with sulphur hexafluoride gas. An assumption in this study was that TEOAE amplitude recorded from an ear depends, in part, on the acoustic load of the ear canal on the tympanic membrane.

As the authors noted, "increasing the external auditory canal loading should reduce the amplitude of the signal, while reducing the load should increase the amplitude" (Stephen & Badham, 1996, p. 191). Following this study of the effect of changes in ear canal acoustic impedance on TEOAEs, the authors concluded that, "the frequency characteristics of the OAEs do depend on the velocity of sound of the gas in the external ear canal. This can only occur if the observed oscillations are generated in the external canal . . . the delayed acoustic components measured in the external canal in response to an acoustic impulse noise arise principally from the passive impedance of the auditory system" (pp. 192–193). This is not to imply that OAEs are independent of cochlear function but, rather, that ear canal impedance is a factor in OAE measurement.

Middle Ear Function and Dysfunction

Animal studies with experimentally produced tympanic membrane or middle ear disorders suggest that they differentially affect inward and outward propagation of energy and consequently OAEs. Simulation of increased mass of the tympanic membrane, for example, was associated with some reduction of inward transmission of energy to the cochlea but appeared to have a greater effect on the outward transmission of energy from the cochlea (Wiederhold, 1993). In contrast, a small experimentally induced tympanic membrane perforation almost exclusively altered inward transmission, rather than propagation of the OAEs from the cochlea to the ear canal.

Neonatal Amniotic Fluid and Mesenchyme

In most neonates, amniotic fluid persists within the middle ear space only for about 1 day. By 48 hours after birth, physical examination usually shows that the middle ear is aerated and the tympanic membrane mobile (Jaffe, Hurtado, & Hurtado, 1967). It is important to point out here that the cellular composition and practical implications of amniotic fluid are distinctly different from the characteristics of the fluid in otis media. In one postmortem investigation, deSA (1973) reported that 55 of 130 infants (42%) had amniotic debris within the middle ear space. Eavey (1993), in another histopathologic study of deceased infants from an NICU population, found amniotic fluid cellular content in 90 of 111 temporal bones (81%).

Mesenchyme is a form of connective tissue, which is usually located between epithelium and bone. The fetal middle ear contains mesenchyme, but the embryonic tissue is either resorbed near the end of pregnancy or dissipates soon after birth. There are, however, a few reports of mesenchyme persisting within the middle ear space for up to a year after birth (e.g., Guggenheim, 1971). Again, citing the historic postmortem portion of the study by Eavey (1993), substantial amounts of mesenchyme (filling more than 60% of middle ear space) were found in 13 of 111 temporal bones (12%).

Neonatal Otitis Media

There is no doubt that otitis media can occur in neonates and is a problem mostly for infants in the NICU, although the actual prevalence is debated (McClellan et al., 1962; Jaffe et al., 1970; Warren & Stool, 1971; Bland, 1972; deSA, 1973; Shurin, Pelton, & Klein, 1976; Tetzlaff, Ashworth, & Nelson, 1977; Berman et al., 1978; Pestalozza, Romagoli, & Tessitore, 1988). One group of investigators (Balkany et al., 1978; Berman et al., 1978) reported abnormal tympanic membrane mobility that was considered compatible with otitis media in 30% of 125 premature infants within the first day to 4 months after birth. Bacterial otitis media was confirmed in 10 of 13 infants who underwent tympanocentesis. The other babies in this series were receiving antibiotics already, and tympanocentesis was viewed as unjustified clinically. These authors concluded that "otitis media occurs frequently among premature infants who are hospitalized in an NICU" (p. 193). deSA (1973) confirmed otitis media histologically (in stillbirths and neonatal deaths) for a lower proportion of 13% of infants ($N = 30$). However, Warren and Stool (1971) documented evidence of otitis media for 3 of 127 premature infants, or only 2%. Some perinatal factors putting an infant at risk for hearing impairment (e.g., prematurity and asphyxia) are also mentioned as contributing to higher proportions of otitis media. There is general agreement that otitis media is rare in healthy term infants (Pestalozza et al., 1988). However, even in this population middle ear status and function are not necessarily normal by the usual standards. For example, using pneumatic otoscopy in a study of 81 healthy, full-term babies, Cavanaugh (1978) found that "tympanic membrane dullness, decreased light reflex, and diminished translucence occurred in more than 90% of the infants during the first 3 days of life and declined to 26% or less by 4 months of age" (p. 520). He attributed these findings in part to the presence of unresorbed amniotic fluid within the middle ear space.

The definitive investigation of neonatal middle ear status, including the presence of amniotic fluid, mesenchyme, and otitis media, is reported in a monograph by Dr. Ronald Eavey (1993). The paper is subdivided into two clinical sections, one on clinical otoscopic observations and the other on temporal bone histologic observations, and one section describing findings for an animal model. Clinical data were limited to 44 infants admitted to a neonatal intensive care unit, but these subjects were otoscopically examined daily. An abnormal otoscopic appearance was reported for 97.7% of the neonatal ears. Furthermore, postmortem histopathologic study revealed purulent otitis media in 24 of 111 temporal bones (22%). And, in three cases, because this observation was made within hours after birth, there was the suggestion of intrauterine otitis media. Eavey (1993) concluded that, "the otoscopic appearance of the neonate in the neonatal intensive care unit is nearly universally abnormal" (p. 1). These findings argue against exclusive reliance on OAEs as a screening tool of auditory function, at least in the NICU population.

Developmental Changes in Middle Ear Function

The middle ear is not functionally mature even in term infants. This point was noted in Chapter 3 when developmental changes in SOAEs were reviewed. However, the robust OAEs that characterize the normal-hearing term infant are evidence that middle ear immaturity is not a critical limitation clinically.

Negative Middle Ear Pressure (Natural)

In contrast to the reports of experimental manipulations of ear canal pressure on OAEs (noted above), several investigators have examined the effects of negative middle ear pressure on OAEs in selected patients (Trine, Hirsh, & Margolis, 1993; Marshall, Heller, & Westhusin, 1997). The results of the systematic investigation of a subject with fluctuating middle ear pressures reported by Marshall and colleagues (1997) will be summarized here. Relatively modest amounts of negative pressure (e.g., even as little as −40 daPa and more negative) significantly reduced TEOAE amplitude, particularly from spectral regions of about 1000 Hz up to 3000 Hz. For TEOAE response frequencies above 2500 Hz, negative middle ear pressures of −75 daPa and greater also produced a clinically significant decrease in TEOAE amplitude. Such statements based on the single subject in the Marshall et al. (1997) study cannot, of course, be generalized to all persons with eustachian tube dysfunction and middle ear pressure anomalies. These investigators also showed that experimentally induced changes in ear canal (positive) pressure were quite similar to actual negative middle ear pressure.

One issue of interest clinically is whether compensation of naturally occurring negative middle ear pressure by inducing an equivalent negative pressure in the ear canal restores the OAE response to its ambient pressure (normal) state. Marshall et al. (1997) found that compensation of negative midde ear pressure by the introduction of an equivalent negative pressure in the external ear canal was not precise for all TEOAE frequency regions. It produced overcompensation (artificially higher TEOAE amplitudes) for low- and mid-frequency regions. Fortuitously, however, the compensation approach seemed to be effective for higher TEOAE frequencies (approximately 2000 Hz and above). Thus, compensation offers promise as a clinically feasible approach for maximizing OAE amplitude, at least for transient OAEs for those commonly encountered patients (especially children) with negative middle ear pressure. This strategy may have contributed to the accuracy of OAE applications, such as newborn hearing screening.

The clinical studies just mentioned were all limited to TEOAEs. Other investigators have utilized animal models of middle ear transmission to assess the effects of abnormalities on DPOAEs (e.g., Matthews et al., 1981; Matthews, 1983). Zhang and Abbas (1997) developed a surgical animal (guinea pig) model for manipulating middle ear pressure and then assessed the effects of pressure changes on the $2f_1-f_2$ DPOAE. In a rather clever research design, the authors included simultaneous measurement of the cochlear microphonic (from the ECochG) to isolate the effects of middle ear pressure alterations on inward propagation of stimulus transmission.

DPOAE measurement, of course, included the effects of pressure changes on both inward and outward energy transmission, but by utilizing the CM data the authors were able to subtract the contribution of the former. Negative pressure (from –25 to –100 mm H_2O) influenced DPOAE measurements more than positive pressure, and for all frequencies tested. The authors speculated that low frequencies were affected by tympanic membrane stiffness, whereas functional changes in the incudostapedial joint affected higher frequency DPOAE data. Relatively greater positive pressures influenced DPOAEs, but only for low frequencies. The effects of middle ear pressure appeared to be equivalent for the inward transmission of the stimulus and for the outward transmission of the OAEs.

Otitis Media

The likelihood of detecting any OAE response in patients with otitis media decreases markedly with the degree of hearing loss. OAEs are invariably abnormal in patients with flat tympanograms and hearing thresholds exceeding adult normal limits (e.g., greater than 25 dB HL). Without regard to degree of hearing loss, TEOAEs are recordable in less than 1 of 10 children with the diagnosis of otitis media (Van Cauwenberge et al., 1995). Similarly, most children with Down syndrome and related middle ear dysfunction have very reduced DPOAE amplitudes or lack detectable DPOAE responses (Hasten, Skotnicka, Midro, & Musiatowicz, 1998). As expected, OAEs in otitis media are observed only if hearing sensitivity is reasonably normal, and even then amplitudes are abnormally small.

Ventilation (Pressure Equalization) Tubes and Grommets

Given the widespread practice of ventilation tube insertion in clinical otolaryngology, it would be very useful clinically to understand the potential effect on OAEs. The general conclusion is that OAEs are recordable with ventilation tubes or grommets in place, but amplitude may be reduced (Daya et al., 1966; Owens et al., 1993; Amedee, 1995;

Tilanus et al., 1995; Richardson et al., 1996). If OAEs are reliably present and, in particular, within the normal region, one can conclude that: (1) the tubes are patent, (2) there can be little or no middle ear dysfunction, and (3) significant cochlear (outer hair cell) dysfunction is effectively ruled out. However, OAEs are less likely to be detected (from 10 to 20% of ears) immediately after insertion, while the patient is still under anesthesia. Cullington, Kumar, and Flood (1998) performed TEOAE measurement following grommet insertion for 108 children (aged 1 to 11 years). None of the subjects had undergone adenoidectomy or tonsillectomy at the same time. The presence of middle ear effusion was documented at the time of surgery. TEOAEs were categorized simply as a pass if overall reproducibility exceeded 50% and the TEOAE amplitude minus noise difference was 3 dB or greater for frequency bands in the 1600, 2400, and 3200 Hz regions. Most of the children had pure-tone thresholds of 20 dB or better by behavioral audiometry. Among 209 ears for cooperative children (5% of the series did not cooperate), 46% of the ears yielded pass outcomes. As the amount of effusion decreased (based on surgeon's estimates), there was a slight tendency for the OAE pass rate to increase. Still, only 32% of the children passed the TEOAE screening bilaterally. As a result, most patients would have required additional auditory assessment efforts. There was no clear explanation for this low pass rate. In another recent study of TEOAE before and after ventilation tube placement (N = 56 ears of 33 children), Chang, Jang, & Rhee (1998) reported significant postoperative increase in OAE amplitude for children with middle ear effusion, whereas a group of children without middle ear effusion showed no changes in TEOAE amplitude with tube insertion. Further study of the effects of tubes and grommets with DPOAEs is warranted, including DPOAE measurement with relatively high frequency stimuli (above 2000 Hz). In any event, ventilation tubes and grommets certainly do not preclude OAE recording. If OAEs are present, then significant cochlear (outer hair cell) impairment and middle ear dysfunction can be quickly and easily ruled out.

Sedation and Anesthesia

Some anesthetic agents, such as nitrous oxide, alter middle ear pressure as gases diffuse into the middle ear space (e.g., Thomsen et al., 1965; Waun et al., 1967; Singh & Kirk, 1979; Richards et al., 1982). Reduction of OAE amplitude during anesthesia with these drugs has been documented (Hauser et al., 1992). Abdul-Baqui (1991) reported that use of a common conscious sedative, chloral hydrate, also appears to be associated with an increase in middle ear pressure (of from +19 to +219 mm H_2O). Tympanometric data were collected from 34 infants and young children before and 40 and 60 minutes after the drug was administered. Presumably, then, the effect of these sedation-related middle ear pressure changes on OAEs would be similar to those of experimentally induced negative pressure changes in the external ear canal described earlier. Given the popularity of chloral hydrate as the sedative of choice during auditory brainstem response (ABR) assessment of hearing sensitivity in very young and difficult-to-test children, this factor should be considered in the clinical interpretation of OAEs in pediatric populations.

Comments

Elimination of middle ear disease or dysfunction at the time of OAE measurement is rarely a viable option. However, at least three modifications in clinical OAE protocols can, in some cases, minimize the negative influences of some minor, yet very common, middle ear disorders. First, as in other audiologic procedures employing air-conducted signals, increasing stimulus intensity level in OAE measurement will produce increased inward (forward) transmission of energy through the middle ear. Studies of TEOAE input/output functions show a characteristic flattening or saturation of amplitude as stimulus intensity levels exceed 50 dB SPL (see Chapter 4 for details). For types of middle ear dysfunction having a relatively greater influence on inward versus outward propagation, increasing stimulus intensity to reach this saturation point may contribute to the emergence of detectable OAEs. For example, in persons with experimentally induced negative or positive middle ear pressures of up to +200 or −200 daPa, Naeves et al. (1992) reported augmentation of TEOAE amplitude by 5 to 6 dB as stimulus intensity was raised from 60 to 90 dB SPL.

Second, OAE measurement is enhanced with a deep and snug probe fit in the ear canal. This point was stressed in Chapter 4. In addition to increasing the attenuation of unwanted ambient (environmental) sounds, the optimal probe placement reduces ear canal volume between the tip of the probe and the tympanic membrane. A reduction in the volume of this ear canal cavity contributes to OAE measurement by both maximizing the effective stimulus intensity level and maximizing the OAE acoustic energy generated (actually transduced from mechanical energy) by the tympanic membrane. This point was also noted in the discussion of developmental characteristics of OAEs (in Chapter 5). This is an example of a well-known principle in acoustics: The smaller the volume of a cavity, the greater the sound pressure level.

The final modification in the test protocol, which is not yet possible with most clinical OAE devices, involves adjusting ear canal pressure prior to OAE measurement. This is routinely done prior to acoustic reflex testing. Tympanometry is completed, and then acoustic reflexes are stimulated at the point of maximum compliance (minimum immittance/impedance), or the "tympanogram pressure peak." Although not an effective strategy for all middle ear pathologies, alignment of external ear canal and middle ear pressures might very well enhance OAE recordings for patients with commonly encountered middle ear disorders due to eustachian tube dysfunction and/or serous otitis media. Formal investigation of this concept with TEOAEs, that is, compensation of clinically deviant middle ear pressure with an appropriate ear canal pressure, demonstrated consistent increases in amplitude values (Trine et al., 1993). Given the reduction in OAE amplitude (4 to 6 dB) associated with even slight deviations from normal ear canal pressure from 0 to −200 daPa (e.g., Naeve et al., 1992), and the prevalence of such negative middle ear pressure (type C tympanograms) clinically, routinely making adjustments for middle ear pressure would presumably play an important role clinically in optimizing OAE findings.

COCHLEAR DYSFUNCTION AND SENSORY HEARING LOSS

The objective in most clinical applications of OAEs is to describe cochlear function. There are a number of variations of this general theme. With newborn hearing screening, for example, OAEs are used in isolation with the goal of distinguishing infants with normal hearing sensitivity from those with at least some degree of sensory hearing loss. On the other hand, in pediatric diagnostic audiologic assessment, OAEs are applied within a test battery in an attempt to either document normal auditory functioning or describe precisely the site of auditory dysfunction. The results of OAE measurement are an important piece of the diagnostic puzzle, but alone they cannot be relied on to define "hearing." Only behavioral audiometry procedures, especially those involving complex speech signals, really evaluate "hearing." Hearing requires the ongoing integration of a host of behavioral auditory processes (see Table 6–3). Other audiologic procedures, such as immittance measures, ABR, and OAEs, provide information on specific auditory functions. While this information contributes importantly to screening for hearing impairment and to describing the site of auditory dysfunction associated with hearing impairment, especially for patients who cannot be easily assessed with sophisticated behavioral audiometry (e.g., infants and young children), clinicians cannot use the results of these electrophysiologic procedures directly to make statements about hearing. In addition to inadequately describing hearing, in the all-inclusive use of the term, there are multiple reasons why OAEs will not ever replace the basic audiogram as a measure of hearing sensitivity (Table 6–4). Discrepancies between OAEs and the audiogram need not be viewed with concern or suspicion. Rather, they provide evidence of the unique contributions of OAEs to assessment of the auditory system. That is, OAEs complement the pure-tone audiogram, providing enhanced sensitivity to cochlear (outer hair cell) dysfunction and, usually, an electrophysiologic confirmation of behav-

Table 6–3. Selected auditory processes or behaviors that are involved in hearing.

- ■ Intensity
  - ✔ threshold (absolute sensitivity)
  - ✔ intensity discrimination
  - ✔ loudness and dynamic range (perceptual maps)
- ■ Frequency
  - ✔ resolution (cochlear tuning)
  - ✔ discrimination (difference limens)
  - ✔ representation (tonotopic and perceptual maps)
- ■ Temporal processing
  - ✔ resolution (detection of gaps between sounds)
  - ✔ duration discrimination
  - ✔ temporal integration
  - ✔ amplitude-envelope coding
- ■ Binaural processing and localization
- ■ Attention
  - ✔ responsiveness and preference
  - ✔ habituation
  - ✔ distraction and selective attention
- ■ Speech processing
  - ✔ voice discrimination
  - ✔ phonetic discrimination
  - ✔ phonetic identification
  - ✔ stress and prosody
  - ✔ speech processing in noise
  - ✔ degraded speech processing

---

ioral responses. Prior to discussing selected literature on the influences of cochlear auditory dysfunction on OAEs, a few qualifications are in order. The clinician expecting data quantifying a precise relation between OAE parameters and specific types or degrees of sensory hearing impairment will, no doubt, be disappointed. For the results of a study to be generalized with confidence to routine clinical application of OAEs, at least three criteria should probably be met: (1) OAE data were collected with commercially available devices (in the United States the devices must be FDA-approved); (2) OAE data were not collected in a sound-treated room but, rather, in a quiet clinic room, as it is not feasible to always perform OAE measurement in a sound booth; (3) noise floors during OAE measurement were adequately low (i.e.,

Table 6–4. The relation between OAEs and the audiogram, and reasons for discrepancies between these two clinical measures of auditory function. In short, OAEs will never replace the audiogram as a measure of hearing thresholds.

- OAE measurement is not a substitute for pure-tone audiometry. Clinical audiologists should not be concerned or discouraged, but, rather, excited and encouraged by differences in patient findings for pure-tone audiometry versus OAEs. Indeed, if OAEs and pure-tone audiometry findings were consistently in agreement, there would be little clinical value in recording OAEs.

- OAE findings are an almost direct measure of outer hair cell functional integrity—"almost" because middle ear function is also a factor in OAE measurement, whereas pure-tone audiometry is dependent on status of the cochlea, eighth nerve, central auditory system, and auditory perceptual factors, as well as the middle ear.

- OAE stimuli typically include many frequencies that are not assessed with pure-tone audiometry. In fact, in comparing findings for OAEs and pure-tone audiometry, it is possible that none of the test frequencies are the same for both measures. For example, none of the OAE test frequencies f_2 or geometric mean of f_1 and f_2) fall on an audiometric frequency (e.g., 1000 or 2000 Hz).

- Dysfunction (versus destruction) of some outer hair cells is likely to be reflected by less than normal motility and reduced OAE amplitude, without affecting hearing sensitivity for steady state (pure tone) signals at audiometric frequencies. Abnormal OAE findings may be recorded in a variety of patient populations with normal audiograms yet some cochlear dysfunction, including patients with:
  - ✔ tinnitus
  - ✔ excessive noise/music exposure
  - ✔ ototoxicity, including aspirin use
  - ✔ vestibular pathology.

- Abnormal OAE findings may also be recorded in a very small proportion of persons with normal audiograms and no apparent history or clinical signs of cochlear dysfunction.

- Normal OAEs may be recorded in patients with abnormal audiograms, including patients with:
  - ✔ functional or nonorganic hearing loss (malingerers)
  - ✔ reduced attention or attention deficits
  - ✔ psychogenic hearing loss (e.g., conversion hysteria)
  - ✔ eighth nerve (neural) auditory dysfunction
  - ✔ central auditory nervous system dysfunction.

- Normal OAEs are also recorded in patients with hearing loss due exclusively to inner hair cell damage or dysfunction secondary to, for example, carboplatin ototoxicity or genetically determined factors.

- The relation between OAEs and pure-tone audiometry findings is highly dependent on the intensity level of the stimuli used to evoke OAEs. That is, for high stimulus intensity levels, OAEs will be detectable despite a mild-to-moderate degree of hearing loss. At low stimulus intensity levels, however, OAEs may be abnormal even with slight decreases in hearing thresholds and an overall suggestion of "hearing within normal limits."

- OAEs are not typically recordable when sensory (outer hair cell) hearing impairment exceeds 40 to 50 dB HL. In other words, hearing loss ranging from this degree to profound (no response to signals at equipment intensity limits) is similarly associated with the simple absence of detectable OAEs.

- OAE response parameters (e.g., amplitude) are characterized by considerable intersubject and interpatient variability, even among persons with very similar pure-tone audiometric findings.

- OAE findings cannot, at least now, be reliably correlated with pure-tone audiometric threshold levels nor used for accurate estimation of any degree of hearing loss.

below the level of even a very small OAE amplitude); (4) etiologies for sensorineural hearing loss were defined; and (5) OAE response parameters (e.g., amplitude) were described as a function of varying degrees of hearing loss. OAE findings are often profoundly influenced by test protocols and conditions, and even characteristics of the recording equipment, some of which might not be obvious or known to the tester (Table 6–5). Other limitations to clinical relevance apply uniquely to studies of either TEOAEs or DPOAEs, as detailed below. Because each of these criteria can substantially influence OAE outcome, and relatively few studies meet all of the criteria, the accumulated experience with OAE in cochlear auditory dysfunction leads only to general, rather than specific, conclusions. Clearly, sensory hearing loss due to outer hair cell damage or dysfunction, and defined by audiometric thresholds poorer than 15 dB HL, is strongly associated with abnormally low OAE amplitudes, and valid OAEs are, for moderate intensity levels, rarely recorded when sensory hearing loss exceeds 35 to 40 dB HL (Probst et al., 1987; Bonfils & Uziel, 1989; Collet et al., 1991; Probst, Lonsbury-Martin, & Martin, 1991; Bonfils & Avan, 1992; Collet et al., 1992; Avan & Bonfils, 1993; Collet et al., 1993; Johnsen, Parbo, & Elberling, 1993). However, given the often noted intersubject variability in OAE amplitudes for normal hearers, and even more so for persons with hearing impairment, confident and consistent prediction or description of auditory sensitivity by OAEs is not feasible (Bonfils & Avan, 1992; Moulin, Bera, & Collet, 1994; Suckfull et al., 1996).

The following review is limited to the general relation between OAEs and cochlear dysfunction as defined by the audiogram. OAE findings in specific cochlear pathologies and etiologies, such as ototoxicity, noise-induced hearing loss, age-related hearing loss, and others, are described in children and adults in Chapters 8 and 9, respectively.

TEOAEs

With the possible exception of newborn hearing screening with TEOAEs, there are more papers describing the relation between TEOAEs and sensory hearing loss than any other clinical topic. For 3 decades, clinical investigators have described OAE findings for children and adults as a function of sensorineural hearing loss, as quantified by the audiogram (e.g., Kemp, 1978; Rutten, 1980; Kemp et al., 1986; Probst et al., 1987; Stevens, 1988; Bonfils & Uziel, 1989; Collet et al., 1989; Spektor et al., 1991; Avan, Elbez, & Bonfils, 1997). The usefulness of this accumulated clinical experience with TEOAEs, however, is rather limited because the technology has evolved substantially during this time period. Most of the early studies were conducted with specially designed and constructed (custom) equipment, and rudimentary software for TEOAE response analyses, because there were

Table 6–5. Examples of equipment and test protocol parameters that may influence the relation between OAE findings and hearing thresholds as measured with the audiogram. Differences in equipment and these test parameters among published studies limit the conclusions that can be made about this relation from accumulated clinical experience.

General

■ Manufacturer of OAE device

■ Probe assembly design
  ✔ type, size, style, weight
  ✔ location of microphone
  ✔ fit within the earcanal

■ Stimulus calibration strategy

■ Noise reduction algorithm and stopping criteria

TEOAEs

■ Stimulus
  ✔ spectrum
  ✔ intensity
  ✔ number of stimuli presented (e.g., 260 versus 520 versus 780)

■ Noise conditions
  ✔ noise level during measurement (as a function of frequency)
  ✔ maximum acceptable noise floor (cutoff for rejection)
  ✔ number of quiet versus noisy averages

■ Analysis criteria
  ✔ criteria for presence versus absence, for example:
    ✦ amplitude or reproducibility?
    ✦ TEOAE- noise floor difference or absolute amplitude?
    ✦ Minimum difference or amplitude defining presence?
  ✔ criteria for normal versus abnormal (e.g., which normative database?)
  ✔ values representing whole response (not frequency specific, or for a frequency band(s) that does not represent a single audiometric frequency, but multiple frequencies)

DPOAEs

■ Stimulus
  ✔ absolute intensity of f_1 and f_2 (e.g., L_1 = 65 dB or 80 dB or 40 dB)
  ✔ relative intensities of f_1 versus f_2 (e.g., $L_1 > L_2$ = 0 or 10 or 15 dB)

■ Noise conditions
  ✔ maximum acceptable noise level for analyses (e.g., 0 or −10 or −20 dB)
  ✔ noise related stopping rules for averaging (e.g., absolute noise or DP–NF difference)

■ Analysis
  ✔ as a function of f_2, f_1 geometric mean (GM) or DP ($2f_1-f_2$)?
  ✔ criteria for presence versus absence, e.g., DP–NF difference of 3 or 5 or 10 dB?
  ✔ minimum absolute DP amplitude accepted as a response, e.g., −10 or −20 dB?
  ✔ criteria for normal versus abnormal (e.g., which normative database?)

---

no commercially available devices. These instruments were by no means inferior. On the contrary, many of the custom OAE systems were constructed with very high quality components, carefully calibrated, and offered considerable flexibility for manipulation of stimulus and acquisition parameters. Differences in the instrumentation used among studies, however, precluded confident and exact comparison of findings. Even with the first clinical device introduced in 1988 (the ILO88), analysis was typically limited to overall measures of response amplitude and correlation, rather than more precise spectral analysis of the response.

Despite the equipment differences, and sometimes constraints, one conclusion is clearly apparent: OAEs are a sensitive measure of cochlear auditory dysfunction. OAEs are typically observed in persons with completely normal audiograms and, in particular, emissions are rarely recorded from ears with sensory hearing loss greater than 35 to 40 dB HL (e.g., Bonfils & Uziel, 1989; Collet et al., 1989; Johnsen, Parbo, & Elberling, 1993).

A particular trend among these papers is the performance of TEOAEs in differentiating normal versus sensory-impaired ears (Collet et al., 1991; Gorga et al., 1993; Prieve et al., 1993; Hurley & Musiek, 1994; Herer, Glattke, Pafitis, & Cummiskey, 1996; Lichtenstein & Stapells, 1996; Vinck, Van Cauwenberge, Corthals, & de Vel, 1998; Harrison & Norton, 1999). For a sizeable sample of subjects, TEOAE response parameters, such as amplitude level, the TEOAE-noise floor difference, or reproducibility values, are graphed in a scatterplot for different frequencies as a function of audiometric threshold at a corresponding frequency. Normal versus impaired hearing is then defined by some audiometric criterion, such as 20 dB HL. Data may next be displayed in the form of ROC curves or with false alarms and misses (for OAE data versus audiometric data) for each of the above response parameters. Examples of these approaches for displaying and analyzing TEOAE findings in normal and sensory hearing loss, as reported by Beth Prieve, Mike Gorga, and colleagues are shown in Figures 6–1 and 6–2 (Prieve et al., 1993). TEOAE data recorded with an ILO88 device used at default settings were described for 113 subjects ranging in age from 4 to 81 years at four frequencies. The test site was not specified. These illustrations show graphs for up to four test frequencies (500, 1000, 2000, and 4000 Hz). In the paper by Prieve et al. (1993), data were also plotted in the form of ROC curves. These graphs are not reproduced here.

A practical and clinically relevant way of viewing the scatterplots (graphs in Figures 6–1) is to assume that one of the little symbols (circles) represents a patient, let's say a 3-month-old infant, you have just tested with TEOAEs. Naturally, you do not have audiometric data for the little patient. If you were able to obtain a valid audiogram, you would be an incredibly talented pediatric audiologist and TEOAEs

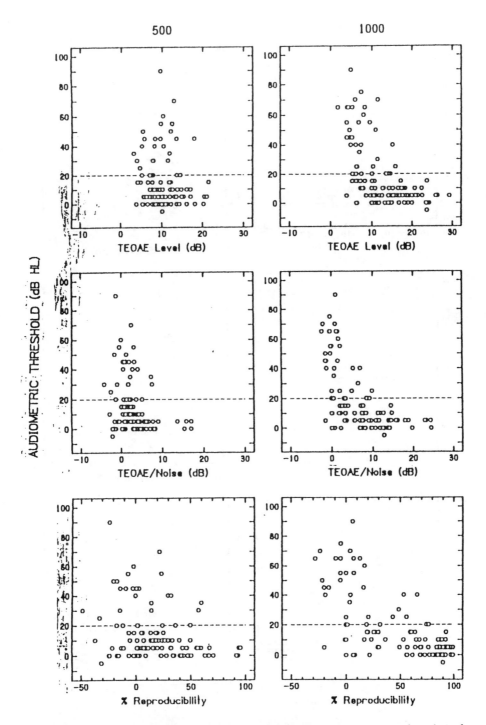

Figure 6–1. Hearing sensitivity (audiometric threshold) shown as a function of three different TEOAE response parameters for four different stimulus octave band frequency regions (500, 1000, 2000, and 4000 Hz). From top to bottom, the parameters are absolute TEOAE amplitude (in dB SPL), the TEOAE minus noise floor difference (in dB SPL), and reproducibility (in %). The cutoff or decision criterion for normal versus abnormal hearing threshold is *(continued)*

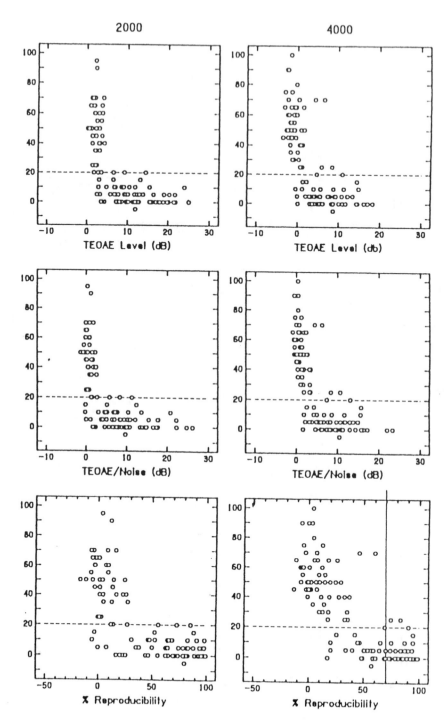

Figure 6–1. *(continued)* represented by the dashed horizontal line in each panel. (Reprinted with permission from Prieves B, Gorga M, Schmied A, Neely S, Peters J, Schultes L, Jestead W. Analysis of transient evoked otoacoustic emissions in normal-hearing and hearing-impaired ears. *Journal of the Acoustical Society of America, 93:* 3308–3319, 1993. Copyright 1993 Acoustical Society of America.)

would not be essential (although still very useful to cross-check the behavioral findings). Does the child have a communicatively significant hearing loss (e.g., greater than 20 dB HL) that warrants more detailed, diagnostic audiologic assessment? To help you answer these questions, for each test frequency a horizontal line indicates an audiometric threshold of 20 dB HL (drawn by the authors). Various criteria can be, and have been, reported for a "pass" versus "fail" TEOAE outcome. The horizontal line drawn in each graph (I drew the line, not the authors of the paper) represent previously reported criteria for TEOAE screening outcome. The pass/fail criterion for the absolute TEOAE amplitude measure (top graphs labeled "A") is 5 dB SPL. That is, TEOAE amplitude values exceeding 5 dB are considered a "pass." For a relative measure (TEOAE amplitude minus noise floor, labeled "B"), the pass/fail criterion is 3 dB SPL (again a value greater than 3 dB indicates a "pass"). In the lower graph ("C"), a "pass" outcome is defined as reproducibility value of 70% or higher. Finally, the four quadrants in each graph, created by the horizontal and vertical lines representing decision criterion for hearing loss and TEOAE response cutoff values are identified (after Harrison & Norton, 1999) as: CR = correction rejection (TEOAE correctly rejects a hearing loss, predicting normal hearing sensitivity correctly, i.e., a true negative outcome); FA = false-alarm (hearing loss predicted but hearing sensitivity actually normal, i.e., a false-positive outcome); Miss = a false-negative outcome because TEOAE predicts normal hearing but there is really a hearing sensitivity loss; and Hit = TEOAE data correctly identify a hearing sensitivity loss (a true positive outcome).

Even cursory inspection of the graphs in Figure 6–1 reveals that TEOAE data for 500 Hz are virtually useless in differentiating normal versus hearing impaired ears. Data points for subjects are widely scattered, with little apparent relation among audiometric threshold and TEOAE parameters. There are a substantial number of errors in all directions. Most concerning is the high rate of false negative errors (misses). A typical limitation in the analysis of data for 500 Hz is the tendency for hearing sensitivity to be within normal limits (<20 dB HL) in an adult population. As expected, hearing loss due to a variety of etiologies (e.g., noise exposure, aging, ototoxicity) is more common in the higher audiometric frequencies. Consequently, the majority of data points fall below the 20 dB HL cutoff (within the normal hearing region).

As also seen in Figure 6–1, TEOAE test performance improves for the higher frequencies. For example, for the absolute amplitude parameter with the 2000 Hz frequency, when amplitude values exceed 5 dB SPL, hearing sensitivity is better than 20 dB HL and when TEOAE amplitude is small (<5 dB SPL or less and indicated by the horizontal line), hearing sensitivity usually exceeds 20 dB HL. The same rather clear-cut relation exists for a TEOAE minus noise floor difference of less than 3 dB (middle set of graphs). For each of these two amplitude-based TEOAE response criteria for pass/fail errors tend to be mostly false positives (lower left quadrant). There are no examples of false negatives (i.e., an incorrect "pass" outcome when there is a hearing loss). This is fortuitous as a miss is the least desirable error because it will contribute to a delayed identification of hearing impairment and to diminished confidence in the value of a screening program. The reproducibility criterion (lower graphs in Figure 6–1) is most widely used clinically to determine pass versus fail outcome in newborn hearing screening programs relying on the TEOAE technique (see Chapter 8 for details). Specifically, a pass outcome is defined by reproducibility values of >70% for two or three different frequencies (octave bands). When this approach is applied for the 2000 Hz frequency alone, the majority of data points fall into the quadrants to the left of the TEOAE criterion. Approximately half of the outcomes are correct true positives, but false failures (false alarms) are also commonplace. In fact, the number of false alarms actually exceeds the number of correct rejections. Notably, there are no false-negative results.

Prieve et al. (1993) recast data for these three TEOAE parameters (absolute amplitude, TEOAE-noise difference, and reproducibility) for analyses of false alarms and misses, or error probabilities, as shown in Figure 6–2 for a low frequency (500 Hz) and a higher frequency (2000 Hz). The criterion for hearing loss is still 20 dB HL. This format clearly shows the inevitable tradeoff between these two types of error. That is, by making the TEOAE criterion for a "pass" outcome more rigorous, for example, a TEOAE-noise difference of 5 dB versus 3 dB or a reproducibility value of 70% rather than 50%, it is possible to eliminate the likelihood of a miss. One can be sure that all hearing loss is identified, and there are no false-negative or false-positive errors, or a high failure rate. The tradeoff is less costly for higher versus lower frequencies. The proportion of false alarms and misses are, of course, equal at the crossover point for these curves. The unacceptably poor test performance for the 500 Hz signal is clearly evident. Prieve et al. (1993) cited as an example of the accuracy of TEOAE data in estimating hearing loss the crossover point of 10 to 12% for the 2000 Hz frequency, using any of the three parameters (top, middle, or lower graphs). At first glance, the accurate identification of 88 to 90% of normal hearers and hearing impaired subjects is attractive. However, when considered in the realistic clinical context of a large newborn hearing screening program, these statistics are rather discouraging. If 1000 babies were screened, then at best 100 babies with hearing sensitivity within normal limits would fail the screening (false positives) and, more concerning, the same number of babies with some degree of hearing loss would pass the screening (false negatives).

It is perhaps inappropriate to make the leap from these data for mostly adults to speculations about TEOAE test performance in neonates and older children. The distinctions between a largely adult versus

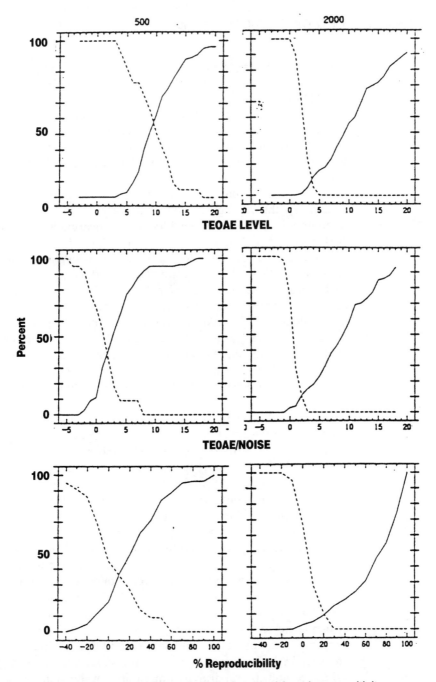

Figure 6–2. Test performance for prediction of normal hearing sensitivity versus sensorineural hearing loss as described by false alarms and misses for three TEOAE response parameters. From top to bottom, the parameters are absolute TEOAE amplitude (in dB SPL), the TEOAE minus noise floor difference (in dB SPL) and reproducibility (in %). Data are shown for the 500 and 2000 Hz octave-band frequency regions, as recorded with the ILO88 device. The point at which the two lines cross over is used to estimate the proportion of false-alarm outcomes (i.e., false falures) and misses (i.e., false-negative outcomes). (Reprinted with permission from Prieves B, Gorga M, Schmied A, Neely S, Peters J, Schultes L, Jestead W. Analysis of transient evoked otoacoustic emissions in normal-hearing and hearing-impaired ears. *Journal of the Acoustical Society of America, 93:* 3308–3319, 1993. Copyright 1993 Acoustical Society of America.)

neonatal patient population are many and quite substantial. Certainly, test conditions and subject status may vary dramatically, usually in favor of the adults. Etiology of the hearing loss is a potentially important factor, however, which appears to be overlooked in most studies. A tacit assumption in the comparison of adult versus neonatal data for TEOAEs and hearing loss is that patients with sensorineural hearing loss are a homogeneous population. That is, the underlying specific cochlear dysfunction is equivalent among the various patients regardless of etiology. Even among adults, this assumption is easily challenged. Are the mechanisms for cochlear dysfunction, and the nature of outer hair cell involvement, identical for hearing loss secondary to perhaps dozens of different pathologies? And, does subtle cochlear dysfunction that can be detected by OAEs always result in hearing sensitivity deficits? The literature clearly produces a "no" response to each question, as summarized below. Yet hearing loss etiology is almost never described for adult subject populations (see Table 6–6), and understandably unknown for most neonatal populations. Thus, the inaccuracies in the relation among TEOAEs and audiometric data evident in graphs such as those just described are quite predictable for adult populations. It is not possible to estimate whether or not data for neonates are equivalent or different in some unpredictable way.

Inferences on the relation of TEOAEs to hearing loss in children are, of course, best investigated in children. A recent TEOAE study provided data for an older pediatric population (Harrison & Norton, 1999). Subjects were 44 children (15 female and 29 male) ranging in age from 4 to 13 years (average of 7.5 years). Data were reported for a total of 59 ears with either normal hearing (hearing levels (15 dB HL from 500 to 4000 Hz), sensorineural hearing loss (hearing thresholds exceeding 15 dB HL with absence of air-bone gaps), or mixed hearing loss (only 4 ears with air-bone gaps for frequencies lower than 1000 Hz). Click and tone burst evoked transient OAEs were recorded in a sound-treated booth with the ILO88 device utilizing a lower frequency filter option. Stimulus intensity levels ranged from 32 to 86 dB SPL. Synchronized SOAEs (see Chapter 3) were also recorded. Data analyses for specific frequency bands included OAE overall power, the OAE-to-noise floor difference (signal-to-noise ratio), and reproducibility. In addition, data were analyzed in the form of receiver operating characteristic (ROC) curves using decision criteria drawn from traditional signal detection theory techniques. In the authors' words, "the ROC curves show actual data for a 30 dB HL decision criterion for hearing loss, as well as idealized curves (represented by dotted lines) for data derived from two populations having Gaussian distributions with equal variance. The sensitivity measure, d', is the distance between the means of the two populations divided by their common standard deviation. Thus, $d' = 0$ indicates no difference between the means . . . as the overlap between the distributions decreases, the curves move up on the graph" (Harrison & Norton, 1999, p. 79). Selected data from this study are displayed in Figure 6–3. Stimulus intensity was 86 dB SPL for data shown in these

Table 6–6. Summary of studies of otoacoustic emissions in cochlear hearing loss. Etiologies for cochlear dysfunction were not specified for studies, unless Indicated.

Study (Year)	N Patients (Ears)	Equipment*	Test** Site	Stimulus***	Intensity	
DPOAEs						
Spektor et al. (1991)	26 (??)	custom	??	GM	$L_1 = L_2$: 35 to 80 dB	not specified
Bonfils & Avan (1992)	(75)	custom	SB	GM	$L_1 = L_2$, 42 to 72 dB	not specified
Gaskill & Brown (1993)	83 (109)	custom	SB	f_1 and f_2	$L_1 = 60$; $L_2 = 45$ dB	mean −10 dB
Avan & Bonfils (1993)	75 (75)	custom	SB	GM	$L_1 = L_2$, 42 to 72 dB SPL	≤20 dB
Moulin et al. (1994)	105 (205)	custom	SB	GM	$L_1 = L_2$, 40 to 80 dB	not specified
Kim et al. (1996)	(142)	???				
Suckfull et al. (1996)	61 (102)	ILO 92	SB	$2 f_1 - f_2$	$L_1 = L_2 = 70$ dB	not specified
Gorga et al. (1997)	806 (1267)	Bio-Logic Scout	CR	f_2	$L_1 = 65$; $L_2 = 55$ dB	≤30 dB
TEOAEs						
Bonfils & Uziel (1989)	(137)	custom	SB	click	0 to 30 dB HL	not specified
Spektor et al. (1991)	26 (??)	ILO 88	? ?	click	82 dB	not specified
Johnsen et al. (1993)	28 (55)	custom	SB	click	0 to 70 dB peSPL	not specified
Collet et al. (1993)	470 (931)	ILO 88	SB	click	81 dB SPL	not specified
Suckfull et al. (1996)	61 (102)	ILO 88	SB	click	83 dB SPL	not specified
Prieve et al. (1993)						
Vinck et al. (1998)	432 (157)	ILO 88/92	SB	click & TB	80 dB SPL	

*ILO92 and ILO88 = Otodynamics, Ltd.

**SB sound booth; QR = quiet (not sound-treated) room.

***GM geometric mean between f_1 and f_2

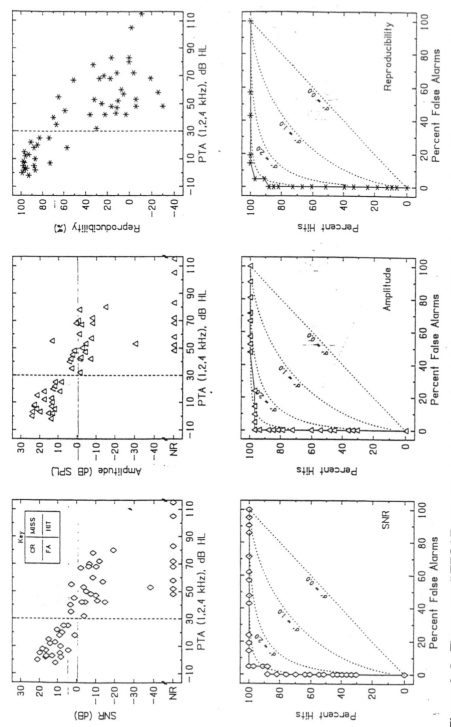

Figure 6–3. Three overall TEOAE response parameters, from left to right, TEOAE minus noise floor difference or signal-to-noise (SNR) ratio in dB SPL, the absolute TEOAE amplitude (in dB SPL), and the reproducibility value (in %) shown as a function of hearing sensitivity (a high-frequency pure-tone average). The stimuli were clicks at 86 dB SPL. Hearing loss criterion is 30 dB HL (vertical dashed line in upper panels). The upper panels show data in the form of a scatterplot, whereas data in lower panels are plotted as receiver operator characteristic (ROC) curves. (From Harrison and Norton, 1999).

figures. As with the previously reviewed study by Prieve et al. (1993), this format permits the visual inspection of test accuracy and test errors, although the orientation of the figures for the two studies is different. In the Prieve et al. (1993) paper, audiometric data were shown on the vertical (Y) axis, whereas in these Harrison and Norton (1999) figures, hearing loss is on the horizontal (X) axis. Also, decision criteria for a hearing loss (vertical line) was, in these figures, a hearing threshold of 30 dB HL, rather than 20 dB HL used by Prieve et al. (1993). Test performance is, however, described with the same terminology for this adaptation of figures from both of the studies (i.e., correct rejection, hit, false alarm, and miss).

The ROC curves (lower set of graphs in Figure 6–3) confirm statistically that with an intensity level of 86 dB SPL, TEOAE data for absolute amplitude, SNR, and reproducibility effectively distinguish normal hearing versus hearing impaired ears. Hit rate was 97% and false alarm rate was 5% for a 30 dB HL decision criterion for hearing loss. These rates worsened, respectively, to 87% and 6% when a hearing loss criterion of 20 was selected and to 97% and 13% for a hearing loss criterion of 40 dB HL. Of the three TEOAE response criteria, SNR yielded the highest rate, whereas the clinically popular reducibility response criterion was associated with the poorest test performance. The hit rate (sensitivity) of the TEOAE SNR criterion was 100% when the false-alarm rate was set at 5% or better (for a stimulus intensity level of 80 or 86 dB SPL and a hearing loss cutoff of 30 dB HL). After discussing their findings in the context of those reported by Lichenstein and Stapells (1996) and Prieves et al. (1993), Harrison and Norton (1999) pointed out that, based on their data, the use of a 3 dB SNR is preferable to a reproducibility value of 50 or 70% for hearing loss prediction from a single data point. This observation can be confirmed by even casual inspection of the data displayed in the scatterplots (upper graphs) in Figure 6–3. In fact, reliance on absolute TEOAE amplitude (center top graph) would be ill-advised because of the possibility of a serious "miss" error. Notice, for example, the symbol indicating a robust TEOAE amplitude of 15 dB SPL for a patient with a hearing loss of 50 dB HL. Test performance improved for higher test frequencies, consistent with earlier reports (Prieve et al., 1993; Hurley & Musiek, 1994; Lichtenstein & Stapells, 1996). Test performance was equivalent for filtered click frequency bands and tone burst signals (i.e., tone burst stimulation did not provide an advantage in classifying hearing loss with TEOAE.) Finally, Harrison and Norton (1999) reiterated the clinically important point that, although TEOAEs can separate normal from sensory impaired ears with reasonable accuracy, TEOAE data do not provide information on the degree of hearing loss.

Finally, it is important to note that, although several papers describe characteristics of TEOAEs in normal hearing infants and young children (e.g., Prieve, Fitzpatrick, & Schulte, 1997), as reviewed in

Chapter 5, there are (to date) no systematic published investigations of the relation between TEOAE and hearing loss in a young pediatric population.

DPOAEs

Increasingly, especially as clinical instrumentation is introduced, the relation between DPOAE and sensory hearing impairment is also being investigated (Spektor et al., 1991; Bonfils & Avan, 1992; Nelson & Kimberley, 1992; Avans & Bonfils, 1993; Gaskill & Brown, 1993; Gorga et al., 1993; Bera & Collet, 1994; Gorga et al., 1996; Kim et al., 1996; Stover et al., 1996; Suckfull et al., 1996; Gorga et al., 1997; Dorn et al. 1999; Gorga, Neely, & Dorn, 1999). In addition to these five criteria cited at the beginning of this section, two factors specially influencing the clinical relevance of investigations of DPOAEs and sensory hearing loss are: (1) the absolute and relative levels of the primary stimuli (L_1 and L_2) and (2) whether the DPs were reported as a function of f_2, or other stimulus features (e.g., f_1 or the geometric mean of f_1 and f_2). In early clinical studies, DPOAEs were often evoked with relatively high stimulus intensity levels (e.g., above 70 dB) which, at the least, rendered the measurement less sensitive to cochlear dysfunction. It is also possible that the apparent DPOAEs detected at these high stimulus levels were the product of exclusively passive cochlear responses, or even produced by equipment artifacts. Another problem encountered in any attempt to extract clinically relevant conclusions from studies published until about 1995 was the tendency to report DPOAE amplitude as a function of the geometric mean, or less often the f_1 frequency, rather than the f_2 primary. We now know that during DPOAE measurement with moderate intensity levels and $L_2 > L_1$, the cochlea is mostly activated at the f_2 place on the basilar membrane (see Chapters 2 and 4 for details). Finally, as with TEOAEs, the relation to the audiogram was described often for DPOAE presence or absence, rather than the magnitude of the DPOAE amplitude. Commonly, DPOAE presence was defined at the observation of a DP at least 3 dB above the noise floor for the $2f_1$-f_2 frequency region. With this simple analysis strategy, however, two serious problems are possible. The absence of a DPOAE may be incorrectly concluded when the noise floors are unacceptably high and DPOAEs do not rise above the noise. Or, apparent DPOAEs will be detected with very low noise floors (e.g., –30 dB SPL) when, in fact, the measured sound is only equipment noise or an unreliable and invalid artifact with an absolute amplitude far lower than expected for a cochlear response. The consequence of this latter misinterpretation was the assumption that DPOAEs could be recorded from patients with moderate to severe (40 to 80 dB HL) cochlear hearing loss.

Inspection of the studies listed earlier in Table 6–6 reveals that few meet the criterion of "commercially available instrumentation." A series of papers describing in detail, and with sophisticated statistical analysis, the relation between DPOAEs and hearing loss has been published by Michael Gorga and his colleagues from Boys Town National Research Hospital in Omaha, Nebraska (Gorga et al., 1993a, 1993b; Gorga et al., 1996; Stover et al., 1996; Gorga et al., 1997; Dorn et al., 1999; Gorga, Neely, & Dorn, 1999). Among these excellent studies, one authored by Gorga, Neely, Ohlrich, Hoover, Redner, and Peters (1997) will be singled out because it describes DPOAEs recorded in a rather typical test environment (a quiet, but not sound-treated room) from a large population of subjects (1,267 ears of 806 subjects) using a clinical device (Bio-Logic Scout system with Etymotic Research ER-10C probe) and conventional test parameters (e.g., $f_1 = 65$ dB, $f_2 = 55$ dB, and a f_2–f_1 ratio of 1.22). This study, in fact, illustrates the positive and negative aspects of utilizing OAE findings to describe hearing loss. Middle ear abnormality for all subjects was ruled out by tympanometry and, in some cases, also by otoscopic inspection. The authors acknowledged that this precaution does not entirely eliminate the possibility of subtle middle ear dysfunction that could affect OAE measurement. The audiogram (obtained with 5 dB intensity increments) was taken as the reference point for hearing status, although again the authors noted the potential insensitivity of this routine measure for cochlear dysfunction. Stimuli were calibrated within the ear with the approach used by the manufacturer, with the recognition that for higher frequencies the accuracy of conventional calibration strategies used with clinical devices has been questioned (Siegel & Hirohata, 1994). Notably, these authors required that signal averaging during DPOAE measurement continue until either noise levels adjacent to the f_2 primary signal were below 30 dB SPL or 32 seconds of averaging time (without artifacts) for the stimulus was reached. The goal was noise level of -20 dB SPL or lower. Data on test time for subjects was not reported, although a little over 3 minutes would probably be required for each DPgram if averaging continued to the maximum test time for this stopping rule for all test frequencies (half-octave steps from 750 to 8000 Hz).

Data from the study of Gorga et al. (1997) are displayed in Figure 6–4. Audiometric threshold (in dB HL) for the f_2 frequencies (indicated with each graph) is on the vertical axis. The horizontal axis represents the difference (in dB SPL) between DPOAE amplitude and the noise floor. It is clear from these figures that, in general and as expected, DPOAE amplitude decreases with increasing hearing loss, and that this relation is tighter for frequencies within the range of 1500 to 6000 Hz than for lower or higher frequencies. Data were also analyzed by means of clinical decision theory and recast into relative operating characteristics (ROC) curves with an audiometric criterion for normal hearing of 20 dB HL. Accuracy of DPOAE test performance in differentiating normal hearing versus hearing loss was then assessed statistically (e.g., hit and false alarm rates). The certainty of determining

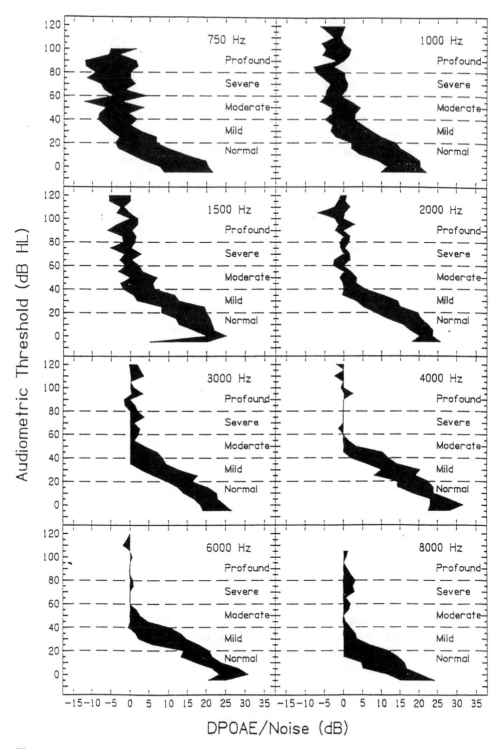

Figure 6–4. Relation between audiometric threshold (in dB HL) to DPOAE to noise floor difference (in dB SPL) for eight different stimulus frequencies (750 Hz to 8000 Hz). Hearing sensitivity is categorized by the horizontal dashed lines.

whether a DPOAE result was from the normal or hearing-impaired population was also calculated. The good news is that DPOAEs have some value in predicting the presence, and even magnitude, of hearing losses of up to 60 dB HL. Unfortunately, as anticipated from the above figures, there is substantial overlap in DPOAE data among normal hearers and hearing impaired subjects. Put simply, for any test frequency there are plenty of normal hearing subjects with small DPOAE amplitudes and, conversely, subjects with hearing thresholds of up to at least 60 dB with apparent DPOAEs. This latter problem is more serious for the DPOAE-noise floor (DPOAE–NF) difference data. A rather large number of subjects with hearing thresholds up to 50 dB and worse had DPOAE-noise floor differences of 20 dB or more (see Figure 6–4). Thus, for an individual patient the clinician cannot estimate with 100% certainty, or even with confidence for many patients, the presence of a hearing loss versus normal hearing thresholds. Gorga and colleagues (1997) displayed their extensive data in a clever fashion which illustrates the relation between DPOAEs and the degree of hearing loss. In this format, the inability of DPOAE data to estimate the degree of hearing loss is readily apparent. Examine, for example, the graph for 2000 Hz. A DPOAE–NF difference of 15 dB or greater is predictive of normal hearing sensitivity (<20 dB HL), and a DPOAE-NF difference less than 15 but more than 0 dB usually implies a mild (20 to 40 dB) hearing loss. However, when the DPOAE–NF difference is 0 dB (i.e., the DP is within the noise floor), the subject could have a hearing loss ranging from moderate to profound.

Summary

What conclusions can be drawn from the substantial literature on TEOAEs and DPOAEs in persons with sensory hearing impairment? Compilation of findings among studies permits the following statements (see also Table 6–6):

■ As typically recorded clinically (i.e., with now-conventional stimulus intensities in non-sound-treated rooms, etc.), both TEOAEs and DPOAEs are reasonably accurate in differentiating persons with normal hearing sensitivity (hearing thresholds (≤20 dB HL) versus those with some degree of sensorineural hearing impairment (20 dB HL). Unfortunately, many early studies of TEOAEs used analysis approaches that, with the advent of more sophisticated software, appear to lack frequency-specificity and, therefore, sensitivity to the presence of mild to even severe hearing impairment within limited regions of the audiogram. Also, findings from most major early studies of DPOAEs have limited relevance to clinicians, as data were not collected in clinical settings with commercially available equipment.

■ Neither TEOAEs nor DPOAEs have value in predicting the actual degree of hearing impairment exceeding 20 to 30 dB HL, although for higher frequency DPOAEs there is a statistical relation with hearing loss up to about 60 dB HL. Also, test performance suffers when normal hearing is defined more rigorously (i.e., a cutoff of less than 20 dB HL) or more loosely (i.e., a cutoff of greater than 30 dB HL).

■ TEOAE test performance is clearly superior for analysis criteria that take into account the signal-to-noise ratio (SNR), that is, OAE amplitude relative to the noise floor (within the corresponding frequency region) than for absolute amplitude measures. The advantage of the SNR approach is not as clear for high as for lower frequencies. For DPOAEs, taking noise levels into account improves the distinction between normal versus hearing impaired subjects, but does not have a major effect on overall test performance (Gorga et al., 1997).

■ In relating OAEs and hearing thresholds, data for large groups of subjects, multivariate analyses strategies are preferable to univariate statistical approaches.

■ The accuracy of hearing predictions by TEOAEs and DPOAEs is relatively higher in the 2000 Hz frequency region (with the exception of 8000 Hz for DPOAEs, possibly due to standing wave factors) and is lower for 1000 Hz. For both TEOAEs and DPOAEs, inclusion of the 500 Hz frequency, as OAE are conventionally recorded, is neither feasible technically nor accurate in terms of test performance, due to greater measurement noise and perhaps middle ear confounding factors (Gorga et al., 1997).

■ False-positive failure rates for adult populations (abnormal OAE outcome in a person with hearing thresholds ≤20 dB HL are excessively high, at least for single stimulus frequency region and when viewed in the context of acceptable test performance for newborn hearing screening. Put another way, even with rather complicated multivariate analyses of data, specificity is far less than ideal, even with cooperative adult subjects when testing was not conducted in a sound booth. Reported false-alarm rates for apparently normal hearing adults (based on the audiogram) are, on the average, in the range of 15 to 25%. That is, up to one fourth of all persons are incorrectly classified as hearing impaired and, for a screening program, would require potentially costly and time-consuming follow-up diagnostic assessment.

In each of the major studies displaying OAE response parameters (reproducibility, amplitude, and amplitude-noise floor differences for TEOAE, and amplitude or amplitude-noise floor differences for DPOAE) as a function of hearing sensitivity in the form of a scatterplot, there are subjects with substantial hearing loss (up to 50 and 60 dB HL) at at least one frequency whose OAE outcome is defined as normal. These are examples of false-negative errors in predicting hearing status. To be sure, the majority of persons with hearing loss meet the criteria for abnormal OAEs. Sensitivity values are usually in the range of 80 to 95%. Still, the false-negative errors are particularly disturbing in the context of newborn hearing screening (see Chapter 8 for a detailed review of test performance). Even if the proportion of serious false-negative OAE outcomes (OAE prediction of normal hearing in a person with hearing thresholds greater than 40 dB HL) was on the order of 2 to 3%, hearing-impaired infants would be "missed" in a large well-baby screening program.

Can the accumulated and somewhat disappointing OAE findings in adult populations be generalized confidently to newborn populations? There are at least three reasons why the answer to this question is probably "no." First, abundant clinical and experimental evidence has confirmed that auditory dysfunction can be present despite a normal audiogram. This critical concept is discussed elsewhere in this chapter and also in Chapters 2, 8, and 9. OAEs are simply more sensitive to most types of cochlear, specifically outer hair cell, dysfunction than the conventional audiogram. Abnormal OAE findings in a rather sizeable proportion of persons with normal hearing thresholds is entirely predictable and, in fact, is an outcome that lends strong support to the clinical usefulness of OAEs in the early detection of cochlear deficits. At the least, persons classified as "normal hearing" should be squeaky clean audiologically and otologically, with no history of middle ear disease or ototoxic medications, including aspirin within a few days of the data collection, no excessive noise exposure, and no tinnitus. Naturally, these strict requirements would not be met by many persons with hearing thresholds of <20 dB HL. In short, the audiogram is not really a "gold standard" for auditory integrity. Second, etiologies for hearing impairment may not be equally distributed among infants and adults. It is possible that some of the adult patients classified as false-negative outcomes have mild, moderate, or even severe sensorineural hearing loss that is not secondary to outer hair cell dysfunction. Hearing loss for some of these patients may be due to inner hair cell dysfunction (perhaps with a genetic basis) or even neural, rather than sensory, dysfunction. As an example, some patients with endolymphatic hydrops (Ménière's disease) may have normal OAEs despite having sensitivity deficits of 40 dB or greater (see Chapter 9). Finally, OAEs are characteristically much larger in newborn infants than in adults. Assuming comparable noise levels, robust OAEs result in better SNRs, and will be more likely to meet OAE pass criteria than smaller amplitude adult OAEs. Stated differently, an infant with no detectable OAEs may be more likely to have a communicatively important sensory hearing loss. For these reasons, minimally, the rather substantial literature on OAEs and sensorineural hearing loss is not entirely applicable to clinical decisions regarding newborn hearing screening, even though the results contribute to our understanding of hearing in general.

CLINICAL RELATION BETWEEN OAEs AND SENSORY HEARING LOSS

The many published papers reporting group data on the relation of OAE findings and sensory hearing loss, including the accuracy of identifying communicatively critical hearing loss with OAEs and statistical analyses of test performance, have produced clinically important information. The accumulated data have been especially useful in the application of OAE findings in newborn hearing screening. For the clinician faced with the challenge of interpreting OAE findings for an individual patient, some general guidelines might be useful for relating OAEs and audiometric information. There are really two relations to consider. With one relation, more often encountered in infants and young children who cannot or will not volunteer a valid pure-tone audiogram, the clinician attempts to make an inference about pure tone hearing levels and sensory auditory status from OAE findings. With the other, an audiogram is available. OAEs are used to confirm the validity of the audiogram, or at least to verify that audiometric hearing loss is sensory and not neural.

Given the imprecise nature between hearing loss and OAE findings, the following should be viewed as clinically useful guidelines, rather than specific rules. There are six fundamental assumptions underlying these guidelines, each of which was introduced in Chapter 1. First, as TEOAEs and DPOAEs are highly frequency specific, they should be analyzed and interpreted for either specific frequencies or, at the least, within rather narrow frequency bands or regions. It is certainly possible, and quite probable, for OAEs to be entirely normal within one frequency region (e.g., frequencies up to 2000 Hz) and abnormal or even undetectable for another frequency region (e.g., frequencies above 2000 Hz).

Second, the noise floor in the frequency of interest is acceptably low (usually below 10 dB SPL). Third, OAE outcome will always fall within one of three general categories: amplitude is normal (relative to an appropriate normative region), abnormal (OAE activity is present but amplitude is below normal limits), or absent (there is no evidence of reliable OAE activity above an acceptably low noise floor). Fourth, the frequency of the stimulus should be aligned with an audiometric frequency. Discrepancies between OAE findings and an audiogram would not be unexpected, of course, if the OAE stimulus frequency did not correspond with the audiometric frequency. If, for example, DPOAEs were plotted as a function of the geometric mean of f_1 and f_2, and DP amplitudes at this mean frequency were compared to a corresponding audiometric frequency, then a disassociation between DPOAEs and hearing thresholds could occur logically. As described in Chapter 4, the DPOAE reflects integrity of the cochlea at the f_2 frequency (when $L_1-L_2 = 10$ dB). Cochlear status at the f_2 frequency might not be equivalent to cochlear status at the geometric mean frequency. Fifth, the relation between OAE and audiometric threshold depends on the sensitivity of OAE to cochlear dysfunction which, in turn, is influenced by OAE stimulus intensity level. Inappropriately high stimulus intensity levels will result in relative insensitivity of OAEs to lesser degrees of hearing loss, whereas very low OAE stimulus intensity levels will sometimes yield abnormal OAE findings despite perfectly normal audiometric thresholds. And, finally, OAE outcome meets criteria for reliability before analysis and interpretation. Always remember the neoclassic principle underlying all OAE and AER interpretation—"If it doesn't replicate, you must investigate" (Hall & Mueller, 1999).

General Relation Among OAEs and Hearing Loss

The overall relation between OAEs and the audiogram is illustrated in Figure 6–5. When OAE amplitude is within normal limits, one would predict hearing thresholds equal to or better than 15 dB HL. Conversely, for persons with audiometric thresholds better than 15 dB HL, we expect normal OAE amplitudes. We typically describe hearing sensitivity as normal if thresholds are somewhere in the 0 to 20 or even 25 dB HL range, mainly because, for adults, communication is not seriously impaired and audiologic management is rarely required. It is important to recall, however, that normal hearing is defined by audiometric zero, and one standard deviation for the distribution of normal hearing thresholds is approximately 5 dB, as measured in SPL at 1000 Hz (Corso, 1958). Therefore, hearing sensitivity worse than 15 dB is statistically not normal. Indeed, in traditional formulae for estimation of hearing impairment, the scale of percentage impairment (deviation from normal) began at 15 dB, using the ASA 1951 standard (Committee on Medical Rating of Physical Impairment, 1958; Committee on Conservation of Hearing, 1959). What does it mean if hearing thresholds are better than 15 dB HL, yet OAE amplitudes are abnormal somewhere within the audiometric frequency region? At the least, this pattern of findings should prompt the tester to ask some simple questions, as summarized in Table 6–7. Based on the experimentally documented high degree of sensitivity of OAEs to cochlear (outer hair cell) dysfunction (see Chapter 2 and earlier sections of this chapter for details), we might conclude that the person has a subtle cochlear deficit that is not detected by the less sensitive audiogram. Before reaching this conclusion, however, one must carefully rule out middle ear dysfunction and ensure that stimulus intensity was appropriate. On the other hand, if OAE amplitudes are entirely normal when hearing thresholds exceed 15 dB HL, assuming an adequately low stimulus intensity level, one must suspect either invalid pure-tone findings (e.g., a malingerer) or, far less likely, neural (retrocochlear) auditory dysfunction.

**RELATION BETWEEN OAE and AUDIOGRAM
(COCHLEAR HEARING LOSS)**

Frequency in Hz

Figure 6–5. A simplified illustration of the relation between sensory hearing loss and OAE outcome. Many factors can influence this relation, as detailed in the text and tables in this chapter.

Abnormal OAE amplitude values, or even the lack of detectable OAE activity, is anticipated whenever there is a mild-to-moderate hearing loss (15 to 40 to 45 dB HL). Within this range, the worse the hearing thresholds the less likely OAEs will be present. As noted above, if OAEs are normal in ears with any degree of hearing loss, then either the validity of the audiogram or the sensory origin of the hearing loss must be questioned. OAE activity is inevitably not observed for sensory hearing loss exceeding 40 to 45 dB HL. Absence of OAEs is, of course, associated with varying degrees of sensory hearing loss, from mild-moderate to profound. Put simply, OAEs are of little or no value in estimating the degree of hearing loss, especially if absent or undetectable. In such cases, to determine degree of hearing loss OAE must be supplemented with pure tone or speech audiometry, if clinically feasible, or an electrophysiologic measure (e.g., ABR).

Another way to approach the relation of hearing sensitivity and OAE outcome and the likelihood of OAE presence is illustrated in Figure 6–6. Similar graphs were helpful in understanding the clinical probability of recording an ABR in neurodiagnostic applications with per-

Table 6–7. Questions you might ask when you record abnormal OAEs from a patient with a normal audiogram. Also, see figures in this chapter which relate OAEs and audiogram findings.

■ Is the audiogram really normal?

▶ Any hearing thresholds that are poorer than about 15 dB HL may be associated with abnormally low OAE amplitude values, even though by clinical guidelines the patient is audiometrically normal.

▶ Cochlear function is different for the patient with hearing thresholds at 0 dB HL versus the patient with hearing thresholds at 15 or 20 dB HL. Remember the standard deviation for pure-tone thresholds is about 5 dB.

▶ Since OAEs reflect cochlear (outer hair cell) status, it is reasonable to expect reduced OAE amplitudes for patients with hearing thresholds at the low end of the audiometrical normal region.

■ Is the patient really otologically normal, even though he or she has a normal audiogram?

▶ Tinnitus. Does the patient have tinnitus? This is a sign of cochlear dysfunction, and could be related to reduced OAE amplitude values.

▶ Middle ear status. Is middle ear function entirely normal? Obtain a detailed otologic history, and closely examine tympanometry findings, to verity that the middle ear is not involved. Remember, OAEs are dependent on the transmission of stimulus energy inward through the middle ear system, and OAE energy outward through the middle ear system. Even under the best of middle ear conditions, energy will be lost coming and going.

▶ Ototoxic medications. Is the patient taking any drugs that could be affecting cochlear (outer hair cell) function, even slightly. Ask about antibiotics, diurectics, and aspirin use.

▶ Noise/music exposure. Does the patient have a history of exposure to high levels of any kind of sound (noise or music)? Cochlear deficits associated with noise/music exposure may produce dramatically reduced OAE amplitudes, or no OAE activity, even though the audiogram is still within the clinical normal region. Be suspicious of noise/music exposure when pure-tone audiometry for a patient shows a very slight notch (e.g., 10 to 15 dB) in the 4000 Hz region.

---

sons having considerable unilateral or asymmetrical hearing loss in the high-frequency region. Likelihood of recording OAEs (in %) is displayed on the vertical axis as a function of the degree of sensory hearing loss (in dB HL). The shaded area toward the left depicts the likelihood that OAE amplitude will be within normal limits, whereas the other shaded area, which is shifted toward greater hearing loss, represents the mere presence of OAEs (e.g., OAE activity clearly exceeds the noise floor but amplitude is below normal limits). Just as in the preceding figure, OAEs are almost always within normal limits for hearing thresholds up to about 15 dB HL (top left of the figure). As hearing loss exceeds 15 dB HL, OAEs are likely to be abnormal and the chances of recording OAEs of entirely normal amplitude becomes virtually nil with hearing loss of greater than 20 dB HL. For patients with mild hearing loss (in the 20 to about 35 dB HL region), OAEs are almost always present, although not normal. Then, for sensory hearing loss of 40 dB HL or more, OAEs are not observed in the majority of patients.

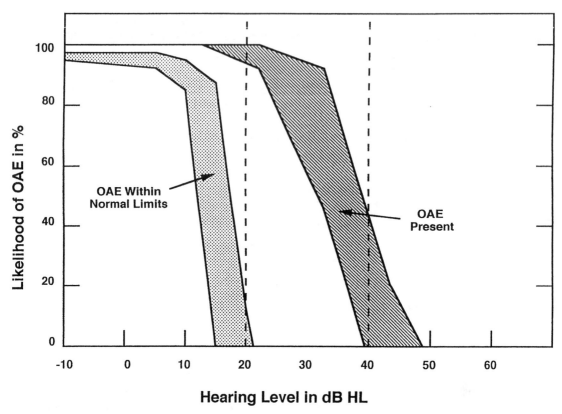

Figure 6–6. The likelihood of recording OAEs within normal limits (left shaded region) or any detectable OAEs (right shaded region) as a function of hearing sensitivity to a comparable frequency region.

Stimulus intensity level, a test parameter under the control of the clinician, may have an important influence on the horizontal (hearing loss) placement of the shaded areas. That is, when OAEs are evoked with a relatively low stimulus level (e.g., less than 80 dB SPL for TEOAEs or less than $L_1 = 65$ and $L_2 = 55$ dB SPL for DPOAE), the odds of an abnormal or absent OAE outcome are increased for any given degree of hearing loss. Put another way, some persons with even normal hearing sensitivity (hearing levels better than 15 dB HL) may have abnormal OAE findings (presumably implying subtle cochlear deficits not reflected in the audiometry) and persons with mild hearing loss may not yield detectable OAEs. The reverse is also true, and OAEs become less sensitive to hearing loss if stimulus intensity is greater than the above-noted values. In fact, with inappropriately high stimulus intensity levels for DPOAE elicitation, an apparent response may appear above the noise floor even for hearing loss exceeding 50 dB HL. As noted in Chapter 4, such responses may include instrument-related artifact and/or passive energy returning from the cochlea, rather than active cochlear processes secondary to outer hair cell activation and subsequent motility.

Cases Illustrating the Relation Among DPOAEs and Audiograms

The following three cases are presented briefly to illustrate the nature of the relation between hearing thresholds and DPOAE amplitudes. One would expect DPOAE amplitudes well within normal limits when hearing sensitivity is entirely normal, as shown in Figure 6–7. In this and the following few graphs, the normal region for DPOAEs encompasses the 10th to 90th percentile region for a group of 30 young, otologically normal adult subjects (60 ears), and the thin solid line in the lower portion of the figure indicates the upper range (90th percentile) of acceptable noise. Methodologic details on the study that produced these normative data were discussed in Chapter 4. The adequate quality of the DPOAE measurements is, in part, confirmed by noise floor values that are below (better than) the upper limit for normal noise. All hearing thresholds, including those for interoctave frequencies are at or close to audiometric zero (0 dB HL). Notice that DP amplitudes are plotted as a function of the f_2 frequency, and that these

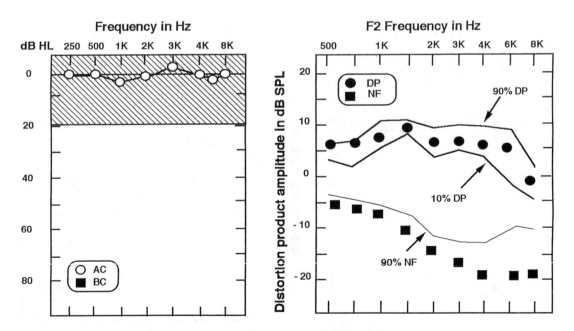

RELATION BETWEEN AUDIOGRAM AND DISTORTION PRODUCT OTOACOUSTIC EMISSIONS

Figure 6–7. An example of a DPOAE gram (right side of figure) for a patient with entirely normal hearing sensitivity, as depicted in the audiogram (left side of figure).

frequencies are aligned with the audiometric frequencies. This approach enhances the possible correlation of audiometric and DPOAE findings. Clinically, these DPOAE findings would be replicated and would meet minimal criterion for reliability (i.e., DP amplitudes for at least two separate repeated recordings within ±2 dB at each test frequency).

Data for another case are shown in Figure 6–8. At first glance hearing looks reasonably good by clinical standards. Almost all thresholds are within or close to normal limits. Certainly, this patient with no air-bone gap would not require audiologic management. Closer inspection, however, reveals that hearing thresholds are well below audiometric zero and, statistically, not normal. It is not surprising, therefore, that DPOAE amplitude values fall below the lower end of the normal range for all but the lowest test frequency (500 Hz). DPOAE amplitudes steadily decrease with hearing levels from low to higher frequency range. This is consistent with expectations reviewed earlier, and illustrated in Figure 6–5. For most of the frequency region, DPOAEs are clearly present (absolute DPOAE amplitude exceeds −10 dB and the noise floor is much lower), but DP amplitudes fall far below

RELATION BETWEEN AUDIOGRAM AND DISTORTION PRODUCT OTOACOUSTIC EMISSIONS

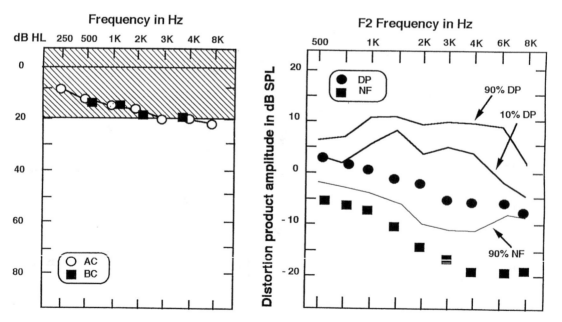

Figure 6–8. An example of a DPOAE gram (right side of figure) for a patient with a very mild sensory hearing sensitivity deficit as depicted in the audiogram (left side of figure).

the normal region, as we would anticipate for a patient with a mild sensory hearing loss (thresholds from 15 to 30 dB HL). An important clinical conclusion highlighted by this case is that an audiogram showing thresholds within normal limits does not necessarily reflect normal cochlear function. To the contrary, these DPOAE findings are evidence of some cochlear (outer hair cell) dysfunction, which is progressively greater for higher frequencies. It would not be unusual for a patient like this to have some audiologic or otologic complaint (e.g., tinnitus, difficulty hearing in background noise, or the general impression that his or her hearing was no longer normal).

An audiogram configuration typically associated with noise-induced hearing loss is shown with a corresponding DPgram in Figure 6–9. As in the previous figure, DPOAE amplitudes fall below the normal region as hearing sensitivity deficits exceed 15 dB HL. Amplitude data in the DPgram can be characterized by each of the three above-noted descriptors for OAE outcome—normal, abnormal, and absent, as

ANALYSIS OF DISTORTION PRODUCT OTOACOUSTIC EMISSIONS (DPOAE)

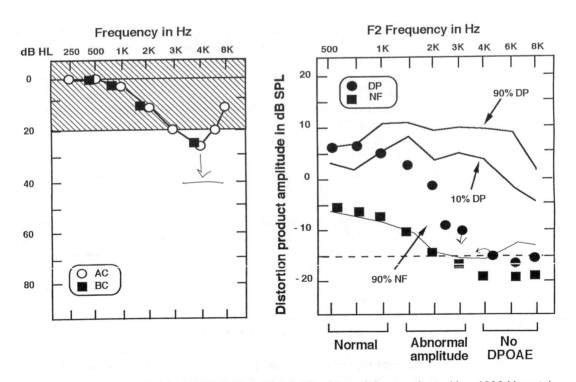

Figure 6–9. An example of a DPOAE gram (right side of figure) for a patient with a 4000 Hz notch characteristic of noise-induced sensory hearing loss as depicted in the audiogram (left side of figure).

defined in the lower portion of the figure. A few other clinically common observations are illustrated by this case. DPOAEs disappear (i.e., amplitudes fall below −15 dB and/or to within 3 dB of the noise floor/NF) as hearing loss exceeds 30 to 35 dB HL. Also, decrements in DP amplitude between audiometric frequencies, for example, from 2000 to 3000 Hz, provide evidence of cochlear dysfunction with a greater degree of frequency specificity than does the audiogram. The degree of frequency specificity or resolution can, of course, be increased further by incorporating more frequencies per octave into the test protocol. Finally, although hearing sensitivity improves for the highest audiometric frequencies (above the notch), DPOAEs remain absent. This finding is evidence that cochlear dysfunction secondary to the noise exposure extends into, or more properly begins in, the higher frequencies (the more basal region of the cochlea). All in all, then, the DPOAE findings serve to not only confirm the audiogram, but also to augment information available in the audiogram—information that may be useful clinically in counseling and otherwise managing the patient.

Cases Illustrating the Relation Among TEOAEs and Audiograms

The final two cases similarly relate TEOAE findings to audiograms. The first, shown in Figure 6–10, is the same patient presented above (see Figure 6–8). Hearing sensitivity is, once again, generally within clinically normal limits, but definitely reflecting a deficit in comparison to audiometric zero, especially for the higher frequency region. TEOAE data are presented in two forms (see Chapters 1 and 4 for detailed explanations of these formats). The upper panel shows the temporal waveform for TEOAE activity in the ear canal. TEOAE activity arising from the base of the cochlea (closest to the middle and external ear) is "emitted" first (with the shortest latency), whereas energy for lower frequencies (more apical cochlear regions) arrives in the ear canal later. The TEOAE spectrum is displayed below, ranging from low to high (about 5000 Hz) frequencies. The shaded region depicts noise within the ear canal during the measurement. TEOAE amplitude, indicated by the solid line, is never robust and decreases further for higher frequencies. There are no detectable TEOAEs for frequencies of 4000 Hz and above, corresponding to hearing thresholds of 20 to 25 dB HL. TEOAE findings for this patient are quantified in the lowest portion of the figure. The correlation between the two temporal response waveforms (or the reproducibility) steadily decreases as a function of test-frequency octave band, as does the TEOAE amplitude-to-noise floor, or signal-to-noise ration (SNR). Thus, TEOAE data confirm the presence of cochlear dysfunction for all but the lowest frequency region despite the unremarkable audiogram.

RELATION BETWEEN AUDIOGRAM AND
TRANSIENT EVOKED OTOACOUSTIC EMISSIONS

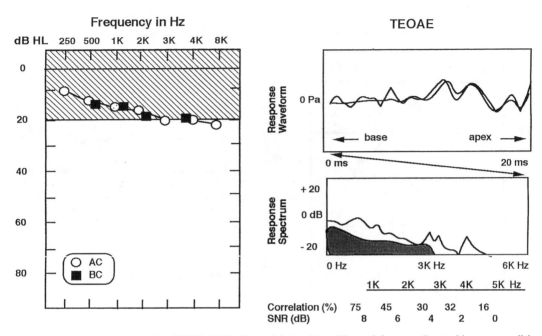

Figure 6–10. An example of TEOAE findings (right side of figure) for a patient with a very mild sensory hearing sensitivity loss as depicted in the audiogram (left side of figure).

TEOAE data for the patient with the noise-induced hearing loss are shown in Figure 6–11. The pattern of the OAE/audiogram relationship is now quite familiar. Regardless of the display format, TEOAEs are entirely absent as hearing loss exceeds 25 to 30 dB HL. With manual control of a cursor, it is possible to perform TEOAE analysis with a high degree of frequency resolution. Thus, one could easily determine at which specific frequency TEOAE amplitude decreased, even though this point was somewhere between two audiometric frequencies. Unfortunately, technologic limitations (see Chapter 4 for an explanation) preclude recording of TEOAE activity for the higher audiometric frequency region (above 5000 Hz), so it is not possible to ascertain with TEOAE cochlear status for frequencies above the notch.

ANALYSIS OF TRANSIENT EVOKED
OTOACOUSTIC EMISSIONS (DPOAE)

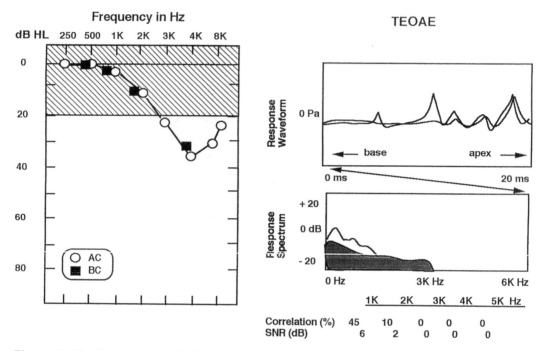

Figure 6–11. An example of TEOAE findings (right side of figure) for a patient with a 4000 Hz notch characteristic of noise-induced sensory hearing sensitivity loss as depicted in the audiogram (left side of figure).

CLASSIC AND NEO-CLASSIC QUOTES

Harold Schuknecht and Robert Patuzzi on Pathophysiology of Loudness Recruitment and Outer Hair Cells

Classic: Schuknecht

"The phenomenon of loudness recruitment appears to be the psychoacoustic expression of the loss of a large component of outer hair cells and the concurrent preservation of a large component of inner hair cells and type I cochlear neurons.

It is well established that the outer hair cells are more susceptable than inner hair cells to almost all types of injury (e.g., inflammatory disease, trauma, ototoxic drugs) and that nerve fibers undergo degeneration only as a retrograde effect following injury to the sustenacular cells, particularly the inner pillar cells and the inner phalangeal cells."

Neo-Classic: Patuzzi

"These data suggest that the compressive growth of vibration of the characteristic frequency (CF) is mostly responsible for the large dynamic range of the inner hair cells and afferent neurons, and ultimately auditory performance in the whole animal. In particular, the absence of the compressive growth of vibration near the CF after cochlear trauma [note: due a reduction in active processes secondary to outer hair cell damage) can produce an abnormally rapid growth in perceived loudness call "recruitment.""

Sources: Schuknecht HF. *Pathology of the Ear* (2nd ed). Philadelphia: Lea & Febiger.

CHAPTER

7

Manufacturers' Forum

Bio-Logic Systems, Corporation
Contact: Kathy Murphy
1 Bio-Logic Plaza
Mundelein, IL 60060
TEL: 847-949-5200 (x230)

Etymotic Research, Inc.
Contact: Laurel
    Christensen
61 Martin Lane
Elk Grove Village, IL 60007
TEL: 847-228-0006

Grason Stadler, Inc.
Contact: Jan Painter
1 Westchester Drive
Milford, NH 03055
TEL: 603-672-0470

**Hortmann AG
    Neuro-Otometrie**
Contact: Bernd Waldmann
Robert-Bosch-Strasse 6
D-72654 Neckartenzlingen
GERMANY
TEL: +49 7127 9299-43
FAX: +49 7127 9299-99

**Intelligent Hearing
    Systems**
Contact: Edward Miskiel
7356 S.W. 48th Street
Miami, FL 33155
Telephone:(305) 668-6102
FAX: 305-595-4175

Madsen Electronics
Contact: Paul Morrison
Maarkaervej 2A
DK-2630 Taastrup
Denmark
TEL: +45 72 11 13 33
Fax: +45 72 11 13 48

Madsen Electronics
Contact: Terry Ross
5600 Rowland Road,
    Suite 275
Minnetonka, MN 55343
TEL: 800-362-3736

Otodynamics Ltd.
Contact: David T. Kemp, Ph.D.
36-38 Beaconsfield Road
Hatfield, Herts AL10 8BB
UNITED KINGDOM
FAX: 44-707-262327

Oz Systems
Contact: Bill Lamm
2730 N. Stemmons
    Freeway, Suite 404,
    West Tower
Dallas, TX 75207
EL: 888-ScreenMe
    (727-3366)
Fax: (214) 631-4231

SonaMed Corporation
Contact: William Dolphin,
    Ph.D.
1250 Main Street
Waltham, MA 02451
TEL: 781-899-6499

Starkey Laboratories
Contacta: Mel Gross,
    Carol Barnett, and
    Patricia Jeng
6700 Washington Avenue
    South
Eden Prarie, MN 55344
TEL: 612-941-6401

INTRODUCTION

This chapter is devoted to a presentation by manufacturers of OAE technology and products. The rapid growth in the application of OAEs in recent years is due, in part, to the the steadily increasing number of different devices designed for clinical OAE measurement. A variety of equipment options is also available, ranging from powerful and flexible diagnostic systems to hand-held automated screening devices. Three types of persons, actually cultures—clinicians, scientists, and manufacturers—must strive to work together in the advancement of OAEs. None of these groups can acheive their goals without an apprecation of, respect for, and support from the other two.

The information found in Chapter 7 was prepared by representatives from most of the manufacturers of OAE instrumentation. Although edited lightly for consistency in style and format, the content within each section, including wording, concepts, and any facts and figures, is the work of the manufacturers. Reproduction of the material does not imply endorsement of content, specific products, or any clinical data or procedures. The chapter will, of course, be quickly outdated with advances in technology and the introduction of new products. The reader is encouraged to contact manufacturers directly for more and current information on any of the products described herein (a listing of manufacturers follows). Each manufacturer's descriptions, of course, extol the virtues of OAE measurement, and most statements can be supported by clinical experiences. It is also reasonable, however, for readers to request references from manufacturers for published clinical investigations in support of claims made for equipment, such as low failure rates for newborn hearing screening, or desirable test performance of OAEs measured with their equipment versus other devices or other technology (e.g., automated ABR). And, of course, readers are strongly urged to devote time to serious study of OAE principles and procedures, as outlined in the remainder of the book, combined with practicum experience, before launching OAE services with patient populations.

BIO-LOGIC SYSTEMS CORPORATION

Products: Scout Sport
                  AuDX

Prepared by: Kathy Murphy

Background

Bio-logic Systems Corporation introduced its first otoacoustic emissions product in 1995. Since the introduction of Scout, continued research and development projects at Bio-logic have resulted in a variety of significant product enhancements affecting both the hardware and the software. Hardware miniaturization is one of the most apparent changes. The current system, Scout Sport, consists of a unit that is similar in size to a standard VCR tape and weighs just over 1 pound. The benefits afforded by this development include enhanced portability and easier, faster system setup. This design change also led Bio-logic to offer AuDX, the first hand-held automated OAE system that functions without connection to a computer (Figure 7–1).

In 1998, the ear probe underwent a complete redesign that resulted in lighter weight, easier to install disposable ear tips, a smaller ear tip size, and the ability to clean debris from the probe. The most notable benefits of the probe design changes have been increased stability of the probe in the ear, especially in newborn ears, and improved reliability.

Bio-logic has also demonstrated continued commitment to software improvement. The original MS-DOS-based Scout software was rewritten as a Windows 95/98 application in 1998. Additional software applications were developed to support a myriad of product enhancements including software that allows the user to define customized test protocols and program the hand-held OAE unit to perform one of these customized protocols. Bio-logic recently introduced database software specifically designed to address data management challenges faced by universal newborn hearing screening (UNHS) programs that is complementary to our OAE products. Cooperative efforts with the developers of other newborn hearing screening data management tools are underway so that Bio-logic's OAE systems are compatible with other commercially available database programs.

Bio-logic offers several different OAE products. Some notable features are common to all of the systems. The variability among the systems relates primarily to the intended use of the instrument and its flexibil-

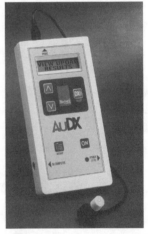

Figure 7–1. Hand-held AuDX from Bio-logic Systems Corp. The AuDX functions without a computer.

ity. After a description of the commonalities among the systems, each system will be described separately with the intent to clarify the differences among them. Keep in mind that by the time you are reading this chapter there undoubtedly will be additional developments that are not described here. Please contact Bio-logic System Corp. or your local Bio-logic representative for up-to-date information about our OAE products.

Features Common to All Bio-logic OAE Systems

Probe Design. One ear probe with a variety of disposable ear tip sizes is used for all of our systems regardless of the type of evoked OAE that is measured, i.e., TEOAEs or DPOAEs (Figure 7–2). Ear tips are available in five sizes that cover the entire range of ear canal sizes. Our unique TreeTip (patent-pending) features flanges of graduated sizes and accommodates newborn and infant ear canal sizes ranging from approximately 3.5 to 5.5 mm in diameter (Figure 7–3). This "one size fits most newborns" design reduces the wastage of disposable ear tips inherent in systems that require trial of more than one ear tip size to achieve a good fit. The flange design also increases the stability of the probe in the baby's ear. An ear tip measuring 6 mm is available for infants with slightly larger ear canals. Compressible foam ear tips in three sizes accommodate the remaining range of ear canal sizes from toddler to adult. Each size serves a broad range of canal diameters because they are compressed before placement in the canal and ex-

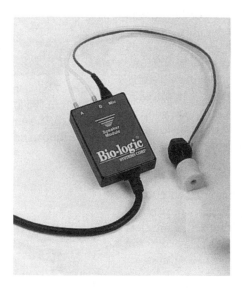

Figure 7–2. One ear probe with multiple tip sizes for performing TEOAE or DPOAE measurement.

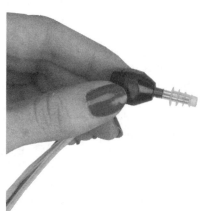

Figure 7–3. The unique TreeTip probe design for Bio-logic OAE devices fits most newborn ears.

pand to conform to the size and shape of the ear canal. Foam tips are very comfortable for the patient and help attenuate ambient noise.

The modular design of Bio-logic's OAE probe allows easy cleaning by the user. The microphone module and silicone speaker tubes can be removed from the probe body, giving the user access to the stainless steel microphone and sound delivery tubes. A cleaning tool is provided.

Hardware Design. All of our current OAE systems are based on miniaturized hardware design that is highly portable. The design includes all of the stimulus generation, response averaging, and signal processing capabilities necessary to perform OAE measurements using either clicks (TEOAEs) or tones (DPOAEs). The system is powered by rechargeable batteries and features an automatic shut-off function that conserves battery life. Fully charged batteries last for several days to a week depending on system usage. A charger/adapter unit recharges the batteries, but also provides power to the unit so tests can be performed when the battery charge is low. The built-in LCD provides status information during testing. Systems that are designed to be used without a computer (AuDX) include buttons on the front panel that allow the user to power the system on, move through and implement the various menu options such as Perform Test, View Data, Print, and so on. Systems that are used with a computer (Scout Sport or AuDX Plus) require only one cable connection from the OAE unit to a serial port on the computer.

Measurement-Based Stopping Rules. The phrase "measurement-based stopping rules" refers to a set of criteria used during an OAE test that determines the duration of averaging. These criteria require online assessment of the OAE response and Noise Floor amplitude and dictate when the software will automatically cease averaging. This type of measurement is superior to a fixed averaging time approach because it helps to achieve measurement of an optimal response (as defined by the user) in the shortest amount of test time. All of Bio-logic's OAE systems utilize measurement-based stopping rules and most systems allow customization of the rules to the user's preferences.

DPOAE measurement, including test protocols, is reviewed in detail in Chapter 4. See, for example, Tables 4–4 through 4–6.

Pass/Refer Indicator. All of our OAE systems can be programmed to assess various DPOAE response parameters automatically and display a pass or refer indicator at the conclusion of a test. This feature is particularly useful in implementing universal newborn hearing screening or other types of screening programs that employ nonaudiologist testers. It ensures consistent interpretation of results from patient to patient and among testers. It reduces the risk of user error in applying the pass/refer criteria. The pass/refer criteria can be customized to the preferences of the program supervisor on some of the systems. The response parameters that can be defined as part of the pass/refer criteria are minimum distortion product (DP) amplitude, minimum difference value between the DP and the noise floor (NF), and the number of stimulus conditions that must meet these criteria for a Pass indicator to display. The pass or refer indicator also prints out as part of the report.

Noise Measurement. The method by which the noise floor (NF) is measured and reported in OAE systems varies from one manufacturer to another. Bio-logic's DPOAE software calculates the NF amplitude by averaging the signal amplitude present in frequency bins surrounding the DP frequency bin. Four 50 Hz wide frequency bins, two above and two below the DP frequency bin, are averaged in the software default mode. Some user definition of this measurement is available in the Scout program. In the TEOAE software, the average noise floor is displayed.

Active Noise Filtering. Bio-logic OAE systems employ a unique, proprietary method of reducing the effects of noise on the DPOAE measurement. This technique improves test performance in noisy conditions.

In-the-Ear Calibration. Measurement of the OAE response is preceded by an in-the-ear calibration phase on all Bio-logic OAE systems. In the case of a TEOAE measurement, the in-the-ear calibration adjusts the overall intensity level of the click stimulus so that it matches the target level. In other words, there is automatic adjustment of the stimulus to account for ear canal size. The in-the-ear calibration data acquired before a DPOAE measurement is used to ensure that the desired stimulus levels of the two primary tones are achieved at each frequency condition regardless of the resonance characteristics of the patient's ear canal.

See Chapter 4 for a discussion of steps important in verifying adequate probe fit in OAE measurement (for example see Figure 4–1) and for troubleshooting probe problems (see Tables 4–1 and 4–8).

Probe Fit Checking. All Bio-logic OAE systems incorporate some method by which the acceptability of the probe fit can be determined and monitored by the tester. Some of these checking methods are automatically performed in the software and result in a message that informs the user if action is required to improve the probe fit. Some of the checking methods, such as a probe stability value expressed in percent during a TEOAE test or the stimulus levels reported during the DP test, present information that the user can interpret and use to make adjustments as deemed appropriate.

Artifact Rejection. Artifact rejection improves overall data quality by rejecting samples of data that are contaminated by excessive levels of background noise. All Bio-logic OAE systems employ artifact rejection as a means of optimizing data quality. The user can manipulate the artifact rejection threshold both in the definition of the default protocol parameters and on-line during data collection.

Bio-logic's Line of OAE Products

Scout Sport. Scout Sport is Bio-logic's computer-based OAE system (Figure 7–4). A functional system includes an IBM-compatible computer that meets minimum requirements, Scout software installed on the computer, the Scout Sport hardware module, a cable that connects the Scout Sport to the computer serial port, the ear probe, and disposable ear tips. Bio-logic sells this product either as a complete system including the computer or as a kit that can be combined with a computer provided by the user. Computer options offered by Bio-logic include notebook, lunchbox, or desktop platforms.

The Scout software is available either as a Windows 95/98 or MS-DOS application. Preprogrammed test protocols are configured to meet the typical clinical diagnostic and screening needs of most facilities. The screening protocols result in a pass or refer indicator that displays on both the computer screen and the printout. Virtually unlimited additional test protocols can be defined and saved by the user. For a DPOAE protocol, some of the stimulus parameters under user control are intensity, F_2/F_1 ratio, frequency range over which the test is per-

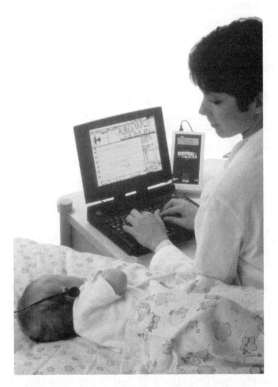

Figure 7–4. The Bio-logic Scout Sport is a computer-based screening or diagnostic OAE system.

formed, points tested per octave, and high to low or low to high frequency test sequencing. The user can also manipulate many of the recording parameters such as sample length (1,024 or 2,048 points), minimum samples collected, number of test replications performed automatically, number of frequency bins on either side of the DP frequency that are included in the noise measurement, and artifact rejection threshold. Protocol creation also allows the user to define the measurement-based stopping rules described previously. Various sets of normative data are available within the software. The user can elect to view clinical data compared to any of these reference data sets.

DPOAE analysis strategies are explained in Chapter 4, summarized in Table 4–6 and illustrated in Figure 4–8. An introduction to the topic is found in Chapter 1.

The standard layout of the DPOAE data in the Scout program allows simultaneous viewing of the complete DPgram as well as a numeric table of measured amplitudes and a spectrum display of the raw data for a specified DPgram data point. The display of DPgram data follows the symbol and color conventions of pure-tone audiometry to the extent that it is possible. Multiple tests can be displayed and printed simultaneously either superimposed on the same DPgram for easy comparison or side by side for convenient reporting of right and left ear data (Figure 7–5).

Scout Sport patient and test information is managed through a database that can be configured to include features specifically developed for the needs of newborn hearing screening programs. Scout Sport operation can also be linked to other commercially available newborn hearing screening database tools.

AuDX. AuDX was the first hand-held OAE system available that functioned without connection to a computer. Operation of the system is very simple requiring only a few button presses to initiate and complete an automated test. On-line messages displayed on the LCD guide the operator and provide helpful messages to ensure a good probe fit in the ear canal. Used as a screening device, AuDX will display a pass or refer indicator at the conclusion of the test. Test results are stored in memory for review on the LCD or printout to the optional Bio-logic label printer that connects directly into the AuDX (Figure 7–6). Self-adhesive labels display all of the test information including a pass or refer indicator and the numeric test details that describe the DP and NF amplitudes. Using DPOAE technology, AuDX is a highly sensitive tool for detecting even mild cochlear hearing loss. Test time is fast as brief as 15 seconds per ear. Of course, when conditions are noisy or the patient's response is poor, testing will take longer because measurement-based stopping rules are employed in an attempt to optimize the response.

Several different configurations of AuDX are available. They are the AuDX II, AuDX Basic, and AuDX Plus. All of the systems function as described in the previous paragraph. However, some systems have additional capabilities either included with the instrument or available as an option.

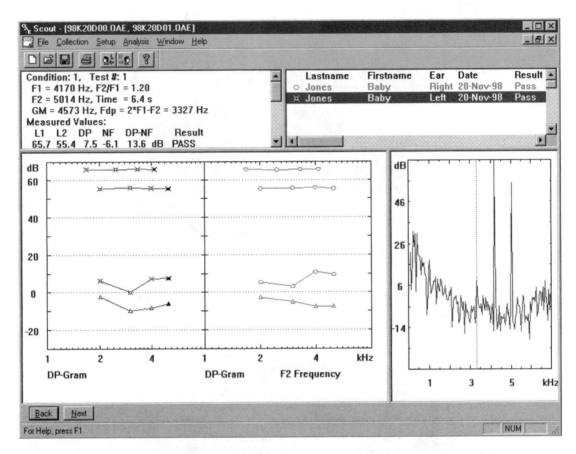

Figure 7–5. Bio-logic Scout Windows 95 software provides flexible data display options.

AuDX II. The AuDX II was configured primarily to meet the variable needs of universal newborn hearing screening programs (Figure 7–7). It may also be appropriate for facilities that need a diagnostic OAE system as well as a screening device.

AuDX Protocol Setup software, routinely provided with AuDX II, allows the user to create customized test protocols and download one of them into the unit. This gives the audiologist the opportunity to create and perform tests that reflect her or his preferences or meet the requirements for a diagnostic DPOAE test rather than a screening procedure. Its programmability also facilitates changing the screening test parameters to meet requirements that may be dictated by the wording of state-mandated infant hearing screening legislation.

AuDX protocol setup software provides user control of virtually all of the test parameters that create the way in which a test is conducted. A protocol can contain up to 10 F_2 frequency conditions (Figure 7–8). Available F_2 frequencies range from 500 to 10,000 Hz in 250 or 500 Hz increments. Other user-controlled parameters include: L_1, L_2, F_2/F_1

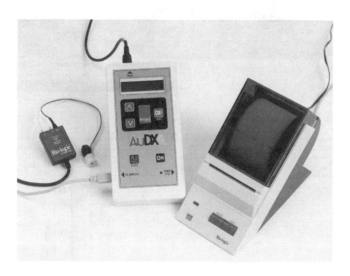

Figure 7–6. The AuDX serial printer prints test results in seconds.

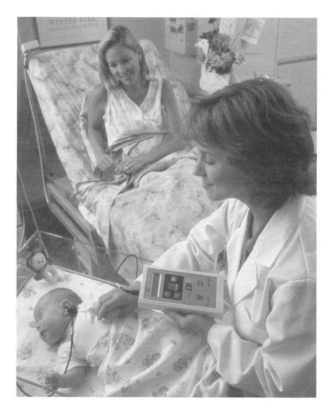

Figure 7–7. The AuDX II is ideal for universal newborn hearing screening.

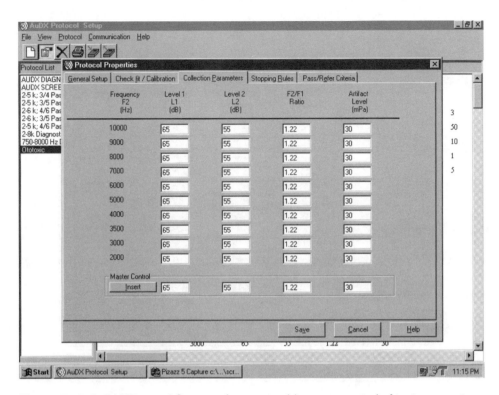

Figure 7–8. AuDX Protocol Setup software provides user control of test parameters.

ratio, default artifact rejection threshold, measurement-based stopping rules, automatic shut-off delay time, and probe checking interval during a test. Additionally the criteria defining a "Pass" versus a "Refer" result can be manipulated by the user (Figure 7–9).

The flexibility of the AuDX protocol setup software allows creation of protocols that may be of interest to those participating in research or more advanced clinical applications. For example, the user can define input/output function protocols or protocols that will measure changes in DPOAE response parameters related to changes in F_2/F_1 ratio.

DPOAE protocols can be specifically created for different clinical applications. Examples are shown in Table 4–4.

The standard configuration of AuDX II includes memory for storing 10 tests and one protocol. However, with AuDX II, functionality can be expanded to include additional memory for storing 50 or 100 tests and for retaining up to 3 test protocols in memory at a time. Another option with AuDX II is the ability to download test results into a computer and use the Scout software for viewing DPgrams and printing reports. The serial label printer that connects directly to the AuDX hardware for printing results on self-adhesive labels is available as an option.

AuDX II is compatible with Bio-logic's database program specifically designed for newborn hearing screening programs. This tool helps to

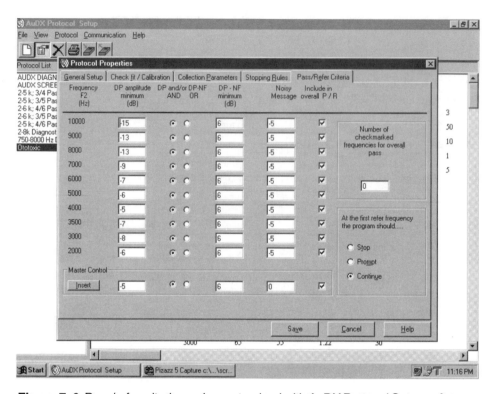

Figure 7–9. Pass/refer criteria can be customized with AuDX Protocol Setup software.

reduce paperwork, facilitates patient follow-up and may be necessary for participation in a statewide program that collects information in a central location. Additionally, AuDX II can be upgraded to interface with some other commercially available database tools.

DPOAEs are now used in some universal newborn hearing screening (UNHS) programs throughout the world. The topic of UNHS is reviewed in detail in Chapter 8.

AuDX (Basic). The AuDX Basic is configured to meet the needs of low volume screening programs that have no need for computerized data management or program tracking and no desire or need to manipulate the test protocol (Figure 7–10). AuDX Basic contains one fixed pass/refer screening protocol and memory capacity for 10 tests. It has no option for user programming, upgraded memory, or additional protocols. It cannot be connected to a computer for transfer and viewing of data or in order to maintain a database. A hard copy of the data can be printed on a self-adhesive label with the purchase of the optional serial label printer. This basic unit is appropriate only for screening purposes.

AuDX Plus. AuDX Plus combines the easy functionality of the hand-held AuDX II with the power of the Scout Sport computer-based system. When the system is connected to a computer that has the Scout Sport software installed, it has all of the capability of Scout Sport. Detach it from the computer and it becomes a hand-held unit that can

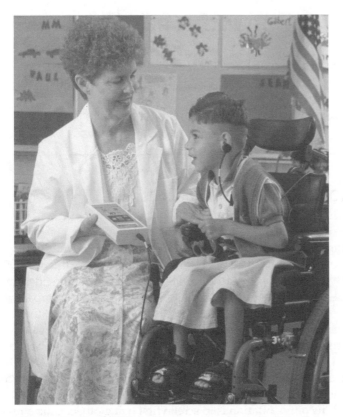

Figure 7–10. AuDX facilitates screening of difficult-to-test populations.

be transported to the patient's bedside. It has all of the capability of the AuDX II and includes increased memory for 50 tests and 3 protocols and the ability to download data to the computer for viewing DP-grams and printing reports. The other AuDX II options are also available including upgraded memory for 100 tests, memory for 3 protocols, and database compatibility.

Because the AuDX Plus embodies all of the functionality of a screening unit as well as a full diagnostic system, it is well suited for programs that want to satisfy both needs with one system.

Manufacturer's Notes

1. The names of compatible newborn hearing screening tools will be provided on request.
2. Patent restrictions preclude the sale of TEOAEs in certain countries by companies other than the patent-holder.
3. Minimum hardware requirements must be met. Call for more information.

ETYMOTIC RESEARCH

Products: ERO SCAN™ Otoacoustic
Emission Scanner

Prepared By: Laurel A. Christensen, Steve Isberg,
Greg Shaw, and David Brown

ERO SCAN™ ER-34 Otoacoustic Emissions Scanner

National birth rate statistics for the United States indicate that approximately 4 million babies are born each year (World Almanac, 1998). In 1993, the National Institutes of Health (NIH) recommended in their consensus statement, "Early Identification of Hearing Impairment in Infants and Young Children," that all babies born in the U.S. be screened for hearing loss within the first 3 months of life (NIH, 1993). In order to carry out this mandate, screening procedures must be both rapid and cost effective. Auditory brainstem response (ABR) testing and otoacoustic emission (OAE) testing are currently the accepted methods for screening infants; however, the NIH consensus statement (1993) recommendation is to screen first using otoacoustic emissions, followed by an ABR if the emission test is failed. This recommendation is based on data showing otoacoustic emission testing to be more rapid and cost effective than ABR for initial screening of infants.

The Etymotic Research Otoacoustic Emissions Scanner (ERO SCAN test system; pronounced arrow-scan) is a quick and easy to use distortion product otoacoustic emission (DPOAE) test unit. The unit may be used by both the technician and the sophisticated professional, depending only on the programming selections made through a user-friendly programmable interface. The unit is suitable for testing patients of all ages in hospital-based neonatal hearing screening programs, pediatrician's offices, school-based hearing screening programs, and by audiologists during diagnostic hearing evaluations.

Product Description

The ERO SCAN is a hand-held distortion product otoacoustic emission (DPOAE) test system. The ERO SCAN system (see Figure 7–11) consists of a hand-held test unit, resting cradle, printer, probe eartips and a pair of lightweight headphones (not shown) that allow the tester to monitor the testing in the patient's ear. An optional watertight carrying case is also available.

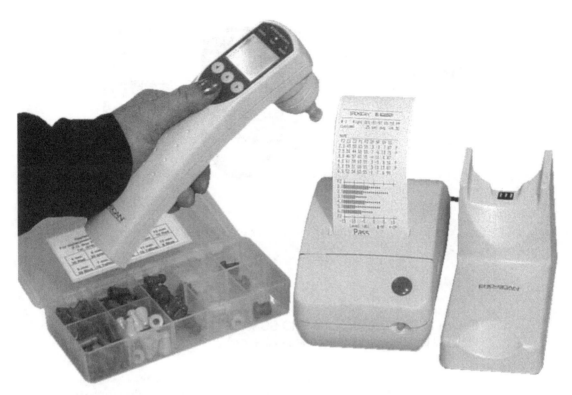

Figure 7–11. The ERO SCAN hand-held DPOAE device from Etymotic Research, with printer and a sample of probe tips.

The ERO SCAN unit is controlled using the arrow keypad. An LCD display with three indicator lights (see Figure 7–12) provides feedback to the tester. The indicator lights inform the tester when the device is ready for use ("READY" light), when a test is in progress ("TEST" light), and when there is excessive environmental noise ("ERROR" light). The four buttons on the keypad allow the user to control testing, customize test protocols, and change the programmable test variables of the system.

The hand-held unit of the ERO SCAN test system elicits a DPOAE by generating two pure tones through a high-quality 18-bit digital-to-analog converter. The frequency ratio (f_2/f_1) of the tones is fixed at 1.20, while the pressures of the tones can be user modified. Nine different sets of test frequencies are available to the user.

The two tones are presented to the ear via speaker tubes located in the probe tip. Disposable eartips (see Figure 7–11) are used to couple the device into the ear of the patient.

The sound pressure in the ear canal is measured by a microphone and digitized by a high-quality 18-bit analog-to-digital converter. The pri-

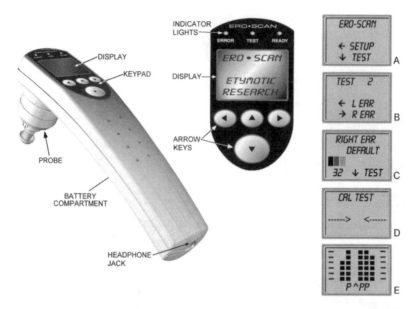

Figure 7–12. Features of the ERO SCAN DPOAE device, including the LCD panel displays (described in the text).

maries at f_1 and f_2, DPOAE at $2f_1 - f_2$, and noise floor pressure are then estimated via a digital signal processor and the discrete Fourier transform (bin resolution = 31 Hz). The ERO SCAN unit estimates the noise floor based on the 4 closest frequency bins to the emission bin.

Ambient and physiologic noise is a major nonpathologic factor in OAE measurement, as reviewed in Chapter 5 and summarized in Table 5–3.

Test results can be downloaded either to the accompanying high-speed printer or to a PC via a serial port. When using the printer, the test results are automatically printed when the unit is placed in the cradle provided and the printer has been turned on. The printer can be powered from built-in rechargeable batteries or from the line. Downloading to a computer is accomplished via a RS-232 port located in the cradle. Screening management software is supplied for this purpose.

Additional features of the hand-held unit include a real-time clock that provides a time-stamp for test results and a nonvolatile memory to store up to 50 tests. The hand-held unit is powered by 4 AA batteries.

One main key to screening using DPOAEs is to obtain a test result with a low noise floor. An adaptive noise-rejection algorithm is used to improve the noise floor of the test result in noisy environments. The ERO SCAN has a built-in sound level meter (SLM) that monitors the ambient environmental noise (see Figure 7–12, LCD panel C). As the unit is placed in the ear canal, a reduction in environmental noise can be observed. Subject (body) noise can also be monitored. Testing is then initiated when the environmental noise is at an acceptable level.

Suggested Test Protocols

In the default setting (Figure 7–13), the ERO SCAN will present test signals at 3 frequencies (2, 3, and 4 kHz) and collect the emission data in approximately 6 seconds. In the "Advanced Set-Up" menu of the device, the user can program up to 3 custom programs to store in the device. The test variables that can be manipulated by the user include the number of frequencies tested and the number of times each frequency is tested, the frequency range of the test signals, the levels of the primary tones, the averaging time of data collection, the signal-to-noise ratio (SNR) required for a "pass", and the number of frequencies

(1) The number of the test.

(2) The ear selected.

(3) The time and date of the test, based on the setting of the internal clock. If the clock is set incorrectly this time and date will be incorrect.

(4) The software version number.

(5) The averaging time used for this test.

(6) The mode selected for this test.

(7) The f_2 frequency.

(8) The calibration response used to set the primary levels.

(9) The levels of the primaries.

(A) The level of the emission in dB SPL.

(B) The percent of samples accepted (based on the noise rejection, low percentages indicate high noise level present during the test).

(C) A "P" indicates that the signal-to-noise ratio for the test was above the Pass criteria.

(D) The noise level in dB SPL.

(E) The signal-to-noise ratio (dp level minus the noise level).

(F) The thick bars indicate the noise level in dB SPL.

(G) The small bars indicate the emission level in dB SPL.

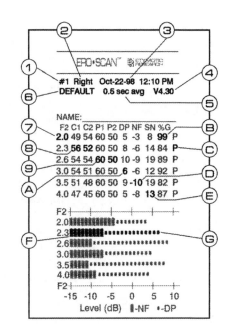

Figure 7–13. Test parameters and variables for the ERO SCAN DPOAE device (see text for details).

that must be at the desired SNR to call the overall test a "pass." Figure 7–13 shows these programmable variables, the system's default settings, and the options the user has to create custom programs.

In addition to the test variables that can be changed via the "Advanced Set-Up" menu, the unit also has other basic options that can be determined by the user. These include the length of unit inactivity before it automatically shuts off, the volume level of the monitoring headphones, and the format of the printed results.

Measurement and Analyses of DPOAEs with the ERO SCAN

To measure DPOAEs with the ERO SCAN system in the default setting, turn the device on by pushing the down arrow button. The display on the unit will look like Figure 7–12 Panel A and the green "READY" light will be illuminated. The user then simply pushes the down arrow key to run an emissions test and the display will show the screen in Figure 7–12, Panel B. Next use the right or left arrow buttons to select the right or left ear. The SLM in Figure 7–12, Panel C will be displayed and the yellow "TEST" light will be illuminated. The ERO SCAN is now measuring the ambient noise in the environment and displaying the levels on the LCD display. Place the unit in the patient's ear, and a decrease of 20–30 dB SPL should be seen on the SLM. Once a seal in the ear is obtained, the ERO SCAN will automatically initiate the test. Figure 7–12, Panel D will be shown on the display while the calibration tones are emitted into the ear canal. If there is a good seal and there is no blockage in the eartip or ear canal, the display shown in Figure 7–12, Panel E will be seen. The bar graphs will fill in as the test proceeds. The number of bars shown is determined by the number of DPOAEs tested. Each bar indicates the SNR at the DPOAE frequency being tested, with the lowest frequency to the left. The blocks in the bar represent one sixth of the pass SNR criteria. A full bar indicates a "pass" at that frequency, and a "P" will be displayed below the bar. If there is no letter under a bar this indicates that the emission at this frequency did not exceed the pass SNR criteria. A symbol will indicate when this frequency had a calibration problem or had 0% of the samples accepted, and no data at this frequency were accepted.

When the test sequence is finished, the "READY" light will illuminate. The ERO SCAN test system will alert the tester via messages on the LCD screen if the probe was blocked or if the seal was inadequate. In addition, anytime the noise level exceeds the noise-rejection level of the unit, the red "ERROR" light will illuminate, indicating too much noise in the ear canal. Following a test sequence, the tester has the option of reviewing the results or returning to the main menu (see Figure 7–12, Panel A). Once the unit is returned to the main menu, the results can be automatically printed by placing the unit on the cradle and turning on the power of the printer unit.

Quick-Test

The ERO SCAN system can be configured for the user to do a "Quick-Test." This setting is different from the normal operation described above and was designed for the technician using the device. In this setting, the ERO SCAN is turned on, the right or left ear is selected, and the unit is placed in the patient's ear. The test will automatically begin when a seal is obtained and the LCD display will print "pass" or "refer" following the test based on the default criteria described above. A special set of keystrokes will allow the unit to switch to normal operation.

An example of a test printout from the ERO SCAN system was illustrated in Figure 7–11. A "full" printout includes both a numeric and graphic display of the test results. The printout format can be modified via the "Basic Set-Up" menu to display just the graphic or just the numeric test results as desired. The top of the printout shows various identifying information including the test number, the ear tested, the date and time the test was performed, the unit setting (Default, Custom A, Custom B, or Custom C) at the time of the test, the averaging time for the data collection, and the current version of software inside the ERO SCAN test system. Note that the printout does not identify patients by name or initials, thus the tester must keep a running list of the patient's name and test number. There is a space underneath the identifying information to write the patient's name, number, or initials on the test printout. Below the name are the results of the test. Moving from left to right across the first row is F2 (the frequency of f_2), C1 and C2 (the calibration response to the signal which is used to set the presentation levels of the primaries), P1 and P2 (the levels of the primaries), DP (the level of the distortion product emission in dB SPL), NF (the level of the noise floor in dB SPL), SN (the SNR calculated by taking DP level minus the NF level), and %G (% Good is the percent of samples accepted based on the noise rejection. Low percentages indicate high noise levels present during the test). A "P" at the end of a row is an indication that the SNR for the test was above the "pass" criteria. The graph at the bottom of the page shows the noise level using the thick bars, and the emission level using the thin bars.

Normative Data

At the time of this writing clinical trials using the ERO SCAN device are underway.

Normative data are required for meaningful interpretation of OAEs. Guidelines for collection and use of normative data are supplied in Chapter 4, whereas normative databases for selected DPOAE devices are displayed in Appendix A.

Summary

The ERO SCAN test system is a quick and easy to use distortion product otoacoustic emission (DPOAE) test unit. The flexible programmable interface will meet the needs of both the screening technician and the trained professional. A screening test can be accomplished in the default setting in seconds by a technician with minimal instruction about the unit. In addition, the trained professional can change the default test settings and accomplish more sophisticated testing with custom settings. The portable nature of the device makes it desirable for DPOAE testing in all possible environments.

References

Early Identification of Hearing Impairment in Infants and Young Children. *NIH Consensus Statement* (1993). March 1–3;11(1):1–24.
The World Almanac and Book of Facts. (1998). New York: World Almanac Books.

GRASON STADLER INCORPORATED (GSI)

Products: GSI 60 DPOAE System
                  GSI 70 Automated OAE System

Prepared By: Jan Painter
                  Grason Stadler Inc.
                  Milford, NH

Overview

Grason-Stadler, Inc. manufactures two different OAE systems. These systems are named the GSI 60 DPOAE System and the GSI 70 Automated OAE System. The GSI 60 DPOAE System is a diagnostic instrument that provides the versatility to work as a screening system for Universal Hearing Screening Programs and/or as a diagnostic system for use in an Audiology Clinic or ENT office setting. The GSI 70 Automated OAE System is designed to be a dedicated screening device for use in Universal Hearing Screening Programs or a physician's office.

GSI 60 DPOAE System

Product Description. The GSI 60 DPOAE System is a flexible, user-friendly instrument that provides testing capability for DPOAEs (distortion product OAEs), SOAEs (spontaneous OAEs), and our patented Simultaneous DPOAE measurements (Figure 7–14). The GSI 60 can be configured as a DSP (digital signal processing) board for insertion into an ISA slot within a desktop computer console or as a stand-alone product that attaches to the parallel port on a notebook computer that supports an 8-bit bidirectional protocol.

The GSI 60 probe consists of a probe box which contains the F_1 and F_2 speakers and a probe tip which contains the measurement microphone and sound delivery tubing. The probe tip is very lightweight and can be disassembled for fast and easy cleaning. The probe is easily connected to the GSI 60 system. Because the system calibration data is supplied on a floppy disk, an operator can easily reload calibration information whenever a probe is changed.

Calibration is performed at our factory using an IEC 711 specified coupler. Reusable and disposable eartips in a wide range of sizes are available for use with patients of all ages. The GSI 60 DPOAE System software is designed to work in Windows 3.1, Windows 95, and Windows 98 formats. This graphic environment allows the user interface to be

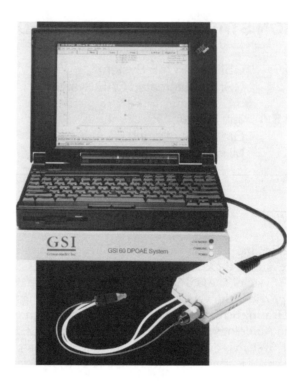

Figure 7–14. The GSI 60 DPOAE System with a Notebook Computer.

easily learned and permits test results to be easily overlaid for comparison purposes. It also permits test results to be printed on a wide variety of Windows-supported printers. The GSI 60 operating system contains a database designed around the Paradox database engine. This enables test results to be stored and later retrieved. It also permits results to be easily exported to another GSI 60 system if the ability to merge test results from a number of GSI 60 systems is needed. Alternatively, test results can be exported in an ASCII format for transfer to a spreadsheet or statistical package.

A variety of test protocols (stimulus and averaging) are included with the system to get the user started in data collection. User-defined protocols can also be developed to meet unique testing needs. These protocols can be easily retrieved for testing as needed. The DP stimulus frequency range available is 500 to 8000 Hz and the intensity range is 20 to 75 dB SPL. Stimulus parameter selections include the number of octaves and number of points per octave to test, the intensities for L_1 and L_2 in dB SPL, and the ratio of F_2 to F_1. The number of additional DP stimulus protocols that can be stored is virtually unlimited, thereby allowing the operator to develop a library of protocols to meet a variety of testing requirements if desired. Similarly, the operator can develop a library of averaging protocols to meet the testing needs of different screening and diagnostic circumstances. The averaging protocol parameters include the setting of the sample rejection criteria (artifact rejection), the minimum and maximum number of averages to perform, and the stopping rules. The stopping rules can be set as a function of the signal-to-noise level, the averaged noise level, or the maximum number of samples collected.

The standard DP stimulus protocols allow stimulus (tone pairs) presentations to proceed from low frequency to high frequency. The Custom Stimulus feature allows the tone pairs to be presented from high to low frequency. This is often helpful when testing newborns as data collection proceeds more rapidly at the higher frequencies. If the DP stimulus protocol is used, the computer calculates the actual frequencies presented for F_1 and F_2 based on the number of points per octave selected. However, it is the operator who determines the actual frequencies for F_1 and F_2 whenever a Custom Stimulus protocol is developed. The Custom Stimulus mode also enables the selection of a different number of data points for each octave to be tested.

Learning to operate the GSI 60 is very simple. Simply select NEW to enter the patient name followed by GO! to begin data collection. The preset stimulus and averaging protocols will proceed automatically. Once data collection is complete, click on SAVE to store the test results in the database. Select the opposite ear followed by GO! to test the second ear. Should you encounter any problems during testing, the test sequence can be PAUSED. Testing can then resume wherever you are ready.

Password protection is available for protocol definitions and default settings. This is especially useful in settings where the actual testing is being performed by assistants rather than by the program administrator. Password Protection provides a good source of audit control for screening programs because the program administrator is able to set and control the protocols used during testing. It is also possible to automate the scoring process by establishing a DP scoring protocol. This is very useful for Universal Hearing Screening programs in which a large number of babies is being tested and where there is a need for timely reporting of test results. (This will be explained in greater detail under the section entitled Measurement and Analysis.)

SOAE measurement and interpretation is reviewed in detail in Chapter 3, whereas the influence of SOAEs on DPOAEs and TEOAEs is summarized in Chapter 5.

The GSI 60 DPOAE System also provides the capability to measure Spontaneous Emissions (SOAEs). This test mode allows the operator to select the frequency range for the measurement (Figure 7–15). Unlike the DP measurement mode where it is possible to predetermine the frequency for the emission measurement, it is not possible to know ahead of time where the spontaneous emission(s) might be measured. The SOAE test mode allows the operator to control the fre-

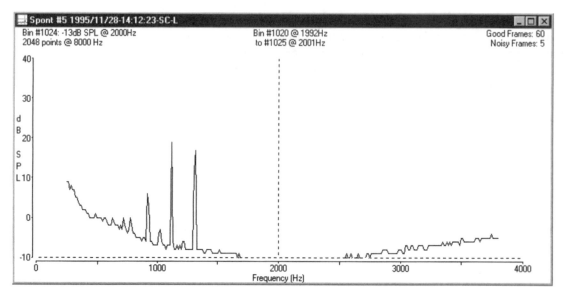

Figure 7–15. Example of a spontaneous emission with the GSI 60 system.

quency range by setting the sampling rate (4000, 6000, 8000, 12,000, or 16,000) and the number of points within the FFT (1024, 2048, or 4096). For example, if the frequency range desired is 0 to 4000 Hz, then a sampling rate of 8000 and an FFT size of 4096 would be selected. This allows the data to be collected into bins that are only 2 Hz wide over the frequency range of 0 to 4000 Hz. The test time is controlled by setting the number of averages needed.

A major challenge during SOAE measurements is eliminating room and computer noise. For this reason, it is highly recommended that the patient be seated in a soundproof room with the computer placed outside the sound room during SOAE testing. The door to the sound room does not have to be closed. The important factor is isolating the computer from the probe.

Suggested Test Protocols

Newborn Setting. When testing newborns, it is suggested that the stimulus protocol cover the frequency range of 2000 to 4000 Hz with $L_1 = 65$ dB SPL and $L_2 = 55$ dB SPL and the F_2 to F_1 ratio set to 1.2(2). The number of points selected within this octave depends on the degree of precision needed from the testing (see Figure 7–16). For example, select 3, 4, or 5 points within this octave. The averaging protocol needs to be fairly robust due to the biological and environmental noise encountered with this newborn population. Selecting a sampling rate of 32,000 Hz allows a larger number of data points to be measured in a shorter amount of time. Set the minimum number of averages to 200 and the maximum to 500. Set the stopping rules to require either a sig-

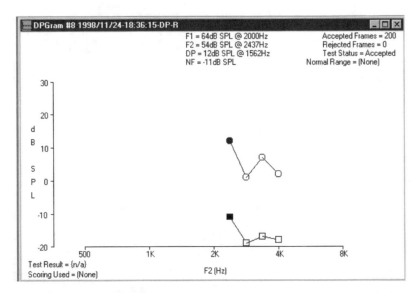

F1 = 64dB SPL @ 2000Hz
F2 = 54dB SPL @ 2437Hz
DP = 12dB SPL @ 1562Hz
NF = -11dB SPL

Accepted Frames = 200
Rejected Frames = 0
Test Status = Accepted
Normal Range = (None)

Figure 7–16. DPgram recorded with the newborn 2K+ protocols with the GSI 60 DPOAE System.

A large section of Chapter 8 (Clinical Applications of OAEs in Children) is devoted to the use of OAEs in newborn hearing screening.

nal-to-noise level (DP dB SPL minus noise floor dB SPL) of 10 dB or the averaged noise floor per DP point to be -20 dB SPL or the maximum number of averages to be 500 whichever occurs first. These DP stimulus and averaging protocols are preset by GSI and are named "newborn 2K+." This averaging protocol will set the test time to be 3 (minimum) to 8 (maximum) seconds per DP point measured. If it is desired to present the tone pairs from high to low frequency, use the Custom Stimulus mode to program this frequency sequence. Another option would be to set the $L_1 = 70$ and $L_2 = 70$ if extreme noise is encountered during testing.

Quick Screening. In settings where a quick screen of cochlear function across a wider frequency range is desired, expand the frequency range to 1000 Hz to 8000 Hz with 3 points per octave selected (Figure 7–17). Set $L_1 = 65$ and $L_2 = 55$ dB SPL. Use a sampling rate of either 16,000 (for testing up to 6000 Hz) or 32,000 Hz (for testing up to 8000 Hz). The averaging protocol used depends on the degree of precision needed. By setting the minimum number of averages to 10 and the maximum to 400 along with stopping rules of either a signal-to-noise ratio of 10 dB or a noise floor of -20 dB or a maximum number of averages of 400 whichever occurs first, it is possible to keep the overall test time fairly short. However, if these settings are used, it is highly recommended that a repeatability check be performed to determine how reliable the test results are. These protocols are included with the GSI 60 and are called SCREEN. This protocol works well when the population being tested is fairly quiet. When testing preschool or primary school children, it would be better to use a more robust averaging protocol such as the one described under the Newborn Setting description. Also, if the setting is very noisy, it may be necessary to set $L_1 = L_2 = 70$ dB SPL.

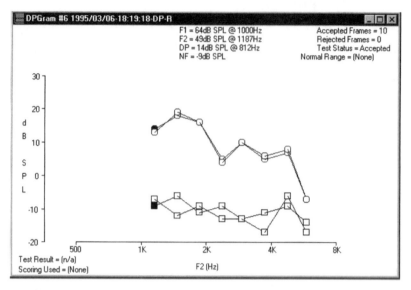

Figure 7–17. DPgram recorded with a screening protocol with the GSI 60 DPOAE System.

A review of ototoxicity, including the effects of specific ototoxic medications on OAEs, is presented in Chapter 8 and summarized in Tables 8–25 through 8–27.

Ototoxic Drug Testing. This is a situation where greater precision is required. *(Note:* a baseline DPGram will be needed prior to the patient receiving the potentially ototoxic drug for comparison purposes. Also, the protocols used for this baseline testing need to be the same as that used during follow-up testing.) Because the toxic effect of some drugs tends to affect the higher frequencies sooner than the lower frequencies, it is suggested that the frequency range for testing be limited to 4000 to 8000 Hz. Set $L_1 = 65$ and $L_2 = 55$ dB SPL. As a means of adding greater precision, select a larger number of data points within this octave, for example, 8 or 10 points. Due to the need for greater precision, a very robust averaging protocol is suggested. Such a protocol might set the sampling rate to 32,000 Hz, the minimum number of averages to 128 and the maximum to 2000 averages. The stopping rules might require a signal-to-noise ratio of 17 dB or a noise floor of -20 or the maximum number of averages to be 2000. This averaging protocol is included with the GSI 60 and is named DIAGNOSTIC (Figure 7–18).

Measurement and Analysis

The GSI 60 performs an ear seal check at the beginning of the test sequence to ensure that an appropriate seal has been achieved. If it is determined that the seal is insufficient, an error message will appear on the screen allowing the operator to check the eartip for any cerumen or to select a different size eartip to achieve a better seal. Once a good seal is obtained, the test sequence can begin. Prior to making any measurements per tone pair presentation, the GSI 60 uses an auto leveling technique to ensure that the desired intensity levels for L_1 and L_2 are

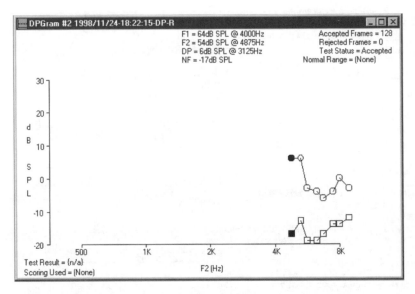

Figure 7–18. DPgram recorded with a diagnostic/ototoxic protocol with the GSI 60 DPOAE System.

met. Thus, the intensity levels used during the stimulus presentation are appropriate for the ear being tested.

The measurement process involves the use of an FFT with 512 points. The test sequence begins with the presentation of the first tone pair set by the stimulus protocol. Prior to accepting a sample of data, each sample is evaluated to determine if the noise level in the frequencies surrounding the DP frequency are below the rejection criteria set in the averaging protocol. If the noise level is not below this value, the spectral data are rejected. (A count of rejected samples and the reason for rejection are stored along with the DPgram.) As good samples of data are collected, they are averaged. Once the minimum number of averages is met, a check is made of the averaged noise floor and the signal-to-noise value to see if either stopping rule has been met. If a stopping rule is not met, the averaging continues. The stopping rules are then constantly monitored until a stopping criterion is met or the maximum number of averages is achieved, whichever occurs first. As the result of each DP point becomes available, it is displayed on the screen along with the text describing the data point values. A red circle is used to plot each DP value from the right ear and a blue X is used to plot DP points from the left ear. The noise floor per DP point is plotted as a green square. If desired, the spectral data for each DP point can be displayed.

DPOAE test protocols, including their rationale, is reviewed in detail in Chapter 4. See for example Tables 4–4 through 4–6.

Analysis of the DPgram can be performed either manually by visual inspection of the test results or it can be scored automatically through the use of the DP Scoring feature (Figure 7–19). The automatic scoring criteria per DP point can be any combination of the following: the

Figure 7–19. The set-up screening for DP scoring protocol selection with the GSI 60 DPOAE System.

absolute intensity level of the DP, the signal-to-noise level achieved, the repeatability of the DP point from the first to the second run, or by meeting/exceeding the value from a Normal range used during testing. Once each DP point has been individually scored, then the overall DPgram can be scored. The overall scoring can be determined by setting the number of points per octave that must meet the scoring criteria per DP point or by setting the number of points within the DP Gram that must meet the scoring per DP point.

Guidelines for collection and use of normative data are provided in Chapter 4, whereas normative databases for selected DPOAE devices, including the GSI 60, are supplied in Appendix A.

Normative Data. Several clinics have provided GSI with their normative data from DPOAE testing for inclusion within the GSI 60. At press time, the following normative data are either programmed into the GSI 60 or included within the instruction manual: Boystown National Research Hospital, Dartmouth Hitchcock Medical Center, University of Miami, and Vanderbilt University. (*Note:* When using these normative ranges, it is important to use the same testing protocols as those used to establish the normative values.) The normative range values can be displayed on the screen either before or after collecting the DPgram. However, if the normal range data are to be used as part of the automated scoring criteria, it must be selected prior to data collection. It is also possible for operators to collect and establish their own normal range data. This template information can then be programmed into the GSI 60.

New Product Innovations/Developments

GSI has entered into a partnership with OZ Systems to provide a Total Solution Package for Universal Hearing Screening Programs. This partnership results in a seamless interface between the GSI 60 and the Screening and Information Management Solution (SIMS) Information Management Program. (*Note:* The Oz Systems product is reviewed later in this chapter). This seamless interface allows the tester to enter patient demographic information only once, and initiate testing and score the DPgram as if these activities were happening within the same program. Scoring is performed by the Interpretive Assistant provided by the SIMS program and is based on a statistical evaluation of data integrity. All test protocols and measurements are performed by the GSI 60. The stimulus and averaging protocols are named the "OZ Templates" within the GSI 60. The SIMS program manages the database of test results along with the patient demographics and reporting functions. In addition, it provides auditing capabilities for each tester along with overall program performance measures.

A unique feature of the GSI 60 is the ability to present multiple primary tone pairs simultaneously and to measure their corresponding DP responses at the same time (Figure 7–20). Either the DP stimulus or the Custom Stimulus mode can be utilized for simultaneous testing. It is important to note, however, that the tone pairs presented simultaneously must be an octave apart to avoid stimulus artifact. This is performed automatically whenever a simultaneous DP stimulus protocol is used. Care must be taken when setting a simultaneous Custom stimulus protocol. The test results from a simultaneous stimulus presenta-

The concept of DPOAE measurement simultaneously for several pair of f_1 and f_2 stimuli is described in Chapter 4. Clinical application of this technique was the topic of a publication in 1997 by Kim and colleagues at the University of Connecticut Health Science Center (see reference list).

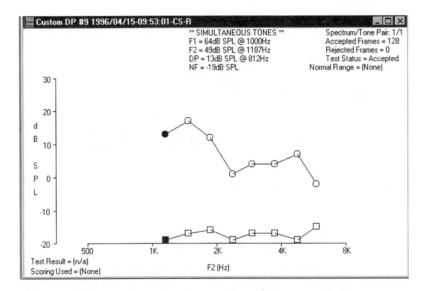

Figure 7–20. DPgram recorded with a simultaneous stimulus presentation feature with the GSI 60 DPOAE System.

tion are plotted as a DPgram. If the spectral data are reviewed, each tone pair and its corresponding emission can be reviewed.

GSI 70 Automated OAE System

Product Description. The GSI 70 Automated OAE System provides a simple and easy-to-use solution for screening cochlear function in Universal Hearing Screening Programs and for fast, accurate DPOAE testing in a physician's office. The GSI 70 is a self-contained DPOAE system that does not require a computer to operate. It is available as a Single or Multiple Patient System (Figure 7–21).

The Single Patient System consists of a battery-operated (rechargeable) screener with a lightweight probe and a printer/charger stand. The GSI 70 probe contains the speakers and microphone necessary for stimulus presentation and measurement of the DP levels. The probe also stores its own unique calibration data. (Should the probe ever need replacement, it is a simple matter of disconnecting the old probe and connecting the new probe.) The test sequence can be initiated via a push-button on the probe assembly or from the screener push-button. The screener contains a graphical display for test results and data storage push-buttons (Figure 7–22). The testing protocol is also stored within the screener. Once the DPgram is completed, it is automatically scored as a Pass/Refer on the display. The test results from the right ear and left ear can be stored and reviewed prior to being transferred to the printer. The printout consists of the scored graphs for the right and left ear along with a table containing the numeric values for each DP point. A template line indicating the Pass/Refer line is displayed on the screener as well as the printout.

The Multiple Patient System contains all of the features of the Single Patient version and adds the ability to enter up to 50 patient names/ID numbers prior to collecting the test results. It also provides storage space for up to 200 test results (400 ears). The patient names/ID numbers can be entered directly via the built-in touch screen with a stylus or they can be typed into the GSI 70 database program on a computer. (*Note*: the computer is an option.) If the names/ID numbers are entered into the database program, they are transferred directly to the screener by pointing the GSI 70 at the IrDA port on the computer. Alternatively, the computer can be attached to the COM port on the printer/charger for this names/ID transfer. The patient name/ID number is recalled from the screener prior to testing. Once the test results are stored within the GSI 70, they can be transferred to the GSI 70 database program by pointing the GSI 70 at the computers IrDA port or by placing the GSI 70 in its charger stand for transfer to the computer COM port. The GSI 70 database is a Windows program based on the Microsoft Access database engine. It provides the ability to enter patient names/ID numbers for transfer to the GSI 70 and to receive test results from the GSI 70 for storage. The stored DPgrams can be sorted by a variety of criteria and retrieved for printout. Any Windows-compati-

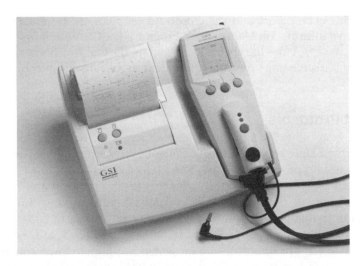

Figure 7–21. The hand-held GSI 70 DPOAE System. The GSI 70 device is fully automated.

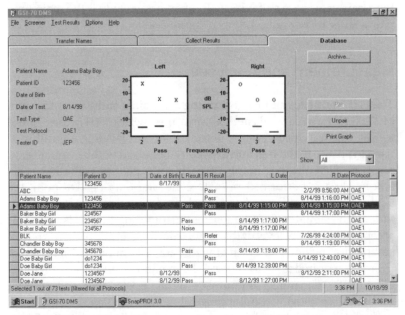

Figure 7–22. The main screen from the Data Management Software program utilized with the GSI 70 hand-held DPOAE device.

ble printer that is capable of printing text and graphics can be used. If multiple test results exist for a particular patient, it is possible to pair the best right and left ear together within the database. In addition to providing the ability to print multiple DPgrams, it is also possible to print a listing of the names/ID numbers of patients who either Passed or need to be Referred for further testing. The results from multiple GSI 70s can be stored in a single GSI 70 database if desired. Stored test results can be exported in a Microsoft Access or an ASCII format to an external Information Management Program. The GSI 70 database program also provides the ability to reprogram the GSI 70. This is important if the screening protocol requirement should change over time.

Test Protocols

Both the Single and the Multiple Patient Systems are shipped with a fixed testing protocol and Pass/Refer template. The Multiple Patient System provides the ability to alter this testing protocol and Pass/Refer template through the GSI 70 database software program. The default testing protocol presents tone pairs at f_2 values of 2000, 3000, and 4000 Hz with $L_1 = 65$ dB and $L_2 = 55$ dB SPL. The f_2 to f_1 ratio is preset to 1.2. The tone pairs are presented in a high to low frequency sequence. If the data collected from the 4000 Hz tone pair presentation do not meet the Pass criteria, the tone pair frequencies are automatically shifted 3/64th of an octave and then retested. The test sequence then proceeds to the f_2 value of 3000 Hz and 2000 Hz. In each case, the tone pair values are shifted 3/64th of an octave only if the main tone pair results are not scored a Pass (Figure 7–23).

Measurement and Analyses

The GSI 70 utilizes an FFT containing 512 points and a sampling rate of 32,000 Hz. An ear seal check is performed with a 500 Hz tone before testing begins. Once a seal is detected, an autoleveling algorithm is used to ensure that the L_1 and L_2 values measured within the ear canal are correct at the beginning of each tone pair presentation. This autoleveling is performed prior to collecting data per DP point for analysis. Each sample of data is evaluated to determine if the amplitude of the signal in the frequencies surrounding the DP is below an acceptable intensity level. If this is not true, this sample of data is rejected and not included in the averaged data. The minimum number of averages required is set to 200 and the maximum number of averages is set to 500. The minimum number of data points averaged must be met before employing the stopping rules. The stopping rules are a signal-to-noise ratio of 10 dB or an averaged noise floor value of -20 dB or a maximum number of samples collected equals 500, whichever occurs first. A DP point is scored as a Pass or Retest based on its amplitude relative to a template line. If the averaged noise floor value is -20 dB without achieving a 10 dB signal-to-noise, this DP point is scored as a Retest. Whenever the maximum number of 500 samples is reached without meeting the targeted signal-to-noise level or the targeted averaged noise floor criterion, this data point is scored as Noisy. If the test sequence is stopped prematurely, the test result is scored as an Abort.

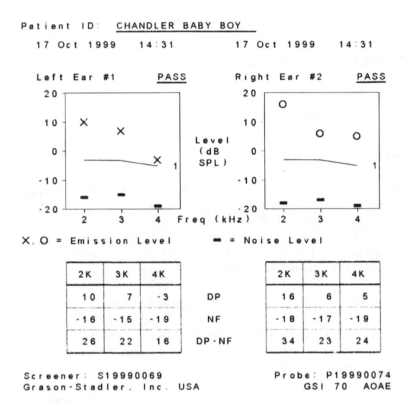

Patient ID: CHANDLER BABY BOY

17 Oct 1999   14:31   17 Oct 1999   14:31

2K	3K	4K			2K	3K	4K
10	7	-3	DP		16	6	5
-16	-15	-19	NF		-18	-17	-19
26	22	16	DP-NF		34	23	24

Screener: S19990069   Probe: P19990074
Grason-Stadler, Inc. USA   GSI 70   AOAE

Figure 7–23. Sample screening DPgrams recorded with the GSI 70 hand-held DPOAE device.

Normative Data and Scoring

The Pass/Retest template line supplied with the GSI 70 default testing protocol is the result of a clinical study conducted by Frank Musiek, Ph.D., and coworkers at Dartmouth Hitchcock Medical Center. This study utilized the results from ABR measurements to determine which DP amplitudes corresponded to a normal ear. Contact GSI for the results of this study.

New Product Innovations/Developments

The GSI 70 is designed to be a screening platform that will support OAE measurements as well as tympanometry and audiometry. The product is being released initially as an automated OAE system. The tympanometry and/or audiometry modules can be added at a later date.

Integration of OAE instrumentation with technology for immittance measurement would be a major advance in the clinical application of OAEs, particularly in children. This topic is introduced in Chapter 10.

HORTMANN

Product: AmDiS-OAE

Prepared by: Bernd Waldmann

Product Description

General. AmDiS-OAE is a PC-based Otoacoustic Emission Analyzer for the audiologist's office, clinic, and research lab. It implements four of the five available OAE recording techniques: spontaneous emissions (SOAE), distortion products (DPOAEs), suppression of DPOAEs, and the newly discovered sgDPOAEs (see below). The fifth method, TEOAEs, may be included in a future release.

Software. AmDiS-OAE software currently runs on computers equipped with Windows 3.1 or Windows 95 and includes all the usual Windows interface elements and capabilities. Multiple test results can be displayed in separate windows (Figure 7–24). AmDiS-OAE includes an open-standard database management system. To accommodate both routine and advanced users, the software can be run in different modes. There is a routine mode for users without permission to modify parameters and an advanced mode for users who need access to many operating parameters and test functions. The screen display includes a toolbar for most frequently used commands, and multiple movable panels for test results.

Hardware. AmDiS-OAE hardware consists of a digital signal processing board and an amplifier module that connect to the computer and to an ear canal probe. The PC is used only for display of results; all real-time signal processing and analysis tasks are performed by a dedicated digital signal processor chip to keep measurement times as short as possible, even on older PCs.

Database. AmDiS-OAE includes a Paradox-compatible database management system for storage of patient data and test results. Patient data include name, date of birth, and medical record and social security number. A special tool supplied with the product converts these results to text files for inclusion in spreadsheet or other analysis software.

Regulatory Affairs. AmDiS-OAE is FDA approved for both DPOAE and new sgDPOAE measurements. It also complies with European Medical Device Directive (MDD) requirements. The product uses a database system that can handle dates beyond the year 2000.

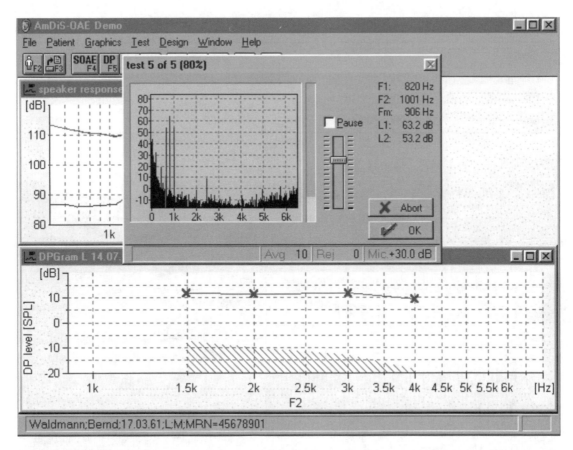

Figure 7–24. Multiple DPOAE test results displayed on the computer screen of the Hortmann AmDiS-OAE system.

Suggested Test Protocols. AmDiS-OAE comes with a number of predefined test protocols that cover most routine applications like a standard DPgram, DP growth function, or screening test. Any number of additional test protocols can be defined by the user and recalled by name. The predefined test protocols are associated with buttons on the programs toolbar for quick access to these functions. These standard protocols can also be modified by the user, the predefined values are shown in Table 7–1.

Measurement and Analyses of OAEs

Checking Probe Fit. For control of probe fit, the system displays an instant spectrum of the ear canal response and an indication of the estimated ear canal volume, both in numeric form and as a simple good/bad indicator light (Figure 7–25). With this display, leaking or

A secure probe fit is crucial to successful OAE measurement. Chapter 4 includes a discussion of steps important in verifying adequate probe fit in OAE measurement (for example see Figure 4–1) and for probe problems (see Tables 4–1 and 4–8).

Table 7–1. Stimulus parameters for predefined tests in AmDiS-OAE.

Name	f_2 [Hz]	$f_2{:}f_1$	L_1 [dB SPL]	L_1-L_2
DPgram	1000, 1500, 2000, 3000, 4000	1.22	65	10
DP growth function	2000	1.22	40, 50, 60, 70	10
Screening test	1000, 2000, 4000	1.22	65	10

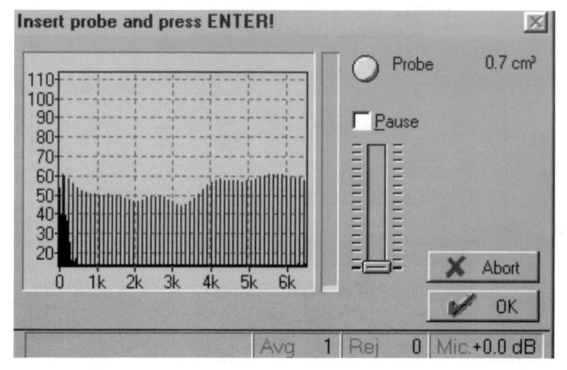

Figure 7–25. Screen used in checking the probe fit of the Hortmann AmDIS-OAE system prior to DPOAE measurement.

occluded probes can be detected. Throughout the program, a multi-sinewave signal is used to gauge ear canal frequency response. Since ambient noise can be seen at frequencies not used by the test signal, the user can simultaneously evaluate ambient noise level and ear canal frequency response.

Ear Canal Response. Before each test, AmDiS-OAE measures the individual ear canal frequency response and uses these values to achieve constant stimulus sound pressure levels at the probe tip. For stimulus frequencies below 5000 Hz, sound pressure at the probe tip has been shown to be a valid and accurate estimate of sound pressure at the eardrum (Siegel JH. *Journal of the Acoustical Society of America* 95:2589-2597, 1994).

Real-Time Display. AmDiS-OAE shows two different views of the test results: During the measurement, a panel that resembles a spectrum-analyzer displays stimuli and highlighted results (pop-up window). The system will automatically set optimum microphone gain and will control stimulus levels, the spectrum display and microphone gain control are available as an additional tool for advanced users.

Real-Time Control of the Measurement. During the measurement, the system will automatically check stimulus levels and will adjust its output if stimulus levels deviate slightly from preset values. It also detects large deviations from preset values (e.g., a slipping probe. In these cases, it will display a warning and offer to abort the measurement. Both emission amplitude and noise level can be evaluated in real-time due to the powerful dedicated digital signal processor. Thus, the system can terminate the averaging process as soon as a preset signal-to-noise ratio has been reached, resulting in the shortest possible test times. A screening test with three test frequencies in a healthy ear can take as little as 15 seconds, including in-the-ear calibration.

Artifact Rejection. In screening applications, it is important that the user does not have to set artifact rejection thresholds manually, because the staff performing the test may not be sufficiently educated to choose a proper setting. AmDiS-OAE includes an algorithm for automatic determination of the optimal threshold, based on ambient noise level, expected emission amplitude and averaging time.

Test Results. During and after the measurement, test results can be viewed as DPgram or DP growth function, depending on the test. The display results consists of a curve showing the emission amplitude in dB SPL, and a hatched area that indicates estimated noise levels during the test. Optionally, the phase of the emission relative to the stimulus frame can be displayed.

Report Sheets. Multiple test results can be combined on a single sheet of paper for comprehensive reports. Again, both routine and advanced users can be accommodated: A standard predefined report sheet can be created by pressing a single button; customized report sheet layouts can be defined by the user.

Screening Evaluation. Automated evaluation of test results for screening application can include several decision criteria:

■ Signal-to-noise-ratio must exceed a certain level. This is the most commonly used criterion to detect a true stimulus-correlated signal in ambient noise.

■ The level difference between emission level L_{DP} and stimulus level L_1 must not exceed a certain limit. This accounts for the fact that any technical instrument will produce distortion products of its own and that these signals must not be mistaken for physiological emissions. Fortunately, these technical emissions are much lower in amplitude than normal physiological ones, so that they can be differentiated from real emissions.

■ The sound pressure of the emission must exceed a certain limit. Some audiologists use this as an additional indicator of emissions.

The "fine points" of OAE microstructure, including theories on its origin, are mentioned in Chapter 4. Fine or microstructure of a DPOAE is illustrated in Figure 4–9.

Normative Data. Because this is a new instrument, normative data were not yet available at the time of printing. Normative data are being gathered at several institutions in the U.S.A. and in Europe. When available, the data will be distributed to users by the manufacturer.

New Product Innovations

High-Precision DPgrams With sgDPOAE. AmDiS-OAE implements a new stimulus paradigm that improves the accuracy of DP amplitude measurements. Conventional DPgrams in normal ears often show large differences in amplitude from one frequency to the next. When recorded at high-frequency resolution, these differences can be seen to be part of a regular fine structure of the DPgram composed of rounded peaks and pointed troughs (Figure 7–26, lower panel). Recent investigations by Heitmann et al. (*Journal of the Acoustical Society of America* 103:1527–1531, 1998) showed that this fine structure can be accounted for by assuming that there are two regions in the cochlea that contribute to the overall emission amplitude. One is the well-known area between f_1 and f_2, where the traveling waves for f_1 and f_2 overlap and where the active cochlear mechanisms produce the distortion product. The second area is in the $2f_1-f_2$ region, where the weak vibration of frequency $2f_1-f_2$ elicits an active cochlear response of the same frequency that travels back to the oval window (Figure 7–27). Depending on the relative phase of the two emission sources, these two signals interfere

The latest thinking on the origin and classification of OAEs is reviewed in Chapter 10, especially a new taxonomy for OAEs offered by Shera and Guinan (1999). As an example, see Figures 10–1 and 10–2.

either constructively or destructively, resulting in alternating zones of high and low amplitude DPOAE. The sgDPOAE stimulus paradigm (patent pending) adds a third stimulus tone close to $2f_1-f_2$, resulting in a suppression of the active process at $2f_1-f_2$. Thus, emission comes only from the region of overlap of f_1 and f_2, the fine structure of the DPgram shows no more ripples (Figure 7–26, upper panel) and emission amplitude depends only on the status of the cochlea in one area. AmDiS-OAE provides for automatic addition of the third stimulus tone to a normal DPOAE stimulus. Frequency and level of the third tone are automatically calculated for optimal results.

Universal Probe for Both Infants and Adults. AmDiS-OAE comes with a unique probe design (patent pending) that results in both small

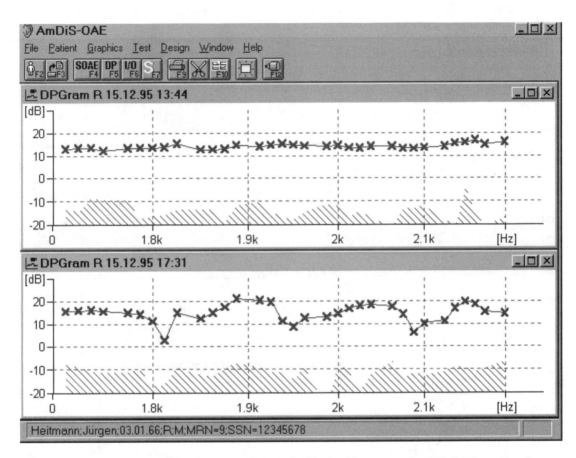

Figure 7–26. High precision DPgrams recorded with the Hortmann AmDiS-OAE system. Lower portion shows fine structure characterized by peaks and troughs. [Note: DPOAE fine stucture is reviewed in Chapters 4 and 5.

dimensions and easy access to areas that may contain debris. One single probe can be used both on infants and adults, adaptation to different diameters of the auditory canal is made via replaceable ear tips.

Automatic Evaluation for Screening. With AmDiS-OAE, DPgram test results can be automatically evaluated according to user-defined criteria. In this way, the clinical audiologist can set up a test protocol and decision criteria for a neonatal screening test and can then delegate the actual test to other staff.

Routine and Expert Modes. AmDiS-OAE was designed to be useful for both routine work in screening or other audiology environments and for advanced clinical and research applications. At first sight, the simple Windows interface contains only a few buttons for standard tests, creation of a standard report, and printing, and every-

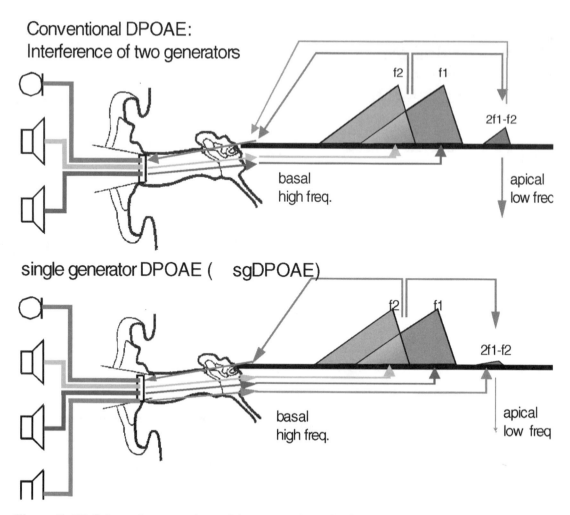

Figure 7–27. Schematic comparison of the conventional DPOAE (top portion) with the single generator (sg) DPOAE (patent pending) available with the Hortmann AmDiS-OAE.

The mechanisms underlying DPOAE generation might be easier to understand with inspection of Figures 4–4 through 4–6, and review of accompanying text, in Chapter 4.

thing from calibration procedures to test result graphics layout is done automatically. However, many operating parameters, from averaging procedures to axis ranges, can be customized via option dialogs or profile descriptions. There is practically no limit on the number of steps per octave or level steps in DPgram or growth function experiments, respectively.

INTELLIGENT HEARING SYSTEMS

Product: SmartOAE

Prepared by: Edward Miskiel, Ph.D.

Product Description

The SmartOAE system from Intelligent Hearing Systems is a complete distortion product otoacoustic emissions (DPOAE) system that has both screening and diagnostic testing features (Figure 7–28). The SmartOAE system uses a Windows interface that allows the user to set testing and analysis parameters with convenient menus and dialog boxes. Default testing and display parameters are automatically loaded, allowing the user to start testing as soon as the system is turned on. Brightly colored DPgram displays make result interpretation easy

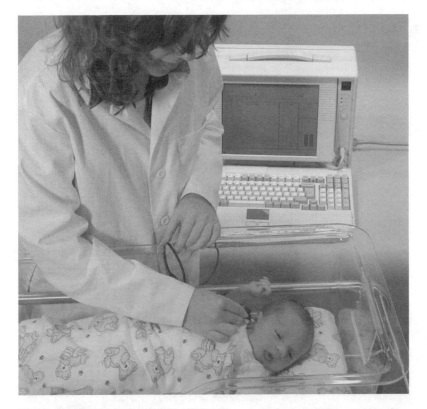

Figure 7–28. The SmartEP DPOAE system from Intelligent Hearing Systems (IHS).

The Oz system for tracking infants in hearing screening programs is described later in this chapter.

(Figure 7–29). The user may also set pass-refer criteria, which determines if a "pass" or "refer" is displayed along with the DPgram information. A complete built-in data management system allows for easy access and retrieval of patient demographics and test results. The system can also be used with the Oz Systems software (Oz Systems) and the Hi*Track (National Center for Hearing Assessment and Management) patient information and data management software packages.

The testing parameter dialog box allows the clinician to set all critical DPOAE acquisition parameters such as L_1 and L_2 values, testing frequency ranges (500–8000 Hz with up to six frequencies per octave), f_2/f_1 ratio, number of presentations, and a low-to-high or high-to-low frequency presentation sequence (Figure 7–30). The user can also choose to enable or disable the in-the-ear stimulus level correction feature and select the artifact rejection level and retry count values. Display options also include the ability to display right, left, or both

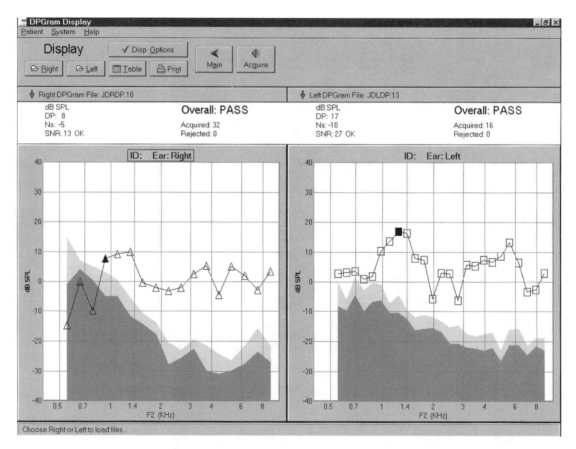

Figure 7–29. SmartOAE DPgram display (Intelligent Hearing Systems).

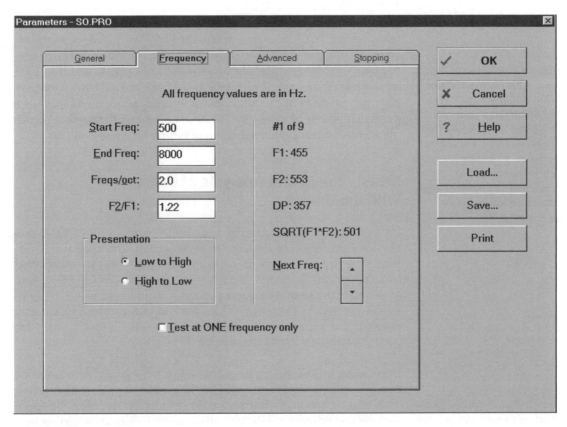

Figure 7–30. Frequency testing parameter options available for DPOAE measurement with the SmartOAE device from IHS.

ear DPgrams, and to display the noise floor, initial noise level, and normative data. The DPgram can be plotted as a function of f_2, f_1, and both the arithmetic and geometric mean of f_1 and f_2.

SmartOAE can be installed in desktop or portable "lunch-box" style computers. The system can also be installed in docking stations available for some laptop computers. When installed in a lunch-box computer or laptop docking station, the system can be easily transported from site-to-site or from bedside-to-bedside for testing. The system itself is composed of a digital signal processing (DSP) board that is installed inside the computer, an OAE amplifier box, OAE amplifier cable, and OAE probe (Etymotic 10C). The small, lightweight, self-contained probe encompasses the microphone and two small speakers avoiding the need for additional external cables or tubes.

A key feature of SmartOAE is its ability to be integrated with SmartScreener, an automated auditory brainstem response (ABR) based infant hearing screening device and SmartEP, a full-featured

Is there a rationale for plotting the DPgram as a function of either the geometric mean, the f_1 or the f_2 stimulus? The answer is yes (the f_2 stimulus). Reasoning is provided in Chapter 4 (and visible in Figure 4–6).

diagnostic evoked potential (EP) system. All three devices share a common IHS hardware component, the DSP board, and therefore can easily be integrated into the same computer without hardware compatibility problems while substantially reducing cost. In addition, having both DPOAE and ABR capabilities in one system allows for easy and immediate verification of results in cases where an infant fails a particular screening modality and thus eliminates the need to schedule additional test sessions that require different equipment.

The combined use of OAE and ABR is essential for the audiologic evaluation of infants and young children, and permits the implementation of current version of the "cross-check principle," as reviewed in Chapter 8 and summarized in Tables 8–19 and 8–20.

Measurement and Analysis of OAEs With the Device

Introduction. SmartOAE can test single or multiple DPOAE frequencies according to the user's specifications. The relationship between the two stimulation frequencies, the f_2/f_1 ratio, can be specified by selecting one frequency and the ratio and then allowing the system to calculate the second frequency value or by entering values for both f_1 and f_2 directly. The exact values for f_1 and f_2 can also be directly entered. The sound level of stimulation signals, L_1 and L_2, are also user-selectable for each test conducted.

Depending on the information entered in the passing criteria dialog box, the patient's test results will be classified as a pass (results met or exceeded the passing criteria) or refer (results did not meet the specified passing criteria and the patient should be referred for further testing). The pass-refer criteria can be specified for each test frequency and for the overall test based on the results obtained with multiple testing frequencies (Figure 7–31). Several choices are available, which can be combined to make the criteria as specific as necessary.

Strategies to employ and factors to consider in establishing pass/fail criteria for newborn hearing screening with OAEs make a big difference in failure rates and program success. Guidelines for selection of these criteria are offered in Chapter 8. See, for example, Table 8–16.

Passing Criteria at a Given Frequency. The user can establish for each frequency tested what criteria should be used to determine if a valid response is present. There are three possible options that can be combined in order to make the criteria as strict or lax as required:

1. *DP − Ns = SNR (dB SPL): Absolute signal-to-noise difference.* This option allows the user to set the passing criteria to a specific signal-to-noise ratio (SNR). The specified SNR is the difference between the (distortion product) DP and the noise level mean (Ns). Results are considered a pass at a specific frequency when this difference is greater than the specified level. (Allowed values: 0 to 50 dB SPL. Recommended value: 5 dB SPL.)

2. *DP − Ns (in units of standard deviation): Relative signal-to-noise difference.* This option allows the user to set the passing criteria to a specific number of standard deviations above the mean of the noise floor (Ns). Results are considered a pass at a given frequency when the difference between the distortion product amplitude and the noise level is greater than the user specified number of

Figure 7–31. Passing criteria selections available for DPOAE measurement with SmartOAE from IHS.

standard deviations of the noise floor. (Allowed values: 1 to 4 standard deviations. Recommended value: 1 standard deviation.)

3. *DP value (dB SPL): Absolute distortion product amplitude value.* This option allows the user to set the passing criteria to a specific distortion product (DP) dB SPL level. Results are considered a pass at a specific frequency when the distortion product is greater than the specified value. (Allowed values: −10 to 50 dB SPL. Recommended value: 0 dB SPL.)

Overall Passing Criteria. The user may also establish the conditions necessary for a completed test to be classified as a pass. The passing criteria can be based on test results for all frequencies or for specified frequency bands. A total of three overall passing criteria options is available. Each of the options can be used alone or in combination in order to make the passing criteria as specific as desired.

1. *Percent passed from all frequencies.* This option permits the user to define the passing criteria in terms of the percentage of frequen-

cies passed from all frequencies tested. The patient is considered to have passed a test when the percentage of frequencies passed across the entire testing range is greater than or equal to the percentage entered. For example, if 80% is entered and the patient passed 9 of 10 frequencies tested, the patient is considered to pass.

2. *Percent passed in every octave.* This selection defines the passing criteria in terms of the percentage of frequencies passed within every octave tested. A test is considered a pass when the percentage of frequencies passed within every octave is greater than or equal to the percentage entered.

3. *Percent passed in specified frequency range.* This choice allows the user to specify the passing criteria in terms of percentage of frequencies passed within a specific frequency range. Up to three different frequency ranges can be specified and each range can have a different percentage passed value. The frequency ranges may also overlap each other. A patient's test results are considered a pass whenever the percentage of frequencies passed within one of the user-specified ranges is greater than or equal to the percentage entered for that specific range. If multiple ranges are selected, then all the selected ranges must meet their respective passing criteria to achieve an overall pass.

To speed the screening process and eliminate the need for unnecessary data acquisition, the SmartOAE software offers the user several options that can be used to stop a test prematurely automatically. The following options are available to stop recording when no additional recording information is required to achieve passing criteria or when it has been determined that the specified passing criteria will never be met:

Stop Acquiring at a Given Frequency. The user may select this option to stop acquiring data for a specific frequency when the recordings at that frequency have met the passing criteria.

Stop Acquiring Altogether. The user can select to stop data acquisition completely using the following two options:

1. *On overall pass.* Selection of this option terminates testing when the specified passing criteria have been met.

2. *On no chance to pass.* Choosing this option stops testing when it can be determined that the passing criteria will never be met.

The selected pass-refer criteria and stopping rules may be saved to a file and recalled at any time, thereby allowing different criteria to be used as desired or as needed depending on testing conditions.

Suggested Test Protocols. For best results, ambient noise should be minimized. Noisy environments or noise generated by the patient such as talking, coughing, and crying may hamper the detection of DPOAEs. Under these circumstances, DPOAE responses may be diminished. A sound booth is optimal for testing but a quiet room with a background noise level below 40 dB SPL is usually suitable. To further minimize noise interference, cooperative patients should be instructed not to move or swallow during testing. A proper probe fit is also critical for successful DPOAE testing. An appropriate ear tip should be selected in order to obtain an adequate seal fit. Debris inside the ear canal may also hamper the recording of DPOAEs. In addition, recordings of DPOAEs are also affected by the state of the tympanic membrane and middle ear. A diagnostic test protocol is displayed in Table 7–2.

General DPOAE measurement is reviewed in detail in Chapter 4. Noise reduction strategies in particular are summarized in Chapter 5 (see Table 5–3 for starters).

Normative Data. SmartOAE employs standard acoustical methods for measuring the amplitude of DPOAEs and noise and therefore all data measurement should comply with standardized published norms (Table 7–3). In general, under normal testing conditions, the averaged noise level above 2000 Hz should be between 10 and 20 dB SPL. The noise level below 2000 Hz will vary depending on ambient noise conditions and patient state. Users can enter normative data that can be displayed as shaded regions on the DPgram displays (Figure 7–32).

Table 7–2. Suggested values for diagnostic testing.

L_1	55 dB SPL
L_2	65 dB SPL
Frequency range	500–8000 Hz
Frequencies per octave	4
f_2/f_1 Ratio	1.22
In-Ear correction	Yes, with a maximum 10 dB SPL
Stimulus presentations	16–32

Table 7–3. Sample data for tests conducted on newborns (less than 5 days old).

Frequency (Hz)	Mean (dB SPL)	Standard Deviation (dB SPL)	N
905	15.80	4.63	23
1409	11.29	5.81	48
2822	9.74	5.61	48
5649	4.00	6.16	48

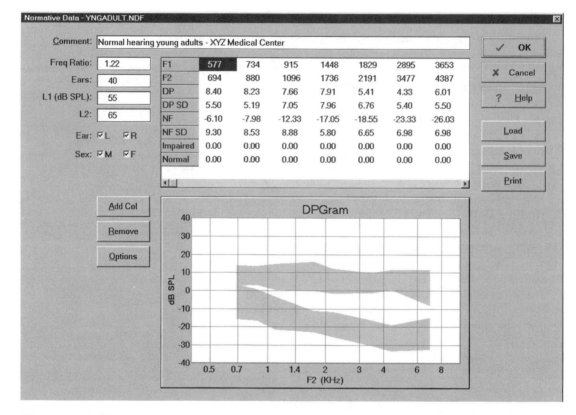

Figure 7–32. Normative data entry screen for DPOAE measurement with SmartOAE from IHS.

Product Innovations

Stimulation of DPs for frequencies up to 20,000 Hz is reported for experiments with animals. Ultra-high frequency DPgrams have potential clinical application, especially in monitoring for ototoxic cochlear damage as described in Chapter 8.

The features offered by the SmartOAE system make it ideal for both clinical and laboratory use. While the system offers numerous testing parameters, the system can be easily set up for quick and easy use by nonaudiological professionals.

The SmartOAE system uses a sampling rate of 40 kHz and an FFT calculation of 8192 points. The spectral resolution of each frequency data point is 4.88 Hz. Intelligent Hearing Systems also offers a high-frequency option for the SmartOAE system. With this option, an 80 kHz sampling rate is used allowing stimulation frequencies of up to 32 kHz. Also with this high-frequency option, an Etymotic ER-10B+ probe microphone and Etymotic ER-2 insert transducers or other sound sources can be used to generate and measure higher frequency DPOAEs.

Over the past several years, Intelligent Hearing Systems has been developing and testing a system that simultaneously tests transient evoked otoacoustic emissions (TEOAEs) and ABRs. The device is expected to be available in the year 2000. This simultaneous testing methodology provides for a robust comparison of both cochlear and retrocochlear function. The device will run on the same hardware circuitry as the SmartScreener and SmartEP systems, thus providing an extremely powerful test instrument at a relatively inexpensive price.

Several manufacturers are introducing combination TEOAE and DPOAE instruments. This technologic advance offers exciting opportunities for research and expanding clinical application and diagnostic exploitation of OAEs in varied patient populations.

MADSEN ELECTRONICS

Product: ECHO-SCREEN

Prepared by: Paul Morrison

Product Information

A New TEOAE Screening Device for the Detection of Hearing Disorders in Infants

Basic Principles. The impact of undetected hearing loss in a child is lifelong in that it interferes with the normal development of communication skills. Early detection of hearing loss allows early intervention, which can reduce the adverse effects of hearing impairment on speech and language development. Sensitivity and specificity for conventional screening procedures carried out in early childhood have been shown to be low. They do not identify all children with significant hearing loss and result in high referral rates. Conversely, diagnostic procedures such as evoked response audiometry are expensive, time-consuming, and require professional expertise to administer the test and interpret the results. Screening based on otoacoustic emissions is widely expected to fill the gap between these two extremes. The Echo-Screen is one of the few emission-based screening devices that can reliably be used by testers without professional training. This makes it ideally suited for use by physicians and nurses in a pediatric or general practice setting, by personnel in well-baby nurseries, and even by health visitors in home settings.

Description. The Echo-Screen is a new miniaturized hearing screening system based upon the measurement of transiently evoked otoacoustic emissions (Figure 7–33). No expertise is required to use the device properly. It is completely microprocessor controlled, and evaluation is done automatically by means of a strict signal statistical criterion. This criterion reduces the probability for a false negative result to less than 1%.

Transient Evoked Otoacoustic Emissions

Introduction. A properly functioning cochlea responds to sound by active movements of the outer hair cells. This mechanism serves two purposes: it increases the sensitivity for low-level sounds, and it increases the frequency resolution of the ear. While the inner hair cells convert the mechanical elongation of the cochlear membrane into the action potentials in about 30,000 nerve fibers, the outer hair cells amplify and tune the incoming sound. The active movement of the

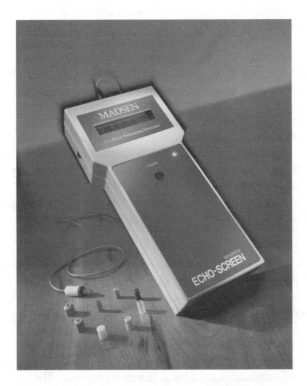

Figure 7–33. The Echo-Screen TEOAE device from Madsen Electronics, with assorted probe tips.

outer hair cells produces results in mechanical energy being transmitted from the inner ear to the outer ear canal via the ossicular chain and the tympanic membrane. The movement of the tympanic membrane creates sound waves in the ear canal. Thus otoacoustic emissions are a byproduct of the active function of the outer hair cells. While otoacoustic emissions often occur spontaneously, they can also be evoked by a transient acoustic stimulus and measured by means of a miniature microphone, which is placed in the ear canal. The amplitude of evoked emissions is quite large in neonates (sometimes corresponding to a sound pressure level of 30 dB) and decreases continuously during the first years of life.

All of Chapter 2 is devoted to a review of the anatomy and physiology underlying OAE measurement. Key references on this very important topic are listed at the end of that chapter.

Signal Processing for TEOAEs. Signal processing is done to detect the emission signals in a noise floor caused by environmental and intrinsic acoustic signals.

Averaging. The most common procedure is averaging: A number of signal intervals following the stimulation ("sweeps") are added synchronously with the stimulus thus improving the signal-to-noise ratio until the emissions are detectable.

Using Signal Statistics. The Echo-Screen uses signal statistics to make the decision as to whether the measured signal will be regarded as an emission automatically. An experienced examiner makes this decision based on a number of objective and subjective criteria, such as the frequency spectrum, typical curve morphology, and time distributions of the measured signals. The danger in using a normal averaging procedure is that any waveform can be produced by chance. To guard against this, other commercial systems have added additional features such as correlation of two quasi-simultaneous measurements. Although this has proven valuable, the amount of correlation depends on the frequency spectrum of noise and signal, which differs from one measurement to another. As a consequence, a given correlation cannot be used exclusively as the criterion for the presence of emissions.

The Echo-Screen Statistics. The Echo-Screen regards each point of the poststimulus signal interval separately. Thus statistical limitations caused by the time distribution of the signals can be avoided. The basic principle is the "history" of a single time-locked point during a number of sweeps. In a random signal its distribution is well defined on the principles of binomial statistics. A statistical test for this single point uses the hypothesis that no time-locked signal is present. When this hypothesis can be rejected on a 99% level of confidence, this point can be regarded to be influenced by a stimulus response. The Echo-Screen can be regarded as a device that measures the signal-to-noise ratio rather than the emission signal only. It calculates statistical distributions for 60 points following the stimulus in a time interval from 6 to 12 ms. A "pass" outcome requires four pairs of alternating positive and negative peaks that meet the significance criterion.

Averaging Versus Signal Statistics. There is an advantage to using signal statistics versus averaging for detection of TEOAEs. A strong emission measured under quiet conditions will be clearly identified using either signal statistics or correlation of the averaged signal. Under noisy conditions, the averaged signal may be unclear, and probably scored as a "refer," whereas using signal statistics, the emission is identified, and the test outcome is a "pass." Both strategies yield equivalent results when no emission is present.

Echo-Screen Test Parameters

Automatic Stimulus Control. The stimulus level is optimized for each ear canal and test run. It should be high enough to obtain a good emission response and low enough to avoid stimulus artifacts. In a calibration run, the stimulus is checked for amplitude as well as time constancy. The measurement will start only if both are okay. During measurement, changes in stimulus amplitude are registered and the test is stopped if it deviates from what was measured during calibration. In this case, a "stimulus instable" message will appear on the display.

Artifact Rejection. Artifacts are defined as signal periods which would lower the signal-to-noise ratio if they were included in the averaging procedure. Conventional devices for OAE measurement require a manual artifact rejection control during measurement. The optimal artifact threshold is not known in advance because the signal-to-noise ratio differs extremely from one individual measurement to another. Because of that the Echo-Screen tests at different rejection levels simultaneously. As a result testing time is reduced dramatically in most of the cases, especially with restless infants.

Follow-Up Procedures

A "refer" condition means that the signal-to-noise ratio has not been high enough to prove the presence of emissions on the required level of significance. Because this could be attributable to a number of pathologic as well as nonpathologic factors, follow-up diagnostics should be carried out as soon as possible. When the measurement has been very noisy, frequent flickering of the red light during the measurement indicates this. In this case, it is worthwhile to repeat the measurement. This is especially true when two or even three pairs of peaks have been detected. This information is displayed on the LCD screen. The further follow-up-procedure should start with the examination of the middle ear status because middle ear dysfunction is the most frequent origin of mild to moderate hearing loss in early childhood.

Diligent follow-up of all "refer" outcomes is mandatory in a newborn hearing screening program. American Academy of Pediatric guidelines for tracking and follow-up steps of a screening program are summarized in Chapter 8, Table 8–8.

10 Clinical Advantages of the Echo-Screen

1. **Size and weight: small, light, and hand-held.** Echo-Screen's modest size lets you test newborns and infants without taking them out of their cribs. This saves time and greatly reduces the risk of waking or disturbing the infants. The fact that you can hold the Echo-Screen in your hand during testing means that you don't even need a table or cart, as is the case with PC-based systems, while the single operation button on the front panel ensures ease of use. The Echo-Screen weighs about 600 g, and its dimensions are only 215 × 54 mm.

   Echo-Screen: The smallest and most lightweight system on the market.

2. **The probe: designed for newborns, easy to clean.** The Echo-Screen probe is designed especially to fit easily and comfortably in newborn ear canals (Figure 7–34). In addition, the detachable probe tip can be replaced in under 15 seconds, saving valuable time during testing. Probe tips can easily be cleaned for reuse. Soft silicone ear tips are ideally sized to fit the ear canals of even prematurely born babies.

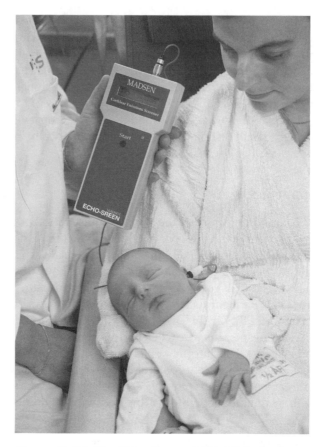

Figure 7–34. The Echo-Screen TEOAE device from Madsen Electronics is automated, and designed for newborn hearing screening.

Echo-Screen: Probe tip is easy to remove, easy to clean.

3. **Artifact-thresholds: flexible, depending on environmental noise floor.** The optimum level for artifact rejection is unknown prior to testing because it is dependent on both the strength of the emission and the amount of environmental noise. The Echo-Screen automatically selects the most suitable artifact threshold during the test. This minimizes test time, improves the sensitivity for weak emissions in quiet, and enables testing under noisy conditions.

Echo-Screen: Different artifact thresholds enable testing in noisy rooms.

4. **Signal statistics and well-defined "pass" criteria (confidence level >99% or ± 3 Sigma).** The Echo-Screen uses signal statistics to make the decision as to whether the measured signal

will be regarded as an emission automatically. An experienced examiner makes this decision based on a number of objective and subjective criteria such as the frequency spectrum, typical curve morphology, and time distributions of the measured signals.

The danger in using a normal averaging procedure is that any waveform can be produced by chance. To guard against this, other commercial systems have added additional features such as correlation of two quasi-simultaneous measurements. While this has proven valuable, the amount of correlation depends on the frequency spectrum of noise and signal, which differs from one measurement to another. As a consequence, a given correlation cannot be used exclusively as the criterion for the presence of emissions.

The Echo-Screen is based on statistically well-defined criteria. It considers each point of the poststimulus signal interval separately. Thus, statistical limitations caused by the time distribution of the signal can be avoided. In a random signal, its distribution is well defined on the principles of binomial statistics. A statistical test for this single point tests the hypothesis that no time-locked signal is present. When this hypothesis can be rejected on a level 99% of confidence (3 Sigma standard deviations), this point can be regarded to be influenced by a stimulus response.

Echo-Screen: Based on binomial signal statistics. Well defined confidence level (>99%) is the criterion for "pass" and "refer."

5. **International validation studies.** The performance of the Echo-Screen in infant hearing screening has been examined in numerous studies, including investigations at the University of Munich (Grosshadern) and the University "la Sapienca" in Rome. Children up to 3 years of age have been tested, and a specificity of up to 96% has been confirmed.

Specificity. Out of 417 newborns tested with normal ABR thresholds, 398 had been confirmed as "pass" with the Echo-Screen. This means that with the TEOAE-based Echo-Screen, an average specificity of >95% can be reached. These numbers are in agreement with international studies of screening with otoacoustic emissions, and reflect the fact that OAEs are sensitive to even minor middle ear dysfunction.

The literature on screening test performance for OAE versus ABR techniques is summarized in Table 8–13, and nearby text in Chapter 8.

Echo-Screen: Specificity = >95%.

Sensitivity. The sensitivity of Echo-Screen with ABR in children up to 3 years of age has been found to be 100%. Because the Echo-Screen probe is optimized for the small ear canal volumes of newborns, reliable test results cannot be expected for children over the age of 6 years.

Echo-Screen: Sensitivity = 100%.

6. **Battery powered with standard cell size: safe and reliable.**
The Echo-Screen is powered by a standard rechargeable battery
for video cameras. A fully charged battery provides enough
power for approximately 100 measurements. The fact that there is
no main connection ensures maximum safety. The output power
of the Echo-Screen is limited to 85 dB SPL.

Echo-Screen: Highest safety due to battery power, 80–100 consecutive measurements guaranteed.

7. **High mobility and ongoing system availability due to spare
battery.** A "low battery" indicator advises the operator to remove
the battery for recharging. It can be replaced with the spare for
uninterrupted testing.

Echo-Screen: No "down time" for battery recharging.

8. **Memory for four measurement results: Two newborns can
be tested consecutively.** The Echo-Screen stores the results for
four complete measurements. This allows repeated testing of the
same ear or consecutive testing of up to four ears without losing
data. The complete result (pass/refer, stimulus stability in %, and
artifact in %) will be stored for each measurement.

Echo-Screen: Memory for four measurements.

9. **Result documentation/print.** After the measurement the complete result (see above) can be printed on almost any type of printer (Inkjet, Laser) in A5 or A4 format.

It is simple to use: simply connect to the printer via the parallel
port and push the button on Echo-Screen's front panel. Fields for
recording patient and operator information are provided on the
printout.

Echo-Screen: Result documentation included (printer connector).

10. **Price.** The Echo-Screen is a complete otoacoustic screening system in a hand-held format. Not only is it simple to use and reasonably priced, but it is economical to run due to the rechargeable
battery and low cost of disposables. It is ideal for use in newborn
clinics as well as by private pediatricians.

Echo-Screen: High-performance for a small price.

Clinical Validation of the Madsen Echo-Screen for Infant Hearing Screening

The Madsen Echo-Screen is a hand-held device that automatically
detects transient evoked otoacoustic emissions (TEOAEs.) It is opti-

mized for use with neonates and infants and is intended for hearing screening of these populations. Many studies have confirmed the value of using TEOAEs for early detection of hearing loss (Kennedy et al., 1991; Kok, Van Zanten, Brocaar, & Wallenberg, 1993; White, Vohr, & Behrens, 1993; Maxon, White, Behrens, & Vohr, 1995), and infant hearing screening with OAE is rapidly gaining acceptance as a routine clinical procedure. Several independent clinical studies have utilized the Echo-Screen, and are briefly described here.

There is substantial literature on newborn hearing screening with OAEs, as reviewed in Chapter 8 (see Table 8–12 for a listing of some of the studies). One recent paper reporting experience in screening over 50,000 babies with TEOAE by Betty Vohr and colleagues in Rhode Island (Vohr et al., 1998).

Schorn and colleagues (1998) studied the performance of automated OAE screening devices in 140 neonates and infants. Their subjects included 56 well-baby nursery neonates, 73 high-risk infants, and 11 infants with known hearing loss. The test battery included TEOAE screening with Echo-Screen and Echosensor (Otodynamics), TEOAE recording with ILO88, DPOAE recording with ILO92, screening tympanometry, determination of acoustic reflexes, and threshold determination using ABR. Sensitivity and specificity with ABR was determined for each of these tests.

The sensitivity for all measures except acoustic reflex was 100%. This means that all of the ears with an ABR threshold greater than 30 dB HL were also detected by all of the OAE devices. The Echo-Screen had the highest specificity, followed by the ILO instruments, the Echosensor, and finally acoustic reflex screening.

Fabiani (personal communication, 1998) used the Echo-Screen in a two-stage screening procedure. In this study, 382 consecutively born babies at the University Hospital in Rome were tested with the Echo-Screen on the second or third day of life. Babies not passing the initial screen were retested within the first 15 days of life. Diagnostic ABR was carried out on the 51 babies who did not pass the second screening. Of these infants, one was found to have a hearing loss. The specificity of the screening in this study was 94%.

Giebel and Trinczek-Gärtner (personal communication, 1998) used the Echo-Screen to investigate the feasibility of universal newborn hearing screening. They attempted to test all newborns in a well baby nursery during an interval of 13 months. The babies were tested between the first and fourth day of life. The investigators attained 97% coverage during this period. Of the 1,240 babies tested, 1,227 (98.9%) passed on both ears, 8 (0.6%) passed on one ear only, and the remaining 5 (0.4%) were referred for diagnostic testing.

Currently, a study in connection with the European Concerted Action on Otoemissions Commission is using the Echo-Screen to test 1,000 babies in Italy and Lithuania. Data from this study are expected to be available soon.

In general, the results of studies using the Echo-Screen lend further support to the merit of using TEOAEs in infant hearing screening. In addition, they suggested that infant screening programs using the Echo-Screen could be expected to have markedly lower referral rates than those using other devices.

References

Kennedy, C. R., Kimm, L., Dees, D. C., Evans, P. I. P., Hunter, M., Lenton, S., & Thornton, R. D. (1991). Otoacoustic emissions and auditory brainstem responses in the newborn. *Archives of Disease in Childhood, 66*, 1124–1129.

Kok, M. R., Van Zanten, G. A., Brocaar, M. P., & Wallenburg, H. C. S. (1993). Click-evoked otoacoustic emissions in 1036 ears of healthy newborns. *Audiology, 32*, 213–224.

Maxon, A. B., White, K. R., Behrens, T. R., & Vohr, B. R. (1995). Referral rates and cost efficiency in a universal newborn hearing screening program using transient evoked otoacoustic emissions (TEOAE). *Journal of the American Academy of Audiology, 6*, 271–277.

Schorn, K., Bauman, U., & Pitzke, K. (1998). Sensitivität undt Spezifität objekktiver Verfahren zur Früherkennung von kindlichen Hörstörungen. *Fortschr. der Akustik*, DAGA Hrsg. B. Hohmann, in press.

White, K. R., Vohr, B. R., & Behrens, T. R. (1993). Universal newborn hearing screening using transient evoked otoacoustic emissions: Results of the Rhode Island Hearing Assessment Project. *Seminars in Hearing, 14*, 18–29.

MADSEN ELECTRONICS

Distortion Product Otoacoustic Emissions: NORMATIVE DATA

Prepared by: Poul Aabo Osterhammel, Arne Norby Rasmussen, and Steen Ostergaard Olsen
Audiological Laboratory
Department of Otolaryngology, Head and Neck Surgery
National University Hospital, Copenhagen, Denmark

Introduction

The purpose of this investigation was to provide normative mean data for distortion product otoacoustic emissions (DPOAE) based on a panel of normal hearing subjects. Distortion product otoacoustic emissions are nonlinear responses consisting of frequencies not contained in the eliciting stimuli and are believed to be generated by or in connection with the outer hair cells in the cochlea. The frequency of the distortion product is related to the frequencies of the primary stimuli or the probes f_1 and f_2. In humans the most prominent distortion product appears at a frequency of $2f_1-f_2$, $(f_1 < f_2)$. It is a third order intermodulation product and also known as the cubic difference tone.

This report comprises DPgrams, i.e., recordings of the amplitude in dB SPL of distortion product otoacoustic emissions measured at the geometric mean of the stimulus frequencies and centred around the audiometric frequencies between 500 and 8000 Hz using a constant stimulus intensity. The present data are represented graphically, but also reported in tables. In the investigations the normative DPgrams were recorded at stimulus levels from 40 to 75 dB SPL in 5 dB steps using the same intensity (equal levels) for the two stimulus tones.

Material and Methods

Subjects. Data were collected from 20 normally hearing volunteers (10 female, 10 male) with pure-tone air conduction thresholds equal to or better than 15 dB HL (ISO 389:1991[E]) as measured at the standard audiometric frequencies (125–8000 Hz) including half-octave frequencies from 750 Hz and up. Only results from one ear of each subject were used, and if any difference, the "better ear" was selected. The mean age for the whole population was 34 years, with a range from 21 to 53 years. For the 10 female subjects the mean age was 32 years (range 21–53) and for the males the mean age was 35 years (range 25–46). All subjects had normal middle-ear function based on tympanometric results and standard otoscopy. Middle ear pressure < ±50 daPa was accepted as normal. Each subject reported a negative history of ear infections, noise exposure, and ototoxic drug administration.

Equipment

For the recording of the distortion product otoacoustic emissions a Madsen Electronics Cochlear Emissions Analyzer (Celesta 503) was used. The analyzer and the Otoacoustic Emission probe (OAE-probe) was placed in the sound booth, and connected to a PC located outside the test booth. The PC was an IBM-compatible (i80486/66 MHz type) including hard disk for data storage. The probe microphone sensitivity at 1000 Hz was calibrated using a Bruel & Kjaer (B&K) type 4230 Sound Level Calibrator fitted with a Madsen Electronics ⅛ inch adapter, and the microphone frequency response was that delivered from the factory on data file for that specific microphone. The stimulus calibration method used was: "Coupler reference without cavity correction" utilizing a Danavox IEC-71 1 coupler, fitted with a ½ inch B&K microphone type 4133, B&K 2639T preamplifier and a B&K 2610 Measuring Amplifier. The Measuring Amplifier was calibrated using a B&K 4230 Sound Level Calibrator fitted with a B&K ½ inch adaptor. Pretest audiograms were obtained by means of a Madsen Electronics OB822 audiometer equipped with TDH39 earphones and MX41/AR cushion. The audiometer was calibrated re ISO 389:1991(E).

Methods

Each subject was seated in a comfortable chair in a double-walled sound-treated test room and the test was initiated by conventional audiometry on both ears to identify the best ear. Tympanometry was performed to check for middle ear pressure, and if > + 50 daPa any further measurement was abandoned. The subject was instructed to remain silent during the measurement of the otoacoustic emissions. The OAE probe was fitted in the outer ear canal using the analyzer's built-in probe fitting function to verify correct fitting.

Input/Output functions with stimulus intensity from 75 down to 40 dB SPL in 5 dB steps were performed on each of the following geometric center frequencies respectively: 500, 750, 1000, 1500, 2000, 3000, 4000, 6000, and 8000 Hz. The ratio between the two stimulus frequencies was 1.22 in all measurements, and the intensity level of the two stimulus tones was always equal. In each measurement, data were collected until the signal was at least 10 dB above the noise floor or until the number of sweeps exceeded 500. The duration of one complete session varied from 30 to 45 minutes depending on the actual signal-to-noise ratio in each case.

Results

The mean results from all subjects are shown graphically in Figure 7–35, where each curve represents a DPgram recorded with the stimulus intensity as the parameter. The same data are shown in tabular form in Table 7–4, which also contains the standard deviations of the 20 measurements. All the data in Table 7–4 are rounded to the nearest half decibel. In Figure 7–36, the mean Input/Output curves for the nine different geometric mean frequencies are depicted and show almost linear functions when displayed in a double logarithmic system. However, if the individual Input/Output curves are considered, quite varying shapes may be seen. See reference for further discussion on Input/Output curves for distortion product otoacoustic emissions. Finally it should be pointed out that all the data in the present report were achieved using "Coupler Reference without Cavity Correction."

OAE input/output functions are described in Chapter 4 and illustrated in Figures 4–10 and 4–11.

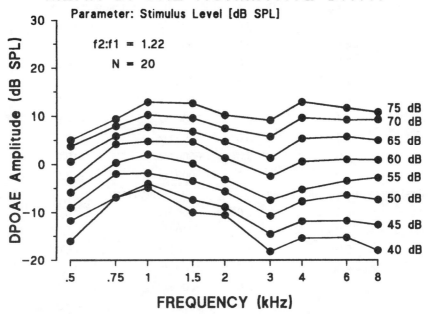

Figure 7–35. DPgrams recorded with a Madsen Electronics DPOAE device at descending stimulus intensity levels (normative data for these intensities are displayed in Table 7–4).

Table 7–4. Normative DPOAE data.

Frequency	DPOAE [dB SPL]	SD [dB]	Frequency	DPOAE [dB SPL]	SD [dB]
Stimulus Intensity ($f_1 = f_2$): 75 dB SPL			Stimulus Intensity ($f_1 = f_2$): 55 dB SPL		
500 Hz	5.0	15.0	500 Hz	−6.0	7.0
750 Hz	9.5	7.0	750 Hz	0.5	7.0
1000 Hz	13.0	7.5	1000 Hz	2.0	8.0
1500 Hz	12.5	6.5	1500 Hz	0.0	7.0
2000 Hz	10.0	8.5	2000 Hz	−3.0	9.0
3000 Hz	9.0	5.0	3000 Hz	−7.5	8.5
4000 Hz	13.0	4.0	4000 Hz	−5.5	8.5
6000 Hz	11.5	6.0	6000 Hz	−3.5	9.0
8000 Hz	11.0	6.0	8000 Hz	−3.0	7.0
Stimulus Intensity ($f_1 = f_2$): 70 dB SPL			Stimulus Intensity ($f_1 = f_2$): 50 dB SPL		
500 Hz	3.5	5.0	500 Hz	−9.0	6.5
750 Hz	8.0	5.5	750 Hz	−2.0	8.0
1000 Hz	10.5	7.0	1000 Hz	−2.0	10.5
1500 Hz	9.5	6.5	1500 Hz	−3.5	6.5
2000 Hz	7.5	7.0	2000 Hz	−5.5	9.5
3000 Hz	6.0	6.0	3000 Hz	−10.5	8.0
4000 Hz	9.5	5.5	4000 Hz	−7.5	6.0
6000 Hz	9.5	8.0	6000 Hz	−6.5	6.5
8000 Hz	9.5	8.0	8000 Hz	−7.5	6.0
Stimulus Intensity ($f_1 = f_2$): 65 dB SPL			Stimulus Intensity ($f_1 = f_2$): 45 dB SPL		
500 Hz	0.5	6.0	500 Hz	−12.0	4.5
750 Hz	6.0	5.5	750 Hz	−7.0	10.5
1000 Hz	7.5	7.0	1000 Hz	−4.0	10.5
1500 Hz	7.0	7.5	1500 Hz	−7.5	8.5
2000 Hz	4.5	7.0	2000 Hz	−9.0	11.0
3000 Hz	1.5	6.5	3000 Hz	−14.5	7.5
4000 Hz	5.5	6.0	4000 Hz	−12.0	6.5
6000 Hz	6.0	8.0	6000 Hz	−12.0	8.0
8000 Hz	5.0	10.5	8000 Hz	−12.5	6.0
Stimulus Intensity ($f_1 = f_2$): 60 dB SPL			Stimulus Intensity ($f_1 = f_2$): 40 dB SPL		
500 Hz	−3.5	6.0	500 Hz	−16.0	7.0
750 Hz	4.0	5.5	750 Hz	−7.0	9.0
1000 Hz	5.0	7.0	1000 Hz	−5.0	7.5
1500 Hz	4.5	6.0	1500 Hz	−10.0	8.0
2000 Hz	1.5	7.0	2000 Hz	−10.5	10.0
3000 Hz	−2.5	7.0	3000 Hz	−18.0	7.5
4000 Hz	0.5	7.0	4000 Hz	−15.5	7.0
6000 Hz	1.0	8.0	6000 Hz	−15.5	7.0
8000 Hz	1.0	9.0	8000 Hz	−18.0	6.0

MEAN DPOAE INPUT/OUTPUT FUNCTIONS

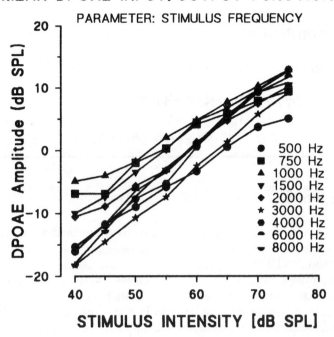

Figure 7–36. Input-output functions recorded with a Madsen Electronics DPOAE device at a variety of stimulus frequencies.

If a different calibration method is utilized, the results will deviate from the data in this report, especially in the high frequencies (>3000 Hz).

References

Popelka, G. R., Osterhammel, P. A., Nielsen, L. H., Rasmussen, A. N. (1993). Growth of distortion product otoacoustic emissions with primary-tone level in humans. *Hearing Research, 71*, 12–22.

MADSEN

**Distortion Product
Otoacoustic
Emissions:** Normative Data in Newborn Infants

Prepared by: Arne Norby Rasmussen
Britt Borgkvist
Poul Aabo Osterhammel

Introduction

The purpose of this investigation was to provide normative mean data for distortion product otoacoustic emissions elicited from healthy full-term neonates. Distortion product otoacoustic emissions (DPOAE) are nonlinear responses consisting of frequencies not contained in the eliciting stimuli, and are believed to be generated in connection with the outer hair cells in the cochlea. The frequency of the DPOAE is related to the frequencies of the primary stimuli or probes, f_1 and f_2. In humans, the most prominent distortion product appears at a frequency of $2f_1–f_2$, ($f_1 < f_2$). It is a third-order intermodulation product and also known as the cubic difference tone. This report comprises measurements performed in a newborn population, and covers mean values at selected frequencies and the corresponding standard deviations. The stimulus level was fixed in all measurements at 70 dB SPL for both stimulus tones.

Materials and Methods

Data were collected from 277 healthy full-term babies aged between 48 and 72 hours. The data were collected in connection with a hearing screening test using transient evoked otoacoustic emissions, and the distortion product otoacoustic emissions were recorded, if permitted by the parents and if the recording conditions were acceptable, i.e., the baby was calm and a good probe fitting could be achieved. A Madsen Celesta 503 Cochlear Emissions Analyzer was used for the recordings, and probe tips were modified by removing the collar in cases where the ear canal opening was too small for a standard eartip. Recordings were performed on both ears if possible, and the starting ear was randomly selected. The geometric mean of the stimulus frequencies tested was: 1000, 2000, 3000, 4000, 6000, and 8000 Hz, and measured in the given order. The ratio f_2/f_1 was fixed at all measurements at 1.22. The stimulus level was adjusted using the "in situ method," i.e., using the probe microphone as the reference. As many frequencies as possible of those preselected were recorded. The subjects were tested in the neonatal department in officelike surroundings, and were tested lying in the cradle or in the arms of the mother, whichever situation created the best conditions for the recording. Each response was considered valid if the level of the DPOAE was greater or equal to the calculated noise floor plus two standard deviations from the mean noise floor calculation. The noise floor was calculated as the mean level of the adjacent 5 FFT-bins on both sides of the actual DP-frequency.

Results

The distribution of the measurements was normal, and the differences between mean and median values were less than 1 dB for all frequencies. The mean level of DPOAE as a function of the geometric mean frequency of the primary tones is shown in Figures 7–37 and 7–38 for the left and right ears, respectively (filled circles). The corresponding mean noise floor and *SD* is also shown (open squares). The number of valid recordings fulfilling the validation criterion for each frequency and ear is shown in Table 7–5.

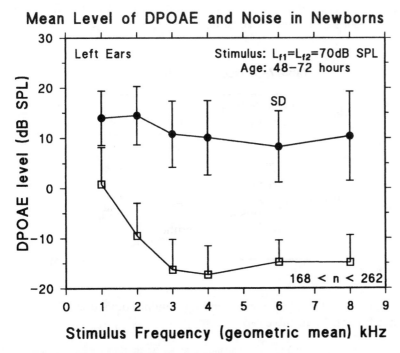

Figure 7–37. Average DPgram (filled circles) and noise floor values (open squares) recorded with a Madsen Electronics DPOAE device from left ears of newborn infants.

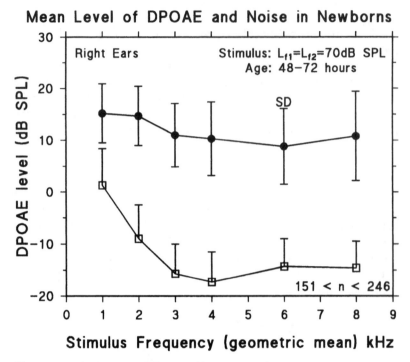

Figure 7–38. Average DPgram (filled circles) and noise floor values (open squares) recorded with a Madsen Electronics DPOAE device from right ears of newborn infants.

Table 7–5. Number of valid responses.

Geometric Mean Frequency	Left	Right
1000 Hz	168	151
2000 Hz	252	238
3000 Hz	262	246
4000 Hz	260	242
6000 Hz	239	226
8000 Hz	237	221

The mean data and the corresponding standard deviations are shown in tabular form in Table 7–6.

Table 7–6. Means (and standard deviations) of DPOAE amplitudes with Madsen device for $L_1 = L_2 = 70$ dB SPL.

Geometric Mean Frequency	Left Ear Mean L_{DP} dB SPL (SD)		Right Ear Mean L_{DP} dB SPL (SD)	
1000 Hz	14.0	(5.4)	15.2	(5.7)
2000 Hz	14.5	(5.8)	14.7	(5.7)
3000 Hz	10.8	(6.6)	11.0	(6.1)
4000 Hz	10.1	(7.4)	10.3	(7.1)
6000 Hz	8.3	(7.1)	8.8	(7.3)
8000 Hz	10.4	(8.9)	10.8	(8.6)

OTODYNAMICS LTD. OAE SYSTEMS

Products: ECHOCHECK; ECHOPORT; ECHOPORT Plus; ILO88DPi; ILO96

Prepared by: David T. Kemp
Institute of Laryngology and Otology (ILO)
University College London

Introduction

Otodynamics' OAE products have a direct link with the Institute of Laryngology and Otology (ILO) research laboratory at University College London where OAEs were discovered and first developed. Starting in 1978, the ILO laboratory designed and built a series of OAE instruments for screening, clinical investigation, and laboratory research purposes under the direction of Dr. David Kemp. Dr. Kemp formed Otodynamics Ltd. as an independent commercial organization in 1988 to produce the first high quality commercial OAE systems for sale in the U.S.A. and Europe. Now in its 11th successful year, the company's products are available and fully supported in every state in the United States and in more than 60 countries around the world through special instrument dealers. Otodynamics' ILO OAE products are the most widely known and used.

Our first ever OAE product, the "ILO88 TEOAE PC kit system" gave thousands of professionals in audiology their first access to OAEs. It caused a revolution in hearing screening policy. The large scale independent trial of the ILO88, supported by the Department of Maternal and Child Health in Rhode Island made the efficiency and low cost of TEOAE screening evident. This helped prompt the National Institutes of Health (NIH) Consensus Conference to declare universal newborn hearing screening a health service target and to recommend OAEs for the initial screen. The ILO88 was followed by the world's first transient and distortion product OAE system, the ILO92, and dramatic improvements in ILO probe, software, and hardware design.

As the most experienced OAE system manufacturer today, Otodynamics offers the widest choice of OAE product formats and the widest range of OAE measurements to meet all requirements. We produce the world's smallest hand-held OAE screener, the world's most powerful stand alone OAE screener/analyzers, and a range of portable and desktop OAE systems, which includes the world's most comprehensive OAE clinical and research instruments. Each of these products is reviewed in Part I below.

Selecting the right OAE system for your application can be difficult. The scientific literature is often loaded with technical jargon of little relevance to the real business of screening or audiological investigation, and promotional literature frequently lacks depth. Otodynamics is an ISO9000 accredited company and to maintain product quality we rely on the expertise of scientists who researched OAEs, on the knowledge of engineers who created OAE technology, and on feedback from users of our instruments for over 10 years. To share this broad experience we have included in Part II a section written by Dr. Kemp which summarizes key facts about OAEs and provides a commentary on OAE technology and usage that we believe will be useful in evaluating OAE systems from any manufacturer.

PART I: Otodynamics Product Review

Introduction. Our new products are carefully designed to cater to very practical needs while drawing on roots in OAE research. The handheld ECHOCHECK is designed for screening with maximum speed and efficiency, and with maximum reliability and simplicity of operation. There are reasons why you could want more. You may need the simplicity of operation of the ECHOCHECK, but also need to inspect and analyze response data later, locally or remotely. Some users also have an additional need for the test results to be logged automatically on a database for management, tracing, or audit. On the other hand many need a flexible, very portable OAE system for screening that must also perform as a clinical instrument directly linked to a PC for full-sized graphic displays. It is the design aim of our newly extended ECHOPORT series to provide all this in various combinations in a portable format, and of our ILO88i series to provide this in a fixed installation. Finally, for those who need the ultimate in OAE analysis for research purposes, there is the Otodynamics' ILO96.

The ECHOCHECK Device. The ECHOCHECK is a hand-held automated otoacoustic emission (AOAE) screening device for use in all hearing assessment programs—from universal newborn screening to pediatric hearing assessment (Figure 7–39). Its design features are absolute simplicity of use, reliability, and convenience; it even slips into your coat pocket. ECHOCHECK provides a rapid objective indication of normal cochlear function obtained via a miniature insert earphone-probe. The ECHOCHECK is suitable for all ages because it automatically senses ear canal size and adjusts the stimulus (Figure 7–40). Healthy newborns with clean dry ears pass in around 6 seconds.

The probe is separated from the body of the instrument for maximum convenience and comfort. It is a standard ILO probe and can be easily disassembled for total serviceability. It is supplied with a wide range of disposable plastic ear tips and replacement sound tubes (Figure

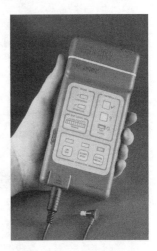

Figure 7–39. The ECHO-CHECK automated OAE screener—light, portable, and easy to use.

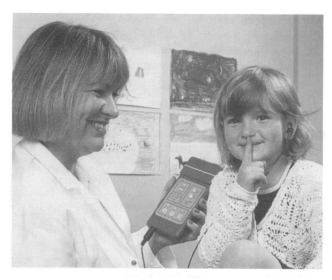

Figure 7–40. The ECHOCHECK is designed for application in the nursery, clinic, home, or school.

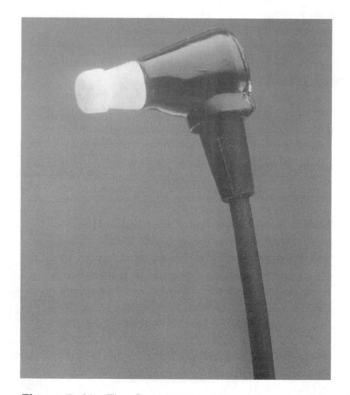

Figure 7–41. The Otodynamics compact serviceable probe design takes disposable tips and is fully disassembleable for cleaning and replacement of the sound tubes. Used with all Otodynamics products.

7–41) and can be fitted to other Otodynamics products with an adapter, so the results on ECHOCHECK can be compared to those on a full ILO system, without even removing the probe! That's how we know it outperforms the ILO Quickscreen in noise.

Touching the START key commences the ECHOCHECK's in-the-ear calibration and OAE test sequence. Probe fit, stimulus, and noise conditions are dynamically indicated by colored lights. The test ends automatically as soon as a confirmed result is obtained. Brightly colored and labeled indicators call out the test result, which can be: Green = OAE confirmed, Yellow = possible OAE, Red/Orange = test invalid, or no lights = no OAE detected. Touching the right-hand control button saves details of the test and the results in memory and optionally prints out a detailed report, including OAE strength, probe fit, and noise levels and test ID on a self adhesive label if required. Up to 100 tests can be stored and recalled. Instrument reliability is ensured by a self-diagnostic test implemented automatically each time the ECHOCHECK is turned on.

Screening with the ECHOCHECK's automated OAE method can be favorably compared to screening with automated ABR. Both use clicks as the stimulus and both objectively test the broad mid-frequency range that is so vital to speech perception. The ECHOCHECK is sensitive to OAE responses from 1000 Hz to 4000 Hz but is maximally sensitive between 2000 Hz and 3000 Hz, similar to screening ABR. Like AABR, AOAE with the ECHOCHECK will not commence recording if conditions are not right, which helps make the results more reliable and training much more simple. Both methods terminate the test automatically and give a clear objective result immediately without the need for interpretation by the tester.

The literature on screening test performance for OAE versus ABR techniques is noted in Chapter 8, with comparative failures for recent studies summarized in Table 8–13.

The ECHOCHECK has powerful noise rejection and signal detection software incorporating the ILO88 Quickscreen nonlinear TEOAE data acquisition and validation system. Technically this method takes replicated dual stimulus intensity responses, combines them to remove stimulus artefacts, then cross-correlates them within the frequency band and assesses their significance against the differential noise level. In practice a green light comes on if there is a good OAE. What is important is that the method has been proved for sensitivity and reliability in hundreds of intensive care and universal newborn hearing screening programs over the last 10 years in the ILO88. The TEOAE method has an exceptionally good false negative record and very high sensitivity for cochlear impairment. ECHOCHECK is designed to have high specificity and sensitivity comparable to AABR.

There are three important differences between AOAE and AABR. ECHOCHECK does not require electrodes to be fitted or any preparation of the skin. There are no expensive disposables. AOAE with the

The many practical components of universal newborn hearing screening (UNHS) programs, and associated costs and benefits, are reviewed in the initial sections of Chapter 8.

ECHOCHECK is therefore easier to use and cheaper to run than AABR. The ECHOCHECK is also cheaper than any currently available AABR system. OAE responses are simply stronger and easier to detect against the body's natural background noise than the auditory brainstem response, so that AOAE with the ECHOCHECK is considerably faster than AABR under comparable conditions. The ECHOCHECK specifically tests the peripheral auditory system excluding the auditory neural pathway. This makes the ECHOCHECK ideal for well-baby auditory screening where the incidence of retrocochlear pathology among the hearing impaired is an order of magnitude below that in the special care baby group. This same property also makes OAEs an essential complement to ABRs in assessment of the at-risk population.

The ECHOCHECK is powered by internal rechargeable batteries that give days of use. A supplementary external alkaline battery pack is provided for when you forget to charge. The standard ECHOCHECK will print a test report on a serial printer. Otodynamics can provide a battery-powered, portable, serial, mini-printer, and computer-link software as options. The printout or PC download includes test sequence number, time and date of test, test result with recommendation for further testing, together with numerical data on the stimulus, OAE response, and noise level during testing.

The ECHOCHECK measures just 7.45 × 3.6 × 0.75 inches rising to 1.15 inches in the upper third. It weighs just 11 oz. There are three connection sockets: one for the probe/charger, one jack for the printer/serial port/PC, and one for the supplementary battery pack. The ECHOPORT is supplied with all accessories including charger power supply, all in a carry bag. Accessories include general purpose fully serviceable TEOAE probe, disposable tips supply, auxiliary battery pack, and preprinted self-adhesive report forms. Options include miniature battery printer, adhesive-label rolls, printer connection kit and PC connection kit, including Windows software. Upgrades are by removable ROM. The ECHOCHECK is manufactured to meet IEC601, EN60601-1, BS5724-1, CSA 22.2 No 601-1, CE, EMC. Classification Type BF. ECHOCHECK has FDA clearance. OAE screening is reimbursable in the U.S.A. under CPT code 92587.

The ECHOPORT Family

The four members of the ECHOPORT family of products are each full featured laptop-sized battery-powered OAE instruments suitable for screening and/or for clinical applications. The ECHOPORT Plus (Figure 7–42) and DP ECHOPORT Plus (Figure 7–43) operate in standalone screener mode or in PC-linked mode. The standard ECHOPORT products ILO288 (ILO88 in U.S.A.) and ILO292 DP ECHOPORTs require a PC connection to operate.

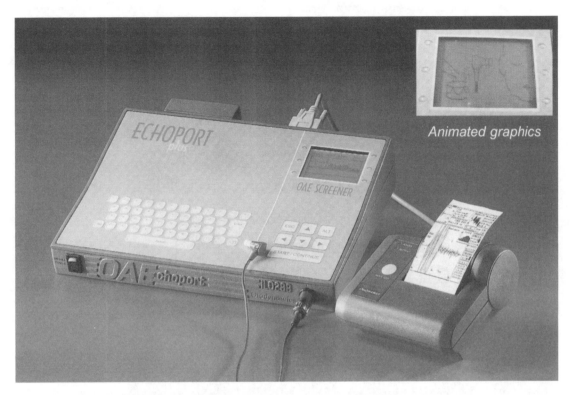

Animated graphics

Figure 7–42. The ILO288 ECHOPORT Plus stand-alone TEOAE screener/analyzer has a keyboard, animated graphic display, and a built-in database. Database transfers data to PC when required, and via modem if needed.

The ECHOPORT Plus product format breaks new ground in OAE technology. The ECHOPORT Plus and the DP ECHOPORT Plus instruments are the first ever full-featured stand-alone battery OAE instruments. Complete with integral keyboard for entering patient data, graphic LCD display, internal PC compatible processor, solid disk data storage, dedicated printer port, and optional battery printer, the ECHOPORT Plus is a complete OAE screening instrument and no larger than a laptop PC. Single keystrokes allow rapid progress through the test sequence. First there is provision for patient data entry into the built-in patient and data management database, then a probe fit check and calibration mode with animated graphic operator feedback via the built-in LCD screen (see inset in Figure 7–39) The graphics are popular with children too, who cooperate to make the baby smile! When probe fitting and stimulation is correct, then the ECHOPORT Plus proceeds with the OAE recording itself. The OAE analysis is immediately displayed graphically during the testing. A Pass/Refer recommendation based on editable built-in protocols is provided on screen at the termination of the test, which itself is automatic following editable rules. Hundreds of patient records can be

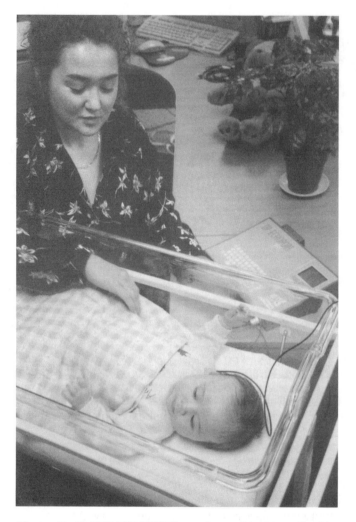

Figure 7–43. ECHOPORT Plus units are ideal for crib-side screening giving an immediate result yet storing all raw data for later analysis, and can upload patient list and download test results remotely. Here the ILO292 DP ECHOPORT is used to test a newborn.

stored internally in enhanced ILO format, which includes complete raw data. Stored data can then be easily recalled or transmitted to a regular PC via a printer cable or serial port, or even remotely via a modem. Once transferred, the raw data can be displayed and reanalyzed as industry standard ILO OAE data files, while the test outcome and demographic details collected with the ECHOPORT Plus can be read by standard patient management packages such as "Oz." (*Note:* The Oz System product is described in the next section of this chapter.)

You do not need a PC to use the ECHOPORT Plus, or any keyboard skills. Switch on and the program is already loaded and ready to screen. But, if you want to operate the ECHOPORT from your PC or laptop, and use the full Version 5.6 or 6.0 ILO software for color display while testing, you can. The ECHOPORT Plus is a fully capable ECHO-PORT ILO88 or 292 and operates identically in computer peripheral mode if required for serious OAE analysis, or use with NCHAM's HISCREEN system.

The ILO288 ECHOPORT (ILO288 EP) Plus (Figure 7–44) is recommended for all screening programs where simplicity of automated operation is essential but with the capacity for detailed supervisory program monitoring. The ILO288 EP Plus is ideal for intensive hospital auditory screens where the provision of a laptop computer would not be appropriate or for mobile screening where a separate computer would be an inconvenience. But the ILO288 EP Plus is equally suited

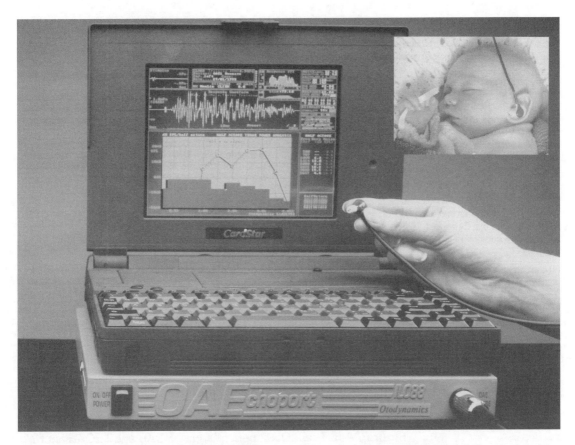

Figure 7–44. The ILO288 classic ECHOPORT in use with laptop and full V5.6 ILO software. Top trace shows TEOAE response waveform and below shows the TEOAE half-octave analysis which parallels the DPgram.

to clinic-based screening where the instrument's additional functionality and analysis will be of value over a simple hand-held device. The ILO288 EP Plus uses TEOAEs for maximally effective screening

The ILO292 DP ECHOPORT Plus (Figure 7–45) is the top of the ECHOPORT range. It provides all the facilities of the ECHOPORT Plus together with full clinical DPOAE screening and analysis in both stand-alone and PC-linked modes. It has comprehensive OAE analytical facilities when used with a PC and can separately provide complex research facilities, including the delivery of contralateral stimulation and binaural recording. Additionally, the ILO292 reads probe ID and performs automatic instrument diagnostic tests for greater all round reliability.

If stand-alone operation is not a priority, the standard ECHOPORT instruments will do the same job with a laptop or desktop computer. ILO88 ECHOPORT was in fact the first ever truly mobile battery OAE

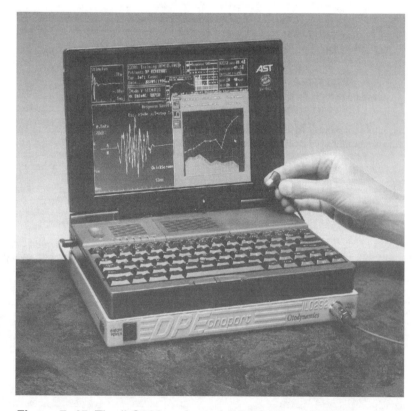

Figure 7–45. The ILO292 performs full DPOAE and TEOAE analysis and intercomparisons including latency measurement and other research functions. It operates as an easy-to-use screener and also as a clinical OAE instrument.

system, and is now widely used across the U.S.A. and Europe (ILO288) for newborn screening. Its most popular feature is the Quickscreen mode with automatic TEOAE detection and analysis. Testers like to see what is happening live on the PC screen and audiologists and program supervisors like to be able to review and reanalyze doubtful test results. The instrument is the size of a slim laptop computer and connects to the printer port (or PC-card auxiliary parallel port) of a laptop or desktop PC. It can be operated using the standard ILO V5.6 full analytical OAE program or the ILO Version 6.0 Windows (c). The ILO88 ECHOPORT cannot be upgraded for DPOAEs.

The ILO292 DP ECHOPORT caters to users needing DPOAE and TEOAE measurements. It is ideal both for screening and clinical applications. TEOAE and DPOAE results can be compared on the same screen. The same size as the first ECHOPORT, the ILO292 has enhanced connectivity, connecting to your laptop or desktop via the parallel port or serial port. The latter is fully electrically isolated. A DPOAE only ILO292 option is available in the U.S.A.

Software supplied with all ECHOPORTs provides easy menu, keyboard, or mouse-driven access to programmable and preset TEOAE and/or DPOAE measurement protocols plus spontaneous emission detection. Also included is the colorful on-screen real-time feedback on probe fit and OAE result for which Otodynamics is famous. Rapid recall, spectral analysis, and intercomparison of data are features of all ILO software. Version 6 software takes the most popular and useful features of Version 5.6, adds essential patient management facilities, and presents them in a familiar Windows environment. ECHOPORT software is downloaded from the PC so updates are easy.

SOAE measurement and interpretation is reviewed in detail in Chapter 3, whereas the influence of SOAEs on DPOAEs and TEOAEs is summarized in Chapter 5.

The ILO88, 288 and 292 standard ECHOPORTs measure 11.78 × 8.5 × 1.25 inches. The ILO292 weighs 4.4 lbs, the others 3.5 lbs. Power is from an internal 6 V 2.5Ah rechargeable battery with intelligent power management. There are fast-charge, standby shutdown, and low-battery indicators on the 292 and a five-segment charge indicator on all systems. There is auto-protective shut down. It provides up to 5 hours typical use on battery or continuous use on charge. Connections on the ILO88 and 288 are a Centronics style computer interface, low-voltage power input socket for the PSU, and the probe socket. For the 292 there is the addition of an isolated serial computer interface and an auxiliary probe socket (second input channel).

The ECHOPORT Plus models are based on the ILO288 and ILO292, respectively, with the addition of a slim contoured processor/keyboard/display unit replacing the standard ECHOPORT top. This unit increases the height of the ECHOPORT to 2.38 inches at the rear and includes an additional printer port. The DP ECHOPORT Plus also includes a headphone noise monitor jack. All existing standard

ECHOPORT products can be upgraded to the corresponding stand-alone ECHOPORT+ operation. All ECHOPORT systems have FDA clearance. ECHOPORT'S are manufactured to meet IEC601, EN60601-1, BS5724-1,CSA 22.2 No 601-1, CE,EMC. They have FDA clearance.

Internally Mounted ILO OAE Systems

For building into a permanent audiological facility, the ILO88DPi (Figure 7–46) is the ideal and most economical system to select. It operates with full ILO V5.6 software or with Version 6.0, providing DPOAE and TEOAE integrated analysis. Screening protocols are included. The system provides all the functionality of the original ILO92 and ILO88XP/DP with state-of-the-art technology and design.

The ILO88DPi hardware is designed for tidy desktop systems. The probe interface slips neatly into a 5-inch disk drive bay of the PC. There are no external cables or power cords. The digital electronics take the form of a small ISA card that fits in the computer's expansion slot. The system is completely self-checking and records probe ID for calibra-

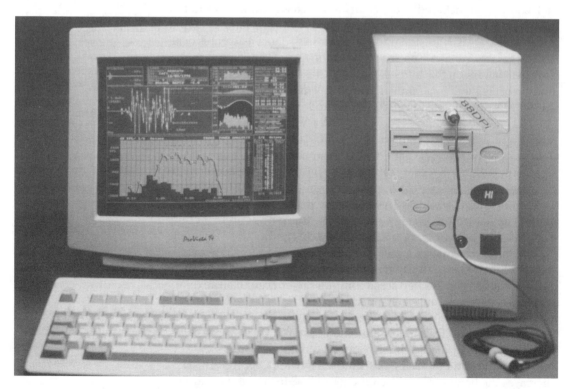

Figure 7–46. The ILO88DPi desktop system performs all screening and clinical functions with TEOAEs and DPOAEs. The system mounts fully inside the PC.

tion and usage control purposes. As an option, the ILO 88DPi can be ordered with an externally mounted amplifier. DP only and TEOAE only versions are available for very specific dedicated usage. Upgrade to 88DPi is possible with both.

ILO88DPi systems are manufactured to meet IEC601, EN60601-1, BS5724-1,CSA 22.2 No 601-1, CE,EMC. All ILO88 internal systems have FDA clearance.

The ILO96 Research System

The ILO96 OAE system (Figure 7–47) is designed to meet the most demanding present, and future clinical, and basic research needs. It offers a range of facilities and functions not available in any other OAE

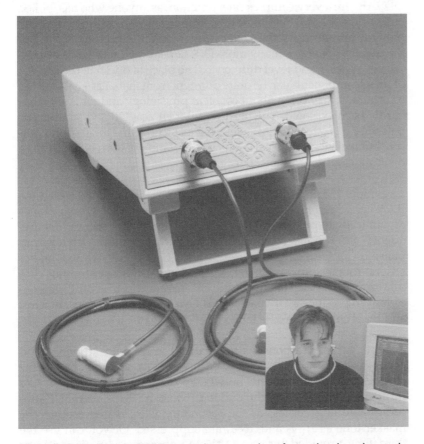

Figure 7–47. The ILO96 research system has four stimulus channels and two microphone channels for elaborate experiments including contralateral OAE suppression, DP tuning curve mapping, and binaural recording. It also runs standard screening and clinical ILO software.

systems. The ILO96 also runs all standard ILO software and performs all the regular screening and routine clinical functions of the ILO88DP and ILO292 instruments. But, additionally, the ILO laboratory at University College London has specified that the ILO96 must also perform laboratory style measurements of OAE phenomena that are not otherwise available commercially and are at the forefront of hearing research.

Contralateral acoustic suppression of OAEs is reviewed toward the end of Chapter 5, whereas anatomy of the efferent auditory system (which mediates suppression effects) is discussed toward the end of Chapter 2.

The ILO96, therefore, has facilities not found on other systems. Take TEOAEs for example. The stimulus may be clicks, tone bursts, or even noise, with optional self cancelling. The ILO96 also can provide monitored contralateral gated masking for cochlear efferent suppression work using either noise or custom stimulation. The hardware is also capable of binaural OAE recording. Not only can data be collected more quickly this way, but any response differences caused by binaural as opposed to monaural stimulation can be studied.

DPOAEs are a very complex phenomenon, as anyone who has looked beyond the $2f_1-f_2$ DP will know. Routine clinical recordings measure only the amplitude of the lower intermodulation product $2f_1-f_2$, but the cochlea generates many more DPs depending on the primary frequency spacing and level difference. The place of origin in the cochlea of these components can be quite different from that of $2f_1-f_2$—and the information they bring about cochlear physiology and pathology has hardly been explored. The most popular clinical DP and stimulation pattern, e.g., $f_2/f_1 = 1.22$, was selected just to give maximal sound output, but we have yet to learn which stimulation pattern of DP components give optimum clinical insight.

The DP at $2f_1-f_2$ is only one of many DPs generated by the cochlea. The concept of linearity, and a bunch of combination tones, is summarized in Tables 4–2 and 4–3.

To explore the ear with DPOAEs you need special tools, which the ILO96 provides. First you need to be able to sweep the primary tones dynamically in predetermined patterns, such as the ratio and DP frequency, etc. You need to be able to track the amplitude, latency, and phase of all DP components—not just $2f_1-f_2$ but $2f_2-f_1$ and higher orders. You need to be able to integrate DP data for one stimulus condition to get the total energy of the DP waveform, or for multiple conditions to produce a DP map. The ILO96 software functions, macros, and Excel compatible data tables allow you to do all of this.

But the cochlear response is not static. The response to one sound changes when another is added. With the ILO96 you can observe the changes in DPOAE production when a masking tone is added. Use this too with the ILO96's three-tone-probe to trace ipsilateral DP suppression tuning curves, or the secondary DPs created around the masker tone as $2f_1-f_2$ and $2f_2-f_1$ are suppressed. Or you can use the third tone provided by the ILO96 to suppress competing sites of DPOAE generation selectively, which results in otherwise confusing interference effects on the DPgram. Also using the third stimulus, contralateral efferent suppression of DPOAEs can be studied.

The ILO96 software features raw data spooling so that, for example, TEOAE data collected during a screening recording can be re-averaged with different artifact reject settings or noise weighting. The statistical validity of the OAE can be computed, not just estimated.

The ILO96 instrument is a full member of the ILO family. It builds on the success of the ILO92. In fact ILO92 and ILO88XP/DP owners can upgrade their machines to the ILO96. The ILO96 requires one full-sized ISA PC slot. You can run standard FDA cleared ILO88 and ILO88DP software on the ILO96 for routine screening and clinical purposes. Use of ILO96 research software with humans requires Institutional Review Board (IRB) approval in the U.S.A.

ILO Software

The design of ILO software and hardware makes it extremely tolerant of its host environment. Standard ILO version 5.6 software will run on all Intel x86 compatible processors of level 386 or higher, with 8 MB of memory and at least VGA graphics. Obviously a high-specification computer is desirable for maximum speed. Version 6.0 requires Pentium I 100 MHz processor or higher, with 32 MB memory. All Otodynamics products are warranted year 2000 compliant.

ILO version 5.6 software is the accumulation of 10 year's experience and embodies a vast array of functions and utilities developed for researchers. Today's Version 5.6 interface is focused on current screening and clinical applications but all the power of the software is there if you need it. Our new Version 6.0 (Figure 7–48) adopts a different philosophy. It's a full Windows program providing just what you need for easy screening OAE patient management. It accepts data from older ILO systems and reads the contents of the new ECHOPORT plus units effortlessly. The screen analysis shows full patient data, test conditions, and the classic ILO displays of stimulus, response waveform, and spectrum.

PART II: Understanding OAE Instruments (by David T. Kemp)

Introduction. This section raises a range of issues that are important to the understanding of OAEs and to the comparison of OAE instruments in general—not specifically Otodynamics instruments. It does not attempt to include a complete description of OAEs or of OAE technology, or even to review uses of OAEs. Rather it aims to be complementary to those descriptions, that can be found elsewhere.

Before starting to judge the claims made for OAE instruments it is essential to be clear about what OAEs are. OAEs are sounds created in

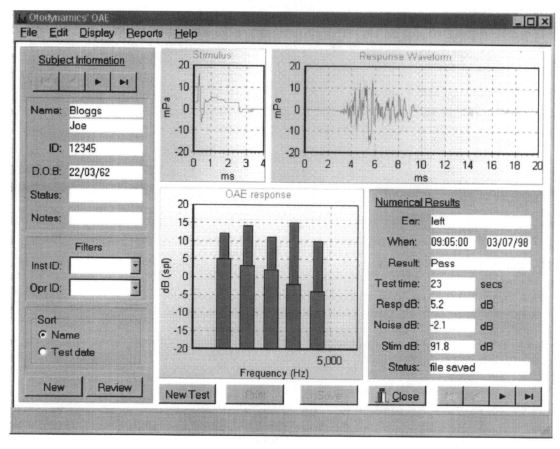

Figure 7–48. The new Version 6.0 Windows software operates on all Otodynamics hardware and provides a choice of environments for ILO users. Version 6.0 will be strongly biased toward ease of use and patient data management, but will retain full computability with data collected on all previous ILO systems.

The critical role of the middle ear in OAE measurement is summarized throughout this book, but especially in the review of anatomy/physiology (Chapter 2) and the detailed discussion of OAEs and auditory dysfunction (Chapter 6).

the occluded ear canal when the eardrum responds to vibrations transmitted from inside the cochlea. This means that the middle ear has to be working normally for vibrations to get out of the cochlea. The size of the OAE recorded depends on the size of the ear canal and the health of the middle ear, as well as the health of the cochlea and how much vibration escapes. The normal range is large. Absent OAEs can indicate pathology of the cochlea, or of the middle ear, or simply a blocked ear canal.

It is vibrations in the cochlea which surround the sensory outer hair cells that give rise to OAEs. These cells are very important for normal threshold and they are very susceptible to damage, but they are not the cells that actually activate the auditory nerve. That is important to remember. Also, only the vibrations that escape from the cochlea contribute to an OAE. Most activity around the motile outer hair cells works to increase the intensity of the stimulation reaching the inner hair cells, which are the cells that activate the auditory nerve. This means that strong OAEs could exist in an ear with elevated threshold, if the pathology was associated with the inner hair cells or was retrocochlear.

How Reliable Are OAEs as Indicators of Normal Hearing? OAEs are objective evidence of healthy cochlear function. But is this enough for hearing screening? To answer this question we need to look at the evidence. TEOAEs have been subjected to the most critical evaluation in hundreds of thousands of routine screening applications in the well baby low-risk population for over 10 years. This is vastly more than the evidence on which the ABR was accepted as the gold standard for hearing screening many years before. Despite this intense scrutiny, OAEs are still highly praised and very widely accepted as a reliable and effective first screening for sensory hearing impairment. Over the last 10 years in the U.S.A. and Europe, many hundreds of hearing-impaired infants have been successfully identified in low-risk populations by TEOAE screening, while documented cases of false negatives (i.e., false passes) remain in single figures. From this we can conclude that on present evidence,

Understanding the relation between OAEs and cochlear status is fundamental for meaningful clinical application of OAEs. An entire section of Chapter 6 is devoted to the relation. Clinical application of OAEs in specific primarily adult cochlear disorders (e.g., noise induced loss, Ménière's disease) is reviewed in Chapter 9, whereas pediatric sensory impairments (e.g., ototoxicity) are covered in Chapter 8.

■ The vast majority of hearing impairment in the low-risk population is a result of malfunction of the cochlear/outer hair cell system, the most sensitive and vulnerable part of the hearing mechanism tested by OAEs.
■ Retrocochlear and auditory neuropathy must be statistically and proportionally very much rarer in the low-risk, well baby population than in the special care population where even there they represent only a small minority.

OAEs are therefore very reliable indicators of normal hearing for universal low-risk screening purposes.

Auditory neuropathy is a hot topic these days. It's discussed in Chapter 8. For a quick summary, inspect the information in Tables 8–21 to 8–23, and in Figures 8–11 through 8–13.

What Is the Useful Frequency Range of OAE Instruments? OAEs have been detected from human ears right up to 18,000 Hz (even higher in animals) and down to below 300 Hz. It is practical and technical considerations that limit the useful frequency range to less than this. Each technique has its own difficulties. The DPOAE technique has difficulty recording the lowest frequency OAEs in noise because the OAE produced is nearly an octave below the test frequency (f_2) and low-frequency noise predominates in the environment. The TEOAE technique suffers from a loss of high-frequency OAE detection above 4 kHz in adult human ears (not so much in infants). This is partly due to the short latency of these signals and their obscurance by the stimulus artifact. DPOAEs do not suffer from such a high-frequency limit. For these reasons DPOAEs are more practical above 1500 Hz. TEOAEs are practical down to 750 Hz.

The ear canal is one of four anatomic regions playing a major role in OAE measurement, as discussed in Chapters 2, and 4 through 6. The topic of standing wave artifact in DPOAE measurment is specifically addressed in the section on "ear canal acoustics" found in Chapter 5.

OAE measurements of both types suffer from serious calibration difficulties above 6000 Hz in adult human ears. This is due to ear canal resonances. Even with the most accurate stimulus control with an insert probe, drum level stimulation and measured response levels may be grossly in error for higher frequencies (by up to 20 dB). DPOAEs are additionally affected by distortions of the $L_1{:}L_2$ ratio which can substantially change the level of DPs.

Overall, then, TEOAEs are practically most reliable between 1000 and 4000 Hz and DPOAEs between 2000 and 6000 Hz. The presence of an OAE response outside these limits is still a good indicator of function but the normative range becomes very wide outside this range and includes undetectable OAEs from many normal ears. The distinction between normal and abnormal becomes blurred, and this is not acceptable for screening.

Can OAEs Really Predict Absolute Hearing Threshold? Absent OAEs can indicate raised hearing threshold because OAEs are not produced at frequencies where the cochlear system is substantially disordered even though there may be only 30 dB hearing-threshold levels. Caution is needed because OAEs can be obscured by noise so their absence in a test is not proof of pathology. The reverse is more true. Their presence in a test is some proof of healthy cochlear and middle ear function.

The audiogram cannot be estimated from OAEs for a variety of reasons. These reasons are summarized in Chapter 1 (see Table 1–3) and detailed further in the discussion of the relation between OAEs and cochlear auditory dysfunction in Chapter 6. Also, numerous examples of OAE results in conjunction with audiograms are presented as case reports in Chapters 8 and 9.

But Can OAEs be Used to Determine Threshold? Hearing threshold is determined by the summed performance of all parts of the auditory system including the middle ear and the outer hair cell system (both of which affect OAEs) and also the inner hair cell system and the auditory pathways (which are not involved in OAEs). OAE intensity is therefore determined by the health of the cochlea and the middle ear, the size of the ear canal and the coupling to the probe, and by the mechanism of escape from the cochlea (largely unknown). All this means that,

■ OAEs cannot be used to determine absolute auditory threshold with any useful accuracy.
■ The normal range of OAE intensity will inevitably be large and differences between individuals within this range probably will not be significant (i.e., may not mean a threshold difference).
■ The practice of finding an OAE detectability threshold against uncontrolled noise is flawed and will not yield reliable estimates of hearing threshold. Finding OAE detection thresholds under controlled conditions is unlikely to yield any more information about threshold than is available from intensity of growth rate data.

In short OAEs cannot and should not be used to replace the audiometer.

OAE Frequency Specificity. Frequency specificity in an audiological test is the desirable ability of a test to predict hearing loss at a particular frequency. OAEs have some capacity for this. It is easy to imagine that every frequency has a very specific place in the cochlea with its own set of cells and nerves, but this is not really the case. Every place in the cochlea responds to least a 30% (⅓ octave) range of frequencies (e.g., 1000 Hz to 1300 kHz) and this broadens at higher levels. If pinpoint place accuracy is not possible with OAEs, frequency specificity is possible, bearing in mind that in practice frequency specific information is normally a requirement of diagnostic tests but not screening tests.

Both TEOAE and DPOAE techniques are capable of providing frequency-specific data and, surprisingly, they have very similar capacities. Despite their precisely controlled frequency, the tones provided for DPOAE measurement typically excite around 20% of the cochlear cells to some degree. The clicks used for TEOAEs or ABR screening excite more than 50% of the cochlea. But the frequency specificity of both TEOAE and DPOAE measurements is not determined by the extent of stimulation. It is a result of the frequency analysis that takes place in the cochlea before emission, and that which takes place in the measuring instrumentation on the emission (particularly with TEOAEs). The limiting frequency specificity of TEOAE and DPOAE measurements is not set by the equipment and it is not set by the stimulus whether it be click or tone, but by the cochlea itself. DPOAE and TEOAE frequency specificity is limited to around ½ octave at best and can be worse due to the fact that there is not one single place responding to each frequency.

Although OAEs provide clinically valuable information on the integrity of outer hair cells, even with OAEs present the cochlea may not be normal. Hearing loss due to inner hair cell dysfunction, secondary for example to carboplatin ototoxicity will not be detected by OAEs alone. This specific point is made in Chapter 8. The anatomic rationale is reviewed in Chapter 2.

Given that OAEs provide objective evidence of healthy cochlear function and that the cochlea treats each frequency of sound separately and maybe differently, how do DPOAEs and TEOAEs provide frequency-specific information and what part does the stimulus play in this? An OAE can tell you anything about the health of the cochlea only at the places that are stimulated. To the extent that each place responds only to its own frequency, and to the extent that its response is in some way characteristic (identifiable) with that frequency, then any sound can be used to test the cochlea (e.g., tones, clicks, even noise). They just tell you about different parts of the cochlea. OAEs in response to a fixed tone(s), such as a DPOAE, tell less about the whole cochlea than the OAE to a click (TEOAE). This is because the tone stimulates a smaller region of the cochlea than a click.

Click-evoked OAEs tell you about a large section of the cochlea but they need to be analyzed by frequency to see which places in the cochlea responded and which did not. That's the function of the TEOAE spectrum, or half-octave band analysis. Tone-evoked OAE (including DPOAEs) measurements tell you about one region responding to one stimulus condition, and need to be repeated at a number of frequencies and levels to build up a picture of the whole cochlear status (the DPgram).

OAE Sensitivity and Specificity. Specificity in a hearing screening test is its ability to pass ears that do not need further investigation. It is costly and wasteful if specificity falls well below 100%. Sensitivity is the ability to refer all those who have a significant hearing problem for investigation. If this falls well below 100%, the screening is not effective.

It is important to remember that in setting OAE pass criteria, increased specificity (i.e., trouble-free, low-cost screening) can be traded for reduced sensitivity (i.e., reduced effectiveness). Because high specificity can be demonstrated in a day on, say 100 ears, while high sensitivity requires at least 100,000 low-risk infants to be screened and followed up, it is clearly prudent to be very critical when accepting instruments demonstrating very high specificity. High specificity can be achieved with OAEs by raising the intensity of stimulus intensity. In standard TEOAE measurement, clicks of around 55–60 dB SL are used (85 dBpeSPL) and this energy is spread over the cochlea. DPOAEs conducted with 60 dB SPL tones represent a higher intensity of stimulation at the frequency-specific place, and DPOAEs collected with 70 dB SPL tones deliver much higher stimulation than TEOAE stimulation. There is evidence that DPOAEs can be less sensitive to elevated threshold than TEOAEs when higher stimulus levels are used, even though this makes for higher specificity.

The maximum length sequence (MLS) technique is described for OAEs by several research groups, notably the British auditory scientist Roger Thornton (see some of Dr. Thornton's publications on this topic in the reference list). The MLS technique is described briefly in Chapter 10.

Several OAE acceleration techniques have appeared in the literature. The maximum length sequence (MLS) stimulation technique was published as a means of enhancing acoustic echo recordings in 1979 and is obviously applicable to TEOAEs. A dense barrage of clicks simulating noise is applied and the response extracted by deconvolution. The ILO96 research software includes this function but improvements in testing speed are practically limited. This is because of the natural saturation of the OAE response and the method's increased vulnerability to nonlinear artifacts. Also the high rate of click stimulation effectively increases the intensity of stimulation many times, raising unanswered questions about its effect on OAE sensitivity.

The simultaneous presentation of several sets of DP stimuli was noted in the section of this chapter prepared by GSI. Also, the concept of DPOAE measurement simultaneously for several pair of f_1 and f_2 stimuli is described in Chapter 4. Clinical application of this technique was the topic of a publication in 1997 by Kim and colleagues at the University of Connecticut Health Science Center (see reference list).

With DPOAEs the use of simultaneous stimulus pairs is a valid way to reduce testing time. Use of stimulus harmonics to achieve this (e.g., GSI 60) is a cost-effective way to measure two points in the time for one. This is probably not enough to make DPOAEs as fast as TEOAEs under the same stimulation intensity. Extenuation to more pairs introduces technical problems. Full analysis of the response of the cochlea to multiple tones can be obtained with the ILO96.

Frequency Resolution in OAE Measurements. An OAE instrument's frequency resolution is the number of data points provided within each octave of frequency range. The ILO TEOAE system simultaneously records around 16 points/octave in the 1500 to 3000 Hz region with the Quickscreen mode, set by the sweep duration. DPOAE frequency resolution is determined by the number of separate measurement steps made in progressing across an octave, from 1 to 8 points/octave is common (the latter taking 8 times as long).

It is doubtful if any more than two values per octave are needed to describe cochlear status adequately. The problem is that both TEOAE and DPOAE responses can vary quite markedly across an octave frequency range so that a single measurement within an octave band width may be quite unrepresentative of the average response over that octave. Oversampling and averaging is required with DPOAEs. Oversampling is inherent in TEOAEs, with averaging provided by the half-octave OAE power analysis.

There are clearly some clinical indications for increasing the number of stimulus frequencies per octave in DPOAE measurement. These are noted in Chapter 4, and illustrated with case reports in Chapters 8 and 9.

Artifact Rejection and Response Validation. Every OAE technique has the potential for artifacts that may be mistaken for a response, which seriously erodes the sensitivity of the technique. With DPOAEs the greatest danger is nonlinear distortion products created in the probe assembly at higher levels. With TEOAEs the greatest danger is long lasting acoustic resonances of the ear canal probe combination.

A valuable control is to run the test with the probe in a test cavity. Although vital, there is a problem with relying solely on test cavity controls. The cavity may not reproduce the exact acoustic conditions that gave rise to the artifact. It is essential to have a method of testing the validity of the OAE recording itself and this should be built into the signal processing as it is on ILO systems.

OAE response validation requires several conditions to be met. First, the response should be well above the noise level and, second, it must be reproducible. OAE instruments differ in the ways they assess noise and response reproducibility (see below). But that is not enough. To guard against artifactual responses, the properties of the response itself need to be assessed and compared to the true responses' properties. Of all the OAE's properties, the intensity of the response is probably the least useful measure here, contrary to much contemporary discussion. It is helpful to remember that the amplitude of the ABR response in microvolts is similarly not considered to be of great importance either!

Two properties are used in validation. True OAEs exhibit smoothly saturating nonlinearity and a latency from 2 to 15 ms. With TEOAEs the latency of the response is directly visible in the waveform. With DPOAEs a detailed phase measurement must be made involving a small stimulus frequency shift. ILO DP instruments incorporate this measurement. Artifacts generally have very little latency (0 to 3 ms). Response nonlinearity is self-evident in the production of DPOAEs but very rapid growth of DP level (>2:1) with stimulus level is an indication of nonphysiological origin. With TEOAEs, multiple level recordings and response subtractions can confirm the physiological nonlinearity and eliminate mechanical artifacts (i.e., the nonlinear stimulation method of the ILO TEOAE system). Otodynamics recording software includes integrated response validation for nonlinearity and latency for both TEOAE and DPOAE measurements.

Noise Level and Quality Issues. Noise level assessment methods differ widely across manufacturers and techniques. TEOAE response levels are expressed per bandwidth, e.g., dB SPL/half octave (see frequency resolution). Each band is a combination of multiple independent measurements at specific frequencies and is a powerful indicator. Otodynamics software displays the response and noise in the same bandwidth which is selectable from 1 to ⅛ octave. Noise contamination in the response is calculated from the difference between two replications of the measurement. More than one octave band response which is 3 dB or more above the noise can be considered a significant result. If the noise level of say "X" dB SPL exceeds the response the result is correct to say "OAE not detected" and certainly less than "X" dB SPL. It is incorrect to report "no OAE" in noise conditions.

DPOAE response levels are single-frequency sound level measurements and must be compared with similar measurements made at the same time at neighboring non-DP frequencies. Otodynamics DP software records the levels found in 10 neighboring frequencies and sets the significant level for the DPOAE at two standard deviations above the mean noise level (for 95% confidence). Some manufacturers quote the mean noise level only. The significance of responses just above the mean noise level is actually quite low. In selecting DPOAE instruments the quoted instrument noise level is less important than how noise levels are calculated and expressed. Remember that the patient and environment noise level will usually far exceed the instrumentation noise. It is the noise computation method that is most important. It is important that a fixed mean noise level is not used as the basis for accepting a valid DPOAE.

Although it is usually the case that noise is acoustic in nature, other sources such as radio frequency and power line interference can also be a problem during OAE recording. ILO instruments have a continuous noise monitoring and waveform indicator. If the probe sound inlet tube is fully occluded, any substantial noise remaining may be an indication of electrical noise.

Workshop Calibration of OAE Systems. An OAE system is primarily a sound measuring system, whereas an audiometer is a sound delivering system. This makes the calibration considerations for the two instruments quite different. Few if any audiometers include direct in-the-ear real-time sound calibration. Audiometer calibration takes the form of workshop adjustment of sound delivery into a reference cavity to equal a reference value. This is not the case with OAE systems. Here the microphone sensitivity is the most important because it is used by the instrument itself to calibrate the sound stimulus levels in the patient's ear. This is a very necessary process because OAE probes are of insert type and are used in such a wide range of ear canal sizes from neonates to adults. A fixed stimulus drive to the probe would otherwise cause up to 10 to 20 dB variations in stimulus level between ears. Measurement of an OAE instrument's sound output into a standard test cavity is not a reliable means of setting up or determining its output into a real ear. It is of course a good means of controlling for changes in the system or probe.

To facilitate calibration, OAE systems should provide a convenient indication of the level registered by the probe and instrument when an external single-frequency sound is applied which has been accurately set using an independent calibrated sound level meter. Because a disagreement could be due to the probe microphone or to an instrument amplification fault, it is also necessary to have a "loop back" test where the instrument records and tests its own internal amplification. This is conducted internally in some of the ILO instruments, and via an external loopback plug in others. Finally, as a control it is useful to measure the electrical drive provided by the instrument to the probe and the ILO test program provides a continuous tone output for this purpose.

Regular Checks With OAE Instruments. Before each test a clean disposable probe tip needs to be fitted. The probe sound tubes need to be inspected for contamination and changed if necessary. Each day a standard test should be run in the supplied test cavity to check for artifacts and general function. Each day any self-test functions recommended by the manufacturer should be run. ILO systems provide a probe calibration check function. The loop back test can be conducted on site by the user. Each day a test should be performed on a known healthy ear and the results compared. At regular periods the probe sound tubes should be changed even if apparently clean.

Probe Types. Two types of probe construction have evolved. The compact form has been favored by Otodynamics Ltd for its ILO systems. In this form the transducers (one stimulator and one microphone for TEOAEs and two speakers and one microphone for DPOAEs) are housed in the inserted unit and are coupled to the ear via rigid tubing less than ½ inch long. The coupler tube assembly is changeable by the tester. The advantages of this construction are better control of stimulus phase (vital for TEOAEs and latency measurement) and a reduction in size and weight. The disadvantage is there is less scope for optimizing probe frequency response and a risk of transducer damage by debris if coupler tubes are not replaced regularly.

The other form employs separating the transducer and ear insert units. The advantage is better control of frequency response, and increased protection of the transducers. The disadvantage is poor control of phase response for TEOAEs and latency measures, possible cross coupling between the long flexible tubing (giving calibration errors), and increased size and cost. Both compact and extended probes require a disposable tip for insertion. There has been some interest in the rigid connection of the probe and the instrument body in hand-held systems. Although attractive for certain pediatric applications, this design does not accord with the lessons on fit quality learned from newborn screening. ILO instruments all use compact insert probes on flexible cables.

Practical Issues in Testing. Probe fit is widely accepted as the single most common cause of poor OAE recordings, especially with newborns. Moist collapsed ear canals and debris are common problems. Tensioning of the pinna, firm but careful probe insertion and slight rotation is recommended by testers who have achieved 95–97% success in universal newborn screening programs. Debris collected by the probe tip and removed on the first insertion often results in the success of the second attempt. Firm fitting reduces noise problems but does not eliminate them. The ILO system allows for the background noise with the probe out of the ear to be measured. This background room noise should be 45 dB SPL or below for good newborn OAE recordings, although, any number of brief, loud disturbances (such as speaking) can be accommodated by the noise rejection system.

Vernix within the external ear canal is one common problem encountered in OAE recording from healthy neonates. Steps in troubleshooting for external ear canal problems are discussed in Chapter 4 (see Tables 4–1 and 4–7). The topic of vernix is specifically addressed in the section on "the external ear" found in Chapter 6.

There are substantial data on test performance of OAEs in newborn hearing screening, and documentation of widely varying failure rates among experienced investigators and clinicians depending on a variety of factors, ranging from test setting to analysis criteria (see Figures 8–7 and 8–9 for example). Failure rates can be reduced by adherence to well-proven steps in OAE meaurement, as summarized in Table 8–4.

Many testers who have not paid attention to these rules typically report excessive failure rates of 30% and more. Do not be influenced by this. Get trained by experienced testers with good track records, and act on what they say. Many hundreds of thousands of infants are tested annually by OAEs with fail rates less than 5%. Take little notice of those who say OAEs do not work for screening in their hands! Those hands are doing the wrong thing, or they are doing it in the wrong environment, or with the wrong equipment! It is true however that in a small percentage of newborns, especially on day one, an OAE recording cannot be made because fluid remains in the middle ear. This can clear spontaneously or after feeding, so a re-try is recommended an hour or two later rather than immediate referral (i.e., a multi-try OAE screen).

Conclusion. OAEs are a powerful new tool for audiological assessment—complementing and not replacing older techniques. They are valuable and successful in universal newborn screening and are indispensable in diagnostic investigations. Amplification should not be decided on without an OAE test, because the cochlea can be normal in a minority of hearing disorders. OAE technology is still evolving. There is lots of choice. Some new OAE technologies will be quickly rejected, others will replace existing systems. TEOAE and DPOAE techniques are both equally well established and complement each other well. Most important for the buyer is that the instrument selected is reliable, comfortable and easy to use, well proven, and provides a correct and appropriate level of interpretation for the purpose in hand.

OZ SYSTEMS

Product: Screening and Information Management
Solution, or SIMS

Prepared By: Misty L. Johnston

Introduction

SIMS is a Windows-based newborn hearing screening information management system. SIMS functions as the operating system that ties all your newborn hearing screening test equipment together in one manageable package. SIMS ensures dependable and consistent screening examinations, accurate information management, and timely distribution of results. SIMS lowers your program costs by reducing labor required for data entry, management, and reporting while eliminating major sources of risk to the patient, staff, and hospital.

Patient Status Identifier

SIMS automatically provides the user with each patient's hearing screening status. This powerful tool helps ensure that no child "falls through the cracks." The seven levels of patient status identification are: birth screening status, follow-up screening status, diagnostic status, status related to incidence based, delayed or progressive loss indicators, early intervention status, high-risk indicators, and the status of patient contact (Figure 7–49).

Program Quality and Performance Indicators

SIMS maintains an extensive series of performance indicators on all screeners and all screening equipment. Key information is maintained for separate screening equipment within a facility, separate screening facilities or nurseries within a hospital, hospital aggregate population and additional populations beyond the hospital such as health regions used by departments of health. These indicators help the program exceed JCAHO and NCQA requirements for quality control and program management.

Accurate, Nonduplicated Patient Information Files

SIMS point-and-click Merge functions allow you to accurately integrate patient information and files from duplicate patient records generated at different testing sites.

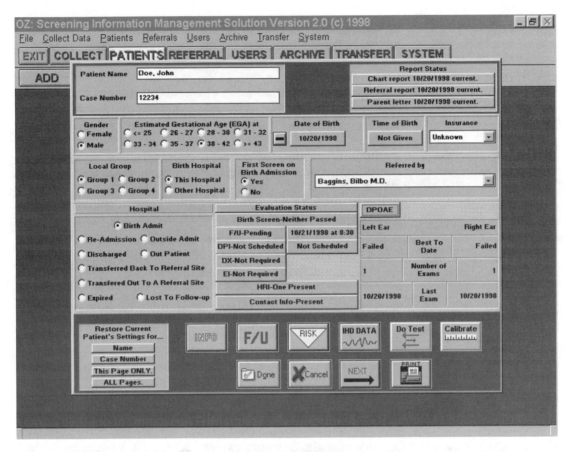

Figure 7–49. Screening and information management solution (SIMS) from Oz Systems patient information page with seven levels of patient status identification.

Integrated Patient Files That Are Easy to Transfer

SIMS transfer function provides the user with the ability to create a central location for newborn hearing records from all your test sites using a variety of media (floppy disk, Zip disk, etc.) modem, or Internet document transfer via e-mail. All transfers are accomplished in a fully secured process that meets the most rigorous standards for patient confidentiality. This data consolidation capability is critical to large hospitals with multiple screening sites and state programs wishing to maintain an aggregate dataset.

Technology Independent

SIMS works with most major brands of AABR, TEOAE, and DPOAE test equipment (Figure 7–50). With SIMS software, you have complete technology independence. The OZ Open Transfer Program (OZ-7) allows any manufacturer to electronically link to the SIMS software. In addition, information from any physiologic screening system, diag-

The reader with questions about the compatibility of OAE equipment with a tracking and database management program for infant screening shouldn't hesitate to pick up the telephone to call (or email) any of the manufacturers at the numbers listed at the beginning of this chapter.

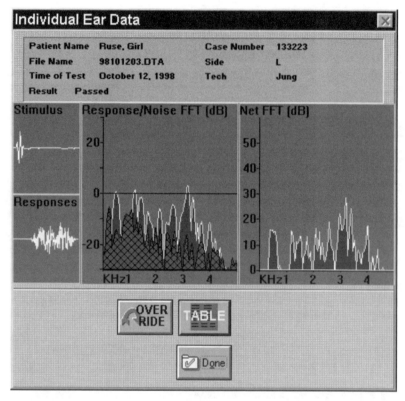

Figure 7–50. Individual patient data screen for TEOAEs from the screening and information management solution (SIMS) product from Oz Systems. SIMS interfaces with AABR, TEOAE, and DPOAE screening or diagnostic equipment.

nostic system, or behavioral audiometry results may be manually entered into SIMS, as illustrated in Figure 7–51.

Easiest to Use

SIMS takes full advantage of the Windows operating environment to provide point-and-click options for most functions. This speeds daily testing as well as new-screener learning. Information may be imported and exported to hospital information systems to further reduce data entry requirements. Standardized program reports are produced with just a click of the mouse. Custom report structures may be saved for repeated use.

Best Document Integrity and Security

SIMS maintains all documentation in individual patient files, with new data entries automatically attached to the patient file. All notes are

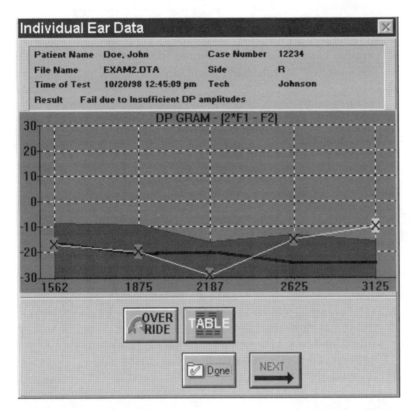

Figure 7–51. Individual patient data screen for DPOAEs from the screening and information management solution (SIMS) product from Oz Systems. SIMS interfaces with AABR, TEOAE, and DPOAE screening or diagnostic equipment.

fully editable, with permanent records of all changes maintained as an audit trail for legal protection. Individually selected access to features assures the program manager of control over each user's security level. Copies of each patient's information is automatically stored in multiple locations on the hard drive and archive copies are written to disk to prevent data loss due to hardware failure.

Customized to Your Program

SIMS allows the user maximum flexibility in program design. Screening criteria, reporting format and frequency, and much, much more can be set locally. The user even has the option to print the letters to the parents in a variety of languages.

Built-In Security Benefits of SIMS

■ Program Manager can assign access limitations for individual screeners.

■ Key patient information changes are noted, creating a permanent audit trail.

■ Original copies of modified patient files are maintained in the "background" for retrieval if necessary.

■ During a Transfer function, patient files are automatically encrypted and compressed to protect confidentiality.

■ Transferred patient files can have limited access to only a specified receiving location and/or user, at sender's option.

■ ID Codes (Passwords) required for each screener.

■ Automatic log-off, system "time-out," requires re-entry of user ID code.

A critical component of a successful newborn hearing screening program—and timely intervention for hearing impairment—is follow-up of all "refer" outcomes. American Academy of Pediatric guidelines for tracking and follow-up steps of a screening program are summarized in Table 8–8.

System Requirements

■ Pentium Processor or equivalent.

■ Windows 95, Windows 98, Windows NT and Windows 2000.

■ Minimum 16 MB RAM (32 MB for best performance).

■ SIMS requires less than 15 MB of hard disc space for program files.

■ Additional hard disc space requirements depends on the testing volume and how long you want to have your data at your finger tips (FAT 32 or NTFS file structure recommended).

■ 56K modem recommended.

SONAMED CORPORATION

Product: Clarity System (OAE/ABR)

Prepared By: William Dolphin, Ph.D.

Introduction

Otoacoustic emissions (OAEs) have become increasingly popular for the initial screening of newborns in recent years. As described in detail elsewhere in this volume, OAEs provide valuable information on a patient's cochlear integrity and, therefore, have a wide variety of applications beyond simple auditory screening.

There is a growing consensus in the United States as well as Europe that all newborns should be screened for hearing impairment within the first few months of life. In 1993 the National Institutes of Health (NIH) Consensus Development Conference on Early Identification of Hearing Loss in Infants and Young Children (NIH, 1993) recommended that all newborns should be screened for hearing loss within the first 3 months of life, and preferably prior to hospital discharge. The preferred model for screening, as suggested by the NIH, should consist of a combined approach using both otoacoustic emissions (OAE) as well as auditory brainstem response (ABR) testing. The NIH model presents a screening protocol that allows for the effective identification of a broad class of hearing impairments while preventing excessive false positive tests from burdening the system for follow-up diagnostic evaluation.

Since the NIH Consensus Development Conference recommendations were issued, there has been a dramatic increase in the number of hospitals conducting newborn screening. Numerous screening protocols are in use. However, the majority of programs follow the NIH recommended model, using OAEs, ABRs, or a combination of the two technologies (e.g., Orlando & Prieve 1998). Due to the rapidity and simplicity of acquisition, OAE is the preferred initial screening test at many sites and was recommended as an initial test by the NIH. By-and-large, programs using OAEs for the initial test use the ABR (manual or automated) in a subsequent screen for those infants who fail to pass their initial test, followed by a manual, diagnostic ABR on an out-patient basis, or, whenever possible, prior to hospital discharge. Such multistage, multisession screening protocols have been demonstrated to be highly effective in reducing the number of false positive referrals for out-patient diagnostic testing (e.g., Dalzell et al., 1996; Orlando & Prieve, 1998).

The Clarity System from SonaMed is the only system designed to comply with NIH recommendations by fully integrating both OAE and ABR technologies. OAE and ABR tests are complimentary and measure different aspects of hearing; the clinician should not be limited to only one or the other. The complimentary nature of the OAE and ABR tests allows for more accurate assessment of a patient's hearing. The incorporation of the two tests into a single screening protocol significantly reduces the number of unnecessary and costly referrals. The Clarity System has been designed to serve as a total screening solution by providing an unequaled range of simplicity, flexibility, and power in a single, simple-to-use device.

An account of the events leading up to the call for universal newborn hearing screening (UNHS) by the NIH panel in 1993, and subsequent research and evidence in support of UNHS, is presented at the outset of Chapter 8 (Clinical Applications of OAEs in Children).

The Clarity System has a number of features that differentiate it from other available screening devices, including:

■ The first and only automated and combined OAE and ABR newborn hearing screening device.
■ Combination of fully automated screening capabilities with manual diagnostic capabilities.
■ Simple, 1,2,3, user interface for automated screener mode.
■ Full manual operation for advanced users and for initial diagnostics
■ Complete data storage and review capabilities.
■ Comprehensive patient information, report generation, and program statistics.

Brief Overview of the Clarity System

The Clarity System was designed to allow operation under two distinct user modes: (1) a fully automated Screening-User Mode, ideal for use by technicians or volunteers for conducting screening tests and (2) a manual Advanced-User Mode, in which the full power and flexibility of the Clarity System is available to the user and is intended for use by knowledgeable clinicians in diagnostic applications. In both modes of operation the user interface is extremely simple to use and highly intuitive.

Newborn hearing screening with OAEs and ABR is reviewed briefly in Chapter 8 (failure rates are summarized in Table 8–13. It warrants restating that the combined use of OAE and ABR is essential for the audiologic evaluation of infants and young children, and permits the implementation of current version of the "cross-check principle," as reviewed in Chapter 8 and summarized in Tables 8–19 and 8–20.

Testing in the Screening-User Mode

In the Screening-User Mode the operator is sequentially lead through a series of three simple instructions displayed on the monitor as shown in Figure 7–52. To conduct a test, the user must complete each of the three instructions displayed on the screen.

1. Enter Patient Information
2. Position Ear Phone and Apply Electrodes
3. Check for Proper Protocol and Begin Testing

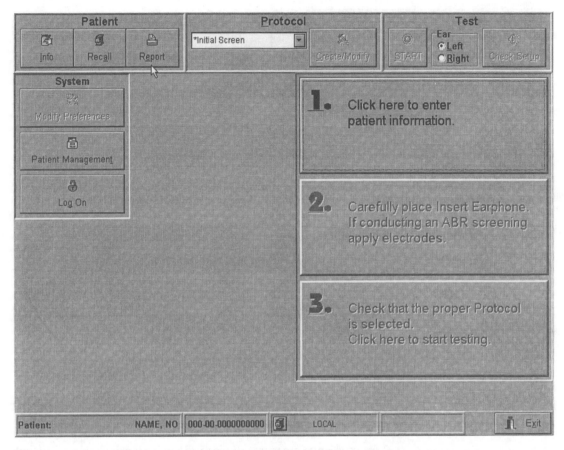

Figure 7–52. The Screening-User Mode main window from the SonaMed Clarity System for combination DPOAE/ABR measurement.

In the Screening-User Mode the user has access to only a limited set of controls, features, and settings of the Clarity System, including entry of Patient Information (e.g., medical record number, name, date of birth, birth weight, etc.), recall of the current patient's information and test results, and printing of the current patient's test reports. To maintain system security and to protect patient privacy, in the Screening-User Mode the user has no access to system parameters, modification or creation of test protocols, or patient information stored in the patient database. Access to these features of the Clarity System are available only with a special security password.

Once patient information has been entered and the test ear has been selected, the system automatically performs a check to ensure that the insert earphone is properly positioned, and, if ABRs are being conducted, that electrode impedances are suitable for testing (Figure 7–53). If problems are found that could potentially result in an invalid or unreliable test, the operator is notified of the situation and prompt-

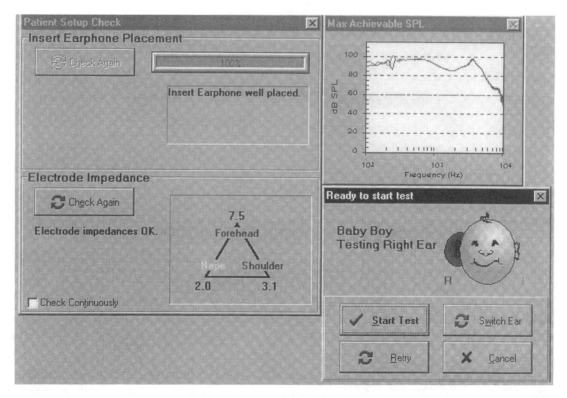

Figure 7–53. The impedance and ear phone position check window from the SonaMed Clarity System.

ed for corrective measures. If electrode impedance values are acceptable and earphone is properly positioned, the test begins when the operator chooses Start Test. Once started, the test automatically proceeds to completion.

During automated screening useful information regarding test progress is displayed for the operator (Figure 7–54). This information includes Pass or Refer results for each individual test as well as an overall result, test progress, including accepted and rejected sweeps, elapsed test time, and other pertinent information. Additionally, to ensure accurate testing, the stimulus level in the ear canal is continuously monitored during the test. If specified stimulus levels are not maintained or achieved, the test is paused and a message box prompts the user to check the ear phone.

Advanced Screening and Manual Test Mode

When operating in the Advanced-User Mode, all the features of the Clarity System are available to the user (Figure 7–55). Access to the Advanced-User Mode is allowed only with the entry of a secure password. If the user does not enter the correct password on log-in, they are

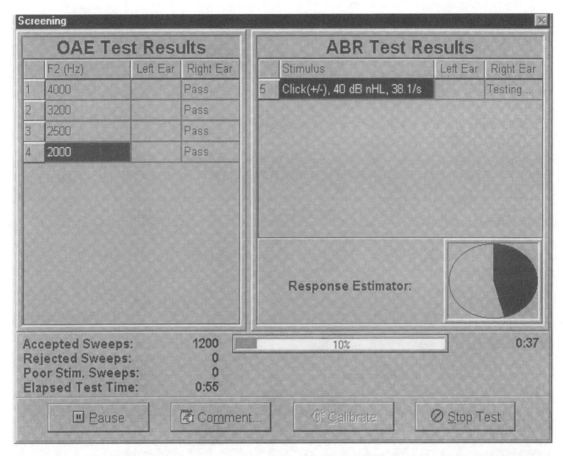

Figure 7–54. The Screening-User Mode test window for displaying test results with the SonaMed Clarity System.

restricted to the Screening-User Mode. The major differences between the two modes is that in the Advanced-User Mode, (1) the operator is able to conduct OAE or ABR tests in either an automated mode or under manual control; (2) the operator is able to create and/or modify test protocols, OAE pass criteria, and system settings; and (3) the operator has full access to stored patient information, including the capability of reviewing all patient data (e.g., screening results, stored OAE and ABR waveforms, etc.) as well as generation, review, and printing of all patient and program statistical reports. Additionally, whereas during a test in the Screening-User Mode the user views only the Pass/Refer display (as shown in Figure 7–54), in the Advanced-User Mode the real time acoustic measures and results are continuously displayed for the user. An example of the display during an OAE test is shown in Figure 7–56.

We briefly review those capabilities not available in the Screening-User Mode in the following sections.

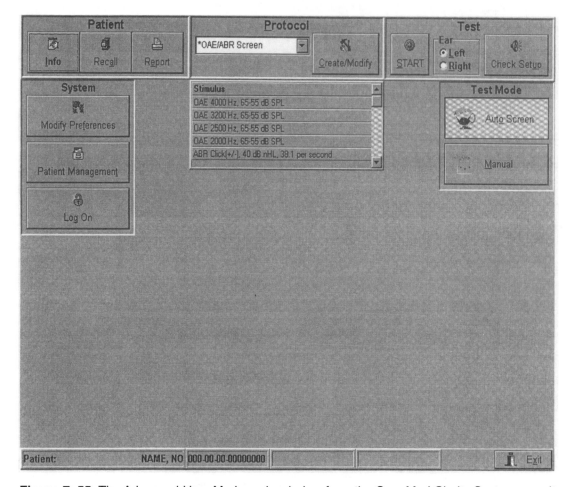

Figure 7–55. The Advanced-User Mode main window from the SonaMed Clarity System permitting the selection of protocols and modification of preferences.

DPOAE measurement, including test protocols, is reviewed in detail in Chapter 4. See for example Tables 4–4 through 4–6. Different clinical application of specific protocols is discussed, and illustrated with case reports, in Chapters 8 and 9.

Creating and Modifying Test Protocols. All tests are conducted using test protocols. Test protocols fully specify the test type (i.e., OAE or ABR), stimulus parameters (frequencies, intensities, durations, etc.), stimulus presentation sequence, as well as OAE pass and refer criteria. During testing it is possible to add OAE or ABR tests to the current protocol at any time.

Setting System Preferences and OAE Pass/Refer Criteria. A wealth of testing parameters and system settings are available to the operator. These have been separated according to logical functional groupings as shown in Figure 7–57. Most pertinent to this discussion is the OAE Pass Criteria page (Figure 7–58). These fields allow the clinician to establish pass criteria for individual frequency DPOAE tests based on their own preferences and experience as well as the latest results from current research and scientific publications. A response will be accepted if it meets the criteria listed. Response signal require-

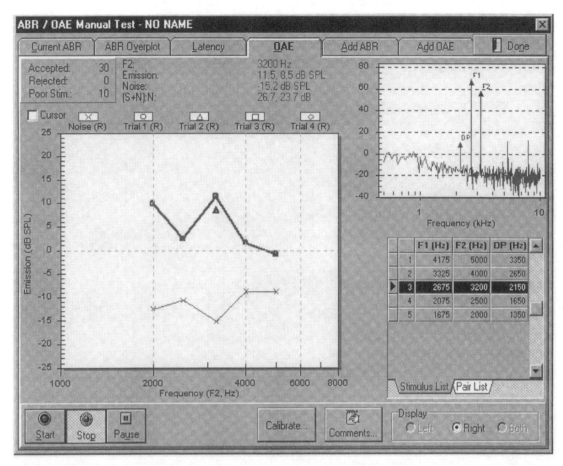

Figure 7–56. The test data form window from the SonaMed Clarity System opened to the DPOAE page.

ments may be set independently for each of the three octave bands which may be tested using the Clarity System. Three signal requirement parameters must be specified: Minimum Noise Floor; the maximum allowable noise floor for a passing OAE; DP Magnitude: the minimum absolute value of the DP in dB SPL; and Signal-to-Noise +Signal (S+N:N): the minimum separation (in dB) between the magnitude of the DP and the average noise floor in a 120 Hz frequency (± 60 Hz) band surrounding the DP frequency. These criteria may also be applied to manual mode OAE testing via the Auto-Stop feature. Additionally, the Replicability option requires that each OAE frequency be tested twice and the user is able to specify the maximum allowable difference (in dB) between the magnitude of the DP in the two responses.

Reviewing Patient Test Results. All data related to the patient and test results are stored on the Clarity System and are available for review, printing, archiving to external media, and export to third-party software.

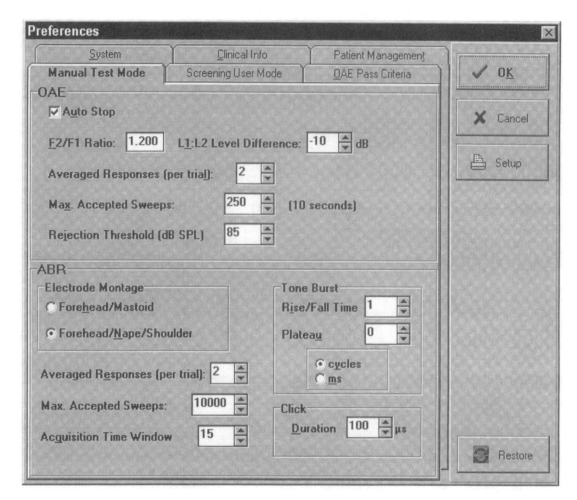

Figure 7–57. The Preferences window with Manual Test Mode page open (from the SonaMed Clarity System).

Generating Patient and Statistical Reports. A range of reports may be generated from within the Clarity System. Immediately following a screening test or when a patient's data has been recalled for review, as shown in Figure 7–59, the user may generate a Patient Test Report which lists the test results for individual and overall test results. Additionally, graphical results may be printed in which plots of OAE "DPgrams" (response magnitude as a function of stimulus frequency) are generated as well as ABR waveforms, if acquired. A variety of statistical and program reports may also be generated based on a range of user-specifiable sort criteria (Figure 7–60). These reports include: (1) Patients Tested Report, which lists all patients tested with the associated test date, tests conducted (i.e., OAE, ABR, screening or manual test), and operator conducting the test; (2) Screening History Report displaying a list of all patients screened within a specified time period

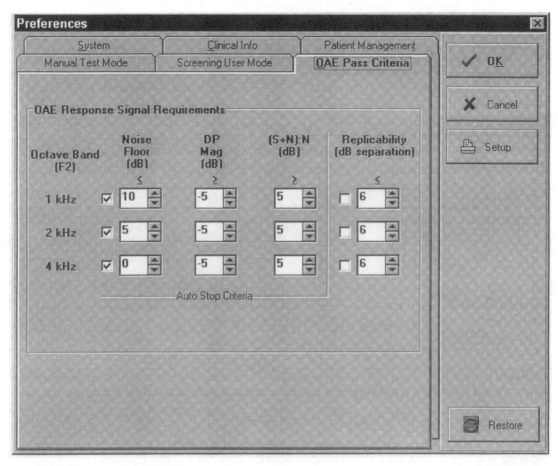

Figure 7–58. The Preferences window with the DPOAE Pass Criteria page open (from the SonaMed Clarity System).

along with the protocols used and Pass/Refer results, which can be sorted based on patient name, physician, test operator, or test date; and (3) Screening Results Reports allow one to obtain administrative data and statistics regarding the screening program.

Screening Results Reports are sorted into three report types: (1) Missing and Referred Screens (Figure 7–61) allows the generation of a list of patients whose test results are missing (i.e., were not tested) or who did not pass the screening test; (2) Screening Statistics generates program monitoring statistics according to the sort criteria chosen, these include number and percent of patients who passed, referred, or were not tested, as well as average test time sorted for overall, for OAE and ABR tests, and by left and right ear. Reports are generated based on specific filter criteria (e.g., date range, operator, physician, insurer, sex). The Report Pass Criteria, shown in Figure 7–61, allows the user to

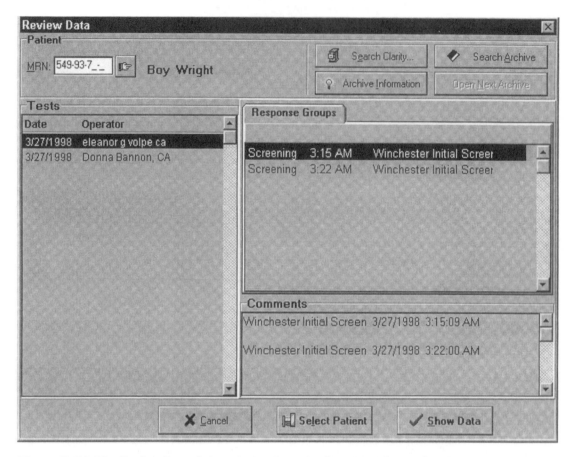

Figure 7–59. The Review Data dialog window from the SonaMed Clarity System.

define the requirements for a patient to pass in terms of test modality (OAE/ABR) and whether one or both ears must pass. For example, in the Screening Statistics report, results may be generated for all operators and patients with the requirement that both ears must pass both an OAE and an ABR test in order to be considered an overall pass; (3) Operator Report (Figure 7–62) allows program administrators to monitor the performance of individual operators within a screening program. The report generates a list of all operators, the total number of babies tested by each operator, their individual refer rates, and average screening times per operator for either OAEs, ABRs or both. These reporting capabilities are unique to the Clarity System and have been found to be extremely useful tools in the implementation and monitoring of newborn hearing screening programs. As an example, the operator report allows the administrator of a screening program a simple and effective means of identifying individual operators who may require further training as evidenced by, for instance, excessively long test times or overly high refer rates relative to other operators of program goals.

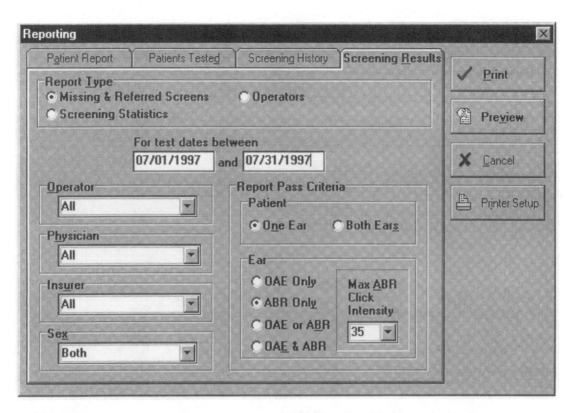

Figure 7–60. The Screening Results report dialog window from the SonaMed Clarity System.

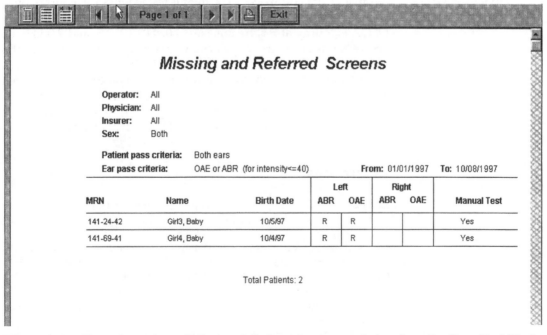

Figure 7–61. The print review of Missing & Referred screens window from the SonaMed Clarity System.

Figure 7–62. The print preview of Operator Statistics Report window from the SonaMed Clarity System.

Normative Data

Normative data from over 2,000 infants tested within 36 hours of birth and are presented in Figure 7–63. These data were derived from DPOAEs testing at 5 f_2 frequencies: 5.0, 4.0, 3.2, 2.5, and 2.0 kHz (¹⁄₆ octave bands). Primary frequencies were set at a fixed frequency ratio of 1.2 (i.e., $f_2/f_1 = 1.2$) with f_2 intensity of 65 dB SPL and f_1 of 55 dB SPL. In the DPOAE test, each stimulus frequency was automatically scored as a pass or refer by the Clarity System. Pass criteria used in the study for each frequency are shown in Table 7–7. Only DPOAE frequencies that met the pass criteria were included in normative data.

References

Dalzell, L. E., Orlando, M. S., & Seeger, C. (1996). *3-stage newborn hearing screening reduces failures at discharge*. Poster presented at American Academy of Audiology, Salt Lake City, UT.

National Institutes of Health. (1993). Early identification of hearing impairment in infants and young children. *NIH Consensus Statement*. 11:1–25.

Orlando, M. S., & Prieve, B. A. (1998). Models for universal newborn hearing screening programs. In L. G. Spivak (ed.). *Universal newborn hearing screening* (pp. 50–66). New York: Thieme.

Notes: Maximum allowable noise floor sets the maximum permissible value of the noise surrounding the DP emission frequency; Minimum

Figure 7–63. DPOAE normative data from over 2,000 newborn infants showing mean DP amplitude. The bars represent one standard deviation around the mean (from the SonaMed Clarity System).

Table 7–7. DPOAE pass criteria with SonaMed Clarity System.

Frequency Band	Maximum Allowable Noise Floor (dB SPL)	Minimum Allowable DP Magnitude (dB SPL)	(Signal+Noise)/Noise (dB)	Replicability (dB Separation)
1 – 2 kHz	10	–5	5	3
2 – 4 kHz	5	–5	5	3
4 – 8 kHz	0	–5	5	3

allowable DP magnitude sets the minimum magnitude of the DP emission for acceptance; (Signal + Noise)/Noise the minimum acceptable difference (in dB) between the magnitude of the DP (the signal) and average magnitude of the surrounding noise floor (noise); Replicability sets the allowable tolerance of difference between the DP magnitude in successive tests.

Summary

The Clarity System was designed as a total solution for newborn hearing screening and it has been clinically demonstrated to be highly accurate and efficacious. The combination of OAE and ABR technologies provides the strengths of both technologies in a single fully integrated, cost-effective, and simple-to-use package. The simplified Screening-User interface presents the ideal solution for screening by technicians and nonaudiologists, while the advanced operation and clinical data review capabilities allows advanced users to perform initial diagnostic evaluations, review all collected data, control over test protocols, pass/refer criteria, and system operation. Additionally, the Patient Result and Statistical Reporting features allow for simplified tracking of infants as well as monitoring of program performance.

STARKEY LABORATORIES, INC.

Product: DP-2000 DPOAE Measurement System

Prepared by: Mel K. Gross, M.A., Carol Barnett, M.A.,
Starkey Laboratories
Patricia S. Jeng, Ph.D., Mimosa Acoustics

DP-2000 DPOAE Measurement System

Introduction. DP-2000 DPOAE (Distortion Product Otoacoustic Emission) Measurement System is currently in it's fourth generation. The latest version is based on the newest multimedia plug and play technology and the well-tested methodology of Bell Laboratory and other researchers. In previous generations, this system has been known by various names including CUBeDIS DPOAE. Over time, continuous improvements in both hardware and software were initiated, culminating in a very user-friendly system. Comparing the current version to previous generations, the physical size and weight have been significantly reduced. There are no heavy isolation transformers or external processing boxes. The high quality hardware allows the system to achieve a very low noise floor, thereby enabling the system to measure lower intensity distortion products. With all these features, the system still remains simple and easy to use in a screening environment, but retains the flexibility that is demanded in a research environment. As a screener, the tester can have the results in just two key strokes or two mouse clicks. As an experimental tool, the Starkey DP-2000 has complete flexibility in establishing various test parameters.

The hardware platform allows for continuous updates of features and expansion of functions. Many new features are in development and will be available on new software releases. Please contact Starkey Advanced Instrumentation Division for up-to-date product information and developments at 800-328-8602, or via e-mail at dp2000@starkey.com.

Hardware Components

DP-2000 DPOAE Hardware Components. *The PC card* (PCMCIA) is the digital signal-processing card. This card creates the electrical signals for the probe. *The Probe Interface Cable* (PIC) amplifies the signal that is received from the microphone of the transducer. The *Probe* is composed of three transducers; one microphone and two speakers. Each individual speaker delivers only one signal, thereby decreasing the distortion of the input signal. *Disposable Single Use Ear Tips* eliminate the possible spread of infections. The ear tips are available in seven different sizes, ranging from 2-mm infant ear tips to an extra-large adult size.

Auxilary Equipment. The DP-2000 DPOAE can be utilized with a palm-top computer, notebook computer, laptop computer, or desktop computer with a PCMCIA slot and operating in Windows 95 or 98 environment.

Total Weight. DP-2000: Less than 6 oz. (not including computer)

Warranty. The warranty is 1 year for hardware components and 2 years for free software upgrades.

DP-2000 System Qualification

■ FDA approval for marketing
■ ETL Approval for Medical Device Safety and Performance
■ Conforms to UL Std. 2601-1
■ Certified to CAN/CSA C22.2 No. 601.1
■ CE Marking

The Starkey DP-2000 as a Screener for Infants

System Setup. The PCMCIA card is inserted into the PCMCIA Type II slot, and the PIC and the probe are connected properly. If the PCMCIA card is installed correctly, the green light on the PIC should be illuminated. The DP 2000 program is selected from the Windows program menu. Patient identifying information and test protocol can be entered at this time.

Preparation. With test ear accessible the infant should be placed into a conformable position. Examine the external auditory canal for any blockage. The angle of the canal should be noted for correct ear tip placement. Mount the disposable ear tip onto the probe. Insert the probe into the test ear canal.

What's a chirp you ask? Chirps and other rather different OAE signals are noted in Chapter 10.

■ STEP 1: Click on the Quick Screen Button to start In-the-ear Calibration. Two consecutive chirp signals will be introduced into the ear canal. The calibration screen will "pop up" showing the frequency responses of the two transducers as measured in the ear canal. These curves verify the system integrity, probe fit, and signal level. Figure 7–64 shows the in-the-ear calibration frequency responses of an infant less than 2 days old.
■ STEP 2: Press the Enter Key or the letter D Key to start the Distortion Product Level measurements. A DP Measurement window will pop up with three plots, as shown in Figure 7–65. The top plot

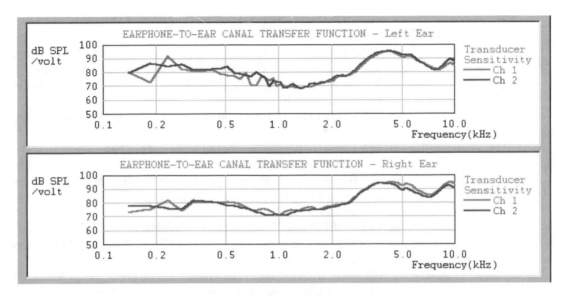

Figure 7–64. In-the-ear calibration with DP-2000 DPOAE Measurement System (Starkey Laboratories Inc). Upper plot shows the in-the-ear calibration for the left ear and the lower plot is for the right ear.

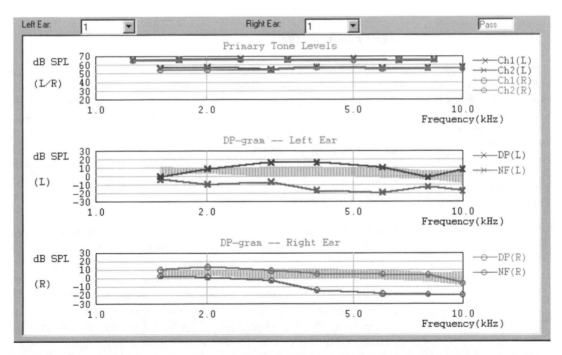

Figure 7–65. DP measurements with DP-2000 DPOAE Measurement System (Starkey Laboratories Inc). Top plot contains the primary tone levels measured at the same time as the DP levels are measured. The middle plot is the DPgram for the left or first ear tested. Lower plot shows the right or the second ear tested. This example used the 7-frequency test parameter protocol and allows a PASS if 4 out of 7 frequency points receive a PASS.

shows the intensity levels of the two primary tones (f_1 and f_2) as measured in the ear canal. As these tones are presented, the Distortion Products and the Noise Floors are measured concurrently and plotted on the DPgrams. The lower two graphs of the DP Measurement window displays the DPgrams for the same infant that is less than two days old.

■ TEST THE OTHER EAR: The same procedure is completed for the opposite ear.

■ TEST RESULT: Located in the upper right-hand corner of the DP-Measurement Window, a field will indicate PASS or REFER. The test results are based upon the PASS/REFER criteria set by the test parameter protocol. *Note: Quick Screen procedure is not ear-specific.*

■ TROUBLESHOOTING WHILE IN-THE-EAR CALIBRATION SCREEN: An acoustic leak can be observed if the ear tip is incorrectly placed in the ear canal. The curves displayed will roll off in the lower frequencies or may have a dip around 200 to 300 Hz. If the curves displayed are far apart either one of the ear tip ports is blocked by cerumen or other foreign matter or the probe is malfunctioning. If the infant is noisy, the curves will appear to have a lot of zigzags. Just calm the infant and repeat the calibration by pressing Space Bar Key or Quick Screen Key.

Test Parameters

DPOAE measurement, including test protocols, is reviewed in detail in Chapter 4. See for example Tables 4–4 through 4–6. Nonpathologic factors influencing OAE measurement are covered in Chapter 5.

Many factors affect the distortion product amplitude. To control these factors the user can set certain parameters in the Test Parameter Window to achieve the best measurement. These factors include time averaging duration, level of f_1 and f_2 as well as the f_2/f_1 ratio. The examiner can also change the f_2 frequency range of the measurement as well as the frequency density (i.e., points per octave). Test parameter manipulation is a very useful tool. Knowing the effect of changing these various parameters will lead to a better understanding of the patient's preneural outer hair cell function.

The DP-2000 allows the examiner to control the various test parameters. Once these parameters have been entered and the protocol has been named, the parameter windows allow easy switching between the various preset protocols. The DP-2000 Test Parameter Window can be divided into four unique areas: protocol name, pass/refer, criteria parameters, and detail table. The Protocol is a set of preselected parameter values that have been entered for the measurement of distortion products. The various protocols can be set for a specific purpose (i.e., infant screening, screening adults, diagnostic testing, examiner's preferences, ototoxic hearing monitoring, and others). The software comes with three protocols, Boys Town 1995 (BT95), Boys Town 1990 (BT90), and Overlook Hospital of New Jersey (unpublished) (OVLKInfant).

The examiner should enter his or her preferred protocol(s) and save it for later use. It is easy to retrieve the various protocols through the drop-down window.

Test Parameters. The following six values can be changed: Minimum f_2, Maximum f_2, f_1 Level, f_2 Level, Points per Octave, Time Averaging, and f_2 to f_1 Ratio.

■ The minimum f_2 defines the lower limit of f_2 frequency range over which DP measurement sweeps across.
■ Minimum f_2: This field defines the lower frequency limit of f_2 frequency range over which distortion product measurements are made. This is expressed in Hz.
■ Maximum f_2: This field defines the upper frequency range over which Distortion Product is measured. This is expressed in Hz.
■ f_1 Level: This field defines the input stimulus level (L_1) of f_1 primary tone, expressed in dB SPL.
■ f_2 Level: This field defines the input stimulus level (L_2) of f_2 primary tone, expressed in dB SPL.
■ Points per Octave: This field allows the examiner to set the number of sampling distortion product points per octave.
■ Time Average: The recorded signals are time-averaged before analysis to provide noise reduction (i.e., lowering the noise floor). The amount of time one averages should be predicated on the amount of noise (electrical, environmental, and internal) present in the test environment. In a quiet office, a 2-second signal duration should provide a noise floor around 20 to 30 dB SPL between 1000 to 10,000 Hz in a cooperative adult's ear. To achieve the same noise floor in a noisy environment, the time averaging may have to be increased to a 4-second time frame.
■ f_2/f_1 Ratio: Current literature suggests the best ratio for a human is around 1.2 to 1.22.

Other Applications: Advanced Features

■ **High frequency:** Maximum f2 = 16,000 Hz.
■ **Independently defined frequency point.**
■ **Different distortion product definitions:** $2f_1-f_2$, $2f_2-f_1$, f_2-f_1, $3f_1-2f_2$, $3f_2-2f_1$, $4f_2-3f_3$, $4f_3-3f_2$.
■ **Input/output functions**
■ **Pass/Refer Criteria:** Three criteria can be set for automatic decision making on pass/refer of the individual points and the overall measurement. These are DPL (Distortion Product Level)/NFL (Noise Floor Level), the minimum DPL for acceptance of the DPL, the minimum number of individual passes needed to be an overall pass.
■ **Detailed Table:** Displays the various parameter values for each test point that will be measured for the individual protocol. In this

Literature on DPOAE parameters, such as the f_2/f_1 ratio, is reviewed in Chapter 4. For an example of how changes in the f_2/f_1 ratio can alter DP amplitude, inspect Figure 4–7. The many mathematically predictable DPs are listed in Table 4–3.

screen one can also modify test point parameter values. An individual test point can be added or deleted. After changes have been entered, one has the option of sorting the various test points in a descending order. If unsorted is selected, then multiple sweeps of frequency test points at various levels can be measured.

■ **DP Measurements:** For each frequency test point defined by the test parameters, four values are measured, calculated, and plotted. The four values are the primary tones, f_1 and f_2, the distortion product level (DPL), and the noise floor level (NFL). The data points are measured and plotted in a descending order. The primary tones are plotted on the top graph, the left ear test results are plotted in the middle using a blue "X," and the right ear test results are plotted on the lower graph using a red "O."

■ **Single-Frequency Mode (SFM):** Single-Frequency Mode allows the tester to test individual frequency test points. After one completes the Distortion Product sweep one or more single-frequency test points can then be measured individually, (i.e., where one obtained an unsatisfactory measurement). The examiner can then click on the SFM button or press "g" to enter the SF mode and test individual frequency point.

■ **Artifact Rejection:** Artifact Rejection Mode is helpful in the evaluation of the difficult-to-test patients. In this mode, the test results will be accepted or rejected based on user-defined criteria.

■ **Numerical Table:** The exact numeric values of each individual test point measurement are displayed. Just click on the Numerical Table bottom on the toolbar, the numerical table window will pop open revealing the results.

■ **Save Data or Not Save Data:** Patient information and test results can be saved into a database. When the Save Button is clicked or "S" key is pressed, the Save Window is displayed and tester's name and comments can be entered. If the user opts to not save data, the default option on the menu can be activated to prompt the tester to save or not to save the data. The same default option can also be activated to save the data automatically. Comments can be entered at the time of saving or entered latter.

■ **Test Summary Report: Manufacturer Default format.** This report contains the report title, clinic's name and address, patient information, test information, results, DP plots, numerical values, and comments.

■ **Other Printouts:** Patient Lists, Test History of a specific patient, In-the-ear Calibration, DP Measurement, and Numerical Table of a single test session.

DATAbase

■ **Microsoft ACCESS:** Currently, the data are saved in ACCESS compatible databases. This program allows the user to; create new databases, open an existing database for measurements, or to export data from single session or multiple sessions; for single or multiple patients. The data are shared using a comma delimited format.

- ■ **Other Database:** At the time of this printing, other databases are being incorporated. Among these are HiScreen, SIMS, NOAH, and StarBase.

The Oz product which interfaces with the DP-2000 and other OAE devices is introduced earlier in this chapter.

References

Gorga, M. P., Neely, S. T., Bergman, B. M., Beauchaine, K. L., Kaminski, J. R., & Liu, Z. (1994). Towards optimizing the limits of distortion product otoacoustic emission measurements. *Journal of the Acoustical Society of America, 96*, 1494–1500.

Gorga, M. P., Neely, S. T., Bergman, B., Beauchaine, K. L., Kaminski, J. R., Peters, J., & Jesteadt, W. (1993). Otoacoustic emissions from normal-hearing and hearing-impaired subjects: Distortion product responses. *Journal of the Acoustical Society of America, 93*, 2050–2060.

Gorga, M. P., Neely, S. T., Bergman, B. M., Beauchaine, K. L., Kaminski, J. R., Peters, J., Schulte, L., & Jesteadt, W. (1993). A comparison of transient-evoked and distortion product otoacoustic emissions in normal-hearing and hearing-impaired subjects. *Journal of the Acoustical Society of America, 94*, 2639–2648.

Gorga, M. P., Neely, S. T., Ohlrich, B., Hoover, B., Redner, J., & Peters, J. (1997). From laboratory to clinic: A large scale study of distortion product otoacoustic emissions in ears with normal hearing and ears with hearing loss. *Ear & Hearing, 18*, 440–455.

Hall, J. W., III, & Mueller, H. G., III. (1997). *Audiologists' desk reference. Volume I.* San Diego: Singular Publishing Group.

Kimberley, B. P., Brown, D. K., & Allen, J. B. (1997). Distortion product emissions and sensorineural hearing loss. In M. S. Robinette & T. J. Glattke (Eds.), *Otoacoustic emissions: Clinical applications* (pp. 181–204). New York, NY: Thieme.

Kimberley, B. P., Hernadi, I., Lee, A. M., & Brown, D. K. (1994). Predicting pure tone thresholds in normal and hearing-impaired ears with distortion product emissions and age. *Ear & Hearing, 15*, 199–209.

Kimberley, B. P., & Nelson, D. A. (1989). Distortion product emission and sensorineural hearing loss. *Journal of Otolaryngology, 18*, 365–369.

Nelson, D. A., & Kimberley, B. P. (1992). Distortion-product emissions and auditory sensitivity in human ears with normal hearing and cochlear hearing loss. *Journal of Speech and Hearing Research, 35*, 1141–1159.

Smyrzinski, J., Leonard, G., Kim, D. O., Lafreniere, D. C., & Junk, M. D. (1990). Distortion product otoacoustic emissions in normal and impaired adult ears. *Archives of Otolaryngology—Head and Neck Surgery, 116*, 1309–1316.

Stover, L., Gorga, M. P., Neely, S. T., & Montoya, D. (1996). Towards optimizing the clinical utility of distortion product otoacoustic emission measurements. *Journal of the Acoustical Society of America, 100*, 956–967.

Stover, L. J., & Norton, S. J. (1993). The effects of aging on otoacoustic emissions. *Journal of the Acoustical Society of America, 94*, 2670–2681.

CHAPTER

8

Clinical Applications of Otoacoustic Emissions in Children

OAEs are a powerful new addition to the pediatric audiology test battery. Although initially proposed mostly as a technique appropriate for newborn hearing screening, in recent years OAEs have assumed many other valuable roles in various pediatric populations. Selected clinical applications of OAEs in children, with a brief rationale, are summarized in Table 8–1. Each of these applications is reviewed in some detail below. Clinical experience is confirming that, among these multiple clinical pediatric applications, the most unique and essential is the information provided by OAEs during pediatric diagnostic assessment. Confirmation and diagnosis of auditory dysfunction in infants and young children, or in children who yield incomplete and/or inconclusive behavioral hearing test results, is often a considerable clinical challenge; and the outcome of such assessments greatly influences the timing and nature of audiologic, habilitative, and medical management. Decisions based on the findings of

Table 8–1. Major pediatric clinical applications of OAEs, and their rationale.

Application	Rationale
Newborn hearing screening	✔ OAEs can be recorded reliably from newborn infants. ✔ OAE recording can be performed in nursery setting (test performance may be affected by noise). ✔ Normal OAEs are recorded in persons with normal sensory (cochlear) function. ✔ OAEs are abnormal in persons with even mild degrees of sensory. hearing loss; the main objective of screening is to detect sensory hearing impairment. ✔ OAE recording may require relatively brief test time. ✔ OAE measurement may be performed by nonaudiologic personnel (e.g., at reduced cost).
Diagnostic pediatric audiometry	✔ OAE recording is electrophysiologic and not dependent on patient behavioral response. ✔ OAEs assess cochlear function specifically (behavioral audiometry and ABR are also dependent on the status of the central auditory nervous system). ✔ OAEs can be recorded from sleeping or sedated children. ✔ OAE recording requires relatively short test time. ✔ OAEs provide ear-specific audiologic information. ✔ OAEs provide frequency-specific audiologic information. ✔ OAEs are a valuable contribution to the "cross-check principle."
Diagnosis of CAPD	✔ OAE recording is electrophysiologic and not dependent on patient behavioral response. ✔ OAEs are a sensitive means of ruling out cochlear (outer hair cell) dysfunction.
Assessment in suspected functional hearing loss	✔ OAE recording is electrophysiologic and not dependent on patient behavioral response. ✔ Normal OAEs invariably imply normal sensory function. ✔ OAEs provide frequency-specific audiologic information.
Monitoring ototoxicity	✔ OAEs are site-specific for cochlear (sensory) auditory dysfunction. ✔ Ototoxic drugs exert their effect on outer hair cell function; OAEs are dependent on outer hair cell integrity. ✔ OAE recording is electrophysiologic and not dependent on patient behavioral response; can be recorded from patients who, due to their medical condition, are unable to perform behavioral audiometry tasks; or from infants and young children. ✔ OAEs can detect cochlear dysfunction before it is evident by pure-tone audiometry. ✔ OAEs provide frequency-specific audiologic information.

pediatric diagnostic audiologic assessments conducted within months after birth often profoundly impact the child's lifetime potential for communication abilities, academic success, employment, and financial status. For these reasons, OAEs are now considered to be "standard-of-care" by many clinicians charged with the serious responsibility of identification and intervention of hearing impairment in young children.

This chapter includes discussion of major pediatric applications of OAEs, with reference to both the published literature and the author's clinical experiences. Each section begins with background information on the general application or clinical population. Then, the literature on OAEs for that application and/or population is reviewed briefly. Next, test protocols and strategies are described, with an emphasis on how OAE results are incorporated into the diagnostic test battery and can contribute to shaping overall patterns of auditory findings. Finally, selected case reports are occasionally presented to illustrate major points.

NEWBORN HEARING SCREENING

Historical Overview

Newborn hearing screening was the first clinical application of OAEs back in the mid-1980s.

Early identification of hearing loss in infants can be traced back to the tireless work of Dr. Marion Downs in the 1960s. Well ahead of her times, Dr. Downs developed and then applied behavioral screening techniques in hearing screening of thousands of newborn infants. For an introduction to Marion Downs, see the Biographical Sketch in this chapter, accompanied by a flattering photograph (Figure 8–1). Almost singularly, she reported her newborn hearing screening experiences at professional meetings and published findings in the literature (Downs & Sterritt, 1964; Downs & Hemenway, 1969; Downs, 1970), all the while collaborating with and encouraging her colleagues in the United States to do likewise. During this period, a similar effort was underway in Europe (e.g., Froding, 1960; Feinmesser & Tell, 1976). By 1970, Dr. Downs had organized the first Joint Committee on Infant Hearing (JCIH) and a risk registry approach to identifying infants most likely to have hearing impairment. The use of risk factors or indicators to identify infants with a greater than normal likelihood of having permanent sensorineural hearing impairment was quickly adopted by audiologists in hospital settings, especially hospitals with intensive care nurseries (ICNs), sometimes also called neonatal intensive care units (NICUs). The majority of infants "at risk" for hearing impairment are not entirely healthy at birth and are, therefore, found in the ICN. Risk registers were also applied on a larger scale during the 1970s. Departments of Health in some states, such as Utah, incorporated risk indicators on birth certificates and systematically tracked at-risk infants in an attempt to implement early detection, assessment, and intervention of serious hearing impairment. Risk factors developed by the Joint Committee on Infant Hearing were widely accepted by audiologists and public health personnel and utilized, to a lesser extent, by pediatricians. The JCIH risk indicators are discussed in

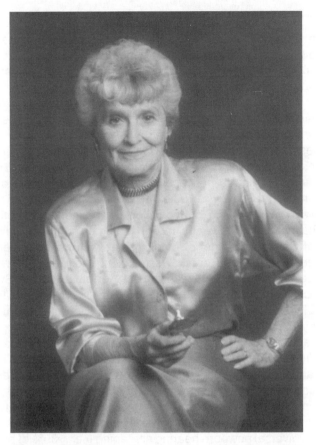

Figure 8–1. Marion Downs, the mother of newborn hearing screening.

Biographical Sketch

Marion Downs, "Mother of Newborn Hearing Screening"

Marion Downs received her B.A. from the University of Minnesota in 1935, and her M.A. from the University of Denver in 1951. Several years later, in 1979, she earned a Doctorate in Human Services at the University of Northern Colorado. Marion Down's entire career has been devoted to early screening, diagnosis, and intervention for children with hearing loss. Her first attempts at newborn screening were reported in 1964. In 1970,

(continued)

she organized and chaired the original Joint Committee on Infant Hearing. This committee announced the first guidelines for newborn screening. Since then, the JCIH has piloted the course of newborn screening and follow-up.

Dr. Downs collaborated with Jerry Northern in publishing *Hearing in Children*, which in now in its fourth edition. She also co-edited *Auditory Disorders in School Children* with Ross Roeser, now in its third edition. She has consulted with various foreign governments on pediatric hearing assessment. These contributions led to her receipt, in 1994, of the Honors of the International Society of Audiology. Other honors awarded to Dr. Downs include the Gold Medals for Achievement from both her alma mater, the University of Minnesota, and from the University of Colorado School of Medicine, as well as the American Speech-Language-Hearing Association. She is also the recipient of the Howard House Award of Sertoma and the Sylvan Stool Award of the Society for Ear, Nose, and Throat Advances in Children (SENTAC). Dr. Downs remains active in promoting early identification and intervention, while regularly playing tennis and teaching her 13 great-grandchildren to ski. She is integrally involved in the Marion Downs National Center for Infant Hearing, funded by a grant from the U.S. Public Health Service to coordinate statewide systems for screening, diagnosis, and intervention for newborns and infants who are deaf and hard-of-hearing. The overall objective of the Center is to facilitate universal newborn hearing screening (i.e., >85% of births), involving audiologists, parents, and consumer groups. More information is available on the Center website at: www.colorado.edu/CDSS/MDNC

Even a very efficient high-risk registry only identifies about one half of the hearing impaired infants born every year. Universal hearing screening is the only effective strategy for early identification of hearing loss among the remaining infants.

greater detail later. Although the risk registry is, in effect, a form of newborn hearing screening, and played an important role in the identification of many hearing-impaired infants during the 1970s, by the early 1980s it became clear that approximately half of children who were eventually diagnosed with communicatively important, permanent, sensorineural hearing impairment were, in retrospect, born as healthy infants in well baby nurseries, with none of these risk indicators (e.g., Stein, Clark, & Kraus, 1983; Elssmann, Matkin, & Sabo, 1987; Stein et al., 1990; Mauk, White, Mortensen, & Behrens, 1991; Pappas, 1993). In other words, the risk registry approach, even when applied very successfully, failed to identify about 50% of children with significant hearing loss. And, the solution to this problem would not be solved by simply increasing the number of risk indicators.

During the 1970s, nonbehavioral techniques for diagnostic auditory assessment in general, and infant screening in particular, were introduced. Most popular among these techniques were the Crib-O-Gram or Linco-Bennett type devices (Simmons & Russ, 1974; Bennett, 1980) and auditory brainstem response (see Hall, 1992, for review). Despite it's noble objective and apparent clinical advantages, the test performance of these "computerized crib" techniques was woefully inadequate. Because these devices were designed to sense generalized physiologic and physical responses to sound stimulation (e.g., change in respiration or bodily movement), they were in some ways a variation of behavioral audiometry. Stimuli were rather intense and frequency-nonspecific sounds (noise bands sometimes over 90 dB SPL) presented via a speaker (i.e., not ear-specific). As a result of these and other technical limitations, newborn hearing screening with the cradle devices was plagued by unacceptably high false-positive (failure of normal-hearing infants) *and* false-negative (missed hearing loss) outcomes.

The direction of newborn hearing screening was altered dramatically by the publication of, first, Jewett and Williston's (1971) classic ABR article, and within a few years the germinal paper by Hecox and Galambos (1974) demonstrating the clinical feasibility and value of ABR in auditory assessment of infants and young children. These publications, in turn, were followed almost immediately by studies characterizing maturational changes in ABR latency, amplitude, and morphology and documenting that ABR was a viable technique for infant hearing screening, even among premature neonates (Salamy et al., 1975, 1976; Schulman-Galambos & Galambos, 1975, 1979; Mokotoff, Schulman-Galambos, & Galambos, 1977). In the early 1980s, there was a flurry of clinical reports of newborn hearing screening of at-risk infants with ABR published by audiologists and others at hospitals and medical centers around the United States (see Hall et al., 1988, and Hall, 1992, for review). Initially, these investigators applied neonatal hearing screening diagnostic equipment and test protocols developed mostly for neurodiagnostic auditory assessment of adults. Not suprisingly, failure rates were rather high (e.g., over 20%) in some of these early studies (Marshall et al., 1980; Jacobson & Morehouse, 1984; Cevette, 1984; Dennis et al., 1984; Swigonski et al., 1987). Even at this formative period in the application of the ABR technique, however, other authors reported remarkably modest failure rates (e.g., 10 to 13%) for at-risk infants screened in the ICN (Dennis et al., 1984; Ruth et al., 1985; Hall et al., 1988). As the decade progressed and clinical experience accumulated, equipment, techniques, and strategies were modified, the learning curve quickly developed, and reported failure rates decreased to less than 10% (e.g., Gorga et al., 1987, 1988; Hall et al., 1987). Finally, modifications of instrumention and transducers and recognition of test factors such as noise and electrical interference were incorporated into automated devices designed specifically for infant hearing screening.

The "learning curve" for newborn hearing screening with ABR occurred during a 10-year period from the late 1970s to the late 1980s, resulting in automated technology and sufficiently low failure rates. A decade later, from the late 1980s to the late 1990s, there has been a similar experiential trend for OAEs.

Why include references to old articles about ABR in a new book about OAEs? This historical perspective of ABR in newborn hearing screening is highly relevant to the discussion of OAEs. To quote former United States Supreme Court Associate Justice Oliver Wendell Holmes, Jr. (1841–1935): *"Upon this point a page of history is worth a volume of logic"* (*Bartlett's Familiar Quotations*, 1980, p. 645). We can minimize the learning curve and substantially enhance the test performance of newborn hearing screening with OAEs by taking to heart the lessons learned from the accumulated experiences with ABR screening.

Rationale for Newborn Hearing Screening

The latest reincarnation of the Joint Committee on Infant Hearing publishes in the year 2000 its influential position statement in audiology, otolaryngology, and pediatrics bulletins and journals.

If this were a novel—perhaps a who-done-it mystery, a shoot-'em-up cops-and-robbers tale, or a power-hungry, lawyers-in-love, cliff-hanger —rather than an ordinary textbook, the reader would be kept in suspense until the story finally unfolded and the plot resolved in the closing pages. Because this exciting book is all about OAEs, however, it is appropriate to get right to the main point. In much of the United States, universal newborn hearing screening (UNHS) is now either a reality, or about to be implemented. Concerted multinational efforts to implement universal hearing screening are also underway in a variety of other countries, particularly in Europe. Within recent years, universal neonatal hearing screening (UNHS), or at least early detection of hearing impairment, in infants was recommended by an NIH-appointed panel (NIH, 1993), and endorsed by the Joint Committee on Infant Hearing (1994) and the American Academy of Pediatrics (Task Force on Newborn and Infant Hearing, 1999). A European Consensus Statement recommending universal neonatal hearing screening was approved in May 1998. The clinical and policy debate is no longer concerned with conceptual questions on the appropriateness of UNHS. Instead, the emphasis is now on other more practical questions, such as: How should we screen all babies for hearing impairment? Do we have a system in place for tracking those who fail the screening? Are there enough audiologists in the right locations with clinical experience in the diagnosis of pediatric hearing impairment and amplification of very young children? And, of course, Is third-party health insurance coverage available for well baby screening, and subsequent diagnosis and intervention for hearing impairment?

For a variety of reasons, as summarized in Table 8–2 and articulated clearly by some prominent persons in the audiology community (Northern & Hayes, 1994; White & Maxon, 1995; Jerger, 1997; Northern, 1998) and feature articles (e.g., Nemes, 1998), the time for universal newborn hearing screening has come. The support for hearing screening of all babies within the first few months after birth is not, however, universal. Less than 1 year after the NIH-sponsored Consensus Conference on the Early Identification and Intervention for Hearing Loss in Children, Fred Bess (an audiologist) and Jack Paradise

Table 8–2. Fact sheet on universal newborn hearing screening (UNHS).

- The prevalence of congenital, bilateral, permanent, and communicatively important hearing loss occurs in 3/1000 live births (0.3%).
- The prevalence of any degree of childhood hearing loss (exceeding 15 dB HL) in a school-aged population is 4.5%.
- Failure rates for newborn hearing screening with automated ABR range from 0.9% (bilateral) to 4% (either or both ears), whereas OAE screening failure rates range from approximately 6% upward.
- The likelihood of parental anxiety regarding newborn hearing screening is very small, and not statististically significant.
- Without newborn hearing screening, the average age that a hearing-impaired child receives intervention is approximately 2 years.
- The cost of newborn hearing screening is less than $25 per infant.
- When hearing is screened at birth and appropriate intervention occurs within 6 months, language development is normal.
- The time for universal hearing screening has come.

(a pediatrician) published an essay in the widely read journal *Pediatrics* entitled "Universal Screening for Infant Hearing Impairment: Not Simple, Not Risk-free, Not Necessarily Beneficial and Not Presently Justified" (Bess & Paradise, 1994). From the title of the paper, the authors' position on UNHS is obvious. It is beyond the scope of this discussion to itemize the concerns raised by Bess and Paradise. Their paper generated an immediate and emotional response, as evidenced by numerous letters to the editor of *Pediatrics* from audiologists, parents, an occasional pediatrician, and even a lawyer, as well as editorials addressing the Bess and Paradise (1994) assertions point by point, and stating the case for UNHS (e.g., Northern & Hayes, 1994; White & Maxon, 1995). Without doubt, the Bess and Paradise (1994) essay served as a catalyst for some carefully conducted investigations of the test performance, cost, and feasibility of well baby screening, and the benefit of early intervention, which together have provided ample data in support of universal newborn hearing screening. These studies will be noted throughout the remainder of the discussion of newborn hearing screening with OAEs. To complete the story, even as the implementation of UNHS is taking place throughout the Unites States and Europe, Bess and Paradise remain steadfast in their plea to refrain (Paradise, 1999; Bess, personal communication, 1999).

The importance of hearing integrity in the first 3 to 4 years after birth for normal aquisition of speech and language has long been appreciated (e.g., Lenneberg et al., 1967). During this sensitive (often called "critical") period, speech and language will almost always develop rapidly, and normally, if the auditory and language regions of the brain are adequately stimulated by sound and, especially, the sounds of communication. Most of us did not need to be formally taught speech or language. Unfortunately, by the time hearing loss in infancy and early childhood is suspected, audiologically evaluated, and appropriately managed, two or more of these communicatively important years have elapsed, and the child has lost an enormous developmental advantage. Clinical experience, and longstanding clinical research (Stein et al., 1990; Stein, Clark, & Kraus, 1983; Harrison & Roush, 1996) have shown repeatedly that, without systematic newborn screening, the average age of identification of hearing loss is often 2 years, or older (Table 8–3). Selected findings from a recent comprehensive study are displayed in Table 8–4. Delays between parental suspicion and each step of the assessment and management process differed for children with known risk factors for hearing impairment versus those

Table 8–3. Useful quotes on the effect of hearing impairment on communication development.

■ "Reduced hearing acuity during infancy and early childhood interferes with the development of speech and verbal language skills. Although less well documented, significantly reduced auditory input also adversely affects the developing auditory nervous system and can have harmful effects on social, emotional, cognitive, and academic development, as well as on a person's vocational and economic potential."

■ "The most important period for language and speech development is generally regarded as the first 3 years of life . . . The average age of identification in the United States remains close to 3 years. The result is that for many hearing-impaired infants and young children, much of the crucial period for language and speech learning is lost."

■ "There is general agreement that hearing impairment should be recognized as early in life as possible, so the remediation process can take full advantage of the plasticity of the developing sensory system and so that the child can enjoy normal social development."

Source: National Institutes of Health Consensus Statement on "Early Identification of Hearing Impairment in Infants and Young Children," March 1–3, 1993.

Table 8–4. Average ages in months for suspicion, diagnosis, hearing aid fitting, and intervention of hearing impaired children with and without known risk factors.

Hearing Loss	*Suspicion*	*Diagnosis*	*Hearing Aid Fitting*	*Intervention*
No Known Risk Factor				
Mild-to-moderate hearing loss (*N* = 42)	15	22	28	28
Severe-to-profound hearing loss (*N* = 118)	8	13	16	16
Known Risk Factor				
Mild-to-moderate hearing loss (*N* = 39)	8	12	22	18
Severe-to-profound hearing loss (*N* = 132)	7	12	15	16

Source: Harrison M, Roush J. *Ear and Hearing 17*:55–62, 1996.

without risk factors. When Harrison and Roush (1996) questioned responders about the reasons for the delays, explanations included: (1) third-party payment factors or determination of eligibility, (2) the health of the child (e.g., otitis media), (3) more audiologic assessment was recommended, and (4) delays associated with either getting hearing aids or the fitting of amplification. Harrison and Roush (1996) provided an excellent review of previous work on the age of identification and intervention for childhood hearing impairment.

One of the more interesting papers supporting this common observation described responses to a questionnaire completed by families of 49 hearing-impaired children (Thompson & Thompson, 1991). For 48 of these children, the parents (not their pediatrician or family doctor) first supected a hearing loss (at an average age of 10.5 months). Earlier authors reported later ages of suspicion, ranging from an average of 12 (Luterman & Chasin, 1970) to 28 months (Williams & Darbyshire, 1982). For the only other child, the pediatrican suspected a hearing loss at age 33 months! Following the parent's first expression of suspicion to the physician, approximately 9 to 10 months slipped by before hearing loss was confirmed. Intervention (e.g., amplification) was then further delayed for a variety of reasons. As noted by Thompson and Thompson (1991): "Ironically, parents find their first contact physician to be a major obstacle to adequate medical care for their child" (p. 79). Sadly, parents who express suspicion are uniformly given inappropriate advice by the child's physician, such as "wait and see, don't worry, he or she will grow out of it," which, quite understandably, leads to parental frustration, stress, and even guilt that they (the parents) did not do more to facilitate prompt intervention. Consensus on the crucial impact of early auditory experience on language development has now been reached and unequivocally articulated (e.g., NIH, 1993). Screening the hearing of all infants within the first 3 months after birth, with equally prompt and appropriate intervention, is the only way to ensure that all children receive a rich and adequate auditory experience.

Parent/caregiver concern about a child's hearing should be the number one reason for prompt audiologic assessment. A child is never too young for a hearing test because they just "won't grow out" of a hearing loss.

Is the outcome of children with congenital hearing loss improved if intervention is initiated in infancy versus later in their children? This question, raised by Bess and Paradise (1994), is fundamental to the rationale for universal newborn hearing screening. Although untold numbers of clinical audiologists, young and old, would readily reply "yes" based on their experiences with individual patients, the published evidence in support of intervention within 6 months after birth was, until recently, anecdotal or limited to a modest number of case studies (e.g., Robinshaw, 1995). Formal studies of the benefits of intervention, often not published in peer-reviewed journals, tended to focus on hearing-impaired children aged 1 year and older. Christy Yoshinaga-Itano and colleagues at the University of Colorado are conducting the definitive investigation of the benefits of early intervention on language abilities of children with hearing impairment (Yoshinaga-Itano et al., 1998). The findings of this very thorough and detailed study (at least through 1998), are summarized in Table 8–5. In addition, one small portion of the data, relating language benefit of early intervention and degree of hearing loss, is illustrated in Figure 8–2. The reader with an interest in newborn hearing screening is strongly encouraged to review the entire landmark article (available from Dr. Christine Yoshinaga-Itano at the Department of Speech, Language,

Table 8–5. Selected features and findings of a study of the language benefits of early intervention (within 6 months after birth) by Yoshinaga-Itano and colleagues at the University of Colorado.

Methodology

■ Subjects were 150 hearing-impaired children (72 of whose hearing losses were identified between birth and 6 months and 78 identified later).

■ Intervention included amplification and ongoing individualized family-oriented communication/language intervention strategies implemented within 2 months after identification.

■ Demographic characteristics for subjects in the early and later identified groups were carefully documented, including:

  ✔ Gender

  ✔ Ethnicity

  ✔ Mother's education

  ✔ Medicaid status

  ✔ Degree of hearing loss (all subjects had congenital, bilateral, sensorineural hearing loss)

  ✔ Mode of communication (oral only or oral and sign language)

  ✔ Multiple handicaps

  ✔ Cognitive ability (quantified with a cognitive quotient)

  ✔ Age at data collection (between 13 and 36 months).

■ Children underwent a comprehensive developmental evaluation (Minnesota Child Development Inventory, or MCDI), which included standardized scales for expressive (54 items) and comprehension-conceptual (67 items) language function. Language status was summarized by a composite language quotient (LQ).

Findings and Conclusions

■ Children with hearing loss, who were identified by 6 months after birth, showed significantly better expressive and receptive language skills (higher LQs) than later identified children.

■ The effect of age of identification was found across all of the demographic variables (noted above).

■ The benefits of early identification were found for all degrees of hearing impairment, from mild to profound (see Figure 8–2).

■ There was no significant difference in language performance among four groups of later identified subjects (from 7 to 25 months of age). That is, the benefits of early identification occur only before 6 months (early intervention <6 months).

■ For children with hearing impairment, the first 6 months after birth are very important, even critical. For children with congenital hearing impairment of any degree, language can develop on a normal schedule if intervention is begun by 6 months.

Source: Yoshinaga-Itano C, Sedey AL, Coulter DK, Mehl AL. Language of early- and later-identified children with hearing loss. *Pediatrics 102*(5): 1161–1171, 1998.

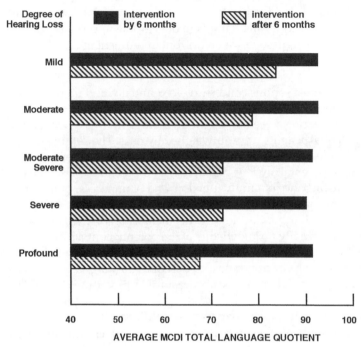

Figure 8–2. Language outcome for hearing impaired children identified at birth with early intervention (before 6 months) versus children with intervention after 6 months. (Adapted from Yoshinaga-Itano et al., 1998).

and Hearing Sciences, University of Colorado-Boulder, CDSS Building, Campus Box 409, Boulder, Colorado 80309).

Related to the communicative benefits of early intervention, and perhaps more compelling when presented to administrators, legislators, and business types, is the economic impact of hearing impairment. Costs associated specifically with the hearing screening of newborn infants, and with entire hearing screening programs (including secondary screenings and follow-up diagnostic assessments) are discussed later. The issue here is the overall financial drain or liability of late identified hearing loss on the individual, the community, the state he or she resides in, and the country. Calculation, or estimation of these statistics must include a wide variety of factors, ranging from the cost of education (perhaps at a residential school for the deaf and hard-of-hearing) and ancillary personnel required for education or everyday communication (e.g., interpreters) to the inevitable increase in unemployment and decrease in wage-earning ability. The economic impact of congenital, severe, late-identified hearing loss has been estimated at $2.5 billion annually (Downs, 1994). This statistic, coupled with the finding that early identification and intervention (by 6 months after birth) can lead to normal language development, provides practical and powerful arguments for an upfront investment in universal newborn hearing screening.

One of the most serious concerns voiced initially, and then reiterated, by Bess and Paradise (Bess & Paradise, 1994; Paradise, 1999) was that universal hearing screening might do more harm than good, and that any potential benefits were outweighed by risks. The authors referred, for example, to "the human and probably more consequential costs of attendant parental anxiety, distraction, and potential misunderstanding, or disturbance of family function, and of unnecessary or harmful procedures or treatments carried out on children" (Bess & Paradise, 1994, p. 332). Further developing this theme, Paradise (1999) claimed, "We have virtually no knowledge of the potential impact of false-positive identifications on either subsequent parent-child relationships, the performance of unnecessary subsequent testing, or the carrying out of inappropriate therapeutic measures or procedures" (p. 671).

Based on the landmark paper by Christy Yoshinaga-Itano, the definition of "early identification" of hearing loss is before a child is 6 months old.

Among the thousands of papers at scientific meetings and articles in peer-reviewed journals reporting accumulated clinical experience with ABR screening and diagnostic assessments of millions of babies during the past quarter of a century, and more recently similar applications of OAEs, documentation of risk or damage to patients is conspicuously lacking. But what about concerns of parental anxiety secondary to hearing screening failures? This concern is not prompted by anecdotal or data-based reports suggesting a substantial and common link between hearing screening and parental anxiety. There are none. Rather, it is based on literature, dating back to at least the 1960s and the early efforts in New York City to screen for a serious metabolic disorder, phenylketonuria or "PKU" (Rothenberg & Sills, 1968). Immediately following the enaction of PKU screening legislation, failure rates were at the rate of 1 in 10 or 11 tests, even though at that time the estimated incidence of the disorder was only 1 in every 10,000 to 25,000 births. Letters sent to parents of babies failing the PKU screening generated anxiety and, understandably, much consternation on the part of the physicians caring for the babies. At Bronx Municipal Hospital Center, the term "PKU Anxiety Syndrome" was coined for those parents "suffering from . . . acute and chronic anxiety ranging in degree from mild, periodic bouts to acute anxiety hysteria" (Rothenberg & Sills, 1968, p. 691). This pattern was also reported in the early 1980s when screening was introduced in Sweden for PKU and congenital hypothyroidism (e.g., Fyro & Larsson, 1982; Fyro & Bodegard, 1987, 1988) and described by various authors for these disorders and others, among them cystic fibrosis (e.g., Sorenson et al., 1984; Tluczek et al., 1992). This time period also saw increased formal study of the attachment or bonding of mother to baby, the negative effects of acute illness of mother or baby, and of mother/baby separation, on this relationship, and the increased vulnerability of new parents to stress.

There is a clear and major distinction between the reported experience with screening for such metabolic disorders versus hearing screening. Hearing loss, while very important, is not potentially fatal or even life-shortening. Whether the information gleaned from this extensive literature on the impact of screening failures for metabolic disorders can or should be generalized to screening for hearing impairment is therefore open to serious question. Nonetheless, close review of the early literature on metabolic screening provides some worthwhile guidelines for interacting with parents whose children have undergone hearing screening. For example, Rothenberg and Sills (1968) commented that,

> We have attempted to outline a practical and immediate approach to the prevention and management of psychiatric complications. Two major steps have been initiated: first, a pediatric resident tells every mother, after she has been with her baby and just before she leaves the hospital, that the PKU Screening Test has been done on her baby and that a number of false positive reactions has been appearing; secondly, an intensive follow-up program has been started which . . . provide opportunities for the parents whose babies have false positive tests to ventilate their feelings and receive support and reassurance until their anxiety has been properly controlled. (p. 692)

Clemens and Neumann (1989) noted, with regard to hypothyroid screening failures,

> We inform the parents of the predictive value of the result of their infant. In our experience, the families—as well as the family doctors—gratefully accept this statistical knowledge, because these data enable them to handle the information more rationally. (p. 447)

Similar precautions and policies, adapted for hearing screening, would be very useful in reducing any possible, even transient, parental concerns about hearing screening refer outcomes. Even the Swedish authors of papers describing some of the more serious concerns about false positive outcomes in metabolic screening subsequently pointed out that

> Families with persistent 6 to 12 month anxiety probably belong to the segment of the population with a habitual maladjustment which makes them more susceptible to stresses of life . . . There is no simple or causal link between the screening experience, the lasting distress noted at 6 to 12 months and the unsatisfactory integration at the 4-year follow-up. (Fyro & Bodegard, 1997, p. 112)

A prolific British author on newborn hearing screening, with ABR and OAEs, recently turned his attention to the issue of parental anxiety. Peter Watkin and colleagues in London conducted a formal investigation of maternal anxiety among 288 mothers whose babies underwent a TEOAE screening before hospital discharge (Watkin et al.,1998). The motivation for their study was, in part, recent British publications describing possible parental anxiety and psychological effects following screening for chromosome abnormalities and genetic disorders, such as Down syndrome. All 288 mothers were given an abbreviated version of the Spielberger's State-Trait Anxiety Inventory following an initial TEOAE screening in the maternity unit, and again 9 months later. Among the group, 27% of the babies failed the screening for one ear and 17% failed for both ears. Six weeks later, 95 babies returned for a retest, including all of the 49 failures. The study also included a control group of 102 mothers, comparable on sociodemographic parameters, who were given the anxiety inventory but whose babies did not undergo hearing screening. The paper includes a detailed description, and discussion, of the results. Briefly, 97% of the mothers viewed the screening as worthwhile initially. Although 15% of the mothers reported that the screening caused some anxiety (they were not dissatisfied with the screening), less than 1% were very worried. Notably, the formal anxiety inventory revealed no significant difference between the screening retest group and the control group whose babies had not been screened. The authors offer a number of practical suggestions or "proactive measures" to minimizing anxiety associated with hearing screening. For example, mothers' worry about their babies being taken away from them for the screening during the first day or two after birth can usually be minimized by performing the screening in the mother's hospital room. In addition, with any universal hearing screening program, professionals should be prepared to respond appropriately to the very small subgroup of mothers who are more vulnerable to anxiety than the general population. Finally, the authors recognized that "Maintaining positive attitudes . . . requires a difficult balancing act, which enables the parents to appreciate the importance of the screen [which is useful to encourage compliance with follow-up visits] in a way that does not undermine their own views and cause anxiety" (Watkin et al., 1998, p. 35).

With an appropriately professional approach, newborn hearing screening is not associated with undue or long-term parental anxiety.

Risk Factors Versus Universal Infant Hearing Screening

Factors contibuting to the movement toward universal hearing screening were noted earlier. Prominent among them is the recognition that at least 50% of children with confirmed hearing impairment, were healthy at birth, with no physical characteristics, health problems, or history suggesting risk for any type of hearing problem. This point is readily apparent in Table 8–6. The use of risk indicators to determine

Table 8–6. Estimated number of infants with hearing loss in the at-risk versus healthy populations born in the United States each year.

Category	Number Born Annually	Prevalence	Total Hearing Impaired
Healthy	3,600,000	3:1000	10,800
At-risk	400,000	30:1000	12,000
Total	4,000,000	5.7:1000	22,800

Source: Northern JL, Hayes, D. Universal screening for infant hearing impairment: Necessary, beneficial and justifiable. *Audiology Today 6:* May/June, 1994.

which children are most likely to have hearing loss is a very efficient approach for finding up to 50% of the children with hearing impairment. In the United States, the most widely used risk indicators are those defined by the Joint Committee on Infant Hearing in 1994 (Table 8–7). This listing is not exhaustive, and additional factors may also be associated with hearing impairment of infants and older children. Some American (e.g., Halpern, Hosford-Dunn, & Malachowski, 1987) and British authors, such as Adrian Davis and colleagues in England (e.g., Davis & Wood, 1992; Davis et al., 1995; Fortnum & Davis, 1997), reported the use of a simpler risk registry strategies that emphasize more generic indicators, such as length of stay in an NICU. As an aside, the British authors (Fortnum & Davis, 1997) thoroughly address, with a database drawn from tens of thousands of children born over a 9-year period, a number of important issues related to permanent childhood hearing impairment, among them prevalence rates for congenital versus acquired hearing loss and the ages of referral, hearing loss confirmation, and audiologic intervention.

Ethnicity can also be considered in determining risk in certain populations (Greville, 1996; Fortnum & Davis, 1997). Three major risk indicators—NICU history, family history, and craniofacial abnormalities—identify almost 60% of all children with permanent hearing impairment. History of an NICU stay, of course, is a handy way of identifying infants with a variety of other risk factors, including most if not all of those recommended by the JCIH in 1994. Identification of childhood hearing loss with risk factors in addition to those recommended by the JCIH are used by audiology centers in the United Kingdom and other European countries (e.g., Thiringer et al., 1984; van Rijn & Cremers, 1991; Davis et al., 1995; Sutton & Rowe, 1997). For example, Sutton and Rowe (1997) confirmed the importance of incorporating as a risk factor length of stay in the NICU (>72 hours) and found significantly higher risk of hearing impairment for babies whose mothers were over 35 years old, for babies whose families originated

Table 8–7. 1994 Joint Committee on Infant Hearing (JCIH) indicators associated with sensorineural hearing loss.

Birth Through Age 28 Days (Neonate)

■ Family history of congenital or delayed onset childhood hereditary sensorineural hearing loss.
■ Congenital infection, such as toxoplasmosis, syphilis, rubella, cytomegalovirus, and herpes.
■ Craniofacial anomalies, including abnormalities of the pinna and ear canal, absent philtrum, and low hairline.
■ Birth weight less than 1,500 grams (3.3 lbs.).
■ Hyperbilirubinemia at level requiring exchange transfusion.
■ Ototoxic medications including but not limited to the aminoglycosides (e.g., gentamicin, tobramycin, kanamycin, streptomycin) used in multiple courses or in combination with loop diuretics.
■ Bacterial meningitis.
■ Apgar scores of 0 to 4 at 1 minute or 0 to 6 at 5 minutes.
■ Mechanical ventilation lasting 5 days or longer.
■ Stigmata or other findings associated with a syndrome known to include sensorineural and/or a conductive hearing loss (e.g., Waardenburg or Usher's syndrome).

Age 29 Days Through 2 Years (Infant)

■ Parent/caregiver concern regarding hearing, speech, language, and/or developmental delay.
■ Bacterial meningitis and other infections associated with sensorineural hearing loss.
■ Head trauma associated with loss of consciousness or skull fracture.
■ Stigmata or other findings associated with a syndrome known to include sensorineural and/or a conductive hearing loss.
■ Ototoxic medications including but not limited to chemotherapeutic agents or aminoglycosides used in multiple courses or in combination with loop diuretics.
■ Recurrent or persistent otitis media with effusion for at least 3 months.

For Use With Infants (Age 29 Days Through 3 Years) Requiring Monitoring of Hearing

■ Indicators associated with delayed-onset sensorineural hearing loss:

✔ Family history of hereditary childhood hearing loss.

✔ In utero infectious (e.g., cytomegalovirus, rubella, syphilis, herpes, or toxoplasmosis).

✔ Neurofibromatosis type 11 and neurodegenerative disorders.

■ Indicators associated with conductive hearing loss:

✔ Recurrent or persistent otitis media with effusion.

✔ Anatomic deformities and other disorders that affect eustachian tube function.

✔ Neurodegenerative disorders.

Source: Joint Committee on Infant Hearing 1994 Position Statement. *Audioloqy Today 6*(6): 6–9, 1994.

from India, and who were born into lower socioeconomic status families. These authors also reported a very practical bit of information for efficient identification of childhood hearing loss. Four factors—NICU stay longer than 72 hours, craniofacial anomaly (including nonear abnormalities), family history of sensorineural hearing loss, and meningitis—were effective in the detection of 70% of all children with permanent sensorineural hearing loss.

Although the only viable option for early detection (within 6 months after birth) of all hearing loss is universal (100%) newborn hearing screening, risk indicators continue to be very important for at least three reasons. First, until universal hearing screening coverage in a country or a state, region, or district within a country is complete, and the goal of screening 100% of infants within the first 3 months after birth is met, a sizable proportion of hearing-impaired children can still be identified early and rather efficiently by use of risk factors determined by chart review in the nursery and/or the child's physician within the first month or two after birth. The use of risk factors is certainly not limited to formal patient chart review in the hospital nursery prior to discharge. Education of parents and pediatricians regarding risk factors and communicative signs of possible hearing impairment by means of brochures and other materials can contribute importantly to early identification of pediatric hearing impairment in the neonatal period and throughout childhood. Attractive, highly informative, and inexpensive brochures for parents and for professionals, in English and Spanish language versions, are available from various sources, such as the American Academy of Audiology. (Contact by telephone at 1-800-AAA-2336 or website: www.audiology.org)

Second, not all hearing loss is present at birth. Risk factors help to identify babies who might pass the initial hearing screening and later develop delayed onset or progressive hearing impairment. With any screening program—at risk or universal—follow-up screening and/or audiologic assessment, and periodic monitoring, is essential for all babies with the factors associated with progressive hearing loss (see Table 8–7).

The cochlea appears to be structurally and functionally mature at approximately 30-weeks gestational age — more than two months before term birth.

Third, risk factors may influence the strategy or technique used for newborn hearing screening. Some factors, such as ototoxicity and craniofacial anomalies, are mostly associated with peripheral (conductive and/or sensory) hearing impairment. Both OAEs and AABR are effective techniques for identification of conductive or sensory hearing impairment. Other health factors, however, unquestionably put a baby at risk for neurologic dysfunction, as well as peripheral hearing impairment. Examples of these "CNS risk factors" are meningitis, cytomegalovirus (CMV), asphyxia, hyperbilirubinemia, and head trauma. Central auditory nervous system dysfunction, which may greatly affect communication, is best detected with an ABR technique, rather than OAEs. The phenomenon now called "auditory neuropathy" is a clear example of this point. Auditory neuropathy is discussed in some detail later in this chapter.

To summarize, UNHS is now a powerful and unstoppable professional and technological movement in the United States. Legislation in support of UNHS has been enacted in almost half of the states, including the four most populous (New York, Texas, California, and Florida).

Moreover, UNHS is endorsed by three well-respected, multidisciplinary bodies with an interest in the early detection of hearing loss in children—the Joint Committee on Infant Hearing (1994), an NIH panel of experts (1993), and, most recently, the American Academy of Pediatrics (1999). The position statement of this latter group, summarized in Table 8–8, provides practical guidelines and objectives for each stage of the process of early identification of and intervention for hearing impairment in infants and young children. UNHS is also a health priority in Europe where the progressive recommendations of a Consensus Conference held in 1998 are being implemented (Table 8–9).

Auditory Development and OAEs

Prior to applying OAEs in newborn hearing screening, one must appreciate the possible influence of auditory development, particularly of middle ear and cochlear function. For example, do changes in middle ear transmission occur from prematurity through term infancy, and perhaps later? At what age are outer hair cells functionally mature? A discussion of the topic is well beyond the scope of this book. Selected developmental events are summarized in Table 8–10. Several research groups in France and the United States have contributed considerably to our understanding of auditory system development using histologic, physiologic, and psychoacoustic techniques (e.g., Lavigne-Rebillard & Pujol, 1986, 1990; Pujol, Lavigne-Rebillard, & Uziel, 1991; Werner & Rubel, 1992; Rubel, Popper, & Fay, 1998). Some of their findings are abstracted in Table 8–11. Exciting advances in the study of auditory development were reviewed recently in an excellent three-part series published in an audiology journal (Peck, 1994a, 1994b; Peck, 1995). The reader is referred also to the sizable literature on peripheral and central auditory development for in-depth information.

Here's a tip if you have access to the internet. Search the topic of interest by key words accessing the National Library of Medicine website located at: www.nlm.nih.gov/databases

Experience With OAEs in Neonatal Hearing Screening

The Early Years

Within a decade after the discovery of OAEs (Kemp, 1978), multiple research groups from around the world began to systematically evaluate clinical applications of OAEs in children, including newborn hearing screening. In Denmark, Johnsen, Elberling, and colleagues published a series of five papers describing TEOAE data collected with specially designed instrumentation in normal and impaired ears of infants, older children, and adults (e.g., Johnsen, Bagi, & Elberling, 1983; Johnsen et al., 1988). Meanwhile, Pierre Bonfils, Paul Avan, Phillipe Narcy, Alain Uziel, and French co-investigators explored the use of TEOAEs, usually recorded with the ILO 88 device, in varied patient populations. A number of their studies yielded information on

Table 8–8. Summary of the American Academy of Pediatrics Task Force on Newborn and Infant Hearing statement on Newborn and Infant Hearing Loss: Detection and Intervention.

■ "ABSTRACT. This statement endorses the implementation of universal newborn hearing screening. In addition, the statement reviews the primary objectives, important components, and recommended screening parameters that characterize an effective universal newborn hearing screening program." (p. 527)

■ Criteria to justify universal screening (for any disorder):

🗸 A test with a high sensitivity and specificity (to keep referrals to a minimum) that is easy to perform.

🗸 No other clinical parameters can be used to detect the disorder.

🗸 Early screening, diagnosis, and intervention improves outcome.

🗸 Screening programs are acceptably cost-effective.

■ Guidelines for the *screening* portion of a universal newborn hearing screening program (UNHSP):

🗸 At least 95% of newborns must be screened using a physiologic measure in both ears (the goal is 100% of the target population).

🗸 Screening must detect bilateral hearing loss ≥35 dB HL.

🗸 The false-positive rate for the screening technique (the percent of infants without hearing loss who fail the screening) should be ≤3%, and the referral rate for subsequent formal audiologic assessment should be 4% or less.

🗸 The screening technique should not miss any babies with hearing loss (a false negative rate of 0%).

🗸 OAEs and ABR, either alone or together, are acceptable screening methods, as both techniques "are noninvasive, quick (<5 minutes), and easy to perform" (p. 527).

🗸 Hospitals where babies are born should set up a UNHSP, designate a medical (physician) director, and assemble an adequate staff (the statement includes a listing of 10 detailed guidelines on the objectives and activities included in the screening program).

■ Guidelines for the *tracking and follow-up* portion of a UNHSP:

🗸 For a program to be considered effective, at least 95% of all babies with a refer screening outcome initially should undergo follow-up diagnostic audiologic assessment (the goal is 100%). The same guideline applies for those infants who are not screened in the hospital and whose parents agreed to the screening.

🗸 In agreement programs required in Part C of the Individuals with Disabilities Education Act (IDEA), state departments of health should (see article for details):
  • Develop and maintain a centralized system for monitoring hearing screening programs (in the state)
  • Track all referral and miss outcomes (see above)
  • Communicate follow-up findings to the child's parents, physicians, audiologists, and speech-language pathologists
  • Verify hearing screening of babies not born in hospitals
  • Provide reports of the screening performance for each hospital
  • Provide reports of individual UNHSPs performance to the Centers for Disease Control and Prevention (CDC) Early Detection and Intervention program.

■ Guidelines for the *identification and intervention* portion of a UNHSP:

🗸 The goal of universal screening is to identify all (100%) of infants who are born with hearing loss (see above criteria) by 3 months after birth, and to intervene appropriately by 6 months.

🗸 The child's physician should direct and coordinate care for the child with hearing impairment, with appropriate support from others.

(continued)

Table 8–8. *(continued)*

- ✔ To provide expert services to infants with hearing loss, a regionalized approach to identification and intervention is necessary.
- ✔ Training and education of additional expert care providers will be needed due to the increased demand associated with the implementation of UNHSPs.

- ■ Guidelines for the *evaluation* portion of a UNHSP:
  - ✔ Quality control should be maintained for each UNHSP by the state monitoring system.
  - ✔ This system should also evaluate regularly the tracking and follow-up components of UNHSPs.
  - ✔ In addition, state departments of health system should evaluate regularly the intervention services within UNHSPs.

Source: American Academy of Pediatrics Task Force on Newborn and Infant Hearing. Newborn and infant hearing loss: detection and intervention. *Pediatrics 103*(2): 527–529, 1999.

Table 8–9. European Consensus Statement on Newborn Hearing Screening (Milano, Italia, May 15–16, 1998).[a]

---

1. Permanent childhood hearing impairment[b] (PCHI) is a serious public health problem affecting at least one baby in one thousand. Intervention is considered to be most successful if commenced within the first few months of life. Therefore, indentification by screening at or shortly after birth has the potential to improve quality of life and opportunities for those affected.
2. Effective programs of intervention are well established.
3. Methods for identification of PCHI in the neonatal stage are now accepted clinical practice. They are effective and can be expected to identify at least 80% of cases of PCHI whilst incorrectly failing 2–3% of normally hearing babies in well-controlled programs.
4. Neonatal testing in maternity hospitals is more effective and less expensive than behavioral screening conventionally carried out at 7 to 9 months.
5. Targeting neonatal testing on only the 6 to 8% of babies at increased risk[c] of PCHI reduces costs but cannot identify more than 40 to 50% of cases. Targeted neonatal hearing screening in parallel with 7 to 9 month behavioral testing is more expensive and less effective than universal hearing screening.
6. Hearing screening in the neonatal period cannot identify acquired or progressive hearing loss occurring subsequently. Surveillance methods are required to identify those cases, which may be 10 to 20% of all PCHI.
7. Risks associated with neonatal hearing screening include anxiety from false positive results and possible delayed diagnosis from false negative results, but these risks are acceptable in view of the expected benefits.
8. Neonatal hearing screening should be considered to be the first part of a program of habilitation of hearing impaired children, including facilities for diagnosis and assessment.
9. A system of quality control is an essential component of a neonatal hearing screening program. Quality control includes training of personnel and audit of performance. The person responsible for quality control should be identified.
10. Although the healthcare systems in Europe differ from country to country in terms of organization and funding, implementation of neonatal hearing screening programs should not be delayed. This will give European citizens greater opportunities and better quality of life into the next millenium.

---

[a]Conference Chairman and Organizer: Fernando Grandori, Ph.D.; Scientific Coordinator: Mark E. Lutman, Ph.D.
[b]Defined as a bilateral permanent hearing impairment greater than or equal to 40-dB nHL, averaged over the frequencies of 500, 1000, 2000, and 4000 Hz.
[c]Examples include neonatal intensive care and family history of hearing impairment.

Table 8–10. Major steps in neonatal middle ear development which may influence measurement of OAEs.

■ Vernix casseous in external ear canal
■ Middle ear mesenchymal tissue dissipates
■ Efficiency of middle ear transmission improves
■ Areal ratio of tympanic membrane to stapes footplate increases
■ Tympanic membrane curvature increases (more efficient)
■ Tympanic membrane thickness decreases
■ Lever function of ossicles improves

Table 8–11. Summary of major steps in human cochlear development. The literature on development of the auditory system and it's relation to OAEs is reviewed in the text of this chapter.

Developmental Event	Time of Emergence (Weeks After Conception)
■ Hair cell differentiation	?
■ Afferent eighth nerve fibers in cochlear epithelium	10
■ Inner hair cells histologically distinguished	10 to 12
■ Outer hair cells histologically distinguished	12+
■ Synapses between hair cells and afferent eighth nerve fibers	11 to 12
■ Development of stereocilia on inner hair cells	12
■ Development of stereocilia on outer hair cells	12+
■ Efferent eighth nerve fiber endings below inner hair cells	14
■ Maturation of inner hair cell–eighth nerve synapse	15
■ Onset of hearing function by structural criteria	20
■ Efferent synapses with outer hair cells	22
■ Maturation of outer hair cell–eighth nerve synapse	22
■ Stereocilia maturation (inner and outer hair cells)	22
■ Outer hair cells and related structures appear mature	30
■ Normal (mature) auditory sensitivity and frequency resolution	?

Source: Adapted from Pujol R, Lavigne-Rebillard M. Development of neurosensory structures in the human cochlea. *Acta Otolaryngologica (Stockh) 112:* 259–264, 1992.

OAE hearing screening of term and, later, preterm infants (e.g., Bonfils, Uziel, & Pujol, 1988; Bonfils et al., 1990; Bonfils et al., 1992; Uziel & Piron, 1991). Not unexpectedly, as OAEs were first reported by an Englishman (Kemp, 1978), British audiologists and hearing scientists almost immediately exploited OAEs in newborn hearing screening, sometimes using the newly developed Programmable Otoacoustic Measurement System (POEMS) device for TEOAEs instead of the ILO 88 (e.g., Stevens et al., 1987; Stevens et al., 1989; Stephens et al., 1990; Kennedy et al., 1991; Webb & Stevens, 1991). The British research designs often permitted comparison of the effectiveness of OAEs versus ABR in well baby and at-risk infant screening. Additionally, in the late 1980s and continuing into the 1990s, the international effort to study OAEs in newborn hearing screening, and other pediatric applications, included contributions from Germany (Pinkert, Arold, & Zenner, 1990; Zwicker & Schorn, 1990; Lamprecht, 1991; Uppenkamp et al., 1992), Italy (e.g., Molini et al., 1991), Belgium (e.g, Decreton et al., 1991; Dohlen et al., 1991), The Netherlands (Kok et al., 1992), Spain (e.g., Canet et al., 1992) Japan (Satoh, 1992), and Singapore (Ng & Yun, 1992).

The early European research initiative was limited mostly to TEOAEs. However, during this time period in the United States of America, studies of the application of DPOAEs (e.g., Lonsbury-Martin & Martin, 1990; Lafreniere et al., 1991; Norton, 1993; Smurzynski et al., 1993) as well as TEOAEs (e.g., White et al., 1992; Norton, 1993; White et al., 1993) in newborn hearing screening were published or presented at the pacesetting International Symposium on Otoacoustic Emissions held in Kansas City, Missouri in May of 1991 or other professional meetings.

"What's past is prologue."
William Shakespeare
(1564–1616), **The Tempest,**
Act II

As noted in the outset of this chapter, statistical data on screening test performance outcome with OAEs in newborn hearing screening reported prior to about 1990 are rather outdated due to major shifts in test protocols and advances in technology, particularly the advent of commercially available automated OAE devices. This is not to say that the accumulated clinical experience with OAE screening is worthless. To the contrary, lessons about how to record OAEs from babies and equipment advances—improved technique and technology—have had a significant impact on the effectiveness, speed, and accuracy of newborn hearing screening with OAEs as reflected, in part, by the progressively lower OAE screening failure rates. The following brief review of selected recent published papers distills experiences with newborn OAE screening in the hospital nursery with equipment designed specifically for clinical use. A more comprehensive listing of published papers on newborn hearing screening with OAEs is displayed in Table 8–12 (full citations of these papers are included in the reference list).

The valuable technical tips gleaned from the entire clinical experience with newborn hearing screening to date are noted mostly in the discussion below of troubleshooting in OAE screening. The vast accumulated clinical experience with OAEs in newborn hearing screening is, of course, grossly underestimated by considering simply the number of articles published in peer-reviewed professional journals. Newborn hearing screening programs around the world now utilize OAEs daily as a clinical procedure. Findings from these screening programs are closely analyzed for the general purpose of early identification of hearing impairment. For most hospital-based programs, however, the screening data are not presented at professional meetings nor pub-

Table 8–12. Studies of newborn hearing screening in the nursery setting with OAE techniques (arranged chronologically).

Author(s), (Year)	Type of OAEs	Number of Subjects (Ears)	OAE Device	Fail Rate	Comments
Newborn Intensive Care Unit (Intensive Care Nursery)					
Stevens et al. (1987)	TEOAE	112	Custom		Early feasibility study
Stevens et al. (1991)	TEOAE	723	Custom		Sensitivity = 93%; specificity = 84%
Bonfils et al. (1992)	SOAE TEOAE	67 (134)	ILO 88		Maturation of OAE by 32 weeks GA
Chase & Hall, (1993)	DPOAE	40	GSI 60	NA	Various test protocols assessed
Maxon et al. (1993)	TEOAE	304 (NICU)	ILO 88 device	27%	Early study with large sample
Smurzynski et al. (1993)	DPOAE TEOAE	61 (118) 65 (65)	Custom (Ariel)		Test performance versus ABR
Jacobson & Jacobson (1994)	TEOAE	67	ILO 88		High false-failure rate in ICN vs. ABR
Hall et al. (1994)	TEOAE DPOAE	20 (40) 20 (40)	ILO 88 GSI 60		Evaluation of protocols;TEOAE vs. DPOAE failures
Bergman et al. (1995)	TEOAE DPOAE	51 51	ILO 88 ER CUBDIS		Test performance vs. older children and adults
Sutton et al. (1996)	TEOAE	100	POEMs		Included tympanometry
Ochi et al. (1998)	DPOAE	36 (67)	Bio-Logic		
Gill et al. (1998)	TEOAE	144	ILO 88		84% pass rate of 66% on initial screen
Hess et al. (1998)	TEOAE	942	ILO 88		Test performance vs. ABR and long-term follow-up
Wood et al. (1998)	TEOAE	862	POEMS device		With ABR; auditory neuropathy
Apostolopoulos et al. (1999)	TEOAE	223 (438)	ILO 88		Test performance vs. ABR and long-term follow-up
Well Baby Nursery					
Stevens et al. (1987)	TEOAE	30	Custom		OAE and ABR are practical screening measures
Lafreniere et al. (1991)	TEOAE DPOAE	23 (35)	Custom		Feasibility of DPOAE hearing screening

(continued)

Table 8–12. *(continued)*

Author(s), (Year)	Type of OAEs	Number of Subjects (Ears)	OAE Device	Fail Rate	Comments
Well Baby Nursery *(continued)*					
Kok et al. (1992)	TEOAE	15 (20)	ILO 88 device		Longitudinal study Day 1 to Day 4
Kok et al. (1993)	TEOAE	1036	ILO 88 device		Prevalence in first few days after birth
Maxon et al. (1993)	TEOAE	1546	ILO 88 device		Early study with large sample but high initial factors influencing screening outcome
Salomon et al.(1993)	TEOAE	304 (545)	Custom		
Jacobson & Jacobson (1994)	TEOAE	52	ILO 88		96.2% pass rate for ABR vs. 52.2% for TEOAE
Hall et al. (1994)	DPOAE	20 (40)	Virtual 330		Failure rate in WBN vs. pediatric clinic weeks later
Maxon et al. (1995)	TEOAE	4253	ILO 88		First stage failure rate of 7%
Dirckx et al. (1996)	TEOAE	Survey of practices	ILO 88 and POEMS		Data for 25 teams (22,356 babies)
Sheppard et al. (1996)	DPOAE	77	Custom		High failure and over-referral rates
Sutton et al. (1996)	TEOAE	100	POEMS device		OAE findings compared with tym-panometry
Welch et al. (1996)	TEOAE	226 (351)	ILO 88		Practical problems and issues addressed
Doyle et al. (1997)	TEOAE	200 (400)	ILO 88		Failure rates vs. ABR and time of screening
McNellis and Klein (1997)	TEOAE	50	ILO 88		High false-failure rate in ICN vs. ABR
Bantock and Croxson (1998)	TEOAE	240	ILO 88		Test performance vs. ABR
Rasmussen et al. (1998)	TEOAE	129	Custom device		Maximum length sequence technique
Salata et al. (1998)	DPOAE	104 (208)	GSI 60		Analysis of various pass/fail criteria
Slaven and Thornton (1998)	TEOAE	270 (514)	POEMS device		Maximum length sequence technique

NA = not applicable; POEMS = Programmable Otoacoustic Emission Measurement System; ILO 88 = Otodynamics Ltd.; ER = Etymotic Research; GSI 60 = Grason Stadler Incorporated.

lished in the scientific literature. A perusal of the abstracts for papers or posters presented at audiology conventions and conferences on early identification of hearing impairment in children will reveal hundreds of unpublished studies of newborn hearing screening with OAEs. To cite just two examples, each year the program for the Convention of the American Academy of Audiology includes numerous papers reporting the results of newborn hearing screening with OAEs. At the European Neonatal Hearing Screening Conference held in Milan in 1998, there were 23 papers on newborn hearing screening with DPOAEs or TEOAEs. Presumably, the more modest published data are representative of the sizable unpublished clinical experience.

At least four recurring themes can be found in the literature on newborn hearing screening with OAEs (1) time of testing, (2) effects of noise, (3) tester experience, and (4) test protocol design.

Time of Testing. First, within the first week after birth, failure rate, on the average, decreases as a function of the time (number of days) when the screening is performed. Indeed, infant age after birth is a major factor in the outcome of OAE screening. OAE failure rate is highest in the first 24 hours after birth, and then decreases markedly over the next 3 to 4 days (Kok et al., 1993; Welch et al., 1996; Levi et al., 1997). The sensitivity of OAE to cochlear (outer hair cell) auditory dysfunction is well-documented and not in question. Less assured is OAE screening specificity—its ability to correctly identify infants with normal hearing sensitivity. That is, in the well baby population, most OAE screening failures are considered "false-positive" outcomes, because the prevalence of hearing loss is about 3 per 1000. The higher the failure rate, the lower OAE screening specificity. There is ample evidence that the test performance of newborn hearing screening with OAEs can meet even stringent requirements for sensitivity (close to 100%) and specificity (greater than 95%) if testing is performed when the baby is at least 3 to 4 days old. In some regions of Europe, this schedule for hospital discharge is typical, and screening can be delayed for several days without negative consequences. However, in recent years, particularly in the United States, the age of hospital discharge for well babies has decreased to less than 48 hours, and sometimes to within 18 to 24 hours after birth. OAEs can certainly be recorded from some infants within hours after birth. Unfortunately, when data are compiled for large groups of infants, failure rates for OAE screening within the first 24 hours after birth are unacceptably high. For example, Levi et al. (1997) reported that TEOAEs were not observed (OAE amplitude did not exceed 3 dB for at least one octave frequency band) in both ears for 32.5% of 65 full-term infants. A pass outcome requires the presence of TEOAEs bilaterally. In a group of 1,036 infant ears and with TEOAE data "visually scored," Dutch researchers Kok et al. (1993) reported absence of a clear TEOAE for 22% of the ears within the initial 36 hours, whereas only 1% continued to show no response at 108 hours (4.5

Whenever feasible, hearing screening of healthy neonates should be delayed until hours before discharge from the nursery. During the first four days after birth, failure rates for OAE screening generally decrease with the passage of time.

days) or more after birth. This excellent paper illustrates the difficulties encountered when attempting to apply the results of relatively early studies to current clinical practice. TEOAE presence (e.g., a pass) was defined subjectively (visually) by reproducibility and response-to-noise strength. Although TEOAE features, such as "echo" levels, reproducibility values, and background noise, were quantified by the authors, the actual determination of response presence or absence remained highly subjective and impossible to re-create precisely by other investigators. In automated TEOAE and DPOAE devices such criteria are highly quantified and can easily be held constant among testers. Nonetheless, the authors' conclusion that, "the prevalence of EOAEs in healthy newborn ears is age related" (Kok et al., 1993, p. 223) is unquestionably valid and has subsequently been repeatedly supported by clinical experience and published reports (e.g., Elberling et al., 1985; White et al., 1993; Welch et al., 1996). It has been appreciated for years that vernix in the external ear canal is the major contributor to the higher failure rate soon after birth (Chang et al., 1993; Thornton et al., 1993; Vohr et al. 1993; McNellis & Klein, 1997). The influence of vernix and other normal anatomic factors in OAE screening outcome is reviewed in Chapter 5. Finally, in contrast to the importance of test time after birth for screening with OAEs, it is not a major factor in automated ABR screening, particularly when the stimulus is delivered via a supra-aural (versus insert) ear coupler design (e.g., Doyle et al., 1997; Hall et al., 1998).

Noise levels in nurseries, which often exceed 60 dB SPL, can exert an important influence on OAE screening technique and outcome.

Effects of Noise. The effects of noise on OAE measurement play an important role in the success and outcome of newborn hearing screening, especially in the nursery setting (e.g., Bergman et al., 1995; Sheppard et al., 1996; Welch et al., 1996; Salata et al., 1997; Ochi et al., 1998). As discussed in detail in Chapter 4, measurement noise can profoundly affect OAEs due to the very nature of the technique. Any OAE is, by definition, detected as a low-intensity sound within the ear canal. In many clinical applications of OAEs, unwanted noise in the ear canal—ambient environmental, and physiologic—can be minimized by patient instruction, by manipulating the test environment, or even conducting the OAE recording in a sound-treated room. These steps are not possible for hearing screening of newborn infants with OAEs in the nursery setting. Noise levels in the nursery setting, especially the NICU, are notoriously high, often averaging 60 dB SPL and occasionally exceeding 100 dB SPL (Philbin et al., 1998). The deleterious influence of noise on OAE screening, and characteristics of the noise, are illustrated in Figure 8–3. Although noise can fill the entire OAEs spectrum (from 500 to 8000 Hz), it predominates for frequencies below 2000 Hz. In fact, clinical experience in many test settings, including the nursery, confirms a sharp decline in noise levels in the ear canal from about 1500 to 2000 Hz, as seen in Figure 8–3. In the NICU or intermediate care unit, average noise levels can exceed 65 dB SPL (Hall, 1992), confounding bedside measurement of OAEs. The top portion of Fig-

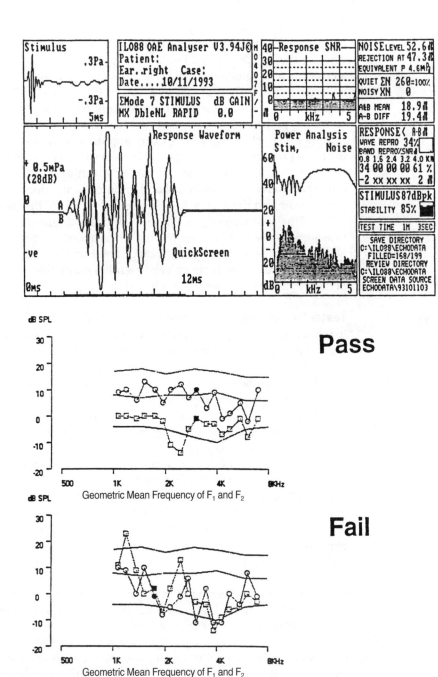

Figure 8–3. In the top portion is an example of TEOAEs recorded with the ILO 88 device from an infant in the NICU . Note the high level of background noise (*shaded area*), especially in the low-frequency region, and the noise level (*upper right box*) exceeding the rejection limit. DPOAE data recorded in two DPgrams with the GSI 60 device from an infant in the NICU is shown in the lower portion. The top DPgram is consistent with a Pass outcome, whereas the lower DPgram is clearly a Fail outcome. Again, noise (□) is most evident for the frequency region below 2000 Hz.

ure 8–3 shows excessive measurement noise (exceeding the rejection limit for the ILO 88 device). The lower portion of the graph illustrates a pass and a fail outcome for DPOAE measurement. These data were collected with a prototype GSI 60 device in 1993 when DPOAEs were being investigated as a screening technique by the author. DPOAE screening protocols are now modified to speed up testing and mini- mize noise effects. Fortuitously, OAE amplitude tends to be larger in the higher frequency regions, probably for a variety of reasons. In any event, the conclusion is apparent. Hearing screening with OAEs can be remarkably enhanced without hampering clinical value by limiting the recording to the higher frequencies. As noted by Bregman et al. (1995), "the vast majority of educationally significant sensorineural hearing loss involves at least the higher frequency region" (p. 160). Strategies for minimizing the effects of noise on OAE measurement (reviewed in Chapter 4) are all very useful in enhancing the outcome of newborn hearing screening with OAEs.

Tester Experience. Tester experience in recording OAEs from infants in the nursery setting profoundly influences newborn hearing screen- ing failure rates (e.g., Maxon et al., 1995). As noted by Karl White, "Probably the most important determinant of whether a TEOAE- based universal hearing screening program is successful is whether screeners have been appropriately trained" (White, 1996, p. 177). Just as behavioral audiometry and, to an extent, ABR assessment is more challenging clinically for infants than older children and adults, OAE recording in infants requires more technical ability and experience. Competence and comfort in performing OAE measures with coopera- tive adults does not necessarily translate to neonates. The reasons are many and varied, among them the small dimensions of the ear canals of neonates, the above-noted problems with vernix, occasionally unco- operative and restless patients, the inability to relocate patients to qui- eter environments, and the ubiquitous sources of noise that influences OAE measurement.

Experience is a critical factor in the success of a OAE newborn hearing screening program. Failure rates are invariably lower if a few testers screen many babies than if many testers screen a few babies.

Optimally, new screeners should acquire preliminary experience un- der supervision, with instruction on appropriate test modifications and troubleshooting to minimize failure-rate and test time. Then, when they have acheived predefined criteria screening adequacy, screeners can be permitted to function independently. An excellent example of the importance of tester experience is provided by the Rhode Island Hearing Assessment Program (RHAP), without doubt the single most ambitious and longstanding universal hearing screen- ing effort in the United States. Begun in the early 1990s as a demon- stration project funded by a federal grant, the RHAP is a joint project of the Women and Infants Hospital in Providence Rhode Island and the Rhode Island Department of Health, coordinated by Betty Vohr, M.D., a pediatrician. In 1998, multiple outcome facets of the RHAP over a 5-year period were thoroughly described in a paper by Dr. Vohr and colleagues. This report is highly recommended for anyone with a professional interest in newborn hearing screening. The initial referral rate for the RHAP decreased from 27% in the early years (White et al., 1993) to 8% in 1996. The overall "first" referral rate for a total of 53,121 babies (47,991 normal nursery and 5,130 NICU) was 10%. Importantly, "only 14.7% of the rescreens failed with TEOAEs when performed at 2 to 6 weeks of age, supporting the efficacy of a two-stage process for hearing screening. This process resulted in an overall 1.2% refer rate, indicating a more than acceptable audiology diagnostic refer rate for a hearing screening program" (Vohr et al., 1998, p. 356).

Test Protocols. OAE test protocols that are appropriate for successful diagnostic measurements in adults should be, and actually must be, modified to be effective in newborn hearing screening. The principles guiding the modifications, reviewed in Chapter 4, are based on accumulated experience with OAE screening. The most obvious modifications in test protocol are a reduction in the amount of OAE data recorded, especially restricting data collection to the higher frequency region (to minimize the effects of noise), and algorithms and stopping criteria which serve to minimize noise and enhance the OAE-to-noise difference, while maintaining reasonable test time. A good example of a modification that has become commonplace in TEOAE screening is the QuickScreen option on the ILO 88 device. Low-frequency filtering lessens the negative influence of noise and shortens the analysis time from 20 to 10 ms. The desired result is quicker TEOAE screening, with little or no loss of valuable data.

Some of the lessons learned from the author's early newborn hearing screening experiences with DPOAEs (Hall et al., 1994) are illustrated in Figures 8–4 and 8–5. For each figure, the stimulus frequency region (for f_1 and f_2) is shown on the horizontal axis, and DPOAE failure rate is displayed on the vertical axis. The data in Figure 8–4 were collected by Dr. Kay Rupp Bachmann from a series of 40 babies in a study of DPOAE screening in the well baby nursery (within 36 hours after birth and before discharge) versus the pediatric continuity care clinic (at 2 to 4 weeks after hospital discharge). DPOAEs were recorded with the Virtual 330 device. For all infants, there was a reliable ABR for intensity levels below 30 dB nHL (recorded with an Intelligent Hearing Systems SmartEP system). Therefore, all failures were considered false-failures, with the ABR serving as the initial reference for hearing status. Failure rates were clearly highest when frequencies in the region of 1000 to 2000 Hz were included in the analysis, reflecting the confounding effects of measurement noise. At first glance, failure rates were optimal (0%) for the high-frequency region (4000 to 8000 Hz). Close examination of data at these frequencies, however, revealed aberrant peaks in the DPgram, which probably represented artifactual energy due to equipment-related distortion (Siegel et al., 1995) and/or standing wave interference (Siegel et al., 1994) rather than

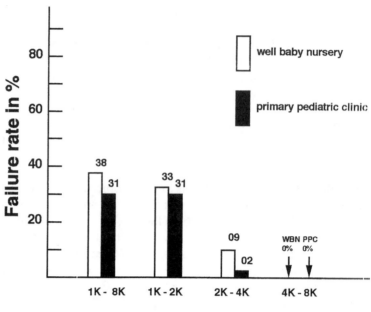

Figure 8–4. Failure rate (%) for DPOAE screening performed in the well baby nursery within 2 days after birth versus the pediatric clinic 2 to 4 weeks after birth with the same series of babies (*N* = 40). Failure rate decreased with stimulus frequency. All infants passed an ABR screening at 30 dB nHL. (Courtesy of K. Rupp Bachmann, Ph.D.)

DPOAE activity. One should be highly suspect of any DPOAE protocol that produces no screening failures, particularly if frequencies above 5000 Hz are included in the analysis. The frequency octave of 2000 to 4000 Hz seemed to offer an appealing option for DPOAE screening, as it was high enough to escape the negative influence of most measurement noise, yet low enough to minimize the likelihood of standing wave interference with calibration and DP detection. Moreover, failure rates were acceptably low for the 2000- to 4000-Hz region. One other point is readily apparent in Figure 8–4. Failure rates were consistently lower for DPOAE screenings conducted in the pediatric clinic weeks after birth versus the nursery within hours after birth. Data reported for both settings and test times were collected from the same group of infants by the same tester (KRB) with the same instrumentation.

The two main variables, therefore, were time after birth and the test environment. Noise levels in the test room (as measured with a sound level meter), and in the ear canal during screening (as documented by the DPOAE device at each test frequency), were not statistically different. The primary factor in the lower failure rate for the pediatric clinic

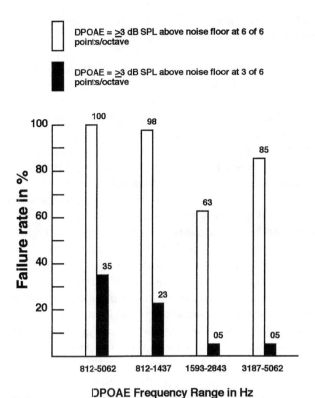

Figure 8–5. Failure rate (%) for DPOAE hearing screening performed in the newborn intensive care nursery (*N* = 40). Failure rate was excessively high for an overly rigorous analysis criteria. Failure rate also decreased with increasing stimulus frequency. All infants passed an ABR screening at 30 dB nHL. (Courtesy of Patricia A. Case, Ph.D.)

was probably time of test after birth which, in turn, eliminated the effect of vernix in the ear canal. These data have two direct implications: First, DPOAE screening is most effective for the frequency region of approximately 2000 to 4000 Hz, and perhaps slightly higher. Second, failure rates for DPOAE screening of healthy babies can be lowered rather substantially by deferring the screening until after discharge. However, because the return rate to the pediatric clinic for well baby visits is invariably less than 100%, and may be much lower, it would be more logical to attempt the OAE screening in the hospital (failure rate in this study was only 9%), and then to make every attempt to have babies with a refer outcome return for their first well baby visit for a rescreen by clinic personnel. With the introduction of hand-held, relatively inexpensive, automated OAE screening devices (see Chapters 7 and 10), this is now a viable option.

Data collected by Dr. Patricia Chase in an intermediate care nursery during a parallel study (see Figure 8–5), similarly provide some practical suggestions for newborn hearing screening with DPOAEs. Subjects were 40 infants at risk for hearing impairment according to JCIH criteria. All infants underwent an ABR assessment (Nicolet Viking II), which yielded a reliable wave V at age-corrected normal latencies for click stimuli at an intensity level of 30 dB nHL or less (Hall et al., 1994). DPOAEs were recorded with a commercially available device (GSI 60) at bedside in the nursery. Several observations can be made from these data. As in the WBN study just described, failure rates were highest when data for lower stimulus frequencies, especially frequencies below about 1500 Hz were included. Also, failure rates were highly dependent on analysis criteria. Almost all babies "failed" the screening when a clear and reliable DP at each of six stimulus frequency pairs was required for a pass outcome. This requirement is unrealistic and not supported by what we know about OAE fine structure (see Chapters 2 and 4). Occasional dips or valleys in DPgrams are anticipated, even in entirely normal ears. Altering the criteria for a "pass" outcome to a clear and reliable DP (a DP-to-noise floor difference of at least 3 dB) resulted in lower failure rates. One could argue that the 3-out-of-6 criteria was too lax, and evidence of a DP at 4- or 5-out-of-6 would be appropriate. Nonetheless, with the less rigorous analysis criterion, failure rates were acceptably low (5%) for the 1500 Hz to 5000 Hz region, and test time was typically less than 2 minutes for repeated DPgrams. In combination, these two preliminary studies, conducted with newly introduced, FDA-approved devices, confirm the feasibility of hearing screening with DPOAEs and offer some practical guidelines on appropriate test protocols for this application of DPOAEs.

Published studies of newborn hearing screening with OAEs represent only a small fraction of the many hundreds of screening programs around the world in operation every day of the year.

Test time for OAE screening is highly variable and dependent on the many factors discussed here. Under ideal conditions and with a normal-hearing infant, OAE screening may require less than 30 s per ear. On the other hand, with excessive measurement noise, a recording algorithm with a rigorous definition for response detection, a test protocol including low-frequency measurement, and/or a hearing-impaired infant, OAE screening may take a long time for a clinical procedure (e.g., more than 30 min per ear). Relatively shorter newborn hearing screening time for OAEs than for ABR is sometimes cited by authors and manufacturers (of OAE equipment) as a reason for favoring the OAE technique. Although OAE screenings do, on the average, require less time, the difference is a matter of minutes. For example, Doyle et al. (1997) reported average test times of 24 minutes for automated ABR (range: 5–90 min) and 13 minutes (range: 4–40 min) for TEOAEs. Salata et al. (1998) compared test times for AABR and DPOAEs with a series of 105 NICU infants. Including the setup time (electrode and ear coupler application for AABR or probe fitting for DPOAE), average total test time was 21 min (range: 2–60 min) for AABR and 22 min (range: 10–45 min) for DPOAE. DPOAE test times can be consistently reduced to less than 10 min, however, by simply limiting data collection to the less noisy 2000 to 5000 Hz frequency region (e.g., Hall et al., 1994; Salata et al., 1997). With technologic advances and increased tester experience, typical test times are diminishing for both AABR and OAEs, often to less than 1 min per ear. Manufacturers of automated OAE devices suggest that test times of less than 1 min can be expected for most infants. And, with one new version of an AABR device (the ALGO-2) which permits binaural stimulation simultaneously, average test times for both ears are less than 5 min in the WBN (Hall et al., 1998).

OAEs Versus ABR

Studies in which both OAEs and automated ABR screenings are performed by the same testers and with the same infants invariably confirm significantly lower failure rates for automated ABR, as performed most often with the ALGO device by Natus, Inc. (e.g., Kennedy et al., 1991; Hall et al., 1994; Hunter et al., 1994; Jacobson & Jacobson, 1994; Doyle et al., 1997; McNellis & Klein, 1997; Hess et al., 1998). The differences in pass/fail rates between the two technologies are summarized in Table 8–13. Athough the absolute values of the pass/fail rates vary among studies and are typically not as impressive as test performance for large-scale established well baby screening programs, the relative advantage for AABR remains quite consistent. The lower failure rates for AABR versus OAEs are most pronounced for screening within the first 24 hours after birth (Doyle et al., 1997; McNellis & Klein, 1997), presumably due to the lesser effect of vernix on ABR than OAE measurement. Keep in mind that vernix will affect inward propagation of the stimulus and the outward propogation of the response for OAE recordings (as reviewed in detail in Chapter 5), whereas only the stimulus delivery to the cochlea will be influenced for ABR. In addition, OAE measurement requires seating a probe within the ear canal, and possible occlusion of stimulus or microphone ports, whereas ABR transducers can be coupled outside of the external ear.

Thus, as summarized in Table 8–14, several factors interact to influence newborn hearing screening performance with OAEs. There is no simple answer to the question: What is the failure rate for OAE screening? However, newborn hearing screening performance can be confidently estimated once the multiple factors in newborn hearing screening are described. The wide variations in test performance, for example, failure rates from less than 7% to over 70%, can be adequately explained by these, and probably other, factors; and this information can be applied by clinicians to minimize failure rates and maximize test performance.

Table 8–13. Studies of newborn hearing screening with OAEs reported in literature, including selected abstracts of papers presented at scientific meetings (listed chronologically). Papers describing hearing screening outcome for a series of infants are listed, with an emphasis on more recent studies. Early studies, developmental investigations, and case reports are noted elsewhere in this chapter.

Author(s) (Year)	Type of OAEs	N (Types)[a] of Subjects	Equipment[b]	Comments
Bonfils et al. (1992)	SOAE TEOAE	67/134 ears (PT)	ILO 88	Maturation of OAEs by 32 weeks GA
Kok et al. (1992)	TEOAE	15/20 ears (FT)	ILO 88 device	Longitudinal study from Day 1 to Day 4
Chase & Hall (1993)	DPOAE	40 (at risk)	GSI 60	Various test protocols assessed
Kok et al. (1993)	TEOAE	1036 (FT)	I LO 88 device	Prevalence in first few days after birth
Maxon et al. (1993)	TEOAE	1546 (FT) 304 (NICU)	ILO 88 device	Early study with large sample but high initial failure rate (27%)
Smurzynski et al. (1993)	DPOAE TEOAE DPOAE TEOAE	61/118 ears (PT) 65/65 (PT) 30/48 ears (FT) 30/48 (FT)	Custom (Ariel)	Test performance versus ABR
Salomon et al. (1993)	TEOAE	304/545	Custom	Factors influencing screening outcome
Hall et al. (1994)	TEOAE DPOAE	20 20	ILO 88 GSI 60 & Virtual 330	Evaluation of protocols; TEOAE vs. DPOAE failures
Jacobson & Jacobson (1994)	TEOAE	52 (FT) 67 (NICU)	ILO 88	High false-failure rate in ICN vs. ABR
Bergman et al. (1995)	TEOAE DPOAE	51 (ICN)	ILO 88 ER CUBDIS	Test performance vs. older children & adults
Maxon et al. (1995)	TEOAE	4253 (FT)	ILO 88	First stage failure rate of 7%
Dirckx et al. (1996)	TEOAE	Survey of practices	ILO 88 & POEMS	Data summarized for 25 teams (22,356 babies)
Sheppard et al. (1996)	DPOAE	77	Custom	High failure and over-referral rates
Sutton et al. (1996)	TEOAE	85 (ICN) 100 (FT)	POEMS device	OAE findings compared with tympanometry
Welch et al. (1996)	TEOAE	226/351	ILO 88	Practical problems and issues addressed
Doyle et al. (1997)	TEOAE	200/400 (FT)	ILO 88	Failure rates vs. ABR and time of screening
McNellis & Klein (1997)	TEOAE	50 (FT)	ILO 88	High false-failure rate in ICN vs. ABR

Table 8–13. *(continued)*

Author(s) (Year)	Type of OAE	N (Types)[a] of Subjects	Equipment[b]	Comments
Bantock and Croxson (1998)	TEOAE	240 (FT)	ILO 88	Test performance vs. ABR
Hess et al. (1998)	TEOAE	942 (at risk)	ILO 88	Test performance vs. ABR and long-term follow-up
Ochi et al. (1998)	DPOAE	36/67 (at risk)	Bio-Logic Scout	Test performance vs. ABR
Rasmussen et al. (1998)	TEOAE	129 (FT)	Custom device	Maximum length sequence technique
Salata et al. (1998)	DPOAE	104/208	GSI 60	Analysis of various pass/fail criteria
Slaven & Thornton (1998)	TEOAE	270/514 (FT)	POEMS device	Maximum length sequence technique
Wood et al. (1998)	TEOAE	862 (at risk)	POEMS device	With ABR; auditory neuropathy
Apostolopoulos et al. (1999)	TEOAE	223/438 (at risk)	ILO 88	Test performance vs. ABR and long-term follow-up

[a]FT = full-term healthy infants usually screened in a well-baby nursery; At risk = infants with one or more risk indicators, usually screened in an intermediate or intensive care nursery (ICN); PT = preterm infants also usually screening in an ICN.
[b]POEMS = Programmable Otoacoustic Emission Measurement System; ILO 88 = Otodynamics Ltd.; ER = Etymotic Research.

TEOAEs in Newborn Screening: Test Principles and Protocols, Analysis and Interpretation

The overriding principles of TEOAE measurement in newborn hearing screening are, in their description, deceptively simple. After verifying that the neonate has recently eaten and is resting comfortably, and after turning on the screening device, entering essential patient demographic data, selecting the appropriate test protocol, and placing the correct size neonatal probe tip onto the probe assembly, the tester must snuggly fit the probe tip into the infant's ear canal, stabilize the probe and probe cord, and begin data collection. Prior to the introduction of automated OAE devices, the tester was very much involved in selecting the test protocol, verifying of the adequacy of the probe fit, determining when to stop the screening (or how long testing should continue), and then, of course, for interpretation of the OAE results. As most newborn hearing screening programs will soon utilize automated OAE devices, step-by-step descriptions of TEOAE measurement in neonates will not be provided here. They are available, for each device, from manuals or other instructional media (e.g., videotapes) supplied by the manufacturer (see also, Chapter 7). Manufacturers also usually

Table 8–14. Differential pass/fail rates for TEOAEs and DPOAEs versus automated ABR in selected studies, arranged chronologically. For each technology in these studies, screening was performed by the same testers in the same test setting with the same population of infants.

Study (Year)	Test Setting	Number of Subjects (Ears)	Device OAE[a]	Device AABR[a]	Failure Rate OAE	Failure Rate AABR
TEOAE						
Stevens et al.(1987)	NICU	(215)	Special	Special	21%	12%
Kennedy et al. (1991)	NICU	377	POEMS	ALGO-1	3%	3.2%
Hall et al. (1994)	NICU	20 (40)	ILO 88	ALGO-1	47.7% and 3.8%	0%
Jacobson & Jacobson (1994)	NICU WBN	67 52	ILO 88 ILO 88	ALGO-1 ALGO-1		
Doyle et al. (1997)	WBN	200 (400)	ILO 88	ALGO-1	21%	11.5%
McNellis & Klein (1997)	WBN	50 (100)	ILO 88	IHS	39%	2%
Hess et al. (1998)	NICU	942	ILO 88	ALGO-1+	26.5%	9.2%
Apostolopoulos et al. (1999)	NICU	223 (438)	ILO 88	Bio-Logic	21%	16%
DPOAE						
Hall et al. (1994)	NICU WBN	20 (40) 20 (40)	GSI-60 Virtual	ALGO-1 IHS	5% 9%	0% 0%
Salata et al. (1998)	NICU	14 (208)	GSI-60	ALGO-2	3%	6%
Ochi et al. (1998)	NICU	36 (67)	Bio-Logic	Synax	31.3%[b]	31.3%[b]

[a]ILO 88 = Otodynamics; IHS = Intelligent Hearing Systems; GSI = Grason Stadler Inc.; ALGO-1 = Natus, Inc.; Bio-Logic = BioLogic Systems Corporation.
[b]Percentage of abnormal findings vs. failures.

provide, at least on request, a skilled trainer or representative for on-site instruction and supervision following purchase of an OAE device.

Test criteria and guidelines for TEOAEs in newborn hearing screening are summarized in Table 8–15. Although this information was meant for the ILO 88, it has general usefulness for TEOAE screening with any device. You may want to practice applying these guidelines with the TEOAE printout shown in Figure 8–6 (TEOAE analysis is reviewed step-by-step in Chapters 1 and 4). Within the past decade, diverse criteria have been used in the analysis of TEOAEs for definition of screening outcome (i.e., what constitutes a "pass" versus a "fail" result). Consensus on acceptable criteria, or minimally data analyzed from sizable population describing outcomes to be expected with different criteria, would be very useful for the meaningful comparison of findings among studies. The impact of TEOAE analyses criteria in newborn

Table 8–15. Criteria and guidelines for newborn hearing screening with TEOAE.

Criteria Required Before Test Interpretation

- ■ >50 low noise samples are collected (rejection level set at about 44 dB SPL)
- ■ Peak click stimulus intensity level of 74 to 83 dB

Criteria for Stimulus Conditions

- ■ Stimulus stability is 75% or higher
- ■ Stimulus spectrum flat across the test frequency region (e.g., 1 to 4000 Hz)
- ■ Stimulus spectrum approaches target of 40 dB SPL

Criteria for Response Interpretation (One Criterion Must be Met for a "Pass")

- ■ Whole reproducibility of 75% or higher
- ■ Reproducibility for octave bands from 1600 to 4000 Hz of 70% or higher
- ■ OAE-to-noise difference for octave bands from 1600 to 4000 Hz of 6 dB SPL or greater
- ■ Overall response level of 23 dB SPL or greater

Common Problems in TEOAE Newborn Hearing Screening

- ■ Inadequate probe fit
- ■ Stimulus intensity too high or low
- ■ Irregular stimulus spectrum
- ■ Noise (either environmental or physiologic)

Sources: Adapted from Vohr et al., 1993; Maxon et al., 1995; Maxon, 1996.

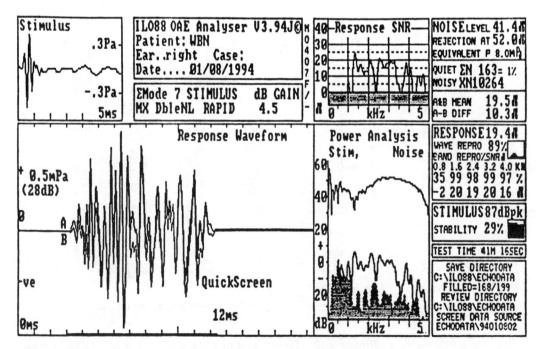

Figure 8–6. Example of TEOAE findings recorded with the ILO 88 device for an infant meeting accepted criteria for a "pass" outcome. For all but the lowest frequency octave, reproducibility values (Response box on the right side) clearly exceeded 70% and signal-to-noise (SNR) differences were well above 3 dB SPL.

hearing screening is quite apparent from even cursory inspection of Figure 8–7.

DPOAEs in Newborn Screening: Test Principles and Protocols, Analysis and Interpretation

A sample protocol for newborn hearing screening with DPOAEs is summarized in Table 8–16, along with rationales for various parameters. The reasons for specific test parameters and analysis criteria, such as the reliance on high-frequency stimuli, have been thoroughly noted elsewhere in this chapter and in Chapter 4. A schematic example of a DPOAE screening outcome is illustrated in Figure 8–8. Although various analysis strategies have been proposed and followed, the most common approach is to judge the outcome as a "pass" or "fail" (refer) based on the DP-to-noise floor difference, an analysis approach very

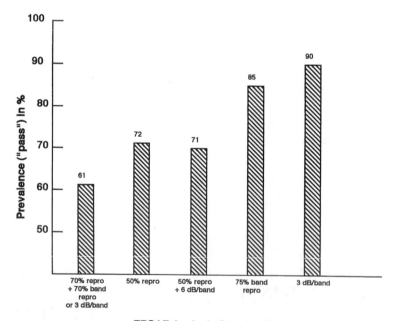

TEOAE Analysis Criterion Category

Figure 8–7. The impact of analyses criteria on TEOAE screening outcome. The proportion of infants "passing" a TEOAE screening varies substantially depending on analysis criteria. (Adapted from Dirckx et al., 1996).

Table 8–16. A DPOAE test protocol and analysis strategy.

Protocol	Rationale
Test Parameters	
■ Stimulus intensity: L_1 = 65 dB, L_2 = 55 dB	See Whitehead et al. (1995).
■ F_2/F_1 ratio: 1.20	Evidence from a number of papers (see Chapter 4).
■ Frequency range: F_2 from 2000 to 5000 Hz	Includes upper end of speech frequencies, but avoids excessive noise of lower frequencies (<1000 Hz) and potential problem of standing wave artifacts of higher frequencies (>5000 Hz).
■ Frequencies/range: 4 or 6	Avoids reliance on limited number of test frequencies.
Recording Technique/Screening Strategy	
■ High noise configuration	Rigorous algorithm and stopping rules for reduction of measurement noise (e.g., noise must reach −20 dB before averaging stops) and the DP − noise floor difference or ratio (e.g., a DP–NF difference of 10 dB is required before averaging stops for each frequency). The time limit for averaging at each frequency should be set so as to produce an acceptable maximum test time per DPgram per ear.
■ Screen from high to low stimulus frequencies	Infant is likely to be most restless at the beginning of the screening procedure. Test time may be prolonged if screening is begun in the low-frequency (high noise) region. However, if the screening procedure begins in low-noise (high frequency) region, screening may progress rapidly and may be stopped as soon as pass criteria are met for first 3 out of 4 stimuli, or 4 out of 6 stimuli, thereby avoiding the need to continue screening in the highest noise condition.
■ Assess reliability	Record two or three DPgrams removing the probe slightly from ear after each run from high to low frequencies (Chase & Hall, 1998). Remember, "if the DPgram does not replicate, you must investigate!" False-negative screening outcomes can be minimized by insisting on two replicable DPgrams for each ear (DIP amplitudes within ±1 or 2 dB for each frequency).
■ Verify stimulus intensity	Verify that the actual stimulus intensity for f_1 and f_2 are within 2 dB of target intensity levels for each frequency.
Analysis Criteria: Detection of Hearing Loss >15 dB HL	
■ DP–NF difference >3 dB *and* DP amplitude within adult normal region	This strategy by definition will detect any degree of sensory hearing loss (essentially eliminate false-negative screening outcomes), but will result in a higher failure rate than more lax criteria for OAE screening, and for automated ABR which is designed to detect hearing loss of about 30 dB HL or greater.

(continued)

Table 8–16. *(continued)*

Protocol	Rationale
Analysis Criteria: Detection of Hearing Loss >35 dB HL	
■ DP–NF difference >5 dB and absolute DP amplitude of at least −10 dB	This strategy will detect mild-to-moderate sensory hearing loss with lower failure rate than the above strategy. A pass, however, does not imply normal hearing sensitivity. The reason for including the criteria of −10 dB for absolute DP amplitude is to minimize the likelihood of passing an infant with no DP activity due to equipment distortion or noise. For example, >5 (dB DP–NF difference with a very low noise floor (e.g., −30 dB) and absolute DP amplitude of −25 dB, which is inconsistent with hearing sensitivity equal to or better than a mild sensory hearing loss.

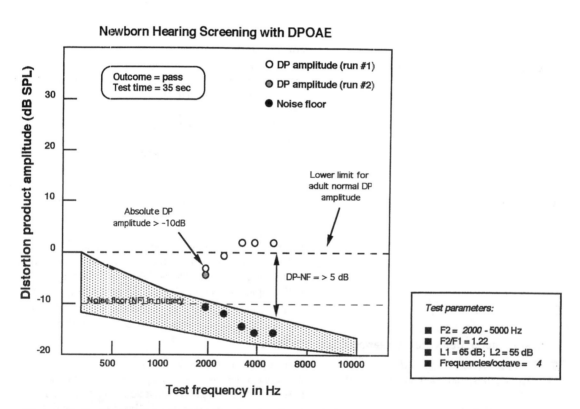

Figure 8–8. Illustration of a "pass" outcome for newborn hearing screening with DPOAEs. DP amplitudes were reliably recorded more than 5 dB above the noise floor for at least four out of five stimulus frequencies. Measured noise was adequately low (within the expected range for quiet newborn infants in the nursery setting).

similar to that described above for TEOAEs. For example, if the DPOAE amplitude is reliably 5 dB or more above the noise floor (NF) for each frequency, or the majority of test frequencies, a serious cochlear (outer hair cell) hearing loss is unlikely. This likelihood can be further reduced (along with false-negative or "miss" test outcomes) by also requiring that noise floor values be below some minimum level (e.g., − 15 dB) and that absolute DPOAE amplitudes exceed a specified criterion (e.g., − 10 dB). Clinical experience shows that these three DPOAE response parameters (i.e., a DP–NF difference of >5 dB, low noise levels within the frequency region of interest, and some evidence of DP activity) are not compatible with sensory hearing loss exceeding 30 dB HL, as confirmed audiometrically. Remember, the objective of newborn hearing screening with OAEs is not to verify that hearing sensitivity is entirely normal but, rather, to identify communicatively significant hearing loss.

Test performance can be manipulated by modifying test analysis criteria and, of course, stimulus parameters. For example, in an investigation of DPOAE screening of infants at risk for hearing loss, with a commercially available device (Grason Stadler 60; Salata, Jacobson, & Strasnick, 1998) demonstrated that sensitivity progressively improved when the pass criterion was shifted from a DP–NF difference of 5 dB to 10 dB to 15 dB (50%, 67%, 83%, respectively). Put another way, the pass rate (or specificity) decreased from 94% for the 5-dB criterion (the DP–NF difference averaged over five frequency pairs), 68% for the 10-dB criterion, and only 38% for the 15-dB criterion. Data are lacking for DPOAE or TEOAE test performance with infants, mostly due to the difficulty in verifying hearing status at the time of the screening (there is no "gold standard") and scarcity of infants with hearing loss, which are necessary for calculation of OAE sensitivity. However, data available for older children and adults suggest that, with the use the DP–NF difference of 5 dB or greater as the pass criterion, close adherence to the requirements for low noise and minimal absolute DP amplitude, and insistence on reliable results (repeated on two different DPgrams), test sensitivity is adequate (hearing-impaired ears will not pass the screening). If the final failure rate for a DPOAE hearing screening program is sufficiently low (5% or less in the WBN), then one can be reasonably certain of success. As the final failure rate approaches 10%, for either TEOAE or DPOAE screening, an alternative approach or the two-step (OAE + ABR) strategy should be considered.

To echo a remark made in the previous section, there is a distinct trend toward automated DPOAE instrumentation of measurement and analysis (see Chapter 7). Therefore, in newborn hearing screening, the tester will have little or no responsibility for selecting a protocol or analyzing DPOAE data.

Troubleshooting in OAE Screening

The numerous techniques and strategies for optimizing TEOAE and DPOAE recording discussed in Chapter 4 are directly applicable in newborn hearing screening. Table 8–17 summarizes some of the important steps contributing to successful newborn screening with OAEs. For example, each of the critical steps in OAE measurement in the clinic—securing an adequate probe fit, meeting target stimulus intensity, minimizing measurement noise, verification of response reliability—must be taken when screening newborn infants in the nursery setting. These guidelines are not repeated here. Importantly, as noted earlier, tester experience is a highly significant variable among studies. As a rule, the smaller the study population, the less experienced the screening personnel. Given the variables that can influence screening outcome, including tester experience, one might expect failure rates to differ substantially among studies. And this is certainly the case, as illustrated in Figure 8–9.

Table 8–17. Major steps in the confirmation and diagnosis of hearing loss, and initial intervention, following newborn hearing screening failure. Diagnostic assessment is discussed later in this chapter.

Step	Objective(s)	Procedure(s)
Follow-up screening	✔Minimize failure rate and associated costs of tracking and diagnostic assessment, and parental concern	✔Repeat screening in hospital with same or different technique (OAE or AABR) *or* ✔Repeat screening at well-baby visit with physician in audiology clinic or other appropriate facility
Diagnostic audiologic assessment test battery (birth to 4 months)	✔Describe type of hearing impairment ✔Define degree of hearing impairment for at least three audiometric frequencies ✔Confirm cochlear site-of-lesion ✔Differentiate conductive vs. sensorineural hearing loss	✔ABR with click and tone burst stimuli, and bone-conduction stimuli as indicated ✔Otoacoustic emissions (TEOAEs and/or DPOAEs) ✔Immittance measures including tympanometry and acoustic reflexes (if possible) with a high-frequency probe tone (e.g., 660 or 1000 Hz) ✔Behavioral audiometry as soon as valid results are possible
Management	✔Obtain medical clearance for hearing aids ✔Provide amplification as soon as possible ✔Make appropriate medical referrals ✔Involve parents integrally in management	✔Refer directly to otolaryngology ✔Use prescriptive fitting technique (e.g., DSL) ✔e.g., Genetics, child development, ophthalmology ✔Parent-infant specialist

After the Screening: Database Management, Tracking, and Follow-Up

Newborn hearing screening is of no value, and is a considerable waste of time and money, if it does not lead to early identification and intervention of permanent hearing loss in infants and young children. Screening is only the first step in an ongoing clinical process that, for some babies, will continue for most of their childhood. Screening is, in many respects, also the easiest step in the process. Major components of a comprehensive newborn hearing screening program are illustrated in Figure 8–10. Each of these components was also summarized earlier (see Table 8–8) with reference to the American Academy of Pediatrics statement (1999). The first follow-up visit after a refer outcome for the initial screening is often a secondary screening, either in the hospital or within weeks after discharge (see Table 8–9). A diagnostic pediatric audiology assessment to confirm and define hearing loss is scheduled after the refer outcome for the final screening. Although this assessment will be performed by audiologists, it is scheduled by or following consultation with the child's primary care physician. By definition, early intervention is initiated within 4 to 6 months after birth. Therefore, the diagnostic pediatric assessment should be conducted

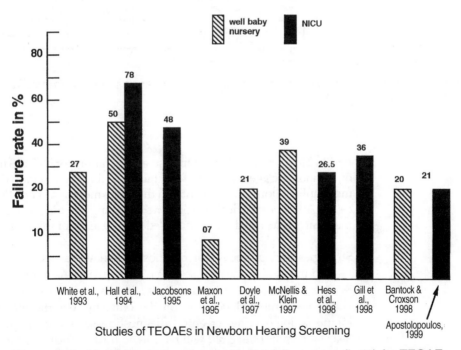

Figure 8–9. Variability in the reported initial failure rates (in %) for TEOAEs among studies over a 7-year period. In some studies, failure rate was defined as all infants not passing the screening. The lowest failure rate (7%) was reported from the Rhode Island Hearing Assessment Program (Maxon, 1995).

NEWBORN HEARING SCREENING OF AT-RISK INFANTS

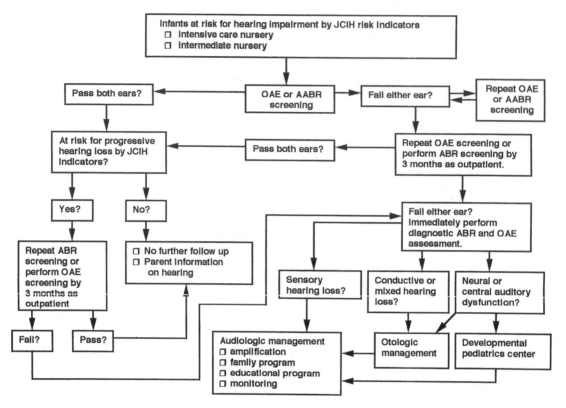

Figure 8–10. Flowchart summarizing major steps in newborn hearing screening (at-risk infant population is illustrated in this figure).

within 2 to 3 months after the final screening failure (or by 2 to 3 months of chronologic age relative to term birth), so that intervention (including amplification) can occur within the first 6 months after birth (Table 8–18). Another practical reason for scheduling the diagnostic assessment early is to avoid the need for sedation, at least for this first session.

Strategies and protocols for diagnostic pediatric assessment are reviewed in detail in the next section of this chapter. As noted in Figure 8–10 and in Table 8–18, what follows the diagnostic assessment may vary considerably depending on the outcome. For the majority of infants failing hearing screening, diagnostic assessment will rule out a hearing loss and the child will require no further audiologic management, unless there is a risk factor for progressive or delayed-onset hearing impairment. Hearing loss will be confirmed, however, for a proportion of infants. It is this small but significant group that requires the prompt and diligent efforts of the child's family and a team of profes-

Table 8–18. Distinctions between early versus late identification of and intervention for hearing impairment in children.

Parameter	Early	Late
■ Age of identification	<6 months	>1 to 3 years
■ Mode of identification	Screening at birth	Parental or MD concern
■ Diagnosis and definition of hearing loss	ABR & OAEs	Behavioral audiometry
■ Hearing aid fitting	Prescriptive techniques	Subjective information
■ Audiologic rehabilitation	Initial and periodic	Intensive and extended
■ Communicative outcome	Good (normal)	Highly variable

sionals, including the audiologist, primary care physician, speech-language pathologist, and often medical specialists (otolaryngologists, geneticists, pediatric neurologist). The many critical details involved in the management of infant hearing impairment are far beyond the scope of this handbook. It is important to point out, however, that maintaining a database of infants requiring follow-up, tracking these infants over time, and verifying that infants requiring diagnostic testing and subsequent management receive it in a timely fashion, is a major undertaking. Fortunately, there are now commercial systems and software designed specifically for this task. These programs begin with a direct electronic linkage between the screening equipment (programs are compatible with almost any brand of OAE device) and a database, for quick and accurate transfer of demographic and screening data. A major manufacturer of a database and tracking system (Oz Systems) is represented in Chapter 7.

PEDIATRIC DIAGNOSTIC ASSESSMENT

The Cross-Check Principle Revisited

In 1976, Jerger and Hayes articulated a clinical maxim for audiologic assessment of children, which they coined "the cross-check principle." The authors effectively presented the rationale for "a test battery approach for evaluation of children," consisting of behavioral audiometry, impedance measurements, and the auditory brainstem response. This classic article should be on the must-read list for all serious students of audiology. Even the experienced audiologist will, by rereading the paper, more fully appreciate the almost prophetic statements scattered throughout the paper and the timeliness of the case reports. A few snippets are reproduced in Table 8–19. One can almost envision likely OAE findings for four of the five patients and how OAEs would have contributed to patient diagnosis and management (bilateral aural atresia would have precluded OAE recording for the

Table 8–19. Excerpts from the classic 1976 paper by James Jerger and Deborah Hayes describing the cross-check principle in pediatric audiology.

"Behavioral observation has been the traditional cornerstone of pediatric audiometry for many years. Some investigators enthusiastically report the success of this method for testing any child, regardless of his level of functioning:

> The trick, if there is any, is to become confidently familiar with the auditory behavior of normal-hearing children regardless of the integrity of their mental processing or central nervous system functioning. Once one knows the hearing level at which these children should respond, as well as the kind of response they will give, the deviation of the deaf child will be patently evident. (Northern and Downs, 1974, p. 137)

We are not so sanguine. We have found that simply observing the auditory behavior of children does not always yield an accurate description of hearing loss. In our own experience, we have seen too many children at all levels of functioning who have been misdiagnosed and mismanaged on the basis of behavioral results alone.

The mishandling of children based on the results of behavioral audiometry is an increasingly alarming problem. In our own audiology service we are evaluating children at much earlier ages than was common in the past. It is not unusual for us to evaluate infants as young as 5 weeks. Physicians and parents are becoming increasingly aware of the possibilities and implications of hearing loss in infancy. We are also seeing more multiply handicapped children . . . And it is just these two groups of children, very young infants and multiply handicapped children, whom we have found are most often misdiagnosed by behavioral results alone.

We discuss a method of pediatric audiologic assessment that employs the 'cross-check principle.' That is, the results of a single test are cross-checked by an independent test measure. Particularly useful in pediatric evaluations as cross-checks of behavioral test results are impedance and brainstem-evoked response audiometry (BSER)." (Jerger and Hayes, 1976, p. 614)

"The basic operation of this principle is that no result be accepted until it is confirmed by an independent measure." (Jerger and Hayes, 1976, p. 620)

Source: Reprinted with permission from Jerger JF, Hayes D. The cross-check principle in pediatric audiometry. *Archives of Otolaryngology 102:* 614–620, 1976.

fifth patient, a 6-month-old girl). A quarter of a century later, it is time to revise and update the cross-check principle, especially for pediatric assessments since OAEs are now an integral component of the pediatric diagnostic test battery. As noted in Table 8–20, OAEs have earned a unique and valued complimentary clinical role along with these other time-tested audiologic procedures.

OAEs in a Current Pediatric Test Battery

The utilization of OAEs in pediatric diagnostic assessment is perhaps more valuable and powerful than any other application in children or adults. Why are OAEs a necessary component of the modern pediatric test battery? The twofold answer is their remarkable sensitivity and

Table 8–20. The new-millenium cross-check principle[a] in pediatric audiology, incorporating otoacoustic emissions (see Table 8–19). The original 1976 pediatric test battery consisted of behavioral audiometry, impedance measures, and the auditory brainstem response.

Procedure	Advantages	Disadvantages
Behavioral audiometry	✔The only true test of hearing.	✔Limited value in infants (<6 months).
	✔Pure-tone audiometry is frequency-specific.	✔Influenced by developmental status.
	✔Measures communication (speech audiometry).	✔Influenced by neurologic (motor) status.
	✔Assesses cortical auditory functioning.	✔Not site-specific.
		✔Often not ear-specific in young children.
		✔Limited value in difficult-to-test children.
		✔Requires sound-treated test setting.
Impedance measures[b]	✔No behavioral response required.	✔Not a test of hearing.
	✔Sensitive measure of middle ear status.	✔Information limited by middle ear dysfunction.
	✔Some information on hearing sensitivity.	✔Does not assess higher (cortical) auditory function.
	✔Provides ear-specific information.	✔Does not assess communication performance.
	✔Provides frequency-specific information.	
	✔Assesses retrocochlear/brainstem auditory function.	
	✔Can record in sleep or during sedation.	
	✔Does not require sound-treated setting.	
ABR	✔No behavioral response required.	✔Not a test of hearing.
	✔Appropriate for all ages, even newborn infants.	✔Does not assess higher (cortical) auditory function.
	✔Objective estimation of hearing sensitivity.	✔Generated only by synchronous firing of onset-neurons.
	✔Provides ear-specific information.	✔May be absent in normal hearing sensitivity.
	✔Provides frequency-specific information.	✔Does not assess communication performance.
	✔Can record in sleep or during sedation.	
	✔Assesses retrocochlear/brainstem auditory function.	
	✔Does not require sound-treated setting.	

(continued)

Table 8–20. *(continued)*

Procedure	Advantages	Disadvantages
OAE	✔No behavioral response required.	✔Not a test of hearing.
	✔Appropriate for all ages, even newborn infants.	✔Does not evaluate neural auditory pathways.
	✔Provides ear-specific information.	✔Invalidated by middle ear pathology.
	✔Provides frequency-specific information.	✔No value in estimating degree of hearing loss.
	✔Highly site-specific (outer hair cells in cochlea).	
	✔Not dependent on neural auditory system integrity.	
	✔Does not require sound-treated setting.	

[a]Jerger JF, Hayes D. The cross-check principle in pediatric audiometry. *Archives of Otolaryngology 102*: 614–620, 1976.
[b]Includes tympanometry and acoustic reflexes (with contralateral and ipsilateral signals).

specificity. As discussed in detail in Chapter 2, OAEs are the product of highly metabolic activity of outer hair cells. Virtually any possible insult to the cochlea, including even subtle disruptions in blood flow to the stria vascularis, will be reflected by OAE changes. There is no more sensitive measure of cochlear function, and OAEs are almost entirely sensory and "preneural." Their measurement does not depend on the functional status of any synapses, nor the rest of the auditory system. This site specificity is a distinct clinical advantage for a component of a diagnostic test battery. In addition to these two essential features—sensitivity and specificity—OAEs are electrophysiologic, requiring no behavioral response from the pediatric patient. These and other characteristics of OAEs are summarized in Table 8–20.

These fundamental features of OAEs take on very practical everyday importance in pediatric audiology. Most audiologic management of children is predicated on the premise that the hearing impairment is sensory, affecting the cochlea. By definition, audiologists are responsible for evaluation and diagnosis of all types of auditory impairment. Conductive hearing loss, however, is traditionally treated medically or surgically by physicians. And, although the audiologist is integrally involved in the detection of eighth nerve (retrocochlear) and central auditory nervous system dysfunction, treatment (if available) is most often a team effort, which may or may not include the audiologist. Determining whether the hearing impairment is sensory or neural (or some combination) depends very much on results of OAE measurement. If the hearing impairment is sensory, then the audiologist is the professional with primary responsibilty for implementing and coordinating management with amplification and a complement of habilitation or rehabilitation strategies and techniques. OAEs are now part of the standard-of-care for pediatric audiology. This serious clinical conclusion is amply supported by the diverse OAE application that are reviewed in this chapter. In short, OAEs are not simply a handy or convenient procedure for assessing auditory function but rather are an essential component of the test battery. OAEs can play a pivotal and critical role in decisions regarding audiologic, not medical management of auditory impairment. The clearest example of this role is in patients with suspected "auditory neuropathy."

AUDITORY NEUROPATHY

Definition and Background Information

Rarely does the introduction of a clinical procedure lead to an almost immediate appreciation of a novel diagnostic entity. Certainly, the discovery of a variety of audiologic tests has facilitated the identification or diagnosis of well-recognized auditory disorders or the refinement of patterns of auditory findings associated with these disorders. Among the audiologic tests or variations of existing procedure that have met these important clinical objectives are variations of speech audiometry (e.g., performance-intensity functions, diagnostic speech materials for central auditory assessment), the traditional site-of-lesion diagnostic audiologic procedures (e.g., ABLB, SISI, tone decay tests), immittance meaures (tympanometry and acoustic reflexes), and the auditory brainstem response. With each of these examples, the development of an auditory procedure led to quicker and more thorough diagnosis of specific auditory disorders, and thereby contributed to more efficient audiologic management. The discovery, or more accurately recognition, of the constellation of auditory findings now called "auditory neuropathy" was due exclusively to routine application of OAEs in patients—in particular infants and young children—at risk for neurologic dysfunction.

Auditory neuropathy is invariably characterized by normal OAEs and/or cochlear microphonic activity. Identification and diagnosis of auditory neuropathy can radically influence audiologic and otologic management, whereas failure to recognize auditory neuropathy can result in mismanagement.

Beginning in the early 1990s, as OAEs were initially incorporated into the pediatric audiologic test battery in leading clinical centers throughout the world, an unusual pattern of auditory findings was independently reported by an international collection of investigators, and observed quietly, and probably with disbelief, by many more audiologists in their daily clinical practice. The scenario being repeated in audiology clinics large and small went something like this:

> An infant or young child did not pass a screening with ABR, or was brought in for an audiologic assessment because someone was concerned about his or her unresponsiveness to sounds. Behavioral audiometry failed to produce reliable responses to tonal or speech signals. A diagnostic ABR was performed to define auditory status. No ABR was observed bilaterally, even at maximum click stimulus intensity levels. At this stage in the diagnostic process, all evidence pointed to a severe-to-profound sensorineural hearing impair-

ment. Plans were underway for prompt audiologic management, including amplification. Then, to confirm that the hearing loss was sensory (cochlear), or perhaps more out of curiosity or to try out a new piece of equipment, OAEs were performed. Someone present during this session might have even protested. "Why do we need OAEs in this case? We already know the child has a severe hearing impairment. The OAEs will just be a waste of time, and be an extra charge to the patient." The audiologist, however, insists on providing a complete assessment, and proceeds with the OAE measurement. Jaws go slack and eyes widen as normal, even robust, OAEs are recorded for one ear, and then the other ear. The resident skeptic immediately exclaims, in a half-question: "Maybe there's a technical problem, or maybe this is just artifact?!" OAE measurement was repeated, with another device if possible, but the results were the same. After the assessment, the audiologist made an attempt to explain the pattern of results to the parents and physician but could not adequately respond to the inevitable queries: "What does this mean? Can the child hear normally? What do we do next? Before this testing, I thought you said my child needed a hearing aid. Will the child's hearing get better?" That night, the audiologist probably stayed awake trying to answer these questions and, even worse, wondered how many pediatric patients she'd seen over the years who might have had the same problem, if OAEs had been available, were fitted with hearing aids or received cochlear implants. The next day, the audiologist started consulting with colleagues at other hospitals and medical centers, asking for advice on test interpretation and case management.

As a result of such cases and professional collaboration, the picture became more clear, and the concept and label of auditory neuropathy began to emerge. OAEs have, in fact, radically altered our approach for assessment and management of pediatric hearing loss. This general pattern of findings is now well-recognized, but numerous variations have been described. And, our strategies for management of auditory neuropathy and our understanding of the long-term outcome for these children, is still evolving. Even the definition of auditory neuropathy is unclear.

Auditory neuropathy is empirically defined as abnormal ABR findings, and often absent or abnormal behavioral responses to sound, despite cochlear integrity. Cochlear function in auditory neuropathy can be documented electrophysiologically with OAE and/or with the cochlear microphonics of the ECochG. Indeed, the presence of cochlear microphonic in the ABR waveforms of children with no subsequent ABR components, and no behavioral response to sounds, was observed clinically long before the discovery of OAEs, although the significance of the finding was not clearly appreciated. Also, the finding of absent ABRs and/or very poor speech audiometry performance in persons with normal or near-normal pure-tone audiograms, has been occasionally reported for decades (e.g., Worthington & Peters, 1980; Kraus et al., 1984; Hildesheimer, Muchnik, & Rubenstein, 1993). Auditory neuropathy is not a new clinical entity but, rather, a newly appreciated pattern of findings. Nonethess, it is attracting considerable attention among audiologists and hearing scientists. A prime example of this interest is the Conference on Auditory Neuropathy held at Lake Arrowhead in California on March 30 and 31, 1998. At this meeting, a multidisciplinary group addressed a range of critical issues and topics related to auditory neuropathy, including genetics and pathophysiology, clinical findings in newborns and older children, potential mechanisms, and rehabilitation strategies. As with most stimulating conferences, more questions were raised than answered. [*Note:* Most of the information from the conference will appear in a forthcoming textbook on Auditory Neuropathy edited by Yvonne Sinninger and Arnold Starr and published by Singular.]

Consensus is lacking on the definition of auditory neuropathy. One eminent group of auditory scientists—including Arnold Starr, Chuck Berlin, Yvonne Sininger, and Linda Hood—describes auditory neuropathy as "due to a disorder of auditory nerve function" (Starr et al., 1996, p. 741). In several papers, these authors described in detail a series of case reports with electrophysiologic and clinical evidence in support of their view that the eighth cranial (auditory) nerve is the site of pathology in patients with hearing impairment secondary to auditory neuropathy (see Table 8–21 for key references on auditory neuropathy). That is, the problem is defined rather strictly as an auditory *peripheral nerve* pathology, involving "auditory nerve dentrites, auditory neurons in the spiral ganglion, and/or axons of the auditory nerve between the cochlea and the pontine brainstem." However, in some publications, these authors also appeared to include cochlear abnormalities involving the tectorial membrane, inner hair cells, and the synapse between inner hair cells and the afferent fibers of the eighth nerve as neuropathy. The group pointed out that "a set of salient features distinguishes these patients from the majority of patients with sensorineural hearing loss or other described syndromes. The symptoms always seen in presumed auditory neuropathy are: (1) mild-to-moderate elevation of auditory thresholds to pure-tone stimuli by air and bone conduction, (2) absent or severely abnormal ABRs to high-level stimuli, *including absence of wave I*, (3) present otoacoustic emissions that do not suppress with contralateral noise, (4) word-recognition ability poorer than expected for pure-tone hearing loss configuration, (5) absent acoustic reflexes to both ipsilateral and contralateral tones at 110 dB HL, and (6) absent masking level differences" (Sininger et al., 1995, p. 10).

Other authors have defined auditory neuropathy more liberally, presenting as examples cases with pathology not limited to, or in some cases not involving, the eighth cranial nerve. With this broad definition

At the least, early identification of auditory neuropathy requires the combined measurement of OAEs and ABR.

Table 8–21. Published reports (arranged chronologically) of patients with normal OAEs* and abnormal ABR findings, a pattern consistent with broadly defined auditory neuropathy.

Author(s) (Year)	Comments
Lutman et al. (1989)	Case report of an 11-year-old child with normal OAEs and unilateral SNHL by ABR
Prieve et al. (1991)	33-year-old with severe-to-profound unilateral SNHL and normal TEOAEs
Baldwin & Watkin (1992)	Infant with normal TEOAEs and abnormal ABR
Katona et al. (1993)	3-month-old infant with OAEs and CM but profound SNHL by ABR and behavioral findings
Konradsson (1996)	Four apparently healthy children (4 and 7 years old) with severe to profound SNHL (ABR and behavioral audiometry) and normal TEOAEs
Laccourreye et al. (1996)	3-year-old child with normal TEOAEs and profound SNHL
Starr et al. (1996)	10 children and young adults with OAEs and CM but abnormal ABRs; detailed neurologic findings
Stein et al. (1996)	Four infants with normal TEOAEs
Watkin (1996)	infant with normal TEOAEs and abnormal ABR
Deltenre et al. (1997)	Three children with normal OAEs and CM and abnormal ABRs and behavioral audiograms
Parker et al. (1997)	Seven patients with normal TEOAEs and abnormal ABR (taken from a large series of children)
Psarommatis et al. (1997)	Two case reports of infants with normal TEOAEs and abnormal ABRs
Berlin et al. (1998)	Five infants with TEOAEs and CM (in ABR), but absent click-stimulus ABRs
Cullington & Brown (1998)	Case report of premature infant (history included jaundice and asphyxia) with Mondini dysplasia with normal TEOAEs and profound SNHL behaviorally
Hall & Bachmann (1998)	Case report of infant with Maple syrup urine disease with normal DPOAEs and abnormal ABR
Starr et al. (1998)	Four children with neurologic disorders with normal OAEs and temperature-related ABR abnormalities
Wood et al. (1998)	Seven infants with normal TEOAEs and abnormal ABR screening results
Miyamoto et al. (1999)	4-year-old with normal OAEs and SNHL who received cochlear implant
Rance et al. (1999)	20 infants and young children with ECochG CM but absent click-stimulus ABRs

*Study by Rance et al. (1999) defined cochlear status with ECochG CM component.

of auditory neuropathy, the term is essentially being used to describe forms of "nontumor, noncochlear" hearing impairment that have been reported previously, before OAE were regularly used clinically (e.g., Hallpike et al., 1980; Worthington & Peters, 1980; Lenhardt, 1982; Stockard, 1983; Kraus et al., 1984; Hildesheimer, Muchnik, & Rubenstein, 1993; Cacace et al., 1994). A finding of normal OAE and/or CM activity, or at least some evidence of cochlear integrity, remains an essential component of the definition. However, the anatomic extent of the auditory neuropathy and the associated patterns of audiologic findings are more variable. In this definition, auditory dysfunction may include the eighth cranial nerve or regions of the central auditory nervous system. Auditory findings are also more variable. For example, behavioral audiometry may produce pure-tone thresholds that are entirely normal or are consistent with varying degrees of hearing impairment (Rance et al., 1999). Patients with this more encompassing definition of auditory neuropathy have, in common, reasonably intact cochlear function with dysfunction of retrocochlear auditory structures that does not result from a mass lesion, such as an acoustic tumor. Actually, one might simply categorize auditory neuropathy as a form of retrocochlear auditory dysfunction of the nontumor type. In the following discussion of assessment and management, auditory neuropathy will be defined as non-tumor-related dysfunction of the neural pathways of the auditory system (eighth nerve or central nervous system) that results in hearing impairment or auditory dysfunction by ABR, and sometimes behavioral audiometry.

What is the incidence of auditory neuropathy? The answer to this logical question has direct bearing on a variety of clinical decisions, ranging from how to screen newborn infants for hearing impairment (OAEs or ABR), to the need for including OAEs in every pediatric assessment, to management concerns. In the author's experience, and based on conversations with colleagues, audiologists in tertiary medical facilities who are reponsible for hearing assessment of NICU graduates and children referred from physicians and other audiologists for definitive diagnosis are encountering auditory neuropathy regularly. This observation is supported by papers presented at national meetings and the published literature (see Table 8–21). Although exact statistics are not yet available, several recent papers provide estimates. Rance et al. (1999) found the pattern of absent ABR and normal outer hair cell function (verified by the ECochG cochlear microphonics) in 12 children among 5,199 who were screened. The proportion with the auditory neuropathy pattern was 0.23% of their at-risk infants. Of the 109 children with permanent hearing impairment, however, the proportion was 11% (1 in 9 cases). Vohr et al. (1998) reported 5 children with hearing impairment out of a total of 111 who had initially passed an TEOAE screening. Two of these infants had the diagnosis of auditory neuropathy.

Auditory neuropathy is more common in the NICU population than in healthy babies.

Assessment and Management Strategies

Risk factors

The prompt identification and thorough assessment of auditory neuropathy is facilitated by heightened vigilance in selected patients. The literature clearly confirms that some patients, particularly children, are at greatest risk. The common denominator, not surprisingly, is neurologic disease or dysfunction. Some of the more common etiologies associated with auditory neuropathy are listed in Table 8–22. Among these, the most commonly reported is hyperbilirubinemia. Indeed, there is a sizable literature documenting the pathology and dysfunction of retrocochlear structures (Levi et al., 1981; Conlee & Shapiro, 1991; El Barbary, 1991; Shapiro & Conlee, 1991) and the relation between retrocochlear auditory dysfunction and serious sensorineural hearing impairment in hyperbilirubinemia (Chisin et al., 1979; Perlman et al., 1983; Nakamura et al., 1985; Vohr et al., 1989), sometimes with reversal of the ABR-documented hearing impairment over time (Wennberg et al., 1982; Ito, 1984; Hall et al., 1985; Stein et al., 1986; Thoma et al., 1986; Deliac et al., 1990; Nwawesi et al., 1994; Graham et al., 1997). A wise clinical policy is to include OAEs in the test battery for any patient with a history of one or more of these factors. Keep in mind that a final medical diagnosis may not be available when the first audiologic signs of auditory neuropathy are recorded. In fact, when the audiologic assessment is first completed, often during the neonatal period, there may be no suspicion of neurologic dysfunction. The audiologic evidence of auditory neuropathy may precipitate the referrals to medical specialists and centers, which will ultimately lead to a definitive diagnosis. Rarely will a child with auditory neuropathy be found otherwise entirely normal after a comprehensive diagnostic workup, including neurologic, neurometabolic, and neuroradiologic studies.

Table 8–22. Selected diverse diagnoses which may be associated with pediatric auditory neuropathy.

✔ Hyperbilirubinemia (kernicterus)

✔ Neurogenerative diseases (e.g., Friedreich's ataxia)

✔ Neurometabolic diseases (e.g., Maple syrup urine disease)

✔ Demyelinating diseases

✔ Hereditary motor sensory neuropathologies (e.g. Charcot-Marie-Tooth syndrome)

✔ Inflammatory neuropathy

✔ Hydrocephalus

✔ Severe and/or pervasive developmental delay

✔ Ischemic-hypoxic neuropathy (e.g., asphyxia)

✔ Encephalopathy

✔ Meningitis

✔ Cerebral palsy (CP)

Detection and Assessment

An approach for detection of auditory neuropathy is shown schematically in Figure 8–11. OAEs play the pivotal role in the diagnostic process. If OAEs are not recorded (right side of flowchart), then the likelihood of observing normal OAEs is minimal and the diagnostic effort is directed to ruling out middle ear pathology and defining the degree of sensory hearing impairment. The outcome of this routine audiologic diagnostic assessment leads to medical management (e.g., for middle ear disease) and/or audiologic management (e.g., hearing aid selection and fitting). OAE presence in the context of abnormal ABR findings, raises the suspicion of auditory neuropathy. ABR assessment at this stage may be relatively straightforward, as in the initial newborn hearing screening. If the ABR abnormality is characterized by elevation of threshold (miminum response) levels and all components are reliably observed and interwave latency values are within normal limits, the pathology may be limited to inner hair cells. Although the term auditory neuropathy has been used to describe this pattern of findings (Harrison, 1998), it is anatomically speaking an uncommon form of cochlear (sensory) hearing impairment (Prieve, Gorga, & Neely, 1991). Possible explanations can include a genetically based inner hair cell disorder (Deol, 1981; Schrott, Stephan, & Spoendlin, 1989); certain etiologies that can affect inner hair cells, such

AUDITORY NEUROPATHY:
Detection

Figure 8–11. Detection of auditory neuropathy, showing the pivotal role of OAEs.

as measles or mumps (Prieve, Gorga, & Neely, 1991); or ototoxicity due to carboplatin (discussed later). OAEs are normal, or at least detectable, because all or some outer hair cells are functionally intact. The ABR, including wave I, is dependent on synchronous firing of afferent eighth nerve fibers in the region of the spiral ganglion secondary to synaptic activation by the inner hair cells. Inner hair cell dysfunction will, to some extent, elevate ABR thresholds. Normal interwave latencies reflect intact retrocochlear pathways. Audiologic follow-up assessments with the inner hair cell pattern should be scheduled often until behavioral thresholds and speech audiometry findings are available. An otologic and genetic consultation would also be indicated. If a hearing loss by pure-tone audiometry is confirmed, it would be appropriate to proceed cautiously with hearing aid selection and fitting. If, on the other hand, ABR interwave latencies are abnormally delayed, relative to age-appropriate normative data, or wave I or other ABR components are not reliably observed, then more extensive electrophysiologic assessment is warranted.

As schematically depicted in Figure 8–12, the finding of normal OAEs or some evidence of OAEs plus a neurodiagnostically abnormal ABR is followed by more precise electrophysiologic evaluation. This diagnostic assessment could be conducted immediately on first evidence of an auditory neuropathy pattern. An alternative approach is to defer the assessment, and management other than audiologic monitoring,

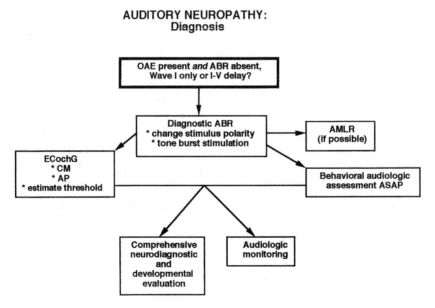

AUDITORY NEUROPATHY:
Diagnosis

Figure 8–12. Diagnosis of auditory neuropathy, illustrating the importance of a broad-based yet highly site-specific test battery approach.

until 2 to 3 months after the initial detection of a possible auditory neuropathy pattern, because it appears that some forms of auditory neuropathy are transient or reversible. The author has documented in infants with a history of, for example, hypoxic insults (asphyxia), meningitis, and hyperbilirubinemia, a complete return of ABRs and/or resolution of ABR abnormalities from the initial assessment to a follow-up assessment 2 to 3 months later. A formal diagnostic test battery for auditory neuropathy consists of an "all-star" collection of auditory procedures, each selected to assess a very specific site within the auditory system or a circumscribed auditory function. Evaluation of auditory neuropathy requires a finely tuned diagnostic approach, utilizing all available techniques for selectively assessing function, whenever possible, of specific structures. Atypical, or expanded, test protocols are followed for each procedure to maximize diagnostic information on auditory status. For example, ABRs are recorded with rarefaction and condensation stimulus polarities to differentiate sensory versus neural responses (e.g., Berlin et al., 1998). Measurement of multiple electrophysiologic responses from the auditory periphery is especially important to differentiate clearly between outer versus inner hair cell dysfunction. For example, one might question the need for including both OAEs and the CM of the ECochG in the test battery, as both are electrophysiologic measures of outer hair cell function. There are at least two reasons why OAEs and CM are complimentary, rather than redundant. CM is thought to reflect receptor potentials (see Chapter 2 for a review of cochlear physiology underlying OAEs) produced at the apical end of outer hair cells when they are activated mechanically. OAEs reflect outer hair cell motility, which results, in part, from electromechanical events subsequent to the receptor potentials. Conceivably, then, CM might be recorded in the absence of OAEs if receptor potentials remained intact yet the complex mechanisms involved in active processes (motility) were disrupted. Second, as detailed in Chapter 2, measurement of OAEs is dependent on outward propogation of energy from the cochlea through the middle ear to the ear canal. Subtle middle ear dysfunction may essentially obliterate OAE detection, without affecting CM recordings. Third, CM generation is not entirely dependent on outer hair cells. There appears to be some inner hair cell contribution to the CM, although considerably less than the portion due to outer hair cell activity (Dallos & Cheatham, 1976). In contrast, the cochlear summating potentials appear to be generated primarily by inner hair cells (Zheng et al., 1997). A subpattern of auditory findings can be inferred from these fundamental distinctions in generation of the CM versus OAEs. CM may be recorded in patients with no detectable OAEs, including some with behavioral evidence of hearing sensitivity deficits. As evidence of this point, Rance et al. (1999) found that about half of their series of 20 patients with auditory neuropathy had CM activity, but no OAEs. Without CM measurement, auditory neuropathy might not have been diagnosed for these patients.

The term "sensorineural hearing loss" is becoming outdated. With a comprehensive pediatric audiologic test battery, it is now possible to differentiate not only between sensory and neural, but also among subtypes of sensory cochlear impairments.

Although each desired or diagnostically indicated audiologic procedure may not be feasible to perform with every patient, the major objective of the assessment should be met, namely the differential evaluation of cochlear, eighth nerve, and central auditory nervous system function with electrophysiologic and behavioral procedures requiring sychronous and less time-dependent activity. The ultimate goal of the diagnostic process is behavioral definition of hearing status with pure tone and speech audiometry.

Diagnosis in auditory neuropathy is challenging in part due to the complexity of this clinical entity. Features of auditory neuropathy contributing to the complexity are summarized in Table 8–23. Clinical presentations are highly varied as "the effects of neuropathy on auditory function appear to be idiosyncratic" (Rance et al., 1999). In most cases, the diagnostic process in auditory neuropathy is ongoing, often for years, until hearing status is completely described electrophysiologically and behaviorally, medical diagnosis is reached, and effective medical and audiologic management is initiated. Deficits in speech perception and understanding, and probably a collection of psychoacoustic auditory functions, are a characteristic finding in auditory neuropathy, if patients survive and are followed until their age and health status permits sophisticated speech audiometry. For some patients, it is likely that changes in medical and/or audiologic status will continue throughout childhood, requiring corresponding alterations in the management plan. And, sadly, a proportion of infants with auditory neuropathy will not thrive or even survive due to widespread and serious disease processes.

The diagnostic process in children with auditory neuropathy is ongoing at least until behavioral audiometry findings are complete.

Management

Management of auditory neuropathy is extremely challenging. Some of the considerations in assessment, and subsequent management, are listed in Table 8–24. At the very least, a team approach involving medical and nonmedical professionals is necessary. During the first months after detection of auditory neuropathy in infants and young children, the most prudent management strategy is to monitor audiologic status periodically until a pattern of findings emerges. Most audiologists, along with some parents and primary care physicians, will be frustrated by this apparent delay in management. In the past, an abnormal or absent ABR with, perhaps, no response to behavioral signals, unquestionably triggered prompt audiologic intervention, especially amplification. Experience has clearly shown, however, that subsequent audiologic assessment for some children with this initial pattern will show normal hearing sensitivity or audiometric contraindications to amplification. Hearing aid fitting would be inappropriate and, possibly, harmful in such children. When hearing aids are fit, cautiously and with low gain, outer hair cell integrity can be verified regularly with OAEs. Although amplification may be withheld, other management steps can and should be initiated (Figure 8–13). These include referral for comprehensive neurologic, developmental,

Table 8–23. Summary of factors contributing to the complexity of assessment and management of auditory neuropathy.

■ Dysfunction is not always auditory or neural.

  ✔ In many cases, there is more diffuse "polyneuropathy" affecting multiple pathways and centers in the peripheral and/or central nervous system rather than pure-auditory neuropathy, which is circumscribed to the auditory system alone.

  ✔ The general audiologic pattern associated with auditory neuropathy can be secondary to inner hair cell dysfunction, and normal function of the eighth cranial nerve and central auditory nervous system function and, therefore, really a form of auditory "sensoropathy" rather than auditory "neuropathy."

■ Multiple potential neuropathophysiologic mechanisms can underlie auditory neuropathy, such as:

  ✔ Delayed or abnormal myelinization in the central auditory system

  ✔ Ischemic-hypoxic insults

  ✔ Metabolic diseases

  ✔ Neurochemical disorders (e.g., neurotransmittor disruption)

  ✔ Neoplasms

  ✔ Pervasive developmental disorders.

■ Dysfunction may be dynamic rather than static, with auditory status worsening or improving over weeks, months, or years.

  ✔ Partial or apparently complete reversal of neural dysfunction and auditory neuropathy

  ✔ Abnormalities can occur, particularly in newborn infants with etiologies such as asphyxia, meningitis, and hyperbilirubinemia.

  ✔ Neural dysfunction and auditory abnormalities can progress.

■ Auditory dysfunction can affect one or more highly discrete levels/regions/structures requiring anatomically and physiologically precise diagnostic procedures. The simple conceptual approach to hearing loss as "sensorineural" is no longer adequate.

  ✔ Cochlear (sensory) disorders must be differentiated into those involving outer versus inner hair cells.

  ✔ Even within a limited anatomic region or structure, there can be distinctions. For example, auditory disorders involving outer hair cells may be differentiated by audiologic diagnosis to those associated with abnormality of receptor potentials (evident in cochlear microphonic abnormality) versus motility (reflected by OAEs).

  ✔ In addition to the traditional afferent (ascending or sensory) explanation for auditory disorders, we must also consider the possibility of efferent (descending or motor) auditory dysfunction.

  ✔ Retrocochlear disorders may be due to disruptions at any level of the peripheral or central auditory system, such as the eighth nerve, brainstem, and/or cerebral pathways and centers.

  ✔ Within any of these pathways or centers, one or more structural and functional subtypes of neurons may be involved in auditory neuropathy (i.e., onset versus other neuron types in the auditory brainstem).

---

and communication evaluation, and perhaps neuroradiologic studies. A child development center is ideal for this multidisciplinary diagnostic effort. Other appropriate referrals include genetics and otolaryngology. Speech-language evaluation, with intensive treatment, is certainly indicated. Cued speech may also be an effective management strategy (Berlin et al., 1998). Alternative forms of communication, such

Table 8–24. Factors contributing to the clinical challenge of audiologic assessment and management of auditory neuropathy.

■ Children may be untestable, or difficult-to-test, using conventional behavioral audiometry due to neurologic involvement (e.g., developmental delay, unresponsiveness to sensory stimuli, motor deficits).

■ Neurologic deficits are often "polyneuropathy" involving other sensory systems (e.g., vision, motor nervous systems, attention, cognition, and other CNS mediated functions).

■ Neurologic and/or audiologic status may be dynamic rather than static, with resolution or worsening of deficits over time.

■ Otoacoustic emissions that are initially normal may later deteriorate, reducing the ability to assess sensory (versus neural) auditory function.

■ Auditory neuropathy may seriously affect multiple auditory measures (e.g., ABR, acoustic reflexes, behavioral audiometry) or may produce apparently isolated auditory dysfunction (e.g., desynchronous ABR abnormalities with normal findings on other audiologic procedures).

■ The mechanisms and pathophysiologic processes underlying auditory neuropathy are poorly understood.

■ Sites of lesion may be multiple in patients with auditory neuropathy, affecting one or more sensory regions (e.g., inner and/or outer hair cells) and multiple CNS regions.

■ There is little information on long-term audiologic, communicative, cognitive, and general neurologic outcome of infants presenting with auditory neuropathy patterns.

■ There is little information on the effects of amplification and cochlear implantation of children with auditory neuropathy and normal otoacoustic emissions.

AUDITORY NEUROPATHY:
Management

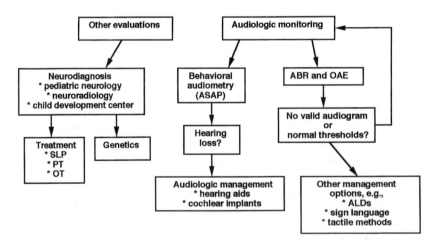

Figure 8–13. Management of auditory neuropathy, which is a multidisciplinary effort.

as sign language, should probably be considered only if responsiveness to auditory stimulation fails to develop with remediation efforts. Assistive listening devices to enhance, but not amplify, speech signals may also be appropriate in some cases. In children with auditory neuropathy, it would be quite reasonable to implement a management approach appropriate for a child with a peripheral (sensorineural) hearing loss, but initially without amplification.

Should children with auditory neuropathy ever be managed with hearing aids or cochlear implantation? There is little doubt that some children with auditory neuropathy have in the past been unwittingly managed with both hearing aids and cochlear implants. Among these children are those who did not obtain benefit from, or simply rejected, amplification. At this time, careful documentation of long-term outcome of children with auditory neuropathy, related to different management strategies, is lacking. Reported experiences suggest that, with evidence of hearing loss by audiometry, careful introduction of mild-gain amplification may be associated with improvement in speech and language development (e.g., Berlin et al., 1998). Berlin, Hood, and colleagues, who have collected considerable experience with pediatric auditory neuropathy note that: "So far we have seen no compelling evidence that hearing aids will help these children, but we are trying them cautiously with some patients whose parents are amenable, on the outside possibility that these problems are related to displaced or pathologic tectorial membranes and that increased displacement of the cochlear partition may lead to more productive shearing forces in the organ of Corti" (Berlin et al., 1998, p. 45). With or without amplification, cochlear status should be monitored periodically with OAEs, keeping in mind that over time OAEs may disappear spontaneously in auditory neuropathy. That is, subsequent absence of OAEs, especially, at all frequency regions, does not necessarily imply excessive amplification. In these children, ECochG measurement to document cochlear status would be helpful. Miyamoto et al. (1999) offered some guidance in stating that: "Although cochlear implantation may offer significant benefits to subjects with auditory neuropathy, caution should be exercised when considering this technology. As with conventional hearing aids, less than optimal results may be seen" (p. 185).

Case Reports

Case 1: Hyperbilirubinemia

A term infant at-risk for hearing impairment due to hyperbilirubinemia underwent ABR assessment in the nursery. ABR waves appeared to be recorded bilaterally (Figure 8–14) with single polarity (rarefaction) stimuli, and an attempt was made to calculate latencies for waves I, III, and V. The morphology of the ABRs, and the periodic nature of the components, was atypical. At a follow-up assessment 2 months later, the ABR was recorded with rarefaction and condensation polarity, and alternating polarity, click stimuli (Figure 8–15). Wave components were clearly opposite in phase for the two stimulus polarities, consistent with ECochG cochlear microphonic activity. An apparent ABR wave V was observed at a delayed latency. DPOAEs were recorded bilaterally on this test date (Figure 8–15), confirming outer hair cell function. On the next test date, at 7 months, (Figure 8–16) ABR measurement continued to show evidence of cochlear microphonic activi-

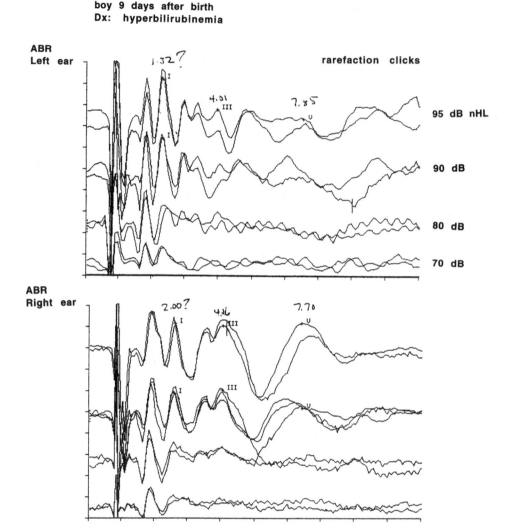

Figure 8–14. Auditory brainstem response (ABR) in the intermediate care nursery at 9 days after birth for an infant at risk for hearing impairment due to hyperbilirubinemia. The stimuli were rarefaction clicks presented to the left ear (*top*) and right ear (*bottom*) at the intensity levels indicated. The waveforms were initially interpreted as consistent with normal brainstem function. Markings of wave component latencies during the initial analyses are hand-written for each ear.

ty with abnormal brainstem functioning, and DPOAEs were observed. Also at 7 months, behavioral audiometry yielded pure tone and speech thresholds consistent with normal hearing sensitivity. DPOAE findings remained normal (Figure 8–17).

Comments. We regularly include OAEs in our pediatric test battery. In fact, OAE measurement is quickly becoming the standard-of-care (i.e., what reasonably prudent clinicians practice) in pediatric audiology. The information provided by OAEs is especially valuable for chil-

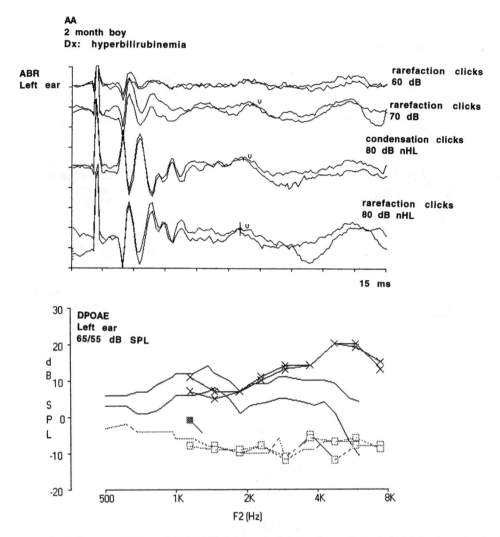

Figure 8–15. Follow-up ABR and DPOAE data at 2 months for an infant at risk for hearing impairment due to hyperbilirubinemia (Case 1). Only data for the left ear are shown (findings were equivalent for right ear stimulation). Waveforms are plotted separately for condensation and rarefaction polarity stimuli. Notice the phase reversal in wave components associated with polarity, consistent with a cochlear microphonic response rather than an ABR. These components were diminished with alternating polarity stimuli. DPOAEs with normal amplitudes (*lower portion*) suggested the diagnosis of auditory neuropathy.

dren with one or more risk factors associated with neurologic dysfunction (e.g., asphyxia, hyperbilirubinemia, meningitis, hydrocephalus, intraventricular hemorrhage). Hyperbilirubinemia is one of the most common diagnoses among children with auditory neuropathy. This case vividly illustrates that the presence of cochlear microphonics should be suspected whenever ABR measurement produces multiple, periodic waves with latencies inconsistent with those for waves I, III, and V, taking into account the patient's age for children 1.5 years and younger. OAE assessment is essential for the diagnosis and manage-

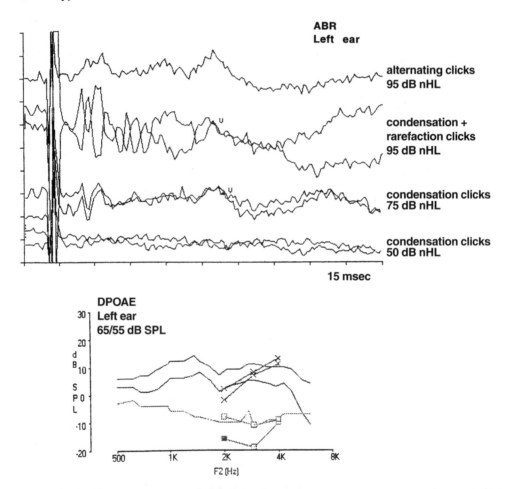

AA
7 month boy
Dx: hyperbilirubinemia

Figure 8–16. Later follow-up ABR and DPOAE findings at 7 months for the infant with hyperbilirubinemia continue to show evidence of the ECochG cochlear microphonic for single polarity stimuli, and a markedly abormal ABR with alternating polarity stimuli (Case 1). No ABR was detected for stimulus intensity levels less than 50 dB nHL. DPOAE amplitude (bottom portion) remained well within normal limits at selected stimulus frequencies, arguing against a sensory hearing loss despite the abnormal ABR findings.

ment of auditory impairment among children with abnormal ABR findings, as in this case. The conclusion that a hearing impairment is sensory cannot be made until OAEs are proven absent, with normal middle ear function. An abnormal ABR is not necessarily compatible with a sensorineural hearing loss. For children with normal OAEs and abnormal ABR findings, it is wise to delay audiologic management with hearing aids or cochlear implants until hearing is defined with behavioral audiologic techniques.

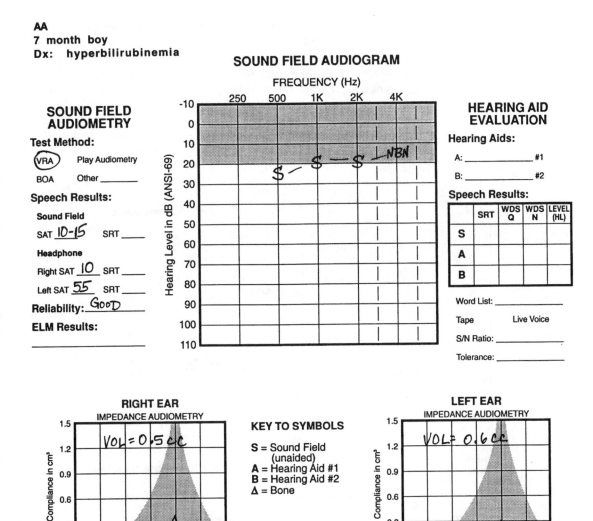

AA
7 month boy
Dx: hyperbilirubinemia

SOUND FIELD AUDIOGRAM

FREQUENCY (Hz)

SOUND FIELD AUDIOMETRY

Test Method:
(VRA) Play Audiometry
BOA Other _____

Speech Results:

Sound Field
SAT 10-15   SRT _____

Headphone
Right SAT 10   SRT _____
Left SAT 55   SRT _____
Reliability: GOOD

ELM Results:
_____

HEARING AID EVALUATION

Hearing Aids:
A: _____ #1
B: _____ #2

Speech Results:

	SRT	WDS Q	WDS N	LEVEL (HL)
S				
A				
B				

Word List: _____
Tape   Live Voice
S/N Ratio: _____
Tolerance: _____

RIGHT EAR
IMPEDANCE AUDIOMETRY
VOL = 0.5 cc

KEY TO SYMBOLS
S = Sound Field (unaided)
A = Hearing Aid #1
B = Hearing Aid #2
Δ = Bone

LEFT EAR
IMPEDANCE AUDIOMETRY
VOL = 0.6 cc

Figure 8–17. Behavioral audiometry findings at 7 months for the child with hyperbilirubinemia (Case 1) confirming hearing sensitivity within normal limits and in agreement with the normal DPOAEs, even though the ABR remained abnormal. The "S" symbols indicate sound-field (not ear specific) responses for warble tone signals. NBN = narrow band noise signal. SATs were 10 dB HL for the right ear and 55 dB HL for the left ear. Tympanometry was normal bilaterally.

Case 2: Multiple Risk Factors

An ABR was requested by pediatrics for an infant girl admitted to the hospital for management of hyperbilirubinemia. She was born prematurely (26-weeks gestational age), but the initial audiologic assessment was conducted at 40 weeks. The patient's history included four risk factors for hearing impairment: low birth weight, hyperbilirubinemia, asphyxia (low APGAR scores), and ototoxic medications (extended courses of treatment with gentimicin and furosemide). The first ABR measurement, made in the patient's hospital room, yielded markedly abnormal waveforms bilaterally for click and 500 Hz tone burst stimulation (Figure 8–18). Although there were no recognizable components, a broad wave was observed in the region of wave I. In view of the risk factors for central auditory nervous system dysfunction (asphyxia and hyperbilirubinemia), OAEs were also recorded at bed-

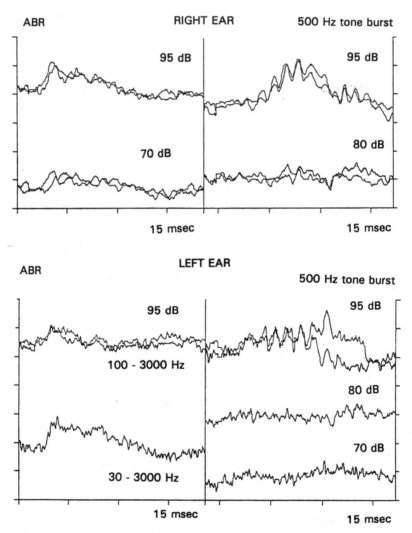

Figure 8–18. ABR results at 40 weeks gestational age for an infant born at 26 weeks gestational age (Case 2). ABR was recorded at bedside in the patient's hospital room. She was at risk for hearing impairment due to hyperbilirubinemia, asphyxia, prolonged mechanical ventilation, and ototoxicity. No clear ABR waves were recorded in either ear for rarefaction click stimuli, with the exception of a poorly formed component in the early latency region. An alternating polarity 500 Hz tone burst stimuli produced evidence of periodic activity, but only at a high intensity level.

side. Noise levels were suboptimal, yet a reliable DPOAEs was detected bilaterally for several stimulus frequencies (Figure 8–19). This admittedly limited information raised doubt about the likelihood of a severe sensorineural hearing loss. A chart note report recommended follow-up audiologic assessment in 3 months to monitor possible changes (improvement or worsening) of auditory status before management was implemented. Dramatic reversal of hearing loss and return to apparently normal auditory function has been documented in infants with the diagnosis of hyperbilirubinemia and asphyxia (Hall et al., 1985). Progression of hearing loss is associated with ototoxicity, as noted in the section on ototoxicity below. Not being familiar with OAEs and the concept of auditory neuropathy, the physicians caring

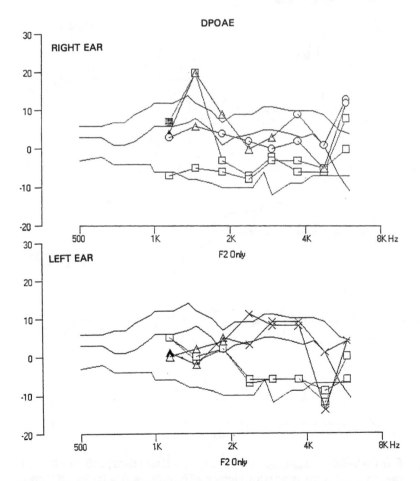

Figure 8–19. DPOAE findings (recorded at bedside) for the premature infant with multiple risk factors (Case 2). Although there was excessive measurement noise, DP amplitudes were reliably recorded within normal adult limits for selected test frequencies, providing some evidence of cochlear integrity and ruling out the severe-to-profound sensorineural hearing loss suggested by ABR results.

for the patient expressed confusion about the report of mixed findings for DPOAE versus ABR assessments, and questioned whether hearing would improve or worsen over time.

The patient returned for audiologic assessment at 3 and then 6 months. ABR and OAE findings for the latter visit are illustrated in Figure 8–20 and 8-21. No ABR was detected, but there was clear evidence of cochlear microphonic responses within several milliseconds after the single polarity click stimulation (Figure 8–20). DPOAEs were clearly

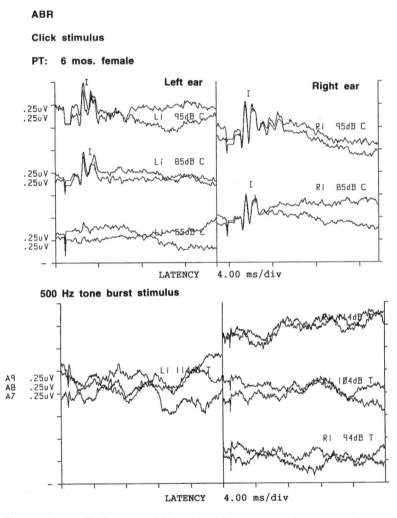

Figure 8–20. Follow-up ABR results (third test date) at 6 months corrected age for the premature infant with multiple risk factors (Case 2) with rarefaction polarity click stimuli, and alternating polarity 500 Hz tone burst stimuli. No ABR was observed in either ear for rarefaction click stimuli or alternating polarity tone burst stimuli. The early latency components were interpreted as cochlear microphonic activity.

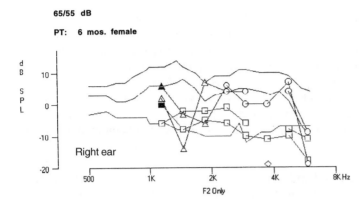

65/55 dB

PT: 6 mos. female

Right ear

F2 Only

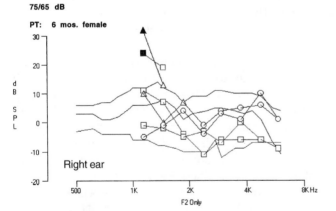

Left ear

F2 Only

A

75/65 dB

PT: 6 mos. female

Right ear

F2 Only

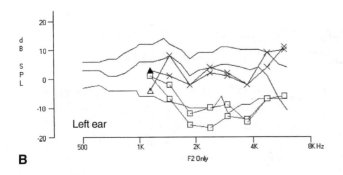

Left ear

F2 Only

B

Figure 8–21. A. Follow-up normal DPOAE findings (at 6 months) recorded with stimuli at $L_1 = 65$ and $L_2 = 55$ dB for the premature infant (Case 2) with multiple risk factors. Findings again offered evidence of cochlear integrity and argued against a sensorineural hearing loss despite the absence of a reliable ABR. However, DPOAE amplitudes for the left ear fell below normal limits. **B.** Follow-up normal DPOAE findings (at 6 months) recorded with slightly higher stimulus intensity protocol a ($L_1 = 75$ and $L_2 = 65$ dB) for the premature infant (Case 2) with multiple risk factors. Findings ruled out serious sensorineural hearing loss despite the absence of a reliable ABR.

recorded bilaterally (Figure 8–21). With the confirmation of the auditory neuropathy pattern of findings, a comprehensive neurodiagnostic and developmental work-up and a speech-language consultation, was recommended. The patient was referred, via her pediatrician, to the Child Development Center. Because behavioral audiometry could not yet be completed, the decision was made to defer audiologic management. Comprehensive and multidisciplinary testing resulted in the diagnoses of cerebral palsy, language impairment, and general developmental delay.

Valid behavioral audiometry findings were obtained when the patient was 13 months (corrected age), as shown in Figure 8–22. Sound field and ear specific thresholds to selected pure-tone signals were within the normal region, as were speech awareness thresholds (SATs). Tympanograms were also normal. Repeat DPOAE assessment continued to confirm normal cochlear (outer hair cell) functioning (not shown). With the support of the child's pediatrician who shared my curiosity about the possibility of a reversal in the abnormal ABR, the mother agreed to one more ABR evaluation with sedation. On this test date, however, ABR findings were markedly abnormal (Figure 8–23), showing no evidence of any waves nor the previously observed cochlear microphonic. Periodic audiologic follow-up continues to confirm normal hearing sensitivity and normal DPOAEs. Cortical auditory evoked response assessment has not been conducted, and sophisticated speech audiometry is not yet possible. The patient receives speech-language and physical therapy services at a local developmental center.

Comments. In years past, this child might have been fit with a hearing aid at 3 to 6 months of age on the basis of the ABR findings, and with the presumption of a sensorineural hearing loss. It is wise clinical policy, however, to delay amplification and other management options (e.g, cochlear implantation) until a hearing impairment is confirmed with behavioral audiometry. Meanwhile, comprehensive neurodiagnostic and developmental evaluations are warranted. In most cases, these efforts will result in one or more diagnoses related to nervous system dysfunction. Pure auditory neuropathy, without associated involvement of other regions of the brain, is probably very unlikely.

HEARING SCREENING: PRESCHOOL AND SCHOOL-AGED CHILDREN

The potential for applying OAEs in screening hearing of preschool and school-aged children is readily apparent from the review of OAEs in newborn hearing screening. Advantages of OAEs include sensitivity to middle ear and cochlear auditory dysfunction (pure-tone screenings may miss middle ear dysfunction), short test time, relative tech-

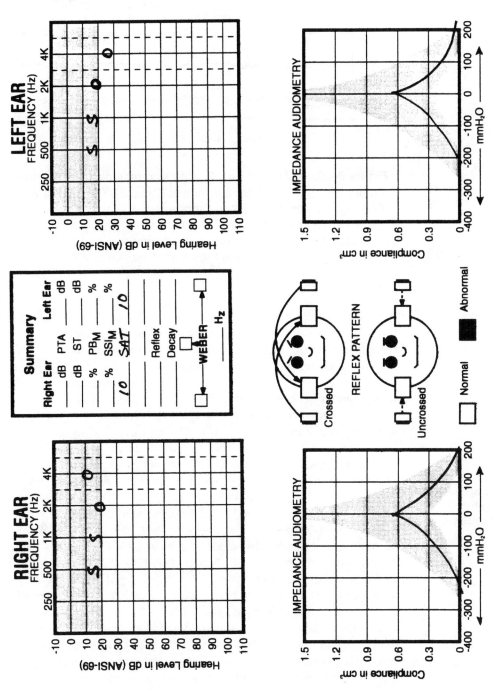

Figure 8–22. Behavioral audiometry findings at 13 months for a premature infant (Case 2) with multiple risk factors. Previous attempts at behavioral assessment of hearing had been unsuccessful. Sound-field ("S") and ear-specific responses to pure-tone signals were observed at intensity levels within normal limits. A speech awareness threshold (SAT) of 10 dB HL was recorded bilaterally. Tympanometry was normal bilaterally. DPOAE amplitudes continued to be observed within normal limits on this test date.

461

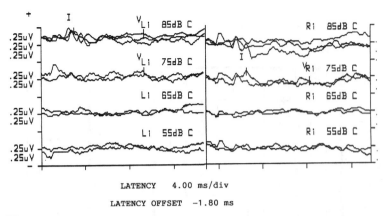

Figure 8–23. ABR results at 13 months corrected age for the premature infant with multiple risk factors (Case 2). The patient was sleeping with sedation (chloral hydrate). No ABR was observed in either ear for rarefaction click stimuli or alternating polarity tone burst stimuli, even though hearing was normal audiometrically and DPOAEs were observed less than 1 week earlier.

OAEs have great potential as an inexpensive and sensitive technique for periodic hearing screening of school-aged children.

nical simplicity of performing the procedure (versus pure-tone hearing screening), and objectivity (no behavioral response). In addition to these features, OAE recording does not require a sound-treated room. According to informal reports of manufacturers representatives in the United States, audiologists are frequently performing hearing screenings in public schools and in preschool settings, such as Head Start programs. However, there are few systematic studies of OAEs in school-aged children (Decreton et al., 1991; Prieve, 1992; Nozza et al., 1997). Nozza, Sabo, and Mandel (1997) assessed TEOAE data in relation to findings for pure-tone hearing screening, tympanometry, and otoscopic examination for a series of 66 children aged 5 to 10 years. After delineating the limitations of tympanometry and pure-tone screening, the authors' noted that "it would be to everyone's advantage if there were a single test that was brief, objective, and easy to administer and tolerate that could identify reliably those who should be referred for further testing" (Nozza et al., 1997, p.237). Many of the findings of this thorough investigation were specific to the TEOAE device (ILO 88) and the test performance of various analyses criteria (e.g., whole reproducibility values of 40 or 50%, or the 5th percentiles of normative data). There was also a detailed analysis and discussion of existing criteria and techniques for hearing screening, in addition to OAEs. The authors discussed factors contributing to false-positive OAE screening errors, including high levels of ear canal noise. Middle ear status was not associated with false-positive OAE outcomes. The possibility of false-negative OAE findings in, for example, children with undedected auditory neuropathy was not noted, although one child who failed the pure-tone screening criterion showed some evidence of TEOAE activity. Preliminary data from school hearing screenings suggest that a small proportion of students will pass OAE screening but fail pure-tone screening, although for most the hearing impairment is longstanding and appropriately managed audiologically. Still, the issue of false-negative OAE screening outcomes should be formally assessed. Also, the combination of tympanometric and OAE technology (see Chapter 10) would appear to have considerable utility in school-age screening, and warrants investigation. In any event, the results of the Nozza et al. (1997) study confirmed that, with proper analysis criteria, OAEs have adequate sensitivity and specificity as a measure of hearing screening in the school-aged population. Test performance for OAEs was, in fact, superior to previously recommended screening protocols (ASHA, 1990).

MONITORING COCHLEAR FUNCTION IN OTOTOXICITY

Because of their sensitivity to disruptions in metabolic processes within the cochlea, OAEs are extremely well-suited for monitoring the cochlear function of patients treated therapeutically with potentially ototoxic drugs. Some of the more common medications with known ototoxicity are listed in Table 8–25. A complete review of ototoxicity would be very lengthy. The reader is referred to the voluminous scientific literature, mostly found in audiology and otolaryngology journals, as well as several excellent reviews published in monographs or textbook chapters (see Table 8–26). At least three principles of ototoxicity are very relevant to the meaningful clinical application of OAEs. The incidence of ototoxic effects varies among drugs and even for specific drugs among patients. A variety of factors can influence the strength or likelihood of ototoxicity, especially concomitant exposure to other drugs, renal function, and age. The latter variable is extremely important clinically. There is a growing body of evidence indicating that sensitivity to ototoxicity is increased during periods when cochlear function is developing. This interesting topic is reviewed in detail by Henley and Rybak (1995). As these authors clearly stated,

The risk indicator for ototoxicity recommended by the Joint Committee on Infant Hearing accounts for almost one third of the newborn infants who are at risk for hearing loss.

> Normal physiological development of resting potentials (the endocochlear potential) and sound-evoked potentials including cochlear microphonics, summating potentials, compound action potentials, auditory brainstem responses and more recently distortion product otoacoustic emissions . . . all of these responses are significantly impaired following acoustic trauma and/or exposure to a variety of ototoxic agents including aminoglycoside antibiotics, loop diuretics, antithyroid and antitumor drugs (α-difluoromethylornithine) and excitatory amino acids. Coupled with physiological and anatomic development is the maturation of specific biochemi-

Table 8–25. Common ototoxic drugs.

Drug	General Therapeutic Application(s)
Aminoglycoside Antibiotics	Treatment of infections
■ Amikacin	
■ Gentamicin	
■ Kanamycin	
■ Livodomycin	
■ Neomycin	
■ Netilmicin	
■ Sisomycin	
■ Streptomycin	
■ Obramycin	
Antineoplastic Drugs	Treatment of cancer and tumors
■ Cisplatin	
■ Carboplatin	
■ Nitrogen mustard	
Diuretics and Loop Diuretics	Treatment of congestive heart failure, pulmonary edema
■ Furosemide (lasix)	
■ Ethacrynic acid	
■ Bumetanide	
Salicylates	Treatment of arthritis, rheumatic fever, and connective tissue disorders
■ aspirin	
Quinine	Treatment of malaria, treatment of leg cramps
Deferoxamine	Iron-overloaded patients who require multiple blood transfusions
Environmental Chemicals	
■ arsenic	
■ mercury	
■ tin	
■ lead	
■ manganese	

cal pathways, which may be vulnerable targets of environmental noise and chemicals, excitatory amino acids, and therapeutic drugs with ototoxic potentials. (p. 68)

Second, the deleterious effects of otototoxic drugs on auditory status, including OAEs, may be delayed after administration, or may persist for days and even weeks after the drug therapy is discontinued. Third, DPOAE abnormalities in ototoxicity, particularly for high-frequency stimuli, may be detected prior to changes in auditory-evoked responses and the pure-tone audiogram. Some fundamental ototoxic mechanisms are summarized for selected major drugs in Table 8–27.

Table 8–26. Selected references and reviews on ototoxicity (arranged topically and chronologically).

Early Studies

Schutz A., Bugie E, Waksman SA. Streptomycin, a substance exhibiting antibiotic activity against gram-positive and gram-negative bacteria. *Experimental Biology and Medicine 55:* 66–69, 1944.

Hawkins JE. Cochlear signs of streptomycin intoxication. *Journal of Pharmacologic Therapy 100:* 38–41, 1950.

Stebbins WC, Miller JM et al. Ototoxic hearing loss and cochlear pathology in the monkey. *Annals of Otolaryngology, Rhinology, and Laryngology 78:* 1007–1019, 1969.

Schwartz GH, David DS et al. Ototoxicity induced by furosemide. *New England Journal of Medicine 282:* 1413–1414, 1970.

Fleishmann RW, Stadnick SW et al. Ototoxicity of cis-dichlorodiamineplatinum (II) in the guinea pig. *Toxicology and Applied Pharmacology 33:* 320–332, 1975.

Fee WE. Aminoglycoside ototoxicity in the human. *Laryngoscope 90:* Supplement 24, 1980.

General References

Stringer SP, Meyerhoff WL, Wright CG. Ototoxicity. In Paparella MM, Shurnrick DA, Gluckman JL (eds). *Otolaryngology* (3rd ed). Philadelphia: WB Saunders, 1991, p. 1653.

Rybak LP, Matz GJ. Effects of toxic agents. In Cumming CW (ed). *Otolaryngology—Head and Neck Surgery* (2nd ed), Volume 4. St. Louis: Mosby Year Book, 1993, p. 2943.

Rybak LP (ed). Ototoxicity. *The Otolaryngology Clinics of North America 26* (5), 1993.

Henley CM, Rybak LP. Ototoxicity in developing mammals. *Brain Research Reviews 20:* 68–90, 1995.

Riggs LC, Matz GJ, Rybak LP. Ototoxicity. In Bailey BJ (ed). *Head and Neck Surgery— Otolaryngology* (2nd ed). Philadelphia: Lippincott- Raven Publishers, 1998, pp. 2165–2170.

High Frequency Audiometry

Jacobsen EJ, Downs MP, Fletcher JL. Clinical findings in high-frequency thresholds during known ototoxic drug usage. *Journal of Auditory Research 9:* 379–385, 1969.

Fausti SA, Rappaport BZ. Detection of aminoglycoside ototoxicity by high frequency auditory evaluation: Selected case studies. *American Journal of Otolaryngology 5:* 177–182, 1984.

Fausti SA, Rappaport BZ (eds). High frequency audiometry. *Seminars in Hearing 6,* 1985.

The primary objective of ototoxicity monitoring is to document early evidence of cochlear dysfunction, preferably prior to the appearance of audiometric hearing loss. In some cases, this information leads to a change in medical management, such as limited doses of the drug, a change in therapy to an alternate drug, and the prevention or reduced severity of ototoxicity. When planned therapy is mandatory, early detection of hearing loss may contribute to more effective parent/patient counseling and prompt audiologic management, including the implementation of amplification and assistive listening device.

Table 8–27. Mechanisms of ototoxicity.

Aminoglycosides

■ Cochlear damage is by a toxic metabolite (with contribution from the liver).

■ Drugs cause calcium antagonism and blockage of ion channels.

■ Maternal inheritance may play a role.

■ Toxic effects may be delayed or prolonged.

■ Some drugs (e.g., Glutathione) may block toxin formation or increase detoxification and prevent aminoglycoside ototoxicity.

Cisplatin

■ Morphologic, biochemical, and electrophysiologic basis of toxicity is not known.

■ Considerable differences in individual susceptability.

■ More severe in pediatric populations.

■ May be inhanced by prior cranial irradiation.

■ Effects documented for stria vascularis and organ of Corti.

■ Outer hair cell degeneration, plus changes in supporting cells and Reissner's membrane.

Loop Diuretics

■ Act on epithelial cells in the loop of Henle of the kidney.

■ Among 8 different types, furosemide (or Lasix) is the most common.

■ Direct effects on the stria vascularis.

■ Changes in outer hair cells.

   ✔ Impairment of oxidative metabolism.

   ✔ Splaying of stereocilia.

   ✔ Breakage of tip links and cross-links between stereocilia.

■ Effects on auditory function include:

   ✔ Reduced sharpness in tuning curves.

   ✔ Reduced cochlear potentials.

   ✔ Depressed ECochG and ABR.

   ✔ Reduced or absent OAEs.

Aminoglycosides

Background

For over 50 years, aminoglycoside antibiotics have been a first-line therapy for bacterial infection, especially for infection due to gram-negative aerobic bacilli micro-organisms. Examples of aminoglycoside antibiotics include netilmicin, amikacin, neomycin, streptomycin, kanamycin, tobramycin, and gentamicin. The later two drugs are quite popular for the medical management of patients often evaluated by audiologists. Gentamicin, for example, is extremely common as a therapeutic agent, or as a prophylatic precaution, for neonatal infections in the NICU. Tobramycin is a standard therapy in children afflicted with cystic fibrosis. Some of these antibiotics, such as streptomycin and gentamicin, are also highly vestibulotoxic.

The general pathophysiologic processes in ototoxicity with aminoglycoside antibiotics are well-appreciated and supported by the findings of hundreds of animal experiments and clinical histopathologic studies. Biochemical changes secondary to aminoglycoside ototoxicity may be acute, affecting calcium and ion channel metabolism of membranes in the cochlea, producing structural damage in the inner ear. The outer hair cells, and supporting cells, show dysfunction and then structural damage beginning in the base and progressing apically. Histopathologic studies and electron microscopy following ototoxicity with some aminoglycoside drugs in neonatal animal models show outer hair cell degeneration, initially in the extreme base of the cochlea (nearest the stapes footplate), with subsequent progression through the basal, medial, and finally apical regions. Among the outer hair cells, degeneration proceeds from the first to the second and then to the third rows (Lerner & Matz, 1979; Leake et al., 1997). As noted below, the ototoxic effects of aminoglycoside are augmented or strengthened by the administration of loop diuretics (e.g., furosemide), cisplatin, and ethacrynic acid, either simultaneously or within a relatively narrow time frame when both categories of drugs remain in the perilymph of the cochlea (Brummet, 1980; Riggs et al., 1996).

There is mounting evidence from industrial investigations that excessive exposure to environmental chemicals, such as solvents, can cause hearing loss with or without concomitant noise exposure.

Parallel to these processes is sensory hearing impairment, beginning with the highest frequencies and extending toward the lower frequencies. The relative strength of ototoxicity, and therefore the incidence of hearing loss with drug administration, varies among aminoglycosides (Fee, 1980). The exact biochemical mechanisms of ototoxicity are now being more clearly delineated. An important new discovery is that some aminoglycosides, such as the commonly used gentamicin, interact with (bind with or chelate) iron, forming an oxidative (redox-active) compound that can then contribute to the formation of free radicals. Free radicals are commonplace during normal biochemical activities in the normal organism, especially respiration. They typically are neutralized or dispensed with by various enzymes and other scavengers (e.g., vitamin E and vitamin C). However, free radicals are also involved in various types of tissue damage in the body through their oxidative activities with proteins (including DNA) and other targets (Halliwell & Gutteridge, 1986). Where there is inflammation, neurodegenerative disorders, neurotoxicity, and many other disease processes, free radicals are usually part of the problem. Currently intensive basic auditory research is being directed toward prevention of ototoxicity by harnessing the potential benefit of the free radical scavengers and the early disruption of the interaction between gentamicin and iron (Song & Schacht, 1996). These research efforts are likely to produce clinically feasible treatments for aminoglycoside ototoxicity. OAEs may play a powerful role in the early detection of such ototoxicity, and the prevention of debilitating auditory deficits.

OAEs

There are numerous animal investigations and clinical studies documenting the detection of aminoglycoside ototoxicity with TEOAEs and DPOAEs, as listed in Table 8–28. These papers also confirm the advantages of OAE over behavioral audiometry in these patient populations. Namely, OAE measurement is typically fast and objective (feasible even with very young or sick patients for whom valid behavioral assessment cannot be performed). OAEs are used to monitor auditory status in patients with a variety of infections and other diseases. An example of a patient group is cystic fibrosis, where *Pseudomonas* chest infections are common (Mulheran & Degg, 1997). The study by Mulheran and Degg (1997) highlights one limitation in the interpretation of clinical findings. It is not always possible to parcel out whether changes in OAEs observed in patient populations are secondary to ototoxicity of a certain drug or, in part, due to the cochlear effects of the disease itself. The possibility that ototoxic effects may extend well beyond (weeks and even months) discontinuance of drug administration, demonstrated previously with ABR (Hall et al., 1986; Hall et al., 1987), is also confirmed by studies with OAEs (e.g., Kakigi et al., 1998).

Vancomycin

Background

This non-aminoglycoside antibiotic, first introduced about 40 years ago, has developed a reputation as ototoxic, although there is no clear evidence that vancomycin acting alone (without concomitant exposure to other ototoxic drugs) causes cochlear damage. This point is illustrated below by a child who received an overdose of vancomycin and underwent auditory monitoring with DPOAEs. Because vancomycin is effective in the treatment of methicillin-resistant *Staphylococcus aureus* gram-negative ("staph-resistant") infections, the therapeutic application of vancomycin has increased in recent years as more micro-organisms have become resistant to some of the more popular antibiotics.

Case 3

There are no published papers describing OAE findings in patients treated therapeutically and exclusively with vancomycin. The author

Table 8–28. Publications on otoacoustic emissions (OAEs) and ototoxicity. Full citations are available in the bibliography.

Drug Category	TEOAEs	DPOAEs
aminoglycosides	Kakiga et al. (1998)	Brown et al. (1989)
		Henley et al. (1990)
		Whitehead et al. (1992)
		Holtz et al. (1994)
		Kumagai (1995)
		Henley et al. (1996)
		Mulheran & Degg (1997)
		Kakiga et al. (1998)
furosemide (Lasix)	Anderson & Kemp (1979)	Martin et al. (1998)
	Anderson (1980)	Frolenkov et al. (1998)
	Ueda et al. (1992)	Mills et al., (1993)
		Whitehead et al. (1992)
		Mills & Rubel (1994)
		Kemp & Brown (1984)
aspirin	McFadden & Plattsmier (1984)	Long & Tubis (1988)
	Johnsen & Elberling (1982)	Weir et al. (1988)
		Long et al. (1986)
		Brown et al. (1993)
		Stypulkowski & Oriaku (1991)
		Kemp & Brown (1984)
		Fitzgerald et al. (1993)
		Kujawa et al. (1992)
quinine	Alvan et al. (1991)	Berninger et al. (1994)
	Karlsson et al. (1991)	Stypulkowski & Oriaku (1991)
	Karlsson et al. (1995)	McFadden & Pasanen (1994)
	Berninger et al. (1994)	
	Berninger et al. (1998)	
cisplatin	Yardley et al. (1998)	Sie & Norton (1997)
	Norton (1993)	McAlpine & Johnstone (1990)
	Lonsbury-Martin et al. (1995)	
	Zorowka et al. (1993)	
	Plinkert & Krober (1991)	
	Allen et al. (1998)	
carboplatin	Yardley et al. (1998)	Trautwein et al. (1996)
		Jock et al. (1996)
		Wake et al. (1996)
		Hofstetter et al. (1997)
ethacrynic acid		Whitehead et al. (1992)

has had the opportunity to perform serial OAE recordings from a preterm infant mistakenly given 10 times the appropriate dose of vancomycin (at an outlying hospital). DPOAE measurement was initially conducted within 24 hours of the drug overdose and then again two and six months later. DPOAE amplitudes for stimulus frequencies of 2000 to 8000 Hz were consistently well-above the adult normal region at the first test session (Figure 8–24). Notice the remarkable reduction in noise levels for the lower frequency region when the infant was quieted by nursing. Sucking and associated muscle movement around the mouth introduces excess measurement artifact during ABR recordings. In contrast, it appears that these activities do not adversely influence OAEs. Follow-up DPOAE measurement (Figure 8–25) confirmed normal cochlear (outer hair cell) functioning bilaterally. Subsequent behavioral audiometry at 6 months (not shown) confirmed normal hearing sensitivity bilaterally throughout the audiometric frequency region. This case suggests that vancomycin is not invariably ototoxic, at least when administered in isolation (with no other ototoxic medications). Over a 13-year period, the author has evaluated with ABR and behavioral audiometry two other children who received excessive dosages of vancomycin, but no other potentially ototoxic drugs. Neither showed any evidence of hearing loss, at least as verified by repeat testing up to 6 months after the initial administration of the drug.

Two ototoxic drugs administered in combination can be more damaging to cochlear function than either drug alone.

Furosemide (Lasix)

Background

The ototoxic effects of the clinically common loop diuretic furosemide (Lasix) on cochlear function are well known, although the exact incidence of hearing impairment is not clear (see Rybak, 1993, for review). Furosemide specifically interferes with stria vascularis physiology with a resulting decrease in the endocochlear potential (e.g., Kusakari et al., 1978). The endocochlear potential is a fundamental source of energy within the cochlea. Consequently, furosemide can have a direct effect on outer hair cell active processes (motility), such as the mechano-electrical transduction (see Chapter 2 for details) and electrophysiologic events, such as OAEs, cochlear microphonics, and the action potentials underlying the ABR wave I (Sewell, 1984; Ruggero & Rich, 1991). Importantly, the disruption of cochlear function by systemic furosemide administration is reversible and is not necessarily associated with permanent damage to the organ of Corti (e.g., Rybak, 1982). As noted above, the combined exposure to furosemide and aminoglycosides can produce a synergistic ototoxic effect, with more cochlear damage than would be predicted for exposure to either drug alone. For example, aminoglycosides in combination with furosemide

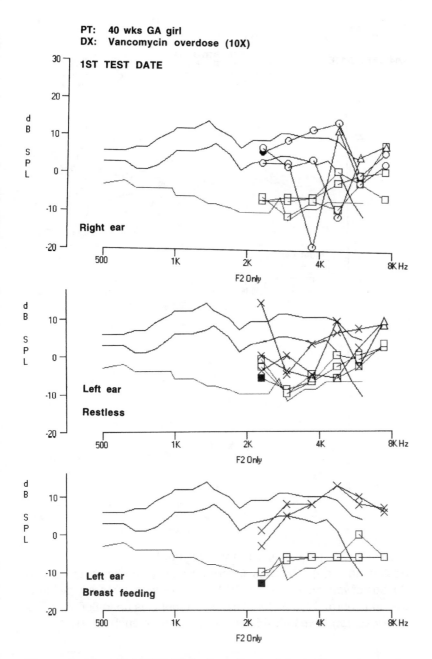

Figure 8–24. Initial DPOAE findings for an infant (40 weeks gestational age) who was incorrectly given 10 times the proper dosage of vancomycin (Case 3). As testing began, the infant was restless and measurement was contaminated by excessive noise. DPOAEs were then discretely recorded as the baby was nursing. Amplitudes (shown for left ear only) were generally within or above the adult normal region for stimulus frequencies up to 8000 Hz. Notice the markedly reduced measurement noise during the first recording when the baby was nursing. Test time was approximately 45 seconds per ear on each test date.

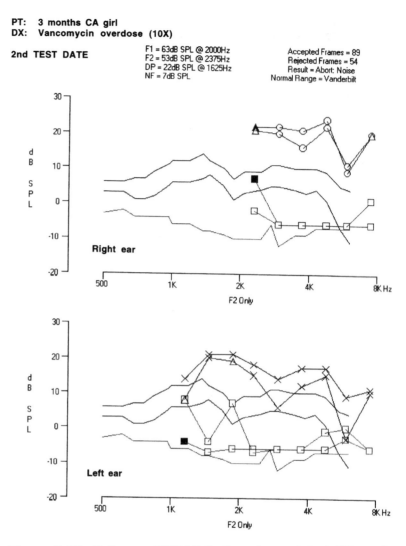

PT: 3 months CA girl
DX: Vancomycin overdose (10X)

2nd TEST DATE

F1 = 63dB SPL @ 2000Hz
F2 = 53dB SPL @ 2375Hz
DP = 22dB SPL @ 1625Hz
NF = 7dB SPL

Accepted Frames = 89
Rejected Frames = 54
Result = Abort: Noise
Normal Range = Vanderbilt

Figure 8–25. Follow-up DPOAE findings for an infant (40 weeks gestational age) who was incorrectly given 10 times the proper dosage of vancomycin (Case 3). Amplitudes were generally far above the adult normal region for stimulus frequencies up to 8000 Hz. Test time was approximately 45 seconds per ear on each test date.

can greatly increase the severity and reduce the time frame of ototoxic auditory dysfunction. There is some evidence that the dual effect of these drugs also contributes to deficits in both inner and outer hair cell function (Mulheran & Harpur, 1998). There is clear evidence that furosemide as administered therapeutically can cause hearing loss in neonates (Brown et al., 1991), and the drug is specified within the ototoxicity risk factor by the JCIH.

OAEs

Experimental investigations confirm the detection of transient fu-
rosemide-induced cochlear deficits with TEOAEs. In a study with
guinea pigs, Ueda et al. (1992) reported that TEOAE amplitude and
reproducibility rapidly decreased with intravenous injection of furosemide, but totally recovered within 60 minutes. Temporary reduction
in amplitude with complete return to normal has also been documented for DPOAEs in rabbits and gerbils (Mills et al., 1993; Martin et al.,
1998). The reversibility of OAE changes appears to be related primarily to the effect of furosemide on the source of the energy supplied to
the outer hair cells (the endocochlear potential generated by the stria
vascularis), rather than direct functional or structural changes in the
outer hair cells. Indeed, DPOAE amplitude reductions parallel those
of the EP (Mills et al., 1993). Consistent with findings for other types of
cochlear insults, such as excessive noise, OAE abnormalities are greatest for relatively low stimulus intensity levels, whereas at least DPOAE
findings may appear normal at very high stimulus intensity levels.
Absence of an ototoxic effect for high intensity stimuli has been attributed to energy from passive versus active processes within the cochlea.
Interestingly, studies of DPOAEs using suppression tuning curve
strategies (see Chapter 4 for details) fail to show changes in tip threshold, best tip frequency, and the Q_{10}, even though DPOAE amplitudes
were reduced by up to 20 dB SPL (Martin et al., 1998). Also, the effects
of furosemide as determined by DPOAEs vary substantially for emissions at different frequency places. For example, the emissions at $2f_1-f_2$
and $2f_1-f_2$ may be more susceptible to effects than those at $2f_2-f_1$ (Mills
et al., 1993), at least in rabbits.

Cisplatin

Background

Cisplatin (cis-diamine-dichloroplatinum II or CDDP) is a major therapeutic weapon for tumors (an antineoplastic drug) of the genitouri-
nary tract, lung, neck, and head. With children undergoing chemotherapy for brain tumors, cisplatin is usually administered in single doses
approximately every 4 weeks. Even a single dose of cisplatin can cause
auditory dysfunction, as detected audiometrically or electrophysiologically (e.g., ECochG, ABR, or OAE). However, despite the unequiv-
ocal ototoxicity of cisplatinum, the reported incidence of hearing loss
is highly variable (Waters et al., 1991), probably in part due to differences in audiometry techniques and sensitivity. Even unilateral hearing loss in cisplatin ototoxicity has been reported (Strauss et al., 1983).
The variable effects on hearing are, in part, because of confounding
factors in clinical studies (e.g., doses, method of administration, cranial radiation, other drugs, and patient age), which probably augment
the effects of the drug or are independently related to cochlear deficits.

There is general agreement, however, that the ototoxicity of cisplatin is rarely reversible. As with aminoglycosides, cisplatin affects outer hair cells, first in the basal turn of the cochlea, with possible damage also to the stria vascularis and spiral ganglion cells (Meech et al., 1998). Thus, cisplatin administration typically produces a high-frequency permanent sensory hearing impairment, although patterns of impairment may vary among individuals, as illustrated in the following case report. As with aminoglycosides, recent basic investigations have yielded some promising evidence that cisplatin ototoxicity can be minimized or prevented with the administration of other drugs (e.g., Church et al., 1995; Rybak et al., 1995; Campbell et al., 1996; Kaltenbach et al., 1997; Kopke et al., 1997; Stengs et al., 1998).

OAEs

DPOAEs are a sensitive measure of cochlear changes secondary to cisplatin exposure (McAlpine & Johnstone, 1990; Sie & Norton, 1997). In some animal experiments and clinical studies, abnormalities in OAEs following cisplatin injection have been detected earlier than those for pure-tone audiometry or ABR (Plinkert & Krober, 1991; Zorowka et al., 1993; Sie & Norton, 1997), although this observation is not invariable (Yardley et al., 1998) and is dependent on the frequency region of the stimulus, the time interval between test sessions, individual differences in susceptability to the drug, and other factors. The type of OAE used to monitor cisplatin ototoxicity may be a consideration, given the progression of deficits from higher to lower frequencies. The use of DPOAEs with high-frequency stimuli (up to 10,000 Hz or higher if possible) appears to offer more sensitivity to cochlear dysfunction than TEOAEs, which have a frequency upper limit of 5000 Hz. Also, there is some evidence that changes in DPOAEs may be delayed or may persist, for days after administration of cisplatin.

Case 4

Following clinical policy established jointly by a pediatric oncologist and audiology, an 8-year-old boy with an inoperable brainstem tumor underwent audiologic assessment immediately before each course of chemotherapy that included cisplatin. Serial monthly audiograms, illustrated in Figure 8–26, initially confirmed normal hearing sensitivity for all audiometric frequencies from 250 to 8000 Hz. DPOAE amplitudes were well within adult normal limits (Figures 8–27 and 8–28). On the third test date, audiometric findings were unchanged, with the exception of a very mild decrease in the threshold for an 8000-Hz signal presented to the right ear. The patient was rather lethargic at this point in the assessment, and the validity of this threshold was questioned. On DPOAE measurement (Figure 8–29), however, the data clearly showed a marked decrease in amplitudes, and a notching deficit pattern, for frequencies above 6000 Hz. The DPOAE pattern was remarkably similar to that for pure-tone audiometry at the next

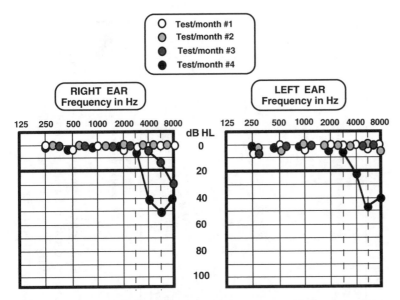

Figure 8–26. Serial audiograms for a 8-year-old boy receiving cisplatin for an inoperable brain tumor (Case 4). Note the slight decrease in hearing sensitivity at 8000 Hz for the right ear on the third test date, and the clear high-frequency notching sensory hearing deficit bilaterally on the fourth test date.

visit (refer back to test 4 in Figure 8–26). Left ear DPOAEs remained normal and unchanged from baseline data. Subsequent audiometric follow-up showed progression of the hearing loss, and total loss of DPOAEs, bilaterally. This case illustrates the sensitivity of OAEs in early detection of ototoxic-induced hearing loss.

Carboplatin

Background

Their names are similar but their effects are distinctly different. Cisplatin damages outer hair cells whereas carboplatin affects inner hair cells.

A sister drug to cisplatin, carboplatin (cis-diamine-1, 1-cyclobutane dicarboxylate platinum [II], or CBDCA) is also an antineoplastic agent used therapeutically for cancerous tumors. At high doses, carboplatin is ototoxic (van der Hulst et al., 1988), causing a high-frequency hearing loss. In sharp distinction to cisplatin, which damages outer hair cells, carboplatin exerts its ototoxic effects on the inner hair cells (Hofstetter et al., 1997).

OAEs

Recent investigations confirm that, even at high doses, carboplatin does not alter OAE parameters. The ototoxic effects are almost entirely limited to inner hair cells, sparing outer hair cells (Jock et al., 1996;

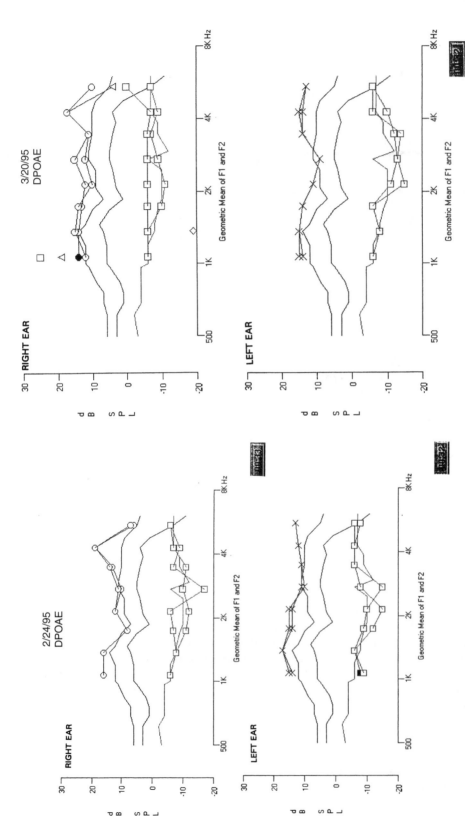

Figure 8–27. DPOAE findings on the first test date for a 8-year-old boy receiving cisplatin for an inoperable brain tumor (Case 4) showing entirely normal amplitude values for stimulus frequencies up to 6500 Hz. Stimulus intensity levels were L_1 = 65 dB; L_2 = 55 dB. Test times are shown for each ear.

Figure 8–28. DPOAE findings on the second test date for a 8-year-old boy receiving cisplatin for an inoperable brain tumor (Case 4), again showing entirely normal amplitude values for stimulus frequencies up to 6500 Hz.

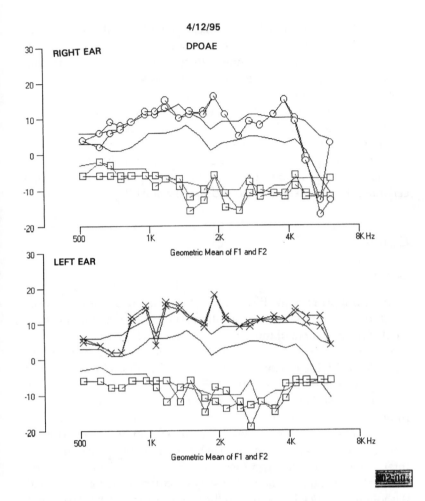

Figure 8–29. DPOAE findings on the third test date for a 8-year-old boy receiving cisplatin for an inoperable brain tumor (Case 4). DPOAE amplitudes for the right ear were decreased in comparison to the previous test for stimulus frequencies about 4000 Hz, producing a notching pattern with no evidence of DP activity at approximately 6000 Hz. Stimulus intensity levels were again $L_1 = 65$ dB; $L_2 = 55$ dB. Note the similarity between these DPOAE data and the right ear audiogram 1 month later (Test 4 in Figure 8–26). DPOAE findings for left ear stimuli remained normal on this test date.

Trautwein et al., 1996; Hofstetter et al., 1997; Harrison, 1998; Yardley et al., 1998). This preferential cochlear effect of carboplatin is, in fact, now being exploited to study in detail the contribution of outer versus inner hair cells to OAE generation (Hofstetter et al., 1997). DPOAEs, at least, appear to be essentially independent of even massive destruction of inner hair cells. Only with very high doses of carboplatin, in animal experiments, are there slight changes in DPOAEs. Histopathologic study of the cochlea in such cases reveals outer hair cell damage limited to the base of the cochlea. There is some suggestion that with carboplatin-induced damage to inner hair cells (and sparing of outer hair cells), TEOAE amplitude might actually be modestly enhanced (Wake et al., 1996). The obvious clinical implication of the almost exclusive effect of carboplatin on inner hair cells is that OAEs are of no value in monitoring potential ototoxicity. Prior to deciding on a protocol for monitoring ototoxicity, it is essential to verify the drug(s) the patient will be receiving. If one of the drugs is carboplatin, then the protocol should include audiologic measures that are dependent on inner hair cell integrity, such as pure-tone audiometry or ABR.

Quinine

Background

Quinine is a primary medical therapy for malaria, although in developed countries this clinical application is now rare. It is still, however, used in the treatment of muscular disorders, such as leg cramps. Documentation of the ototoxicity of quinine dates back hundreds of years. Audiologic/otologic symptoms include tinnitus first and then hearing loss up to a maximum of about 45 dB HL, both of which can be reversed within 3 to 4 days if quinine is discontinued even after administration for up to a week at high doses (Paintaud et al., 1994). Cochlear effects of quinine, which are dependent on plasma concentration, include alteration of basilar membrane mechanics and interuption of the active processes (motility) of outer hair cells (Karlsson et al., 1991). It is unlikely that stria vascularis function is affected. Although superficially similiar in the type (sensory) and degree (mild-to-moderate) of hearing loss, there are clear differences in the ototoxic influences of quinine versus salicylates on cochlear function, and in their effect on OAEs.

OAEs

Although both quinine and aspirin affect outer hair cell motility and, therefore, OAEs, the onset and recovery of OAE changes are faster for quinine than aspirin (McFadden & Pasanen, 1994). The effects of quinine on OAE are apparent within several hours of the initial dose (a standard tablet of 325 mg). Elevations in OAE threshold and decreases in OAE amplitude parallel changes in the shape of psychoacoustic tuning curves, such as increased threshold for the characteristic frequency (Karlsson et al., 1991; Berninger et al., 1998). These alterations in auditory function are associated with increased loudness recruitment (Berninger et al., 1998).

Salicylates (Aspirin)

Everyday aspirin is a drug with known ototoxicity as documented by histopathologic studies, and confirmed by investigations utilizing OAEs. Patient history should always include a question about the use of aspirin, especially when tinnitus is a symptom or OAE findings are abnormal. Aspirin's characteristic effect on hearing is a flat sensory hearing loss, which may be reversible several days after the drug is discontinued (Myers et al., 1965). The author regularly encounters patients, usually presenting with complaints of tinnitus, who are taking aspirin at the recommendation of their primary care physicians or rheumatologists who advise the patients to "increase the dosage until they notice ringing in the ears."

OAEs

There is long-standing evidence that aspirin temporally alters OAEs (see Table 8–28), usually with total reversal within days after the drug is discontinued. Unfortunately, dosage as a factor in OAE alterations has not been systematically investigated clinically. As with other ototoxic drugs, however, the effects of aspirin on auditory function (including DPOAEs) are highly variable among patients (Brown et al., 1993).

OTHER PEDIATRIC APPLICATIONS OF OAEs

For the reasons reviewed earlier in this chapter, OAEs are a valuable component of the pediatric test battery. It is not suprising, therefore, that they are now applied in the audiologic assessment of children with a variety of diagnoses (see Table 8–29). To objectively and precisely define cochlear (outer hair cell) status, the clinician should routinely include OAEs in the audiologic test battery for patients with diagnoses of autism, pervasive developmental disorders (PDDs), central auditory processing disorders (CAPD), along with infants and difficult-to-test children, those receiving potentially ototoxic drugs, and possible malingerers. The result is a more accurate and timely description of auditory status, which in turn contributes directly to more effective management. In addition, as experience with OAEs in children accumulates and findings are closely analyzed in the context of other audiologic and neurodiagnostic data, we will learn more about numerous neuroaudiologic pathologies. To find an example of this dividend of OAEs, one needs to look no further than the literature on auditory neuropathy.

Table 8–29. Reports of otoacoustic emissions in varied pediatric pathologies. Papers describing OAEs in children with auditory neuropathy are noted in Table 8–21.

Pathology	Study (Year)	Comments
Autism	Grewe et al. (1994)	
HIV	Christensen et al. (1998)	
Miliary tuberculosis	Stach et al. (1998)	
Cleft lip/palate	Anteunis et al. (1998)	
Johanson-Blizzard syndrome	Rosanowski et al. (1998)	
Down syndrome	Hassmann et al. (1998)	
Middle ear effusion	Choi et al. (1999)	
Meningitis	Fortnum et al. (1993) Francois et al. (1997) Richardson et al. (1998)	OAEs are highly sensitive but not as specific in detection of hearing loss following meningitis.
Mondini deformity	Cullington & Brown (1998)	OAEs present with later diagnosis of profound SNHL
Cochleosaccular degeneration (Scheibe degeneration)	Lalwani et al. (1997)	OAEs absent consistent with SNHL
Hereditary nonsyndromic autosomal recessive progressive hearing loss	Hall et al. (1997)	OAEs absent in affected family members
Central auditory processing disorder	Hall et al. (1992) Hall et al. (1996) Hall & Mueller (1997)	OAEs effectively rule out peripheral auditory dysfunction

CHAPTER

9

Clinical Applications of Otoacoustic Emissions in Adults

There are varied and valuable OAE applications in adults (see Table 9–1). A major and obvious rationale for recording OAEs in children is the sometimes limited information available from behavioral measures, especially the audiogram. For most adults, in contrast, a valid audiogram is easily obtained. Two clinical advantages of OAEs in pediatric populations—site-specificity of OAEs to auditory dysfunction and the high degree of sensitivity specifically to cochlear impairment—are equally important in adult patients. As an example of the sensitivity advantage, there is now mounting evidence that noise- or music-induced cochlear damage is detectable with OAEs before it becomes apparent in the audiogram. And the many virtues extolled for OAEs as a tool for monitoring ototoxic auditory dysfunction in children extend as well to very sick adults. The site-specificity of OAEs in adults is perhaps most vividly demonstrated by patients with sensorineural hearing loss and suspected retrocochlear pathology. Is the

Table 9–1. Selected clinical applications of OAEs in adult populations with rationales for their use.

Application	Rationale
Assessment in suspected functional hearing loss	✓ OAEs not dependent on patient behavioral response ✓ Normal OAEs invariably imply normal sensory function ✓ OAEs provide frequency-specific audiologic information
Differentiation of cochlear vs. retrocochlear auditory dysfunction	✓ OAEs are site-specific for cochlear (sensory) auditory ✓ Dysfunction in combination with ABR, OAEs can clearly distinguish sensory versus neural auditory disorders
Monitoring ototoxicity	✓ OAEs are site-specific for cochlear (sensory) auditory dysfunction ✓ Ototoxic drugs exert their effect on outer hair cell function; OAEs are dependent on outer hair cell integrity ✓ OAE recording not dependent on patient behavioral response; can be recorded from patients who, due to their medical condition, are unable to perform behavioral audiometry tasks ✓ OAEs can detect cochlear dysfunction before by pure-tone audiometry ✓ OAEs provide frequency-specific audiologic information
Tinnitus	✓ OAEs are site-specific for cochlear (sensory) auditory dysfunction ✓ OAEs can provide objective confirmation of cochlear dysfunction in patients with tinnitus and normal audiograms ✓ OAEs provide frequency-specific audiologic information, which may be associated with the frequency region of tinnitus
Noise/music exposure	✓ OAEs are site-specific for cochlear (sensory) auditory dysfunction ✓ Excessive noise/music intensity levels affect outer hair cell function; OAEs are dependent on outer hair cell integrity ✓ OAEs can provide objective confirmation of cochlear dysfunction in patients with normal audiograms ✓ OAEs findings are associated with cochlear frequency specificity, i.e., "tuning"; musician complaints of auditory dysfunction can be confirmed by OAE findings, even with a normal audiogram ✓ OAEs can provide an early and reliable "warning sign" of cochlear dysfunction due to noise/music exposure, before any problem is evident in the audiogram

loss purely sensory (cochlear), purely neural (retrocochlear), or does it involve both sensory and neural structures? This question can be confidently and quickly answered when OAEs are used in combination with a neural measure (e.g., the ABR). In other almost exclusively adult clinical entities, such as Ménière's disease, it appears that OAEs have value in differentiating among pathophysiologic processes in patients with comparable clinical presentations. In short, there is a clear rationale for the application of OAEs in adults.

NOISE- AND MUSIC-INDUCED HEARING LOSS

Background

Basic Science

A prerequisite to understanding the pathophysiology of noise-induced cochlear dysfunction is an understanding of normal cochlear physiology. The topic is summarized in Chapter 2 or, better yet, review one or more of the key references listed at the end of Chapter 2.

Considerable basic research in small animal models, such as chinchilla, guinea pig, gerbil, rabbit, cat, and chicken, has confirmed the unique sensitivity to noise-damaged cochlea of OAEs, especially DPOAEs (Schmiedt, 1986; Franklin et al., 1991; Kim et al., 1992; Canlon et al., 1993; Subramaniam et al., 1995; Hamernik, Ahroon, & Lei, 1996; Trautwein et al., 1996; Hamernik et al., 1998; Iwasaki, Mizuta, & Hoshino, 1998; White et al., 1998). DPOAEs have assumed an important role as an electrophysiologic index of the cochlear status in experiments involving exposure to noise and other potentially damaging insults, and possible protection of the cochlea by prior noise exposure or drugs (e.g., White et al., 1998). However, the correlation among OAEs, audiometric threshold changes, and cochlear damage as indicated by outer hair cell populations is inexact.

Clinical Applications

Diagnostic Assessment

The relatively greater sensitivity of OAEs to cochlear dysfunction is exemplified clinically by the reports of abnormal or absent OAEs among patients with normal audiograms (Table 9–2). The relation between OAEs and the audiogram was discussed in Chapter 6. The conventional assumption underlying clinical interpretation and certain applications, such as newborn hearing screening, is that the presence of OAEs implies hearing thresholds better than about 30 dB HL. Conversely, absence of OAEs suggests some degree of hearing loss, presuming normal middle ear function. There is clearly, however, a third possibility. An early stage of noise-induced auditory dysfunction is characterized by OAE abnormalities—confirming some cochlear dysfunction or damage—and normal or near-normal hearing sensitiv-

Table 9–2. Clinical papers on miscellaneous applications of OAEs in adult auditory pathologies and dysfunction.

Pathology	Type of OAE	Study, Year	Comment
Noise-induced dysfunction	TEOAE	Fabiani, 1993	Reduced amplitude provides early evidence of loss
	TEOAE	Reshef et al., 1993	OAEs were sensitive measure of cochlear damage
	TEOAE	Attias et al., 1995	OAE abnormalities even with normal audiogram
	TEOAE	Lucertini et al., 1996	Correlation between OAEs and pure-tone findings in NIHL
	TEOAE	Lucertini et al., 1998	Correlation between OAEs and audiogram
	TEOAE	Hatzopoulos et al., 1998	OAEs sensitive to NIHL with sophisticated analysis
	DPOAE	Sutton et al., 1994	Lower stimulus intensities and $L_1 > L_2$ increase sensitivity
	TEOAE; DPOAE	Musiek et al., 1994	Reduced OAE amplitude with hearing loss
	DPOAE	Engdahl, 1996	Exercise increases noise effects on OAEs
	DPOAE	Attias et al., 1998	At high stimulus levels, DPOAEs less useful
	DPOAE	Jurgens et al., 1999	Mathematical model for predicting audiogram from DPOAEs
	TEOAE; DPOAE	Vinck et al., 1999	Sensitivity of DPOAEs and TEOAEs to TTS
	DPOAE	Delb et al., 1999	Study of optimal test protocols for increased sensitivity
Music-induced dysfunction	TEOAE	Perrot et al., 1999	Stronger bilateral efferent influences in musicians
	DPOAE	Hall & Santucci, 1996	DPOAEs in clinical evaluation of musicians
	DPOAE	Hall & Mueller, 1998	Sensitivity of OAEs to music-induced auditory dysfunction
	DPOAE	Hall & Bulla, 1999	Diagnostic value of DPOAEs in musicians and audio engineers
Ménière's disease	SOAE	Haginomori et al., 1998	SOAE in hearing loss region and in contralateral ear
	TEOAE	Haginomori et al., 1995	Lidocaine changed TEOAEs in Ménière's disease
	TEOAE	Fabiani, 1993	OAE changes with glycerol testing
	TEOAE	Harris & Probst, 1992	Findings atypical of other sensory types of hearing loss
	TEOAE; DPOAE	Musiek et al., 1994	Some hearing-impaired patients have robust OAEs
	TEOAE; DPOAE	van Huffelen et al., 1998	Differentiation of Ménière's types with OAEs
	SOAE	Ceranic et al., 1998	High SOAE prevalence and reduced prevalence in Ménière's
	DPOAE	Ohlms et al., 1991	Atypical OAE findings in some patients
	DPOAE	Sakashita et al., 1998	Changes in DPOAE I/O functions in Ménière's disease
	DPOAE	Kusaki et al., 1998	I/O functions more valuable than DPgram
Pseudohypacusis	TEOAE	Musiek et al., 1995	OAEs contribute to objective assessment of status
	TEOAE; DPOAE	Musiek et al., 1994	OAEs are a quick procedure for verification of malingering
	TEOAE	Robinette, 1992	OAEs help confirm malingering

(continued)

Table 9–2. *(continued)*

Pathology	Type of OAE	Study, Year	Comment
Presbycusis	TEOAE	Fabiani, 1993	Decreased amplitude with age-related hearing loss
	TEOAE	Bonfils et al., 1988	
	TEOAE	Collet et al., 1990	Decreased OAE amplitude with age-related hearing loss
	TEOAE	Stover & Norton, 1993	SOAEs and TEOAEs studied
	TEOAE	Castor et al., 1994	Presbycusis and contralateral stimulation study
	DPOAE	Karzon et al., 1994	Correlation between DPOAEs and age-related hearing loss
	DPOAE	Lonsbury-Martin et al., 1991	Decreased amplitude in age-related hearing loss
	TEOAE; DPOAE	Musiek et al., 1994	OAEs are decreased with hearing loss
	TEOAE	Prieve & Falter, 1995	No age effect with normal hearing
	DPOAE	Nieschalk et al., 1998	Signs of potential presbycusis in middle-aged subjects
Sudden idiopathic hearing loss	TEOAE	Hinz & Wedel, 1984	OAEs absent with hearing loss greater than 30 dB HL
	TEOAE	Sakashita et al., 1991	Relation between OAEs and changes in hearing status
	TEOAE	Truy et al., 1993	Correlation between OAEs and hearing loss limited
	TEOAE; DPOAE	Nakamura et al., 1997	Monitoring recovery with OAEs
	DPOAE	Ohlms et al., 1991	OAEs observed in a patient with profound hearing loss
Retrocochlear lesions	TEOAE	Bonfils & Uziel, 1988	Some patients with acoustic tumors have normal OAEs
		Patuzzi, 1993	Review article
	TEOAE	Uziel, 1990	Few patients show normal OAEs
	TEOAE	Cane et al., 1992	Intraoperative monitoring of cochlear function with OAEs
	TEOAE	Robinette, 1992	Mixed TEOAE findings in retrocochlear lesions
	TEOAE	Cane et al., 1994	OAEs can be present with retrocochlear hearing loss
	TEOAE	Hatzopoulos et al., 1998	Normal OAEs in some patients with retrocochlear loss
	TEOAE	Prasher et al., 1996	Suppression effects reduced in retrocochear pathology
	TEOAE	Norman et al., 1996	High rate OAEs different for retrocochlear vs. normals
	TEOAE	Ferger-Viart et al., 1998	79% of 168 patients had no TEOAEs before tumor removal
	DPOAE	Ohlms et al., 1991	Differentiation of cochlear vs. retrocochlear loss with OAEs
	DPOAE	Telischi et al., 1995	Monitoring cochlear function intraoperatively
	TEOAE; DPOAE	Musiek et al., 1994	Discrepancies are noted between audiogram and OAEs
Tinnitus	SOAE	Penner, 1989	Attempt to reduce SOAE-related tinnitus with aspirin
	SOAE	Penner, 1990	SOAE perception as tinnitus

Condition	OAE type	Citation	Finding
Tinnitus *(continued)*	SOAE	Plinkert et al., 1990	SOAE study on origin of tinnitus
	SOAE	Penner & Coles, 1992	Aspirin used to treat tinnitus due to tinnitus
	SOAE	Burns & Keefe, 1991	Unstable SOAEs in tinnitus may be related to perception
	TEOAE	Norton et al., 1990	Relation of tinnitus with OAEs
	TEOAE	Chery-Croze et al., 1994	Abnormal OAEs with normal audiogram in tinnitus
	TEOAE	Chery-Croze et al., 1996	Study of medial olivocochlear system with suppression
	TEOAE	Graham & Hazell, 1996	Increased variability of suppression in tinnitus patients
	TEOAE; SOAE DPOAE	Liu et al., 1996	Most tinnitus patients had abnormal TEOAEs and DPOAEs
	DPOAE	Chery-Croze et al., 1993	Contralateral stimulation and DPOAE in tinnitus
	DPOAE	Janssen et al., 1998	DPOAEs highly varied in tinnitus
	TEOAE; DPOAE	Ceranic, 1995	Review article
	TEOAE; SOAE	Ceranic et al., 1998	Increased TEOAE amplitude in head-injury tinnitus
	SOAE	Ceranic et al., 1998	Higher frequency variability in SOAEs in tinnitus patients
	DPOAE	Shiomi et al., 1997	Abnormal DPOAEs in normal hearing tinnitus patients
	DPOAE	Mueller & Hall, 1998	DPOAEs correlated with tinnitus frequency
	DPOAE	Ruth & Hall, 1999	DPOAEs more sensitive than audiogram in tinnitus patients
Genetic hearing loss	TEOAE	Morell et al., 1998	Hearing loss related to connexin 26 gene in Ashkenazi Jews
	DPOAE	Ohlms et al., 1991	OAE abnormalities consistent with degree of hearing loss
	DPOAE	Hall et al., 1997	OAEs detect subclinical inherited sensory hearing loss
	DPOAE	Cohn et al., 1999	OAEs useful in diagnosis of loss related to connexin 26 gene
	TEOAE	Butinar et al., 1999	OAE in evaluation of hereditary motor and sensory peripheral neuropathy
Critically ill patients	DPOAE	Hamill-Ruth et al., 1998	OAEs are an efficient screening technique in this population
Thyroid hormone depletion	DPOAE	Mra & Wax, 1999	Decreased OAEs with thyroxin depletion
Head injury	SOAE	Ceranic et al., 1998	High prevalence of SOAEs in head-injured tinnitus patients
Myasthenia gravis	TEOAE	Toth et al., 1998	OAE amplitudes were lower in MG
Acquired immunodeficiency syndrome (AIDS)	TEOAE	Soucek & Michaels, 1996	Reduced OAE amplitudes in AIDS
King-Kopetzky syndrome	TEOAE	Zhao et al., 1996	Study of contralateral suppression

ity, implying less than complete outer hair cell damage. This pattern is especially associated with noise- or music-induced auditory dysfunction and tinnitus (e.g., Desai et al., 1999). Animal research confirms that scattered OHC damage, perhaps less than 20% of the total OHC population, is not always evident in pure-tone threshold measurements (Bohne & Clark, 1982). Then, as the proportion of OHCs damaged exceeds some critical level (e.g., 25 to 30%), permanent threshold shift can be documented. Because OAEs are now a rather common clinical audiologic measure, their absence with a normal audiogram can no longer be considered a "subclinical auditory impairment." OAEs in children and adults also offer the desirable feature of objectivity. This feature is an advantage in young and difficult-to-test children where the validity of behavioral measures is sometimes questionable. Not all adults, however, graciously and willingly volunteer valid pure-tone thresholds. Therefore, the feature of objectivity is very much an advantage in selected adults as well. For this reason, it is reassuring to have experimental documentation that OAEs accurately reflect noise-induced changes in patients with behaviorally measured normal auditory thresholds (e.g., Franklin et al., 1991).

Monitoring Noise Damage with OAEs

"Noise-induced hearing loss, although not medically or surgically treatable, is the major preventable cause of hearing impairment in the United States."
Dobie RA. Noise-induced hearing loss. **Head & Neck Surgery— Otolaryngology (2nd ed).** *Bailey BJ (ed). Philadelphia: Lippincott-Raven Publishers, 1998, p. 2162.*

The multiple advantages of OAEs—sensitivity, site-specificity, objectivity, and speed—all come to bear in monitoring for noise-induced hearing loss (e.g, Probst, Harris, & Hauser, 1993). Although the cost-effectiveness of this approach has not been systematically studied, it is reasonable to presume that time saved during, for example, industrial auditory screenings with OAEs versus behavioral testing would translate into cost savings. Data in support of OAEs as a quick and sensitive index of noise-induced auditory dysfunction is mounting (Hotz et al., 1993; Reshef et al., 1993; Attias et al., 1995; Attias et al., 1998). One model for including OAEs in hearing conservation programs as a tool for monitoring cochlear status is illustrated in Figure 9–1. This model assumes that pure-tone audiometry remains the standard, or at least the traditional, measure of hearing sensitivity. That is, calculations of the percentage of hearing impairment, and decisions regarding possible compensation for hearing impairment, are made with audiometric data. OAEs, however, can be employed exclusively to monitor cochlear status until changes are observed. DPOAEs are especially well-suited as a monitoring tool because the frequency range (at least 8000 and sometimes higher) extends up to and beyond the region affected by overexposure to noise. Thus, the lower and higher frequency "skirt" of the classic noise-induced notch in hearing thresholds (in the 3000- to 6000-Hz region) can be confidently defined. At that time, pure-tone audiometry is performed as usual to define the extent and configuration of hearing loss.

In contrast to the voluminous literature on OAEs hearing screening of infants and, to a lesser extent, older children, there are to date few papers addressing the topic of hearing screening in adult populations. Lucertini, Bergamaschi, and Urbani (1996) applied TEOAEs as a measure of auditory function for adult males being evaluated medically for recruitment into the Italian Air Force. TEOAEs were recorded with the ILO 88 device from 30 normal and 83 hearing-impaired subjects. The etiology of hearing loss was cochlear in all cases. As the authors acknowledged, with the ILO 88 device it was not possible to investigate cochlear status for audiometric frequencies higher than 4000 Hz (see Chapter 4 for the explanation), yet a sizable proportion of their subjects had hearing loss above 5000 Hz or, as expected, greatest hearing loss within the 3000- to 6000-Hz region. Unfortunately, the authors limited their analysis of TEOAE to overall intensity (echo level), spectrum, and reproducibility rather than frequency-specific response parameters. Also, most data analysis was limited to whether TEOAEs were simply present or absent, rather than a quantification of TEOAE amplitude or reproducibility as a function of hearing loss. Although the authors did analyze response spectrum, it was, in their words, "a

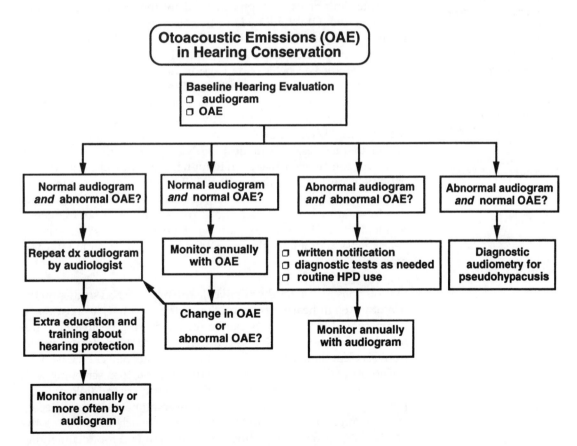

Figure 9–1. A possible approach for integrating OAEs into a hearing conservation program, taking advantage of their sensitivity to noise-induced cochlear dysfunction, their objectivity, and relatively brief test time.

qualitative assessment, based on the visual inspection of the spectral tracings," and only for subjects with reproducibility values of 60% or more. This reproducibility value was selected by the authors as the criterion for response presence. Perhaps because of the analysis strategy taken by the authors, the results of the study were somewhat disappointing in that "TEOAE detectability could not be considered in our population as a valuable method for separating normal from hearing impaired ears" (p. 83).

Attias et al. (1998) investigated the clinical efficacy of DPOAEs as a tool for screening for noise-induced hearing impairment in 76 military personnel. DPOAEs were recorded with an ILO 92 device at a stimulus intensity level of 70 dB SPL for both primaries ($L_1 = L_2 = 70$ dB SPL). DPOAE amplitude was significantly reduced, and DPOAEs more often not detectable, in persons with a history of noise exposure with normal audiograms versus normal hearers with a negative history for noise. The authors did observe apparent DPOAEs in some cases with hearing losses of up to 75 dB HL. However, close inspection of the data collection and analysis approach used by the authors raises some questions about this finding. First, there is experimental evidence that lowering the stimulus intensity levels to 50 to 55 dB, and utilizing a intensity relation in which $L_1 - L_2 = 10$ or 15 dB, sensitizes DPOAEs to the noise-induced cochlear damage in humans (e.g., Sutton et al., 1994). Data were reported for the DPOAE-noise floor difference, rather than absolute DPOAE amplitude. The instances of apparent DPOAEs in serious hearing loss were mostly in the high-frequency stimulus region (4000 Hz and above). Noise floors are invariably lowest in the higher frequencies, so a modest DP-NF difference (5 dB or less, as reported) can be calculated even though the absolute DP amplitude is extremely low (e.g., less than -10 dB SPL). Also, as discussed in detail elsewhere (Chapters 4 and 6), the likelihood of artifactual DPOAE data due to standing wave interference is greatest in the higher frequency region. It would be useful to know whether any subjects with sensory hearing loss audiometry showed DPOAE amplitudes within the normal region.

There are numerous references and sources of information on hearing conservation regulations and guidelines. In the United States, you might contact:
National Hearing Conservation Association (NHCA)
9101 East Kenyon Ave., Suite 3000
Denver, CO 80237
or
The Council for Accreditation in Occupational Hearing Conservation
611 East Wells Street
Milwaukee, WI 53202

One obvious reason for the relative dearth of published studies on the use of OAEs in hearing conservation is the ease and, in most cases, accuracy with which adults can be screened using behavioral puretone-based techniques. Noise-induced hearing loss clearly results from cochlear damage, specifically affecting outer hair cells. Given the sensitivity of OAEs to outer hair cell dysfunction, then screening with OAE would seem to be of potential value in industrial audiology, occupational medicine, and/or hearing conservation programs. Recognized regulations for hearing conservation, such as those of the OSHA-1983, specify the audiogram as the standard for documenting hearing status. These policies were developed painstakingly over a long period of time. The criteria for temporary and permanent threshold shift . . . noise-induced hearing loss . . . have profound and far-reaching vocational, governmental, health, and monetary implications. In all likelihood, these criteria and reliance on the audiogram as the standard of hearing will not be meddled with for many years. As reviewed in some detail in Chapters 2 and 4, OAEs will, for anatomic as well as practical reasons, never supplant the basic audiogram as the conventional measure of hearing sensitivity. There are at least a half-dozen logical and predictable explanations for discrepancies between the audiogram and OAE findings. In some cases, the audiogram can show abnormal hearing threshold levels when OAEs are entirely normal. In other cases, the audiogram may be entirely within clinically normal limits, but OAEs are unequivocally abnormal and consistent with cochlear dysfunction. It is not difficult to imagine the chaos and upheaval in industrial settings or in the military if the finding of abnormal OAEs at one or more test frequencies was accepted as the sole criteria for definition of hearing impairment. The financial implications alone, for calculating compensation and determining disability ratings, are staggering.

Attempts to refine OAEs as an objective measure of hearing sensitivity and hearing loss are futile. However, there is already ample evidence from hundreds of studies that OAEs can be successfully applied as a technique for screening auditory function. In varied pediatric and adult populations, OAEs offer a quick, objective, and very sensitive tool for differentiating normal versus abnormal cochlear (outer hair cell) function. It is quite possible that OAEs will asssume an important role in the early identification of noise-induced hearing loss in various settings and as an objective "cross-check" to the pure-tone audiogram.

Temporary Threshold Shift (TTS)

TTS caused by exposure to moderate-to-high levels of sound is associated with changes in the amplitude and frequency content of TEOAEs (Kemp, 1982) and DPOAEs (Schmiedt, 1986; Martin et al., 1987; Subramanian et al., 1994). Return of OAEs with resolution of TTS is illustrated by a case report at the end of this section.

Noise and Exercise

Temporary threshold shift (TTS) with noise exposure is increased by exercise. The exact mechanism is unclear, but among the factors that might be involved are the amount of metabolic activity (and metabolic exhaustion), body temperature (more TTS with increased temperature), and the release of biochemicals during exercise. The enhancing effects of exercise on TTS are also reflected by greater decrease in DPOAE amplitude. Engdahl (1996) conducted a study of eight normal hearing adults (three women and five men) with DPOAEs recorded for relatively low intensity stimuli ($f_1 = 55$ dB and $f_2 = 40$ dB). Exercise

"DPOAE I/O functions may reveal discrete pathological alterations both in the active cochlear signal processing and the passive mechanisms of the cochlea prior to their detection by clinical audiometric tests" (p. 83). Nieschalk M, Hustert B, Stoll W. Distortion-product otoacoustic emissions in middle-aged subjects with normal versus potentially presbycusic high-frequency hearing loss. **Audiology 37: 83–99, 1998.**

In evaluating the effects of noise on cochlear function, the possible effects of aging should also be taken into account. The literature on OAEs in aging is reviewed in Chapter 5.

on a stationary bicycle produced a heart rate approximating 60% of maximal oxygen update. Third-octave band noise of 102 dB SPL was presented by an audiometer for 10 minutes. DPOAE amplitude was reduced by noise exposure alone, in the frequency region of the noise, with recovery over a 20-minute period. The authors found no significant correlation between TTS and reduced DPOAE amplitude, consistent with TEOAE findings reported earlier from their laboratory, possibly because the TTS was minimal. Physical exercise alone had no effect on auditory threshold or DPOAE findings. Noise exposure during exercise produced more TTS and DPOAE amplitude reduction than noise alone.

Music-Induced Cochlear Damage

"How sweet the moonlight sleeps upon this bank!
Here we will sit, and let the sounds of music Creep in our ears: soft stillness and the night Become the touches of sweet harmony."

William Shakespeare (1564–1616)

The Merchant of Venice [1596–1597]

The Impact of Exposure to Music Versus Noise

Excessive exposure to any sound leads to a shift in hearing threshold. The effect is determined by the intensity, frequency content, and temporal nature of the sound (i.e., intermittent, continuous, etc.), not by whether the sound is appealing and pleasant versus annoying and obnoxious to the listener (Bulla & Hall, 1998; Hall & Bulla, 1999). Music and noise, of course, produce sound-induced auditory dysfunction. A number of investigators have studied audiometrically the effect of music exposure on hearing. The music genre (e.g., rock and roll, classical, or country music) is irrelevant (e.g., Behroozi, 1997). Risk to hearing is as great for orchestral musicians (e.g., Royster, Royster, & Killion, 1991) as for rock and rollers (e.g., Dibble, 1995). For example, Axelsson and Lindgren (1977, 1981) examined pure-tone hearing thresholds in a population that included disk-jockeys, entertainment artist managers, live-sound engineers, and musicians. Sensorineural hearing loss was documented in 13 to 30% of their population, depending on the criteria used to define hearing loss. Similarities among the characteristics of hearing loss in musicians and industrial workers confirms that excessive exposure to music can effect the ear as much as industrial noise exposure. Furthermore, music-induced hearing loss can affect anyone in the industry, not just performing or studio musicians. Most studies of the auditory effects of cumulative exposure to loud music emphasize live-performance musicians and their audiences or conductors of bands and orchestras. Audio engineering professionals employed in recording studio activities are also at risk for hearing impairment. Audio engineers often must listen for prolonged periods of time at sometimes excessive sound levels. These professionals are frequently exposed every day to sound levels exceeding Department of Defense (DOD) criteria for acceptable noise exposure (Bulla & Hall, 1998; Hall & Bulla, 1999). Music-induced hearing loss, and cochlear dysfunction, as documented by DPOAEs, in an audio engineer are illustrated later in a case study.

Audiologic assessment of musicians and other professionals in the music industry should focus on early identification of any auditory dysfunction. OAEs are the most effective tool to meet this clinical objective. The major steps in the early detection and effective management of music-induced hearing loss are summarized in Figure 9–2. OAEs are a key component in this strategy. Patients often come to the

AUDIOLOGIC ASSESSMENT OF MUSIC PROFESSIONALS

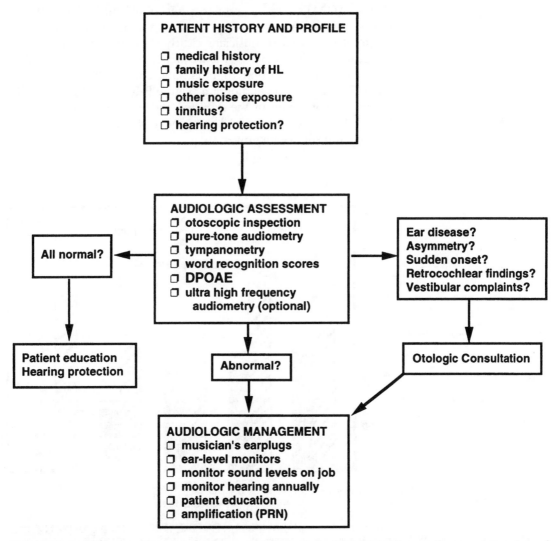

Figure 9–2. Major components of a program for early detection, diagnostic assessment, and audiologic management of music-induced auditory dysfunction and hearing impairment. OAEs play a crucial role in the early identification of cochlear dysfunction, in patient counseling, and in monitoring cochlear status.

hearing care professional expecting a cure—a magic pill—for music-induced hearing loss. However, prevention is the only viable treatment. By closely monitoring professionals at risk for auditory dysfunction with OAEs, rather than the documentation of permanent hearing loss with the audiogram, and with appropriate patient education and hearing conservation strategies (Hall & Santucci, 1995), prevention of permanent hearing impairment is possible. For music professionals, maintenance of normal auditory function not only improves quality of life, it can preserve their employment and, indeed, their livelihood.

Patterns of OAEs in music-industry professionals are illustrated below in case reports. Analyses of audiometric versus DPOAE data for a group of professional musicians clearly show the rationale for this application of OAEs. Across the frequency region from 1000 to 8000 Hz, a higher proportion of musicians shows abnormalities for DPOAEs than for the audiogram (Figure 9–3). Inspection of audiometric findings confirms the expected notching pattern of deficits in the 3000- to 6000-Hz region. The majority of musicians had normal hearing thresholds for lower frequencies (e.g., 1000 Hz). DPOAE amplitudes are less likely to be normal at each audiometric frequency,

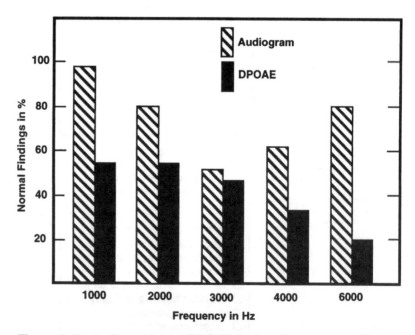

Figure 9–3. Audiometric and DPOAE findings for a group of 35 professional musicians. Note the higher proportion of abnormal findings for DPOAEs at all test frequencies, even lower frequencies (e.g., 1000 Hz) that are removed from the region of maximum pure-tone hearing impairment.

even 1000 Hz. These data lead to at least two important clinical implications. First, cochlear dysfunction may extend beyond the frequency region suggested by the audiogram. Presumably, outer hair cell dysfunction extends basal and apical to region of maximum cochlear damage, as indicated by the notching audiogram. In the author's experience, DPOAEs recorded from the "fringe frequency region" adjacent to a mild-to-moderate audiogram deficit are commonly abnormal, or not detectable. OAE findings may better reflect the seriousness of a patient's clinical complaints of hearing difficulties, especially for music signals. Second, OAE deficits can clearly be documented at frequencies and in ears with little or no audiometric evidence of hearing loss. This information not only permits early detection of sound-induced cochlear dysfunction, it leads logically to more effective counseling and education regarding hearing protection.

The most valuable, even priceless, equipment musicians own is not their vintage guitar, their professional drum set, and their state-of-the-art amplifiers . . . it's their hearing. OAEs can play a crucial role in the protection and preservation of this equipment and, in turn, the musician's career.

Music professionals understand the dimensions of sound and the concepts of frequency and intensity. And they also appreciate the importance of excellent hearing to their professional livelihood and success. At the end of the diagnostic assessment, the author regularly reviews in depth with musician patients their audiometric and DPOAE findings, referring as appropriate to simple drawings of cochlear anatomy and to photomicrographs of normal versus damaged outer hair cells. Data presented above are used as the evidence that the OAE findings are predictive of subsequent deterioration of auditory function, if effective hearing protection is not initiated. A full discussion of the hearing protection options available for professional musicians is beyond the scope of this chapter. The two major options are custom earplugs specifically designed for musicians (ER-9s, ER-15s, and ER-25s) and ear-level monitoring devices (Hall & Santucci, 1995; Mueller & Hall, 1998). For the reader interested in more information on music and hearing, the internet offers a wide array of websites for manufacturers of hearing protection devices and not-for-profit groups involved in professional hearing protection.

CASE REPORTS

Case 1: Industrial Noise Exposure and TTS

The patient was the manager for the building where the audiologic clinic was located. On entering the clinic, I observed and heard the right-handed patient using a powerful rivet gun while repairing some ductwork in a utility room. The sound intensity was dangerously high, even 4 to 5 feet away. In passing, I asked the patient whether he was wearing ear protection. Within 30 minutes, the patient walked into the clinic complaining of tinnitus and decreased hearing in the right ear. After a brief visit with the resident otolaryngologist, with no recommendations for treatment, the patient underwent an audiologic evaluation.

"Early attempts to predict susceptibility to NIHL using nonauditory characteristics of the subject (i.e., gender, eye color, smoking, age, etc.) can only account for minor amounts of variability across the subjects in their susceptibility to NIHL" (p. 165). Henderson D, Subramaniam M, Boettcher FA. Individual susceptibility to noise-induced hearing loss: An old topic revisited. Ear and Hearing 14: 152-168, 1993.

Serial audiograms are plotted in Figure 9–4, along with initial immittance and speech audiometry findings. In Test 1 (within 1 hour after the noise exposure), the audiogram showed a severe notching hearing loss in the 2000- to 4000-Hz region for the right ear and a very slight notch at 3000 Hz for the left ear. TEOAEs, recorded within 1.5 hours of the noise exposure (Figure 9–5), revealed no energy above the 2000-Hz octave for the right ear, or above the 3000-Hz octave for the left ear. Two days later, TEOAE energy for the right ear had returned in the 3000-Hz region, whereas findings for the left ear were essentially unchanged (Figure 9–6). Five days after the noise exposure, we repeated pure-tone audiometry (refer back to Figure 9–4), which confirmed partial reversal of the hearing loss at 3000 Hz and almost total return of hearing thresholds to normal limits at 2000 and 4000 Hz. On this date, we performed both TEOAE and DPOAE measurement. TEOAE energy was then observed in the 4000-Hz octave for the right ear (Figure 9–7). In addition, reduced DPOAE amplitude was noted in the 3000-Hz region, more so for stimulus intensities of $L_1 = L_2 = 65$ than for $L_1 = L_2 = 75$ dB SPL (Figure 9–8). These findings for DPgrams were confirmed by input-output functions in the frequency region of 1000 to 8000 Hz (Figure 9–9). Finally, a follow-up audiogram at 4 months after the noise incident revealed further reversal of the TTS (Figure 9–4 again).

Comment. OAEs can be applied in the frequency-specific documentation of progressive recovery from cochlear (outer hair cell) dysfunction secondary to TTS. DPOAEs can supplement TEOAEs by confirming return of cochlear function for higher frequencies (above 4000 Hz). The sensitivity of OAEs to cochlear dysfunction is enhanced by reducing stimulus intensity level. OAEs provided evidence of cochlear dysfunction for the left ear (contralateral to the noise exposure), which was not apparent in the pure-tone audiogram. In this case, input-output functions confirmed information obtained from DPgrams, but did not contribute to further definition of cochlear status.

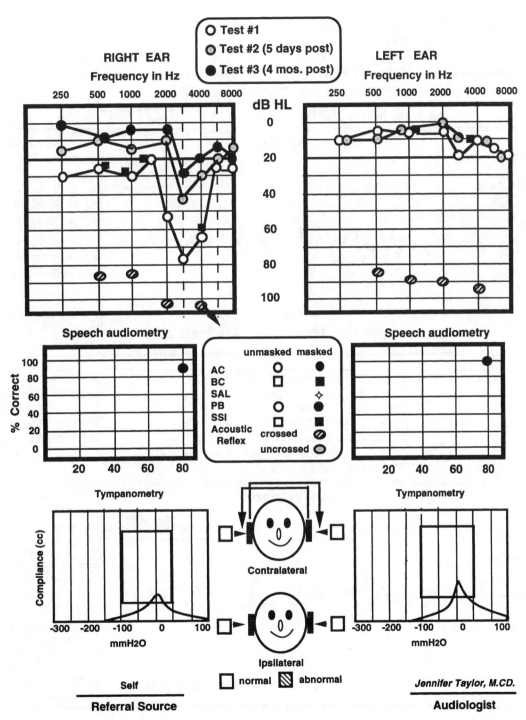

Figure 9–4. Serial audiograms for a 32-year-old male building manager (Case 1). The first test was performed within 1 hour of excessive noise exposure to the right ear (extended use of a rivet gun held with the right hand). Findings for two subsequent pure-tone audiograms document resolution of temporary threshold shift for the right ear, especially in the 3000-Hz region.

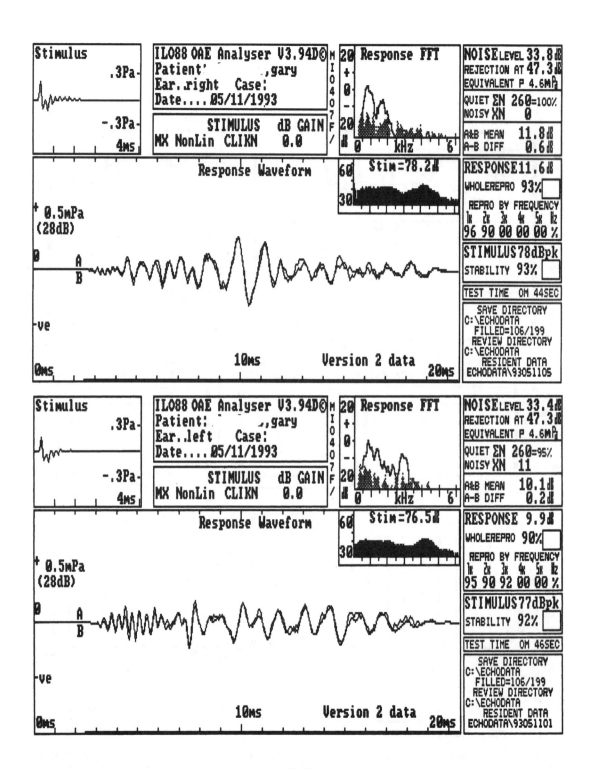

Figure 9–5. Initial TEOAE findings for a 32-year-old male building manager (Case 1), recorded within 1.5 hours after excessive noise exposure to the right ear. For the right ear (in the upper graph), TEOAEs lacked energy for octave bands above 2000 Hz, whereas left ear TEOAEs (the lower graph) lacked energy above 3000 Hz. Audiometric findings are illustrated in Figure 9–4.

498

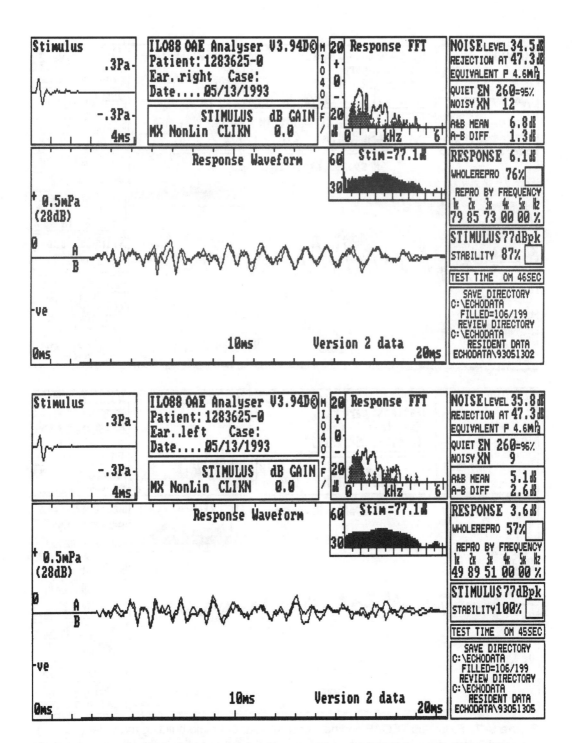

Figure 9–6. Follow-up TEOAE findings for a 32-year-old male building manager (Case 1), recorded within 2 days after excessive noise exposure to the right ear. For the right ear (in the upper graph), TEOAE energy returned for the 3000-Hz octave band, consistent with audiometric evidence of partial reversal of temporary threshold shift. Audiometric findings are illustrated in Figure 9–4 and initial TEOAE findings in Figure 9–5.

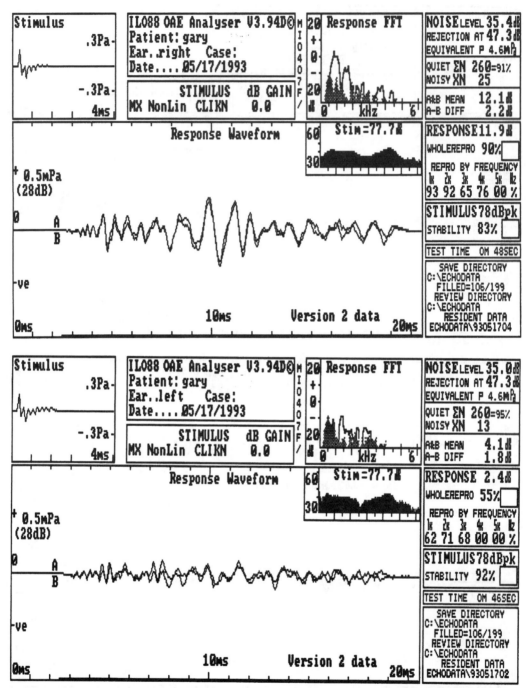

Figure 9–7. Follow-up TEOAE findings for a 32-year-old male building manager (Case 1), recorded 6 days after excessive noise exposure to the right ear. For the right ear (in the upper graph), TEOAE energy returned for the 3000- and 4000-Hz octave bands, consistent with audiometric evidence of continuing reversal of temporary threshold shift in this frequency region. Notice also signs of more robust TEOAEs in the temporal response waveform and the "response FFT." Serial audiometric findings are illustrated in Figure 9–4, and earlier TEOAE findings in Figures 9–5 and 9–6.

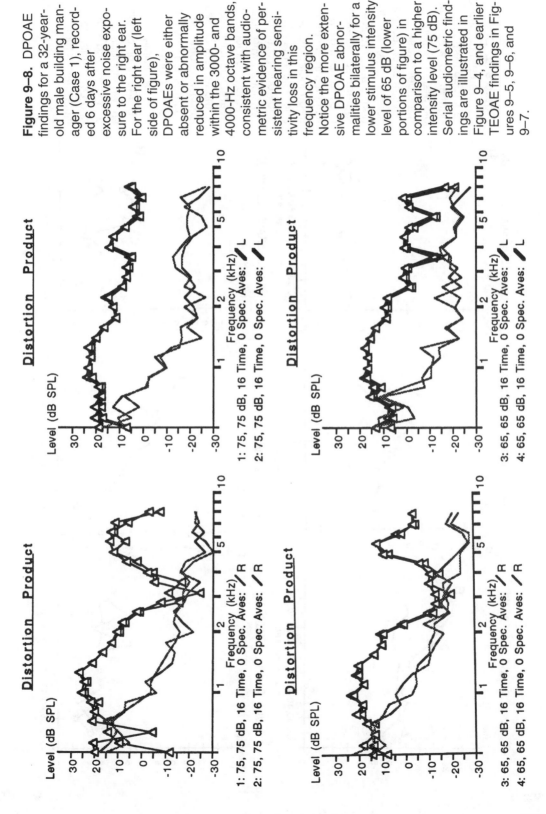

Figure 9–8. DPOAE findings for a 32-year-old male building manager (Case 1), recorded 6 days after excessive noise exposure to the right ear. For the right ear (left side of figure), DPOAEs were either absent or abnormally reduced in amplitude within the 3000- and 4000-Hz octave bands, consistent with audiometric evidence of persistent hearing sensitivity loss in this frequency region. Notice the more extensive DPOAE abnormalities bilaterally for a lower stimulus intensity level of 65 dB (lower portions of figure) in comparison to a higher intensity level (75 dB). Serial audiometric findings are illustrated in Figure 9–4, and earlier TEOAE findings in Figures 9–5, 9–6, and 9–7.

501

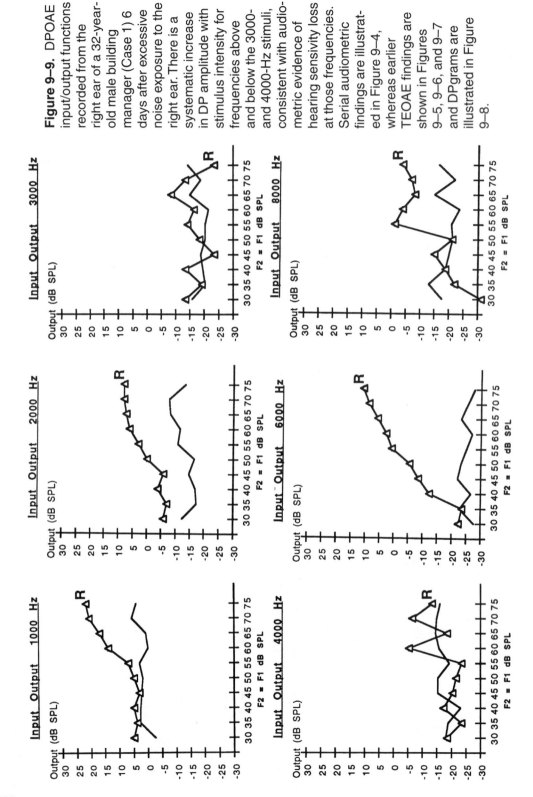

Figure 9–9. DPOAE input/output functions recorded from the right ear of a 32-year-old male building manager (Case 1) 6 days after excessive noise exposure to the right ear. There is a systematic increase in DP amplitude with stimulus intensity for frequencies above and below the 3000- and 4000-Hz stimuli, consistent with audiometric evidence of hearing sensivity loss at those frequencies. Serial audiometric findings are illustrated in Figure 9–4, whereas earlier TEOAE findings are shown in Figures 9–5, 9–6, and 9–7 and DPgrams are illustrated in Figure 9–8.

502

Case 2: Child With Noise-Induced Hearing Loss

A 10-year-old boy was referred to audiology after failing a hearing screening at school. He had a history of deer hunting with his father, although the father was quick to point out that his son usually stood off to the right side of the father (with his left ear facing) as the father fired the shotgun. Audiologic assessment showed a very mild hearing sensitivity loss for the right ear, with a severe notching sensorineural hearing loss in the 3000-Hz region for the left ear (Figure 9–10). Word recognition scores in quiet were depressed for the left ear, even at an intensity level of 80 dB HL. DPOAEs, recorded first with a diagnostic protocol including three stimulus frequencies per octave (Figure 9–11), were characterized by amplitude values within or just below normal limits for the right ear. No consistent DPOAEs were recorded for the left ear, even for the 1000-Hz region where hearing sensitivity remained within normal limits. DPOAEs were then recorded with eight stimulus frequencies per octave (Figure 9–12). For the right ear, there was a distinct notch in the DPgram in the 4000- to 4400-Hz region, which was not apparent in the audiogram or the initial DPgram.

OAEs in a variety of pediatric patient populations are reviewed in Chapter 8.

Comment. OAEs can supplement the audiogram by confirming cochlear (outer hair cell) dysfunction in sensorineural hearing impairment, by providing more frequency-specificity in defining cochlear abnormalities, and by confirming evidence of cochlear dysfunction that is not clearly evident audiometrically (right ear in this case).

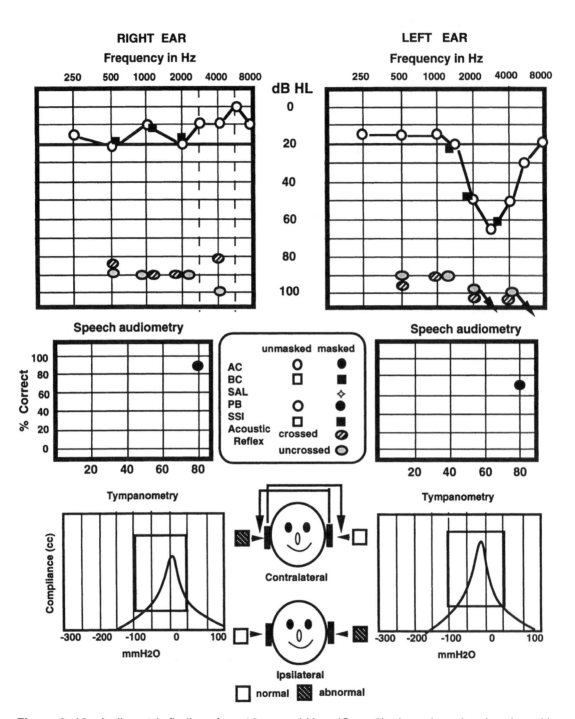

Figure 9–10. Audiometric findings for a 10-year-old boy (Case 2) who enjoys deer hunting with his father (without hearing protection). He was referred to audiology after failing a hearing screening at school.

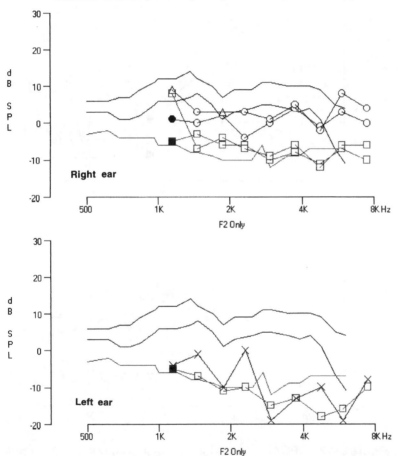

Figure 9–11. DPOAE findings for a 10-year-old boy (Case 2) recorded from each ear for stimuli presented at three frequencies per
octave. Reliability is only fair for DPOAEs with right ear stimulation,
but amplitudes appear to be essentially normal.

505

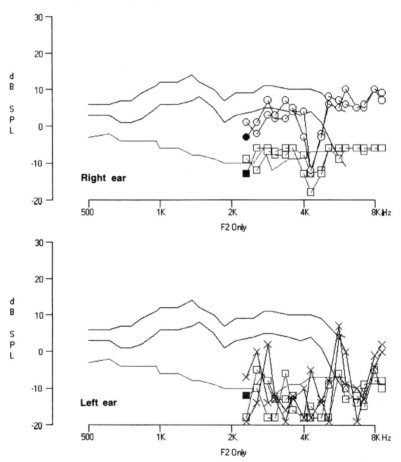

PT: 10 y.o. male
DX: failed school hearing screening

Noise exposure DPgram protocol (8 frequencies/octave 2 - 8 K Hz)

Figure 9–12. DPOAE findings for a 10-year-old boy (Case 2) recorded from each ear for stimuli presented within the 2000- to 8000-Hz region at 8 frequencies per octave. There is a distinct notch in DPOAE amplitudes just above 4000 Hz with right ear stimulation, reflecting cochlear dysfunction contralateral to the severe left ear sensory hearing loss documented audiometrically (see Figure 9–10).

Case 3: Professional Musician

The patient was a 49-year-old leader of, and keyboardist in, a 8- to 10-piece band which plays its own unique, excellent, and loud blend of riverboat blues, rock and roll, and party music. At the time of the evaluation, he had a 30-year history of performing and complaints of difficulty hearing in difficult (noisy) listening conditions. Given this history, the patient's audiogram was rather unremarkable (Figure 9–13), showing only a very mild deficit for higher frequencies, mostly for the left ear. Tympanograms were extremely compliant bilaterally. Word recognition in quiet was excellent (100%). TEOAEs, performed with an early version of equipment software, repeatedly showed little energy for octave frequencies above 2000 Hz for the right ear (Figure 9–14) and essentially no response for the left ear (Figure 9–15). Widespread bilateral cochlear (outer hair cell) dysfunction was further documented by DPOAEs. For stimulus frequencies above 2000 Hz presented to the right ear, DPOAE amplitudes were severely reduced, whereas no DPOAE activity was detectable at any of the test frequencies for the left ear (Figure 9–16).

Comment. This musician vividly illustrates the enhanced sensitivity of OAEs to cochlear deficits not revealed by pure-tone audiometry and the possibility of some outer hair cell dysfunction yet normal hearing sensitivity. Repeated audiologic assessment over a period of years has shown no further decrease in pure-tone hearing thresholds and consistently absent OAEs. Management included the recommendation for custom musician earplugs (ER-15s) during performances.

There is recent evidence from contralateral suppression studies of OAEs that efferent auditory system effects on cochlear function differ for musicians versus nonmusicians. (Perrot X et al. Stronger bilateral efferent influences on cochlear biomechanical activity in musicians than in nonmusicians. **Neuroscience Letters** *262(3): 167–170, 1999.)*

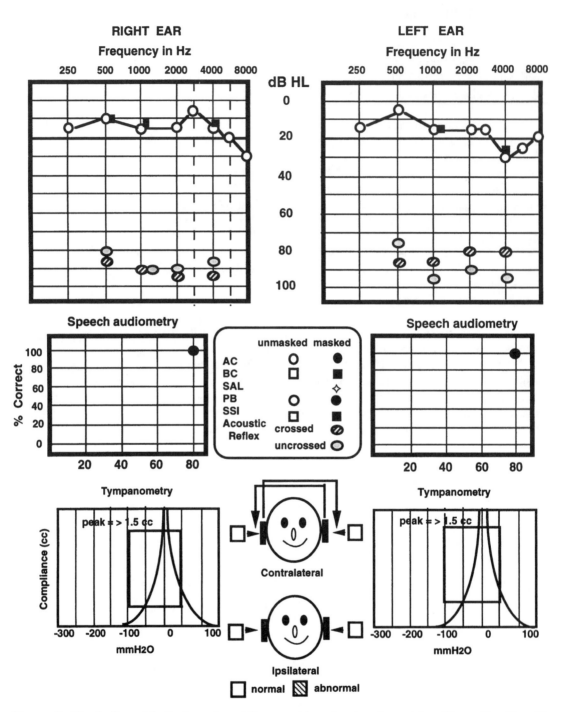

Figure 9–13. Audiometric findings for a 49-year-old professional musician (Case 3) with a 30-year history of playing keyboards in (and leading) a large rock and roll band (without hearing protection). The patient and his wife were concerned about his hearing.

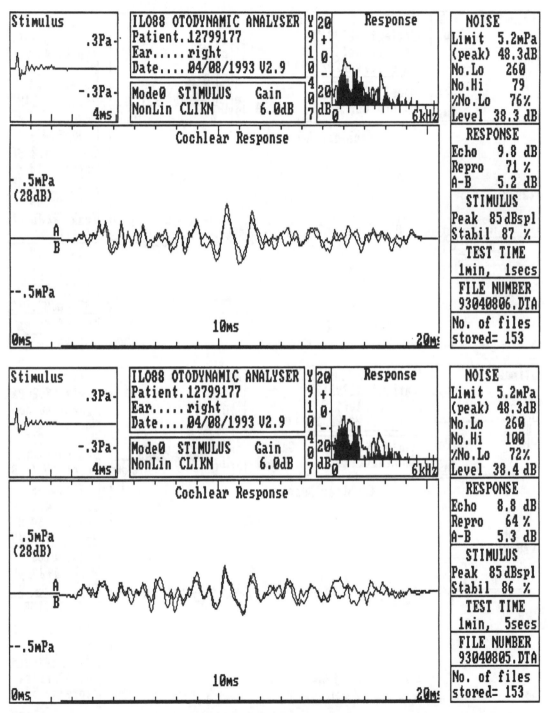

Figure 9–14. Repeatably abnormal right ear TEOAE findings for a 49-year-old professional musician (Case 3). TEOAE energy was abnormally low for octave bands above 2000 Hz, despite reasonably normal hearing sensitivity (see Figure 9–13).

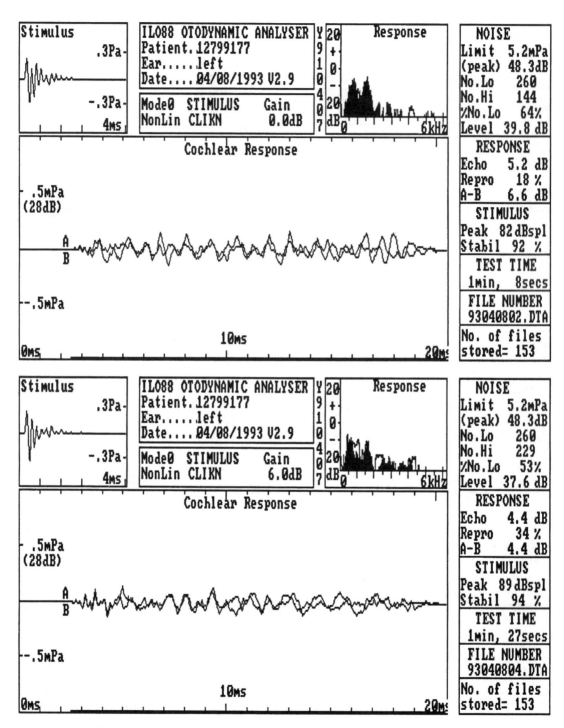

Figure 9–15. Repeatably abnormal left ear TEOAE findings for a 49-year-old professional musician (Case 3). There was little evidence of reliable TEOAEs at any frequency, despite hearing sensitivity within clinically normal limits, except for the 4000-Hz region (see Figure 9–13).

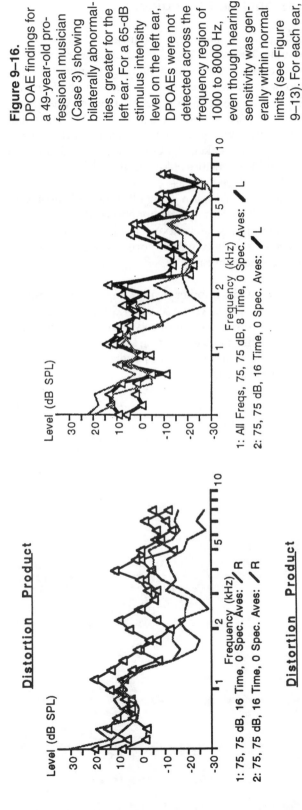

Distortion Product

Level (dB SPL)

1: 75, 75 dB, 16 Time, 0 Spec. Aves: /R
2: 75, 75 dB, 16 Time, 0 Spec. Aves: /R

Distortion Product

Level (dB SPL)

3: 65, 65 dB, 16 Time, 0 Spec. Aves: /R
4: 65, 65 dB, 16 Time, 0 Spec. Aves: /R

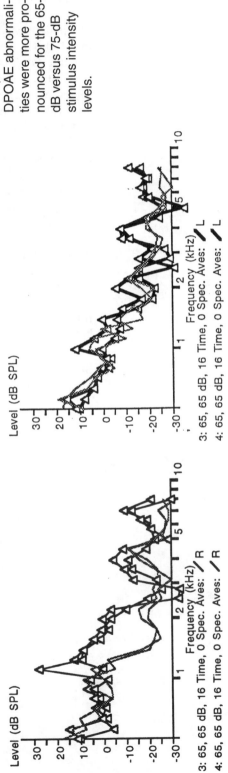

Level (dB SPL)

1: All Freqs, 75, 75 dB, 8 Time, 0 Spec. Aves: L
2: 75, 75 dB, 16 Time, 0 Spec. Aves: L

Level (dB SPL)

3: 65, 65 dB, 16 Time, 0 Spec. Aves: L
4: 65, 65 dB, 16 Time, 0 Spec. Aves: L

Case 4: Professional Audio Engineer

The patient was a 45-year-old male audio engineer at a major recording studio in Nashville, Tennessee. He reported often working 12- to 18-hour days in environments with sound intensity greatly exceeding 90 dB SPL. Audiologic assessment confirmed bilateral high-frequency sensorineural hearing loss, greater for the right ear, which was consistent with exposure to excessive sound levels (Figure 9–17). The patient confirmed that in the studio his right side was typically facing a large bank of amplifiers and loudspeakers. DPOAEs were recorded with a test protocol with stimulus intensities of $L_1 = 65$ dB and $L_2 = 55$ dB, and including eight stimulus frequencies per octave (Figure 9–18). Although the pattern of the DPgram generally followed the audiogram configuration, DPOAE activity was not observed for stimuli at audiometric frequencies immediately above and below the notching loss, even with hearing sensitivity within normal limits at these frequencies, especially for the right ear.

Comment. This case provides another clear example of the sensitivity and frequency-specificity of OAEs to sound-induced cochlear dysfunction. OAEs can confirm noise-induced cochlear dysfunction before it evolves into a noise-induced hearing loss (Attias et al., 1995). The case also illustrates for an individual the pattern of findings for the group of musicians shown earlier in Figure 9–3.

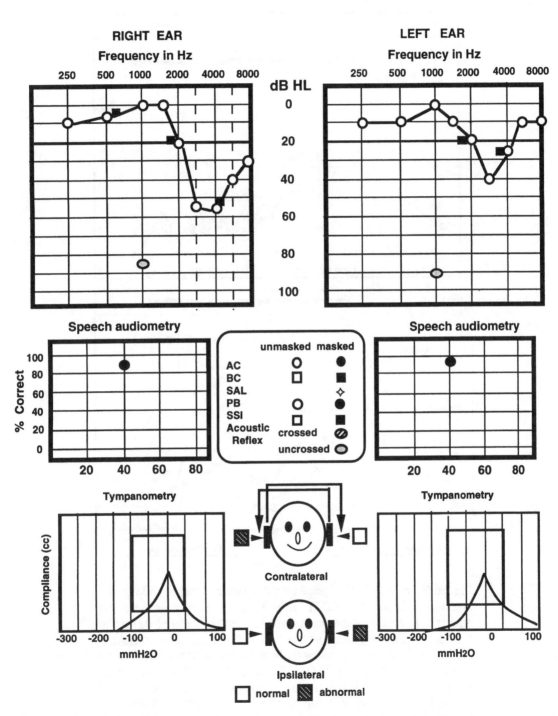

Figure 9–17. Audiometric findings for a 45-year-old male professional audio engineer (Case 4) showing a notching sensory hearing loss in the 3000- to 6000-Hz region, greater for the right ear.

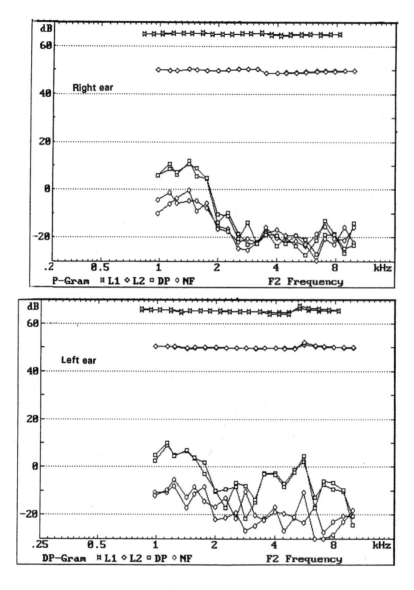

Figure 9–18. DPOAE findings for a 45-year-old professional audio engineer (Case 4). DPOAE amplitudes are indicated by the squares, whereas the diamond symbols represent the noise floor in the ear canal during measurement. With this equipment and protocol, DPOAE amplitudes below 0 dB SPL are considered abnormally reduced. Although the DPOAE findings agree with the audiometric pattern, the DPOAE results provide a higher degree of frequency resolution (8 frequencies per octave up to 10,000 Hz). Furthermore, at "fringe" frequencies around the notching loss, DPOAEs are abnormal even though audiometric thresholds are within normal limits. The patient's audiogram is illustrated in Figure 9–17.

Case 5: Professional Musician (Symphony)

A 46-year-old female harpist at a major symphony underwent audio-logic assessment at the suggestion of a friend. She estimated a total of about 8 hours of exposure to harp sounds each day during rehearsals, teaching students, and performances. As shown in Figure 9–19, there was evidence of only a very mild sloping high frequency decrease in hearing sensitivity bilaterally, with the suggestion of a subtle notch at 6000 Hz for the right ear. DPOAEs confirmed a high-frequency cochlear deficit, but also revealed an asymmetric notching decrease in amplitude values in the 3000-Hz region for the right ear (see Figure 9–20). The patient was fitted with ER-15 musician earplugs and given the recommendation to wear them during all practicing and perform-ing.

Comment. Music-induced auditory dysfunction is not limited to spe-cific genres. This case highlights the ear-specific nature of auditory dysfunction for some musicians. For example, a harp played on the right side will produce an asymmetric deficit on the right, whereas the typical violinist (fiddler) will demonstrate more auditory dysfunction for the left ear. Early detection of cochlear dysfunction by OAEs (ver-sus the audiogram) can contribute to hearing conservation in a popu-lation that depends greatly on their auditory sense.

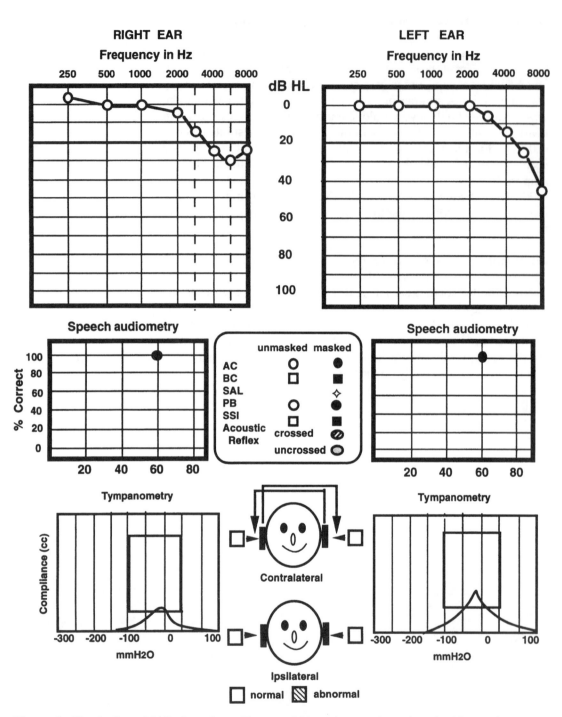

Figure 9–19. Audiometric findings for a 46-year-old female symphony harpist (Case 5) showing a mild notching sensory hearing loss in the 4000- to 8000-Hz region for the right ear and a gently sloping high-frequency sensory hearing loss for the left ear.

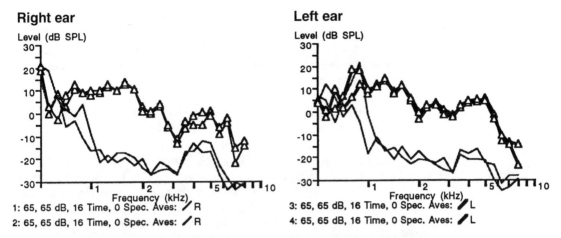

Figure 9–20. DPOAE findings for a 46-year-old female harpist (Case 5). DPOAE amplitudes are indicated by the triangles, and the noise floor by the solid lines. For the right ear, there is a distinct (and abnormal) decrease in DPOAE amplitudes in the 3000-Hz region, confirming cochlear dysfunction. DPOAEs are within normal limits in this frequency region for the left ear.

MÉNIÈRE'S DISEASE

Background

The symptoms of Ménière's disease—vertigo, fluctuating hearing loss, tinnitus, and (often) a sensation of fullness in the ear—are well-known. The pathophysiologic bases of Ménière's disease, however, remain ill defined. Dilation of the endolymphatic spaces in the cochlea (endolymphatic hydrops) is a common histopathologic finding in Ménière's disease, implying either an overproduction or inadequate reabsorption of endolymph. There are numerous theories as to the pathogenesis of the mechanisms underlying the cause and progression of Ménière's disease. A variety of medical and surgical approaches are followed by physicians in attempts to adequately treat the disorder, with widely varying degrees of success.

Although there is agreement that the general anatomic site of lesion in Ménière's disease is the cochlea and that the endolymphatic system (ducts and sacs, or sinuses) are implicated, the precise structures affected are rarely noted. The specific characteristics of Ménière's disease, the natural history or progression of the disease, and its responsiveness to medical or surgical treatment are highly variable among patients. These common observations suggest multiple pathophysiologies, and perhaps differential involvement of intracochlear components. With the application of OAEs in Ménière's disease, at least two patterns of OAE findings have emerged. For the majority of patients with sensory hearing loss secondary to Ménière's disease (typically in

"Ménière's disease remains, in many ways, as much an enigma as it was when Prosper Ménière first reported patients with episodic vertigo attacks in 1861" (p. 1119) . . . "A major limitation in the study and treatment of Ménière's disease is the high variability of the pattern of the disease among subjects and within a single subject over time" (p. 1129). Mattox DE. *Ménière's disease, vestibular neuronitis and paroxysmal positional vertigo and nystagmus. In* Ballenger JJ and Snow JB, Jr. (eds). **Otorhinolaryngology— Head and Neck Surgery (15th ed).** *Baltimore: Williams & Wilkins, 1996, pp. 1119–1132.*

the lower frequencies and, sometimes, also in the higher frequencies), OAEs are abnormal and, with hearing loss greater than 25 to 30 dB, there is no detectable OAE activity. This pattern is clearly expected, based on the extensive literature describing the relation of OAEs and sensory hearing loss. In distinct contrast, some patients with sensorineural hearing loss due to Ménière's disease have TEOAEs or DPOAEs with normal or even greater than expected amplitude values, even with thresholds exceeding 30 dB HL and, in selected cases, up to 60 dB HL (Ohlms et al., 1991; Harris & Probst, 1992; Musiek et al., 1994; van Huffelen et al., 1998). The precise proportion of Ménière's patients with atypically robust OAEs is not yet known. Estimates by authors reporting group data vary substantially. For example, Harris & Probst (1992) found detectable TEOAEs in only 2 of 31 patients with hearing loss exceeding 30 dB HL, whereas others (Sakashita et al., 1991; Bartoli et al., 1992; van Huffeln et al., 1998) have reported the presence of TEOAEs in more than one third of patients with this degree of hearing loss. Similarly, DPOAEs can be recorded in a sizable proportion of patients with hearing impairment, including pure-tone thresholds exceeding 40 dB HL (Ohlms et al., 1991; Lonsbury-Martin et al., 1993; van Huffeln et al., 1998).

The author collaborated with two colleagues (audiologist Donna Schwaber and neurotologist Mitchell Schwaber) in an investigation of DPOAEs in a series of patients who had just been diagnosed with Ménière's disease (according to criteria of the Committee on Hearing and Equilibrium of the American Academy of Otolaryngology—Head and Neck Surgery). Group DPOAE data for normal subjects, patients with non-Ménière's cochlear auditory dysfunction, and patients with diagnosed Ménière's disease are shown in Figure 9–21. DPOAE amplitudes were, as expected, higher for normal subjects than for either group with cochlear hearing impairment. There was no signficant difference in average DPOAE amplitudes between the two groups with hearing impairment. When these data were recast in a scattergraph (Figure 9–22), the findings were considerably more interesting. Most patients with hearing impairment (greater than 20 dB HL) had either abnormal DPOAE findings, or no detectable DPOAE activity, at an equivalent test frequency. There were, however, a small number of patients with Ménière's disease and hearing thresholds of up to 40 dB, and greater, with clear evidence of DPOAEs. Atypically robust DPOAEs were not observed for any patients with other etiologies of cochlear hearing loss. This interesting DPOAE pattern is illustrated below by a case report.

A minority of patients with diagnosed Ménière's disease show normal OAEs, or even OAEs larger-than-normal amplitude, despite hearing threshold levels of 40 dB HL or greater. OAEs can help to differentiate among pathophysiologic processes underlying Ménière's disease.

The divergent patterns of OAEs found in patients with Ménière's disease may be a reflection of more than one specific site-of-lesion. Abnormality or total absence of OAE activity is consistent with involvement of outer hair cells and, in particular, disruption of cochlear mechanics and motile processes. Endolymphatic hydrops can result in structural damage to the stereocilia, the tiplinks connecting them, and/or their attachment to the cuticular plate (Aran et al., 1984; Horner & Cazals,

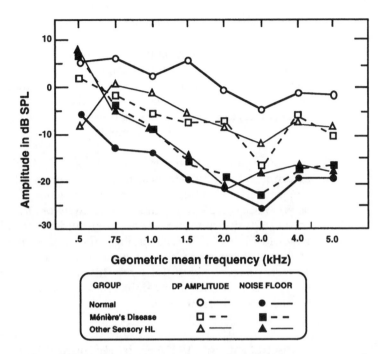

Figure 9–21. Average DPOAE amplitude values for normal subjects, a group of patients with non-Ménière's disease sensory hearing loss, and a group of patients with Ménière's disease. Age, gender, and pure-tone hearing thresholds were equivalent for the three groups. There was no significant difference in average DPOAE amplitudes for the two groups of hearing impaired patients. (Data courtesy of Donna Schwaber, M.CD. and Mitchell Schwaber, M.D., Nashville ENT Clinic.)

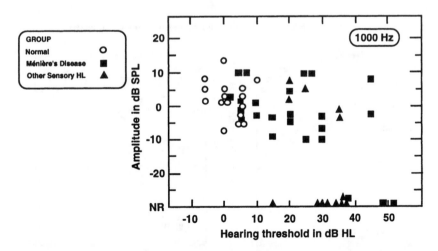

Figure 9–22. Scattergraph of DPOAE amplitude values for normal subjects, a group of patients with non-Ménière's disease sensory hearing loss, and a group of patients with Ménière's disease. The stimulus frequency was 1000 Hz. Age, gender, and pure-tone hearing thresholds were equivalent for the three groups. Two patients with Ménière's disease (out of a total of 24) showed atypically large DPOAE amplitude values despite hearing thresholds exceeding 40 dB HL. (Data courtesy of Donna Schwaber, M.CD. and Mitchell Schwaber, M.D., Nashville ENT Clinic.)

1988; Horner et al., 1988). Another intriguing possibility is the selective involvement of inner hair cells in Ménière's disease, with sparing of the outer hair cells. Unusually robust OAEs can be recorded from ears with outer hair cell integrity, yet damaged inner hair cells (Wake et al., 1996). Some of this literature was reviewed in the dicussion of carboplatin ototoxicity in Chapter 8. Other speculation suggests dysfunction at the level of the afferent synapses to inner and outer hair cells, or efferent auditory system involvement (e.g., Nadol & Thornton, 1987).

For some patients with apparently unilateral Ménière's disease, as determined by a unilateral hearing loss audiometrically, OAEs may be abnormal in the contralateral ear (van Huffelen et al., 1998). This may be another example of the unique sensitivity of OAEs to very subtle cochlear dysfunction not yet apparent audiometrically noted elsewhere in this book. The OAE findings in such cases may offer evidence of early cochlear dysfunction in the "normal" ear and confirm that the Ménière's disease is really bilateral. This finding can contribute importantly to decisions regarding unilateral surgical therapy and estimates of outcome with treatment.

Case 6: Robust DPOAEs in Ménière's Disease

A 51-year-old female underwent audiologic evaluation and DPOAE measurement on the same day she was diagnosed by a neurotologist with Ménière's disease on the right ear. Audiometry (Figure 9–23) revealed the characteristic low-frequency sensorineural hearing loss,

AUDIOGRAM AND DPOAE in a Patient with Ménière's Disease

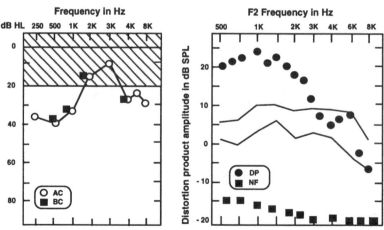

Figure 9–23. Audiometric (left portion) and DPOAE findings (right portion) for a 51-year-old female just diagnosed with Ménière's disease affecting the right ear (Case 6). Only right ear findings are shown. There is a mild low-frequency hearing loss by pure-tone audiometry, yet DPOAE amplitudes are remarkably robust within this frequency region. (Data courtesy of Donna Schwaber, M.CD. and Mitchell Schwaber, M.D., Nashville ENT Clinic.)

and also some high frequency decrease in hearing sensitivity (a peaked pattern). DPOAE measurement was performed immediately after audiometry using a protocol that emphasized first the 500- to 1000-Hz octave and then frequencies from 1000 to 8000 Hz. As seen in the right side of the figure, DPOAE amplitudes were remarkably robust throughout the low-frequency region, despite the presence of an apparent sensory hearing impairment. The two solid lines in the DPgram encompass the normal adult region (10th–90th percentile range). DPOAEs were smaller in amplitude for higher frequencies, which was more consistent with a sensory hearing loss.

Comment. This is one of the patients referred to earlier in the discussion of group data displayed in Figure 9–22. It illustrates a variant of Ménière's disease, described repeatedly in the OAE literature, which apparently spares outer hair cells.

RETROCOCHLEAR AUDITORY DYSFUNCTION

Differentiation of sensory versus neural hearing loss can be facilitated by OAE measurement in combination with other audiologic procedures, especially ABR. At first, one might expect to invariably record normal OAEs in patients with neural auditory dysfunction, as the outer hair cell generators are "preneural." As reviewed in Chapter 2, OAEs are independent of the afferent auditory nervous system, unlike behavioral audiologic measures, ABR, and acoustic reflexes. With purely retrocochlear auditory dyfunction, OAEs characteristically are normal. However, neoplasms (tumors) in the internal auditory canal and/or posterior fossa may, as they grow and occupy more space, impinge on the internal auditory artery and compromise blood flow to the cochlea. Clinical experience confirms that OAEs are abnormal, or even undetectable, in the majority of patients with neoplastic retrocochlear pathology (the literature is summarized in Table 9–2). This finding (i.e., a clear retrocochlear auditory dysfunction with concomitant cochlear deficit) may be associated with relatively large tumors, although a variety of cochear/retrocochlear findings may occur depending on the type of tumor (e.g., vestibular schwannoma, neurofibroma versus meningioma) and its size and location. Thus, the proportion of patients with retrocochlear pathology showing OAE activity varies among studies. For example, in one of the earlier papers, Martin Robinette (1992) recorded TEOAEs in only 20% of a sample of 61 patients with confirmed acoustic neurinomas. Other authors in this era similarly found that abnormal OAEs were a common finding in retrocochlear pathology (Bonfils & Uziel, 1988). More recently, Ferber-Viart and French colleagues (1998) also reported that only about one in five patients with acoustic neurinoma had normal TEOAE findings preoperatively. The finding of normal preoperative OAEs was, however, associated with a higher chance of hearing preservation postoperatively. In contrast, other authors cite a higher proportion of recordable TEOAEs in acoustic tumors. Cane, Lutman, and O'Donoghue (1994) detected TEOAE activity in almost half (47%) of a group of 45 patients with confirmed cerebellopontine angle tumors and hearing loss exceeding 25 dB HL. These authors also demonstrated the feasibility of monitoring cochlear status intraoperatively with OAEs (Cane, O'Donoghue, & Lutman, 1992). A group from the University of Miami (Telischi et al., 1995) similarly applied DPOAEs as a tool for intraoperative monitoring of cochlear function, although recordings were complicated by a number of technical problems. Norman et al. (1996) were able to record (with the POEMs device) "satisfactory" TEOAEs from an even higher proportion of patients (59% of a series of 39) with acoustic neuroma. Interestingly, when these authors increased stimulus rate up to 5000 clicks/s using a maximum length sequence (MLS) technique, TEOAE amplitude decreased less in the patients with retrocochlear pathology than expected for normal subjects, suggesting the possibility of efferent auditory system involvement in at least some patients. Finally, in an early report on the clinical applications of DPOAEs, Ohlms et al. (1991) noted that, "patients with retrocochlear lesions, such as unilateral acoustic neuromas, commonly demonstrated only mildly reduced DPOAEs, even in the presence of appreciable hearing losses" (p. 167). To fully evaluate and differentiate sensory versus neural auditory function, OAEs should probably be routinely measured in patients with retrocochlear signs or symptoms. The presence of normal OAEs provides evidence of cochlear integrity and, therefore, that the neoplasm has not compromised blood supply to the cochlea. In the author's experience, the finding of normal OAEs in a patient suspected of retrocochlear auditory dysfunction, and hearing loss exceeding 30 dB HL also raises the possibility that the lesion was a neurofibroma or meningioma, rather than an acoustic tumor arising from within the internal auditory canal. This point is illustrated with the following case report.

"Distortion-product otoacoustic emissions were very sensitive to brief vascular occlusions . . . within approximately 25 seconds of blockage onset. On alleviation of the occlusion, DPOAEs rapidly and completely returned" Widick MP et al. Early effects of cerebellopontine angle compression on rabbit distortion-product otoacoustic emissions: A model for monitoring cochlear function during acoustic neuroma surgery. **Otolaryngology—Head and Neck Surgery 111: 407–416, 1994 (p. 407).**

Case 7: DPOAEs in Neurofibromatosis

An 18-year-old male college student complained to his parents about headaches, fatigue, clumsiness, and difficulty hearing speech on the telephone with the left ear. The parents attributed these complaints to stress associated with a grueling examination schedule and sleep deprivation. Because of the hearing complaint, however, he was scheduled for an appointment with audiology during the next school break. The results of an audiologic assessment are summarized in Figure 9–24. Acoustic reflexes were not observed with sound presented to the left ear, even though tympanograms were normal. There was an asymmetric rising sensorineural hearing loss (greater for the left ear). Word recognition score was 0% for the left ear. These retrocochlear audiologic signs prompted a neurodiagnostic ABR in our clinic the same day. As seen in Figure 9–25, no reliable ABR was recorded for

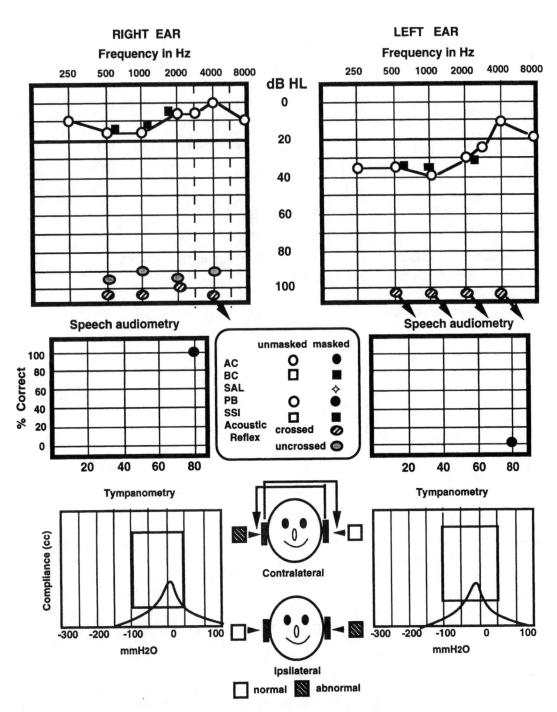

Figure 9–24. Audiometric findings for an 18-year-old male college student (Case 7) with complaints of headaches, ataxia, fatigue, and difficulty hearing the telephone on the left ear. Acoustic reflexes were absent with sound in the left ear, and word recognition was nil on that side.

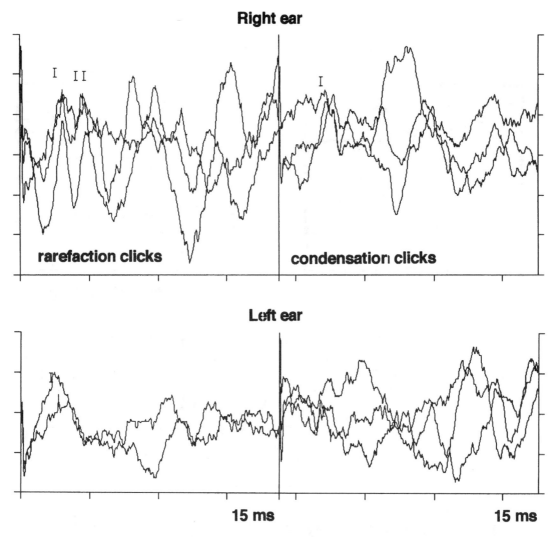

Figure 9–25. Auditory brainstem response (ABR) waveforms for an 18-year-old male college student (Case 7). There was no reliable response for either ear at an intensity level of 85 dB nHL, despite no more than a mild hearing sensitivity loss (see Figure 9–24).

either ear, despite manipulations of stimulus and acquisition parameters (e.g., stimulus polarity, rate, and intensity). Throughout this assessment, the patient was resting comfortably and quietly on a bed. Next, OAEs were measured to clearly differentiate cochlear versus retrocochlear components of the hearing impairment. DPOAEs of normal amplitude were reliably recorded with two different devices (Figure 9–26), confirming cochlear integrity. In view of these consistently retrocochlear findings, the patient was immediately escorted to the neurotologist who ordered an MRI. Within 3 hours after the patient arrived in the audiology clinic, an MRI revealed bilateral neurofibro-

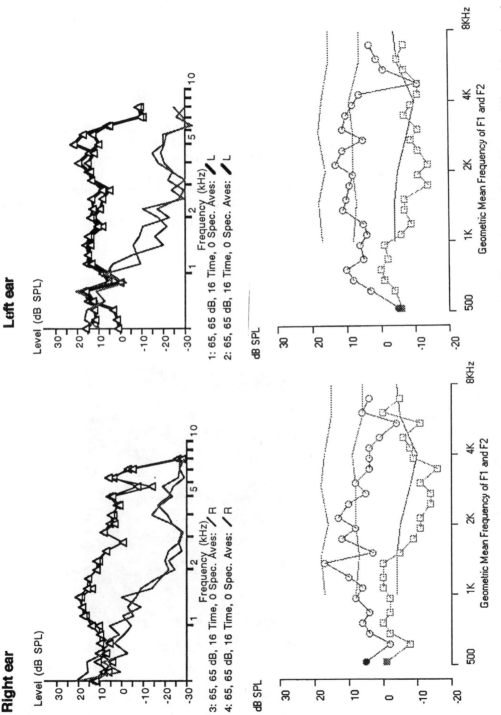

Figure 9–26. DPOAE findings for an 18-year-old male college student (Case 7) recorded with two different brands of equipment. DPOAE amplitudes were within normal limits for each ear as recorded with each device, even though pure-tone audiometry confirmed a sensorineural hearing loss for the left ear (see Figure 9–24).

mas (Figure 9–27). The larger neurofibroma (on the left side) was removed surgically, with total loss of hearing. The smaller lesion on the right side was decompressed with a nonsurgical photon knife procedure. The patient is followed regularly. Hearing has decreased only slightly on the right side. The patient wears a completely-in-the-canal hearing aid successfully on the right ear.

Comment. OAEs are useful in defining possible sensory dysfunction in a sensorineural hearing loss. In this case, OAEs ruled out cochlear involvement, while ABR confirmed retrocochlear dysfunction. Preservation of cochlear integrity in retrocochlear pathology, with sparing of internal auditory artery blood flow, appears to be more likely for a neurofibroma than for an acoustic tumor (vestibular schwannoma). Thus, OAEs are probably apt to be present more often in patients with neurofibromas. Although this case does not fit the definition of "auditory neuropathy," it was instructive to note that, despite a purely retrocochlear hearing impairment, the patient obtained benefit from amplification.

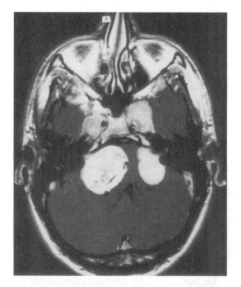

Figure 9–27. Magnetic resonance imaging (MRI) for an 18-year-old male college student (Case 7) within 2 hours after audiologic evaluation (see Figures 9–24 through 9–26) showing bilateral neurofibromas in the posterior fossa.

MALINGERING/PSEUDOHYPACUSIS

The rationale for application of OAEs in patients suspected of pseudo-hypacusis is readily apparent. Even though the malingering patient's audiogram may suggest the presence of a sensory hearing loss, normal OAEs argue strongly, and objectively, for cochear (outer hair cell) integrity. Thus, the clinician has a significant advantage in the diagnostic evaluation of this sometimes challenging and frustrating patient population. Several authors have formally described the use of OAEs, and other electrophysiologic procdures in the revelation of pseudohypacusis and confirmation of true auditory thresholds (e.g., Robinette, 1992; Musiek et al., 1994) . Many others have, no doubt, enjoyed the benefits of OAEs with unsuspecting malingering patients. OAEs are not, however, invariably of value in this population. Some pseudohypacusic patients, such as those seeking compensation for work- or military service-related apparent hearing loss do, indeed, have some degree of organic auditory dysfunction, often secondary to noise exposure. As noted in Chapter 4, degree of hearing loss cannot be predicted confidently with OAEs. Absence of OAE activity implies that hearing thresholds exceed 25 to 30 dB HL, but the OAE findings do not contribute to objective estimation of the extent of hearing loss. The patient may be superimposing a functional hearing impairment on a pre-existing sensory deficit. One must also keep in mind, as summarized above, that OAEs are recordable in some patients with neural auditory dysfunction. This possibility should be ruled out audiologically before pseudohypacusis is assumed.

"If a patient volunteers abnormal thresholds but normal OAEs, the clinician should entertain two possible causes: pseudohypacusis or retrocochlear involvement." (p. 300). Musiek FE, Bornstein SP, Rintelmann WF. Transient otoacoustic emissions and pseudohypacusis. **Journal of the American Academy of Audiology 6: 293–301, 1995.**

Case 8: Diagnostic Application of TEOAEs in Pseudohypacusis

A 49-year-old patient was referred to audiology for definition of hearing impairment as part of a workman's compensation case. He reported a long history of noise exposure, and great difficulty in hearing. Pure-tone audiometry appeared to confirm the patient's complaints (Test #1 in Figure 9–28). These pure-tone thresholds, however, did not agree with acoustic reflex findings, speech reception thresholds, and word recognition scores (over 80% at 40 dB HL despite no pure-tone threshold better than 50 dB HL). TEOAEs were then recorded with the patient closely watching every step of the procedure. As seen in Figure 9–29, there was some evidence of a TEOAE response in the low- and mid-frequency region. It should be noted that these data were collected with an early version of equipment software that did not permit octave analyses of TEOAE reproducibility and signal-to-noise ratio. Nonetheless, these TEOAEs were inconsistent with the degree of hearing loss suggested by the volunteered pure-tone audiogram. The patient was then counseled regarding the reasonably good TEOAE results, returned to the sound booth, and strongly encouraged to

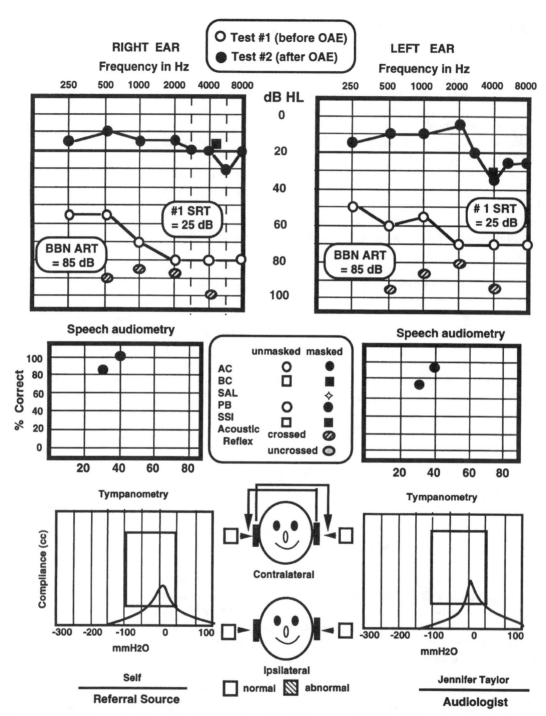

Figure 9–28. Two sets of audiometric findings for a 49-year-old industrial worker (Case 8) with complaints of hearing loss. Initially, the patient's volunteered pure-tone thesholds were consistent with a severe hearing impairment. Speech thresholds, word recognition performance, and acoustic reflex findings, however, put the validity of pure tone audiometry in question. Test 2, conducted after TEOAEs were recorded, was considered a valid representation of the patient's hearing status.

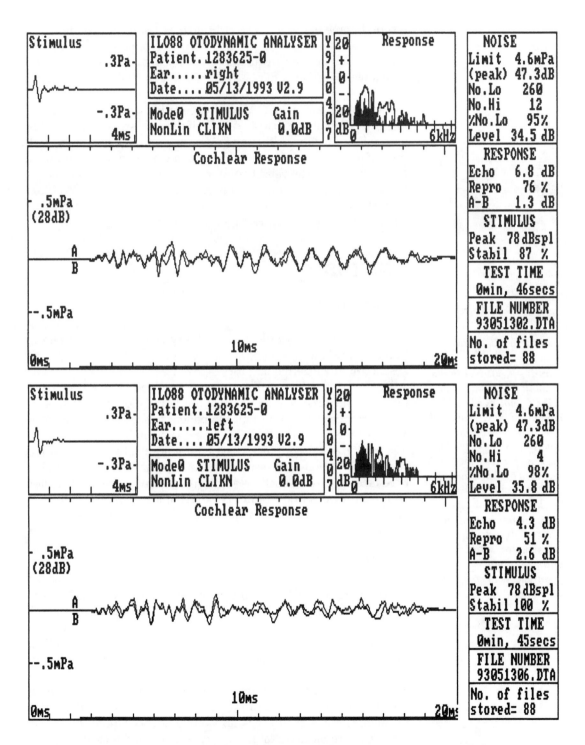

Figure 9–29. TEOAE findings for a 49-year-old industrial worker (Case 8) recorded immediately after the initial audiogram (Figure 9–28). There was clearly TEOAE energy within the audiometric region, arguing against the presence of a severe sensory hearing loss bilaterally.

respond immediately to all acoustic signals. On the second test, after OAE measurement, hearing sensitivity was remarkably improved. There was a mild high-frequency sensory hearing loss bilaterally, consistent with the history of noise exposure and with the OAE pattern.

Comment. Evidence of OAEs is incompatible with sensory hearing loss exceeding about 35 to 40 dB HL, if the loss is secondary to outer hair cell dysfunction. Although OAEs have no value in defining with precision the degree of hearing loss, the information can contribute to the evaluation of the validity of pure-tone audiometry and can assist the audiologist in patient counseling and redirecting audiologic assessment strategies. This case also suggests that OAEs potentially have therapeutic, as well as diagnostic, value.

TINNITUS

Background

Tinnitus is not just found in adults. In a survey of 6,166 school-aged children conducted by Niskar et al. (1998), ringing or buzzing sounds were reported by 3.2% on the test day. And, as noted by Baguley and McFerran (1999) "Tinnitus in childhood is . . . quite common when children are directly asked about the symptom. However, children rarely spontaneously complain of tinnitus" (p. 99).

Tinnitus is defined as a phantom auditory perception, or the perception of a sound (e.g., ringing, buzzing, roaring, cricket sound) in the absence of any external auditory signal. Remarkably commonplace, an estimated 40 million persons in the United States alone perceive tinnitus at some time. For about 7% of this population, tinnitus is sufficiently troublesome to prompt the patient to seek professional care. Many of the theories developed to explain tinnitus begin with the assumption that the original source is an abnormality at the level of the cochlea, even though the seriousness of tinnitus for a patient appears to be mediated by interactions among the auditory cortex (perception) and other regions of the brain (i.e., the limbic system and autonomic system). (See Jastreboff, Gray, and Gold, 1996, for a review.)

SOAEs and Tinnitus

As summarized in Table 9–2, the possible relation between SOAEs and tinnitus has attracted considerable interest. The paper by Ceranic, Prasher, and Luxon (1995) provides a thorough review of the topic. As early as 1980, Wilson demonstrated an interaction among auditory microstructure (presumably related to active processes within the cochlea), changes in body position (upright to horizontal to inverted), and the perception of tinnitus. Tinnitus was typically observed in the inverted position by his normal hearing subjects, but not in the upright position. This observation has, apparently, not been thoroughly investigated, nor replicated. Naturally, there is a strong clinical desire for an objective measure of tinnitus, and SOAEs initially appeared to be a promising candidate for this role. Occasionally, tinnitus can be linked to SOAEs (Probst, 1986; Penner, 1988; Penner, 1989; Norton, Schmiedt,

& Stover, 1990; Plinkert, Gitter, & Zenner, 1990; Penner & Coles, 1992; Zenner & Ernst, 1993). In selected patients, the frequency(ies) of the perceived tinnitus does coincide with frequency(ies) of SOAEs recorded in the external ear canal, and changes in SOAE induced, for example, by aspirin ingestion are related to changes in perceived tinnitus. The vast majority of persons, however, are not aware of their SOAEs, presumably due to adaptation or habituation to the constant low-level sounds. In fact, the presence of SOAEs generally is thought to be a indication of cochlear integrity in the corresponding frequency region. For most persons with tinnitus, the frequency(ies) are not correlated with SOAEs and vice versa (e.g, Liu et al., 1996). Still, there is recent evidence that variable, unstable, or inconstant SOAEs are associated with the perception of tinnitus (Ceranic, Prasher, & Luxon, 1998). These authors found that, "a subject with tinnitus may be considered 7.5 times more likely to have 'on-off' SOAE." And they reported that the prevalence of SOAEs was 100% in patients with tinnitus secondary to head injury (Ceranic, Prasher, & Luxon, 1998; Ceranic et al., 1998).

In most cases, SOAEs and tinnitus are mutually exclusive. The literature on SOAEs is reviewed in Chapter 3.

The Relation of TEOAEs and DPOAEs With Tinnitus

As OAE measurement has been incorporated into clinical audiology, including the diagnostic assessment of persons with tinnitus (see Mueller & Hall, 1998, for review), a clear pattern has emerged. OAEs are characteristically abnormal, or not detectable, in the frequency region of the tinnitus, even among persons with clinically normal audiograms (McGee & Stephens, 1992; Ceranic et al., 1995; Shiomi et al., 1997; Ruth & Hall, 1999). One of the most comprehensive, and recent, studies was reported by Japanese investigator Yosaku Shiomi and colleagues (1997). In comparison to normal hearing and otologically normal subjects (including no tinnitus), DPOAE amplitudes were consistently reduced among tinnitus patients, even those with audiometrically normal hearing. The decrement in DPOAEs among tinnitus patients was most pronounced within the 4000- to 7000-Hz region.

The author routinely records DPOAEs in the diagnostic evaluation of persons presenting with the complaint of tinnitus. As shown in Figure 9–30, the majority of these patients have abnormal DPOAE findings (almost always within the high-frequency region that is matched to their tinnitus). A sizable proportion of the patients with abnormal DPOAEs have pure-tone hearing thresholds within clinically normal limits (20 dB or better). This finding has important diagnostic implications. For almost all patients, it is possible to document abnormal cochlear function in a frequency region corresponding to their perceived tinnitus. The information gained from DPOAEs can also be useful in counseling the patient and convincing them that indeed their problem is real.

Audiometric versus DPOAE Findings

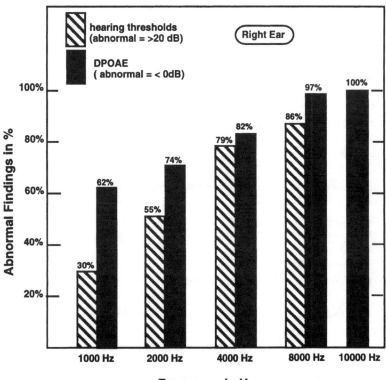

Figure 9–30. Proportion of abnormal findings for pure-tone audiometry and DPOAEs for 162 patients evaluated because of the complaint of tinnitus. Data are shown only for the right ear. DPOAEs were invariably abnormal somewhere in the 1000- to 10,000-Hz region, in some cases even with normal pure-tone hearing sensitivity.

Case 9: Ruling Out Tinnitus With OAEs

A 33-year-old female television reporter presented to the audiology clinic very distressed about ringing tinnitus in her left ear. She associated the onset of the tinnitus with a recent upper respiratory infection and with the presence of a silicone plug in her left ear. Appropriately concerned about hearing protection when she attended a peformance of her brother's rock and roll band, she had inserted malleable silicone earplugs deeply into both ears. When she attempted to remove the plug from her left ear, her rather long fingernails neatly sliced through the silicone leaving most of the plug in her ear canal. Before hearing testing, an otolaryngologist carefully dissected and removed under microscope the remaining silicone from her left ear canal. Audiologic assessment showed normal hearing sensitivity, normal middle ear function, and excellent word recognition scores (Figure 9–31). The patient was very anxious due to the tinnitus, fearing that she had damaged her ears and therefore prematurely ended her television career. OAEs were measured to rule out cochlear pathology. DPOAEs were reliably recorded from both ears (Figure 9–32). Multiple SOAEs were also recorded bilaterally. The patient was assured that these sensitive measures of cochlear function ruled out any significant problem. Her outlook improved immediately, and she no longer perceived the tinnitus. After shaking everyone's hand vigorously and thanking the entire clinic staff repeatedly, she returned to the television station and her career.

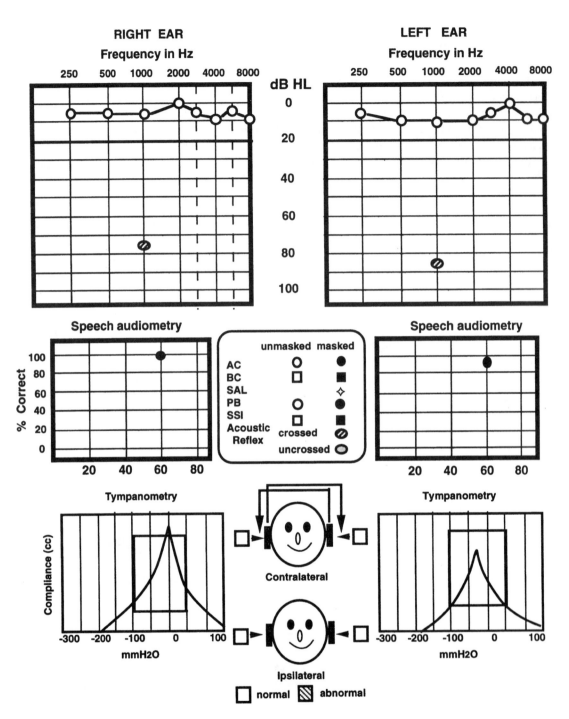

Figure 9–31. Audiometric findings for a 33-year-old female television reporter (Case 9) self-referred to otolaryngology and audiology for removal of a silicone plug in her left ear canal. She was extremely concerned about tinnitus in her left ear. After the plug was removed, a normal audiogram was recorded.

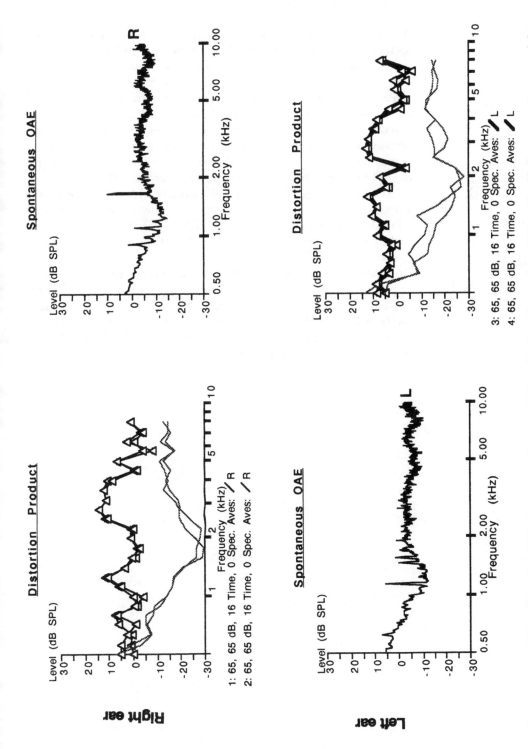

Figure 9–32. DPOAE and SOAE findings for a 33-year-old female television reporter (Case 9) with the presenting complaint of tinnitus in the left ear, prior to the removal of a silicone plug from that ear. DPOAE amplitudes were normal bilaterally, and SOAEs were recorded from each ear. These findings were used to reassure the patient that her cochlear function was normal.

Case 10: Localization of Tinnitus With DPOAEs

A 26-year-old female hospital receptionist came to the otolaryngology and audiology clinics after working all night with the complaint of ringing tinnitus in the right ear. When questioned about noise exposure, she admitted to frequently listening to music at high intensity levels with her new and powerful car stereo system. In fact, she had last enjoyed the sound system less than 12 hours earlier while driving to work. Her right ear was preferentially exposed to the speakers in the system. Audiologic findings were generally normal, although there was some evidence of a very slight decrease in hearing thresholds for the right ear, and the hint of a notching pattern near 3000 Hz (Figure 9–33). DPOAEs were consistent with normal cochlear function on the left ear. For the right ear, however, there was a clear decrease in DPOAE amplitudes in the region of 2500 Hz (Figure 9–34). This notch in the DPgram corresponded to the pitch of the patient's tinnitus.

Comment. OAEs can be helpful in localizing cochlear dyfunction to a specific frequency region and, of course, one or both ears. With this patient, OAEs were correlated with the lateralization of the tinnitus to the right ear and the perceived pitch of tinnitus. OAE findings were used in counseling the patient about risk to her hearing posed by excessive volume of music in her car.

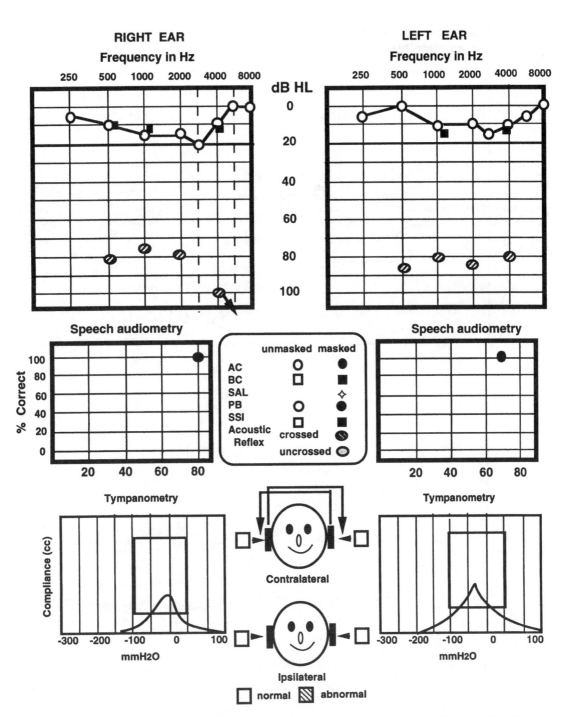

Figure 9–33. Audiometric findings for a 26-year-old female receptionist (Case 10) within 12 hours after exposure to excessive sound levels produced by an expensive automobile stereo system. The patient complained of ringing tinnitus in the right ear.

PT: 26 y.o. female (VUH receptionist)
DX: right ear tinnitus

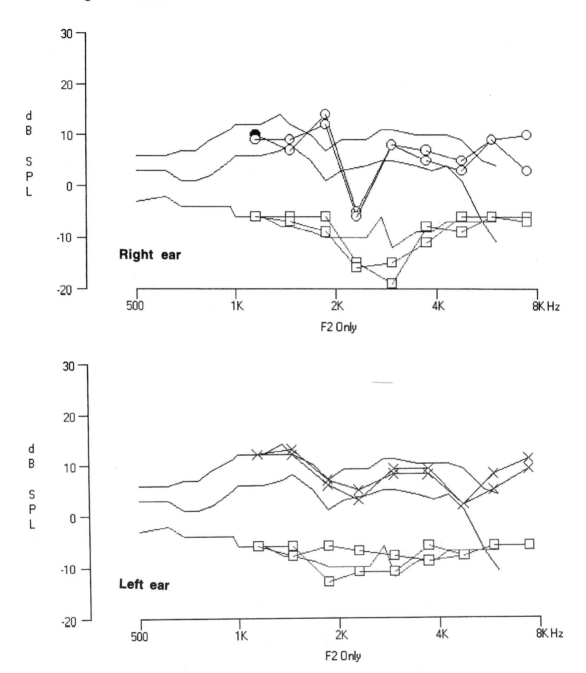

Figure 9–34. DPOAEs for a 26-year-old female receptionist (Case 10) complaining of ringing tinnitus in the right ear, localized to approximately 2200 Hz. Note the dip in the DPgram within this frequency region, even though the audiogram failed to show a marked abnormality (Figure 9–33).

Case 11: DPOAE Abnormalities in a "Normal Hearing" Patient With Tinnitus

A 22-year-old female medical student was referred to audiology directly from the otology clinic because of tinnitus. The patient was extremely distressed about her perception of a high-pitch tinnitus. She expressed concern that, because of it, she would lose her hearing and be forced to drop out of medical school and to abandon her favorite pastime (playing the piano). She expressed thoughts of suicide. After an extensive and highly emotional counseling session, the patient underwent audiologic assessment. Hearing sensitivity was entirely within normal limits (Figure 9–35). Middle ear function was also normal. Although DPOAE amplitudes were normal for the frequency region of 1000 to 4200 Hz, they were abnormally decreased for higher frequencies (Figure 9–36).

Comment. OAEs showed evidence of cochlear dysfunction, which was associated with the patient's perception of tinnitus. This information was invaluable in counseling the patient about the origin of her tinnitus and helped to convince her that "she was not crazy." Abnormal OAEs are an almost invariable finding in persons with tinnitus, as shown earlier in Figure 9–30.

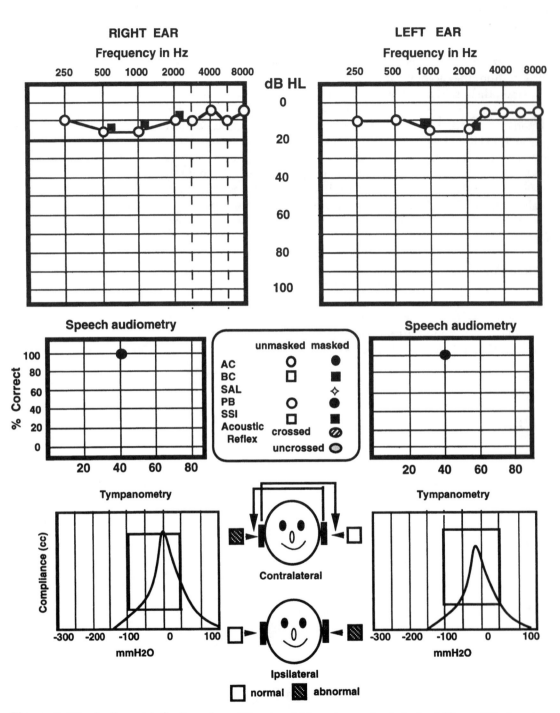

Figure 9–35. Audiometric findings for a 22-year-old female medical student (Case 11) showing hearing sensitivity within normal limits. The patient was extremely distressed, and depressed, because of high-frequency ringing tinnitus in each ear.

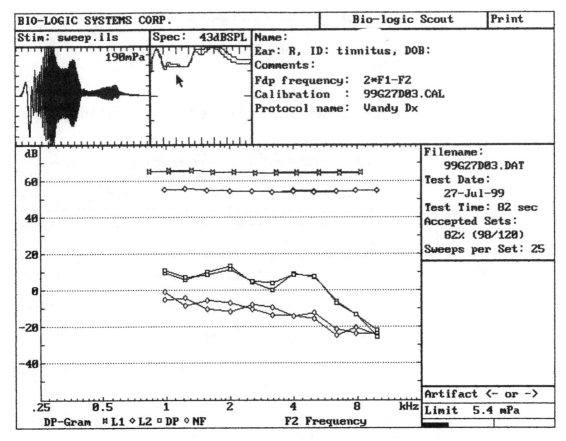

Figure 9–36. DPOAEs recorded from the right ear of a 22-year-old female medical student (Case 11) with tinnitus. With this device, DPOAE amplitudes below 0 dB are considered abnormal. DPOAEs provided evidence of cochlear dysfunction bilaterally in the high-frequency region, despite the normal audiometric findings (Figure 9–35).

MISCELLANEOUS APPLICATIONS IN ADULTS

Published reports of other clinical uses of OAEs were summarized in Table 9–2. Most are variations of the applications described in detail in this chapter. For example, the paper by Hamill-Ruth and colleagues (1998) is an excellent demonstration of the clinical feasibility and value of OAEs as a quick and sensitive tool for screening cochlear function in adults who are at risk for hearing impairment but, for various reasons, are not candidates for behavioral audiometry. The subjects in this study were 133 critically ill persons admitted to the surgical intensive care unit. Risk factors for hearing impairment included metabolic and electrolyte abnormalities, ototoxicity, and even noise exposure secondary to the ICU environment.

OAEs can contribute to the identification, diagnosis, and delineation of auditory dysfunction in myriad pathologies afflicting adults. The reader can periodically monitor published accounts of OAE in adult populations by consulting the MedLine system on the internet at: www.nlm.nih.gov/databases

The literature on OAEs and age-related hearing loss—presbycusis—was reviewed previously in a discussion of factors influencing OAEs (Chapter 5). A handful of studies devoted to this topic are listed in Table 9–2.

Case 12: Reversal of Sudden Onset of Hearing Loss

A 48-year-old male physician dropped by the clinic early one morning after noticing a dramatic decrease in his hearing for the right ear the night before. The initial audiogram showed a severe sensorineural hearing loss (Figure 9–37). OAEs were not recorded (right portion of the figure), with amplitudes less than 15 dB (and within the noise floor). The patient was immediately evaluated by an otolaryngologist and treated with steroids. Over the next 12 days, hearing sensitivity progressively improved until thresholds for most frequencies were within normal limits. DPOAEs were recorded first at Test #4 (12 days postonset), when hearing was within normal limits, but amplitude values remained outside of the adult normal region. On the final test date, there was a decrease in pure-tone thresholds and DPOAE amplitudes for frequencies above 3000 Hz.

Comment. OAEs can confirm cochlear pathology in sudden onset of sensorineural hearing loss, but they do not contribute to the definition of degree of hearing loss. Even with an apparent total reversal of hearing loss audiometrically, OAE abnormalities may persist, suggesting the presence of residual cochlear deficit.

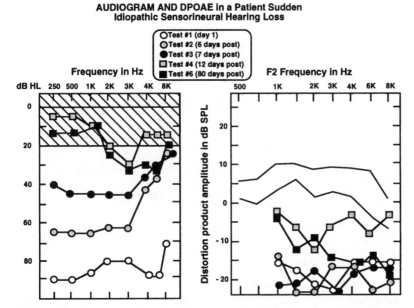

Figure 9–37. Serial pure-tone thresholds (right portion) and DPOAEs (left portion) for a 48-year-old male physician with sudden onset of sensorineural hearing loss (Case 12). Pure-tone thresholds for selected frequencies returned from the severe region to within normal limits, whereas DPOAE amplitudes, although showing some increase, remained consistently abnormal.

CHAPTER

10

Future Clinical Directions

My crystal ball is not any better than yours. All of us, however, can get a glimpse at the future of clinical OAE measurement by surveying current trends in basic OAE research. How can one determine what's hot in basic hearing science (usually research utilizing animal models) and in human experimentation (performed often with laboratory instrumentation and normal subjects)? The simplest way is to regularly monitor the work presented at annual meetings of, for example, the Association for Research in Otolaryngology (ARO) and papers published mostly in a select group of journals (listed at the end of Chapter 2). To periodically discover what is being studied and reported at these meetings, and in the literature, anyone can access websites for organizations (e.g., www.aro.org) or public databases such as the National Library of Medicine (www.nlm.hih.gov).

Creative thinking is a common denominator in most of the papers cited herein. For example, Christopher Shera and John Guinan of the Eaton-Peabody Laboratory of Auditory Physiology at Harvard University Medical School and the Massachusetts Eye and Ear Infirmary challenge the traditional system for classification of OAEs (outlined in Chapter 1). Referring to the typical opinion that each of the different categories of OAEs arises from nonlinear distortion secondary to outer hair cell motility, these authors boldly "argue that the common view cannot be correct" (Shera & Guinan, 1999). This open-minded and unorthodox approach to OAEs at the end of the second half of the 20th century is reminiscent of the forward thinking Thomas Gold, toward the end of the first half of the century. Fortunately, it's highly unlikely that Drs. Shera and Guinan will turn their attention from hearing science to astrophysics or some other field of study.

The reader will have no problem anticipating potential clinical applications of some of the research reviewed in this chapter. Indeed, the desirability of further clinical research of some rather basic OAE measurement approaches (e.g., input-output functions for TEOAEs and DPOAEs) was stressed earlier in Chapter 4. Certain technologic advances in OAE equipment have obvious clinical advantages and usefulness. A good example is the trend toward hand-held and automated OAE devices. In fact, the first generation of OAE instruments with these features is already being marketed to clinical audiologists and others involved in newborn hearing screening. Highly sophisticated measurement techniques, such as maximum length sequence (MLS), also have immediate inherent appeal for increasing the speed and accuracy of newborn hearing screening and are now undergoing field assessment with commercially available equipment. Other research findings will no doubt be studied and then applied clinically before long. An example is analysis of the phase of DPOAEs. To date, DPOAE analyses strategies have almost exclusively utilized amplitude information. There are, however, a number of basic investigations of DPOAE phase in animal models and normal human subjects. When

After his prescient work on cochlear physiology in the late 1940s (see Chapter 1 for details), Dr. Thomas Gold pursued an illustrious career in astrophysics at Cornell University in New York. There he was Professor and Chairman of the Department of Astronomy. He also founded the Cornell Center for Radiophysics and Space Research and served as its director for 20 years. Ironically, prior to his Cornell years Dr. Gold was a Professor of Applied Astronomy at Harvard University — the very institution where George von Békésy had unceremoniously dismissed the auditory scientist Gold's innovative cochlear findings. During his long and productive academic tenure, Dr. Gold amassed 280 publications on topics ranging from hearing to the origin of planetary hydrocarbons. He even served as a member of the United States President's Space Science Panel. (Source: Cornell University website: www.people.cornell.edu).

will we begin reading about the clinical value of DPOAE phase? Two events could provide the impetus for clinical investigatons. A user-friendly option for measurement of phase could be included on a variety of clinical DPOAE devices. It would then be only a short time before clinicians began to explore the potential value of this new DPOAE response parameter, versus amplitude, in different patient populations. Or, some of the investigators who have developed instrumentation for measuring DPOAE phase could take the equipment into a clinical setting and, with Institutional Review Board approval for human research, systematically evaluate the effects of auditory pathologies on DPOAE phase. Chances are quite good that one or both events will occur soon. Thus, the recurring theme of this chapter is the actual or pending transition of certain OAE measurements and analysis strategies from the laboratory to the clinic, or from the "bench to the booth."

RETHINKING THE CLASSIFICATION OF OAEs

The conventional system for classifying OAEs was described at the beginning of this book and summarized in Table 1–1. In this system, both TEOAEs and DPOAEs are in the category of evoked OAEs, and the generation of both types is related to nonlinearity in cochlear function involving outer hair cell activity. It is reasonable to assume, therefore, that TEOAE and DPOAE findings will be in close agreement for normal subjects and various patient populations. Yet clinicians systematically applying both DPOAEs and TEOAEs report occasional discrepancies in findings. That is, TEOAEs may be abnormal or not detected in some persons with quite normal appearing DPOAEs, and vice versa. The organizational schema for OAEs introduced by Shera and Guinan (1999) provides a natural explanation for divergent findings of TEOAEs versus DPOAEs (Figure 10–1). These authors state that "at low sound levels stimulus-frequency and transiently evoked emissions must arise by mechanisms fundamentally different from pure distortion products" (p. 782). Therefore, "As a consequence of their different origins, reflection- and distortion-source emissions presumably manifest different dependencies on cochlear pathologies" (p. 792). The new OAE taxonomy further explains some of the OAE "paradoxes," such as the variable differences in amplitude and prevalence for TEOAEs and DPOAEs among animal species and the differential effects of certain drugs (e.g., aspirin) on these two types of OAEs. Shera and Guinan (1999) hastened to point out that, with the usual techniques for measurement of either type of OAE, which are dependent in part on stimulus parameters (intensity level and frequency, or the f_2/f_1 ratio), there will likely be a "mixing" of both types of OAEs in the external ear canal. Innovative measurement strategies clearly permit the isolation or separation of two distinct sources for DPOAEs, one

The traditional approach for categorizing OAE types is reviewed in Chapter 1, and detailed also in review articles such as the comprehensive 1991 paper published in the **Journal of the Acoustical Society of America** *by Rudi Probst, Brenda Lonsbury-Martin, and Glen Martin.*

REVISED TAXONOMY FOR OTOACOUSTIC EMISSIONS

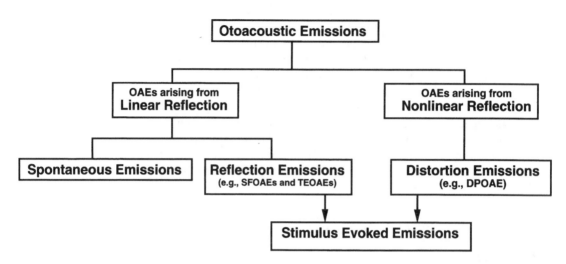

Figure 10–1. A classification system or taxonomy for OAEs proposed by Shera and Guinan (1999). Transient OAEs and spontaneous OAEs are categorized as originating in linear reflection (left portion of the figure) whereas distortion product OAEs are produced by nonlinear distortion (right portion of the figure).

near the f_2 place and the other near the f_{dp} place within the cochlea (Gaskill & Brown, 1990; Fahey & Allen, 1997; Heitmann, 1998; Siegel et al., 1998; Talmadge et al., 1998). For most DPOAE measurements in humans, the f_{dp} place is at $2f_1$–f_2. These are designated as "D" and "R" in Figure 10–2. The relative contribution of these two sources to DPOAE findings can be assessed with various strategies, such as ipsilateral suppression of either source or minimization of the reflection "R" component by presenting a third primary tone with a frequency close to the f_{dp}. Strategies may also be employed for isolating reflection versus nonlinear contributions to TEOAEs. Shera and Guinan's (1999) fresh view of OAEs opens up a plethora of research opportunities, and perhaps clinical applications.

INTEGRATION OF ABR, IMMITTANCE, AND OAEs (TEOAEs & DPOAEs) TECHNOLOGY

The importance of the cross-check principle in pediatric diagnostic assessment was repeatedly stressed in Chapter 8. For infants and young children, the major test battery procedures are electrophysiologic. Wouldn't it be convenient and powerful diagnostically to be able to seamlessly perform immittance measures (tympanometry and

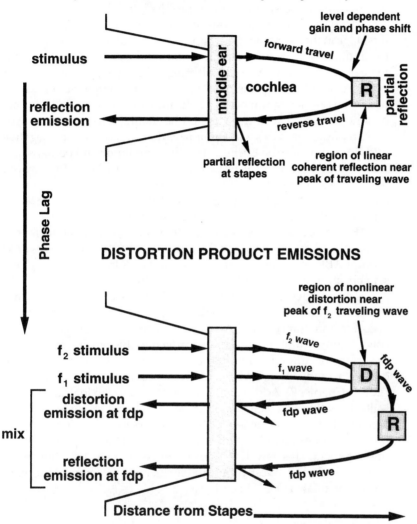

Figure 10–2. A schematic illustration of the generation of distortion product OAEs at relatively low stimulus intensity levels (from Shera & Guinan, 1999, p. 790). According to this schema, DPOAEs measured in the ear canal include a mixture of reflection and distortion emissions. Nonlinear distortion (**D**) occuring at or about the maximum amplitude of the f_2 wave on the basilar membrane produce energy (waves) at the DPOAE frequency that reaches the ear canal via direct outward propagation (upper f_{dp} wave arrow) or by first traveling further forward until it is reflected (**R**) backward (the lower second f_{dp} wave arrow). See also Figure 10–1.

acoustic reflexes), OAEs, and ABRs with the same piece of equipment? A three-in-one instrument would be especially handy for newborn hearing screening, and pediatric assessment in general. A combination measurement protocol in a young child might go something like this. A probe would be snuggly fitted into the ear canal. Tympanometry would be performed first. Acoustic reflexes might also be an option at this stage in the assessment, perhaps with a broad band noise stimulus to simultaneously verify normal middle ear status and roughly estimate hearing sensitivity (e.g., Hall et al., 1982). Then, with external ear pressure maintained at the point of maximum compliance or admittance (the tympanogram peak), OAEs measurement would be immediately performed with the same probe. Taking into account tympanometry findings in this way minimizes the effects of slightly negative middle ear pressure on OAEs, enhancing amplitude and perhaps permitting the detection of OAEs in some patients for whom OAEs would not otherwise be recorded. If tympanometry confirmed clearly abnormal middle ear function (e.g., restricted mobility as reflected in a flat or type B tympanogram), then OAE measurement might be deferred, or if OAE measurement was conducted, their absence could be attributed to middle ear versus cochlear dysfunction. Absence of OAEs would prompt ABR estimation of hearing sensitivity. Or, if OAEs were present but auditory neuropathy suspected, ABR assessment for neurodiagnosis and threshold estimation would also be conducted. In either event, recording electrodes would be applied first. The same probe used for immittance and OAE measurement would be used for air-conduction stimulus presentation during the ABR. Several major manufacturers of ABR and immittance instrumentation also market OAE devices. Combination OAE and ABR devices are already on the market (see Chapter 7). Adding immittance measures is a logical and clinically attractive next technologic advance. Another recent technologic advance is the introduction to the marketplace of variety of OAE instruments designed for both transient and distortion product OAE measurement. This new development opens up many possibilities for innovative clinical investigation and further enhancement of the diagnostic potential of OAEs in cochlear pathologies.

Combination OAE and ABR systems are now available, and described by manufacturers in Chapter 7. In addition, as also noted in Chapter 7, the integration of immittance and OAE technology into a single system is currently under development by at least one manufacturer.

AUTOMATED OAE TECHNOLOGY

We have witnessed rapid introduction of algorithms and intrumentation for OAE stimulus presentation and response analysis. A variety of automated OAE devices are commercially available (see Chapter 7). This trend will no doubt continue for both desktop and hand-held units. The pressing need for newborn hearing screening devices that do not require a highly trained person for data collection, analysis, and interpretation provided the initial motivation for research and development of automated technology. Other potential clinical applications of automated OAE equipment might include industrial and school programs for hearing screening. Although automated technology is a reality, much research needs to be conducted on its test performance in clinical settings, and validation of findings with conventional OAE measurement, along with other auditory test findings.

NOVEL STIMULI FOR OAE MEASUREMENT

Chirp Stimuli

The common types of stimuli used to evoke OAEs are clicks and tone bursts for TOAEs and pure tones for DPOAEs. There is some evidence that the TEOAEs can also be evoked by other signals, including noise (Maat, van Dijk, & Wit, 1996) and short frequency sweeps, or chirps (Neumann, Uppenkamp, & Kollmeier, 1994). Clicks (produced by rectangular pulses) are acoustic signals with brief duration (e.g., 0.1 ms or 100 μs) and broad frequency spectrum. Energy is distributed over a wide range of frequencies. Also, because of their very brief duration, transduction by miniature earphones is somewhat inefficient. Unwanted distortion is produced also at high stimulus intensity levels. Therefore, maximum stimulus levels are limited and, of course, stimulus frequency specificity is compromised. Each chirp signal generated by Neumann and colleagues (1994) was described by its instantaneous frequency and its envelope. OAEs were recorded for chirp signals over a frequency range of 500 to 6000 Hz. OAEs evoked by chirp versus conventional click signals were compared for 25 subjects ranging in age from 24 to 71 years. Chirp and click stimulation produced OAEs that were similar in the time and frequency domains. However, chirp-evoked OAEs were higher in amplitude, and characterized by better signal-to-noise ratios, than those for click stimulation. Currently, no commercially available OAE devices offer chirp signals as an option.

Most manufacturers of OAE instrumentation are now marketing hand-held and fully automated devices, designed mostly for newborn hearing screening. Descriptions and photographs of these devices can be found in Chapter 7.

Bone-Conducted Stimuli

The comparison of findings for air- versus bone-conducted stimuli is a fundamental technique in the assessment and analysis of auditory function. Bone-conduction stimulation of the cochlea, of course, bypasses the external ear canal and middle ear system. Normal pure-tone hearing thresholds, or a normal auditory brainstem response, can be recorded even from persons with middle ear pathologies and sizeable conductive hearing impairments, since the response is recorded proximally (centrally). OAEs are dependent on the external and middle ear system for outward propogation of the response as well as inward presentation of the stimulus. Therefore, bone-conduction stimulation for OAEs does not offer the same clinical advantage. We would expect that bone-conduction stimulation in OAE measurement of patients with middle ear pathology would fail to produce a response.

Bone-conduction stimulation has attracted a modest amount of research attention for TEOAEs (Rossi & Solero, 1988; Rossi et al., 1988; Collet et al., 1989) and, more recently, for DPOAEs (Xu et al., 1991; Purcell et al., 1998).

At least three features of bone-conducted stimulation in OAE measurement argue for at least attempting this innovative test technique. As noted by Purcell and colleagues, in reference to DPOAEs (1998, p. 362):

> Through application of the stimulus directly to the head, the immediate source of the stimulus has been removed from the ear canal, where a microphone picks up the DPOAE. Emissions are very small in magnitude, and better use of the digitizer dynamic range can be achieved with any reduction in ear canal magnitude. A second unique property of bone conduction is that both cochleae are stimulated simultaneously. A clinical screening can be imagined in which both ears are tested at the same time. (Xu et al., 1991)

Finally, and most obvious, the influence of the external and middle ear systems on stimulation is essentially eliminated.

In the study by Purcell et al. (1998), DPOAEs were stimulated with two customized piezo-electric transducers, one for the f_1 signal and another for the f_2 signal. These authors concluded that DPgrams, and input-output functions, were similar for air- versus bone-conduction stimulation when stimulus intensity levels were carefully equalized. Bilateral stimulation of the cochleae with bone-conduction was verified. And, occlusion of the ear canal did not produce a substantial effect on DPOAEs. Previous reports of bone-conducted TEOAEs noted similar conclusions. In fact, Rossi et al. (1988) were able to record bone-conducted TEOAEs from a patient with unilateral otosclerosis. Based on the outcome of these studies, further investigation of the bone-conduction DPOAE approach in patients with middle ear dysfunction seems to be warranted.

MULTIPLE LENGTH SEQUENCE (MLS) TECHNIQUE

The MLS technique is the very rapid and quasi-random presentation of a sequence of stimuli, and silent periods separating stimuli. Rates of presentation may exceed 2000 stimuli per second, in contrast to stimulus rates for conventional electrophysiologic measures that are typically well under 100/s, often as slow as 10 or 11 stimuli/s. The problems of conventional stimulus presentation at rapid rates, namely, the occurrence of multiple stimuli within the time period of a response to one of the stimuli and "distortion" or "corruption" (Thornton, 1991; Hine & Thornton, 1997) of the waveforms, are circumvented with the MLS technique by the mode of presentation and the analysis approach. The relationship between stimuli and interstimulus intervals, or silent periods, is not predictable and constant. Also, a sequence-specific analysis strategy permits deconvolution and extraction of multiple overlapping responses (see Burkhard et al., 1990 for a detailed discussion of the MLS technique). The major clinical advantage of MLS is the collection of more data in less time. Consequently, the MLS technique would appear to be well-suited for clinical applications that require minimal test time and maximum effort to achieve an adequate signal-to-noise ratio, such as newborn hearing screening (Thornton, 1993; Johannsesen, Rasmussen, & Osterhammel, 1998). For a number of years, auditory evoked responses have been recorded with MLS averaging (e.g., Burhard, Shi, & Hecox, 1990; Eysholdt & Schreiner, 1992; Thornton & Slaven, 1993) with both experimental and clinical instrumentation (e.g., Nicolet Spirit device). There is now abundant evidence that TEOAEs can be recorded with the MLS technique from adults (Picton et al., 1993; Thornton, 1993a, 1993b; Thornton, Folkard, & Chambers, 1994; Thornton, 1996; Thornton, Slaven, MacKenzie, & Phillips, 1996; Hine & Thornton, 1997), and also neonates (Johannsesen, Rasmussen, & Osterhammel, 1998a, 1998b). This literature confirms that absolute amplitude of TEOAEs decreases with the MLS technique as the stimulus rate increases above about 40/s, but morphology and the characteristics of input-output functions do not differ for conventional versus MLS methods.

NEW STRATEGIES FOR MEASUREMENT AND ANALYSIS OF OAEs

Latency (and Phase)

Clinicians familiar with the ABR will appreciate the irony of the almost exclusive reliance to date on analysis of OAE spectral characteristics and response amplitude. In contrast, ABR analysis is heavily dependent on temporal characteristics, especially the calculation of absolute latencies for wave components and interwave latency values. ABRs for tone burst stimuli illustrate clearly the influence of cochlear travel time on latency values. That is, latencies are shortest for high frequency stimuli as ABRs are generated in more basal region, whereas latencies for lower frequency stimuli (e.g., 500 Hz), generated in more apical regions, may be up to twice as long. Actually, the analogy of ABR and OAE latency was directly investigated years ago by Steve Neely and colleagues at Boys Town National Research Hospital (Neely et al., 1988). In addition, cochlear traveling time has for years been investigated with ECochG and ABR (e.g., Elberling, 1974; Don & Eggermont, 1978; Parker & Thornton, 1978; Don et al., 1993). ABR amplitude is highly variable and therefore assumes a relatively minor role in clinical analysis and interpretation. Both TEOAEs and DPOAEs are, course, recorded after the presentation of stimuli. For TEOAEs displayed as a waveform within the time domain during the first 20 ms

There is considerable basic research on OAE phase, at least in normal subjects. Application of OAE phase analysis may well be one of the exciting new clinical research frontiers. Keep monitoring the literature for the latest developments.

after the click stimuli, the latency feature is obvious but not precisely quantified (see Figure 1–8 in Chapter 1). There is longstanding evidence that TEOAE latency invariably decreases as frequency increases (e.g., Kemp, 1978; Kemp & Chum, 1980; Rutten, 1980; Wit & Ritsma, 1980; Bonfils et al., 1988; Collet et al., 1989. Recently, the interaction of TEOAEs at different latencies with systematic changes in stimulus intensity have been specifically studied (e.g., Kruglov et al., 1996).

At this juncture a distinction should be made between latency and phase, although some authors cited below use the two terms interchangeably. Latency, described in a unit of time (milliseconds or seconds), is the delay between stimulus presentation and measurement of an OAE response. Changes in phase, described in degrees, may be irregularities in the OAEs secondary to noise in the recording, but are also consistently (inversely) related to the stimulus frequency.

Several major research groups are investigating DPOAE latency in humans (Brown et al., 1984; Kimberly et al., 1993; Madeira da Silva, Reis, & Penha, 1994; Whitehead et al., 1994; Brown et al., 1995; O'Mahoney & Kemp, 1995; Kemp, 1996; Moulin & Kemp, 1996a, 1996b; Stover, Neely & Gorga, 1996; Wable, Collet & Chery-Croze, 1996; Bowman et al., 1997; Bowman et al., 1998). One reason for this interest is the appreciation that "DPOAE phase responses can be utilized to estimate round-trip phase delay [travel time] in the adult and neonatal cochlea" (Bowman et al., 1998, p. 15). The underlying assumption is that the time required to reach the place of maximum stimuluation during inward propogation is equivalent to the travel time outward from this place to the external ear canal (Neely et al., 1988) and does not include any time for the actual generation of the DPOAE. Another viewpoint of the inward-outward travel time also takes into account properties of the cochlea, which may independent of stimulus intensity and the time utilized during a filtering process at the place of stimulation (Hall, 1974; Ruggero, 1980; Bowman et al., 1998). That is, with this model, three different components are involved in DPOAE latency—stimulus travel in, cochlear filter response (or buildup) time, and OAE travel out (Bowman et al., 1998).

Techniques for measurement of DPOAE latency are rather sophisticated, although clinically feasible. Briefly, DPOAE round-trip latency is estimated by holding one stimulus constant and sweeping the other. Thus, the f_1 stimulus may be fixed as the f_2 is swept across a range or vice versa. For either measurement paradigm, DPOAE latency decreases as the f_2 frequency increases (Figure 10–3). This is not unexpected, because higher f_2 frequencies correspond to more basal cochlear places (closer to the stapes footplate) and require shorter travel times. Latencies, however, are shorter when f_2 is swept than when f_1 is swept. Stimulus intensity also plays a role in DPOAE latency measurement, especially for higher frequencies (above 2000 Hz) and with

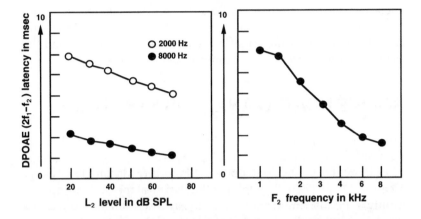

Figure 10–3. A highly schematic representation of the relation between stimulus frequency (f_2) and intensity (L_2) and latency of the prominent DPOAE in humans ($2f_1-f_2$). DPOAE latency decreases as a function of increases in stimulus frequency and intensity. (Adapted from the work of Moulin & Kemp, 1996a, 1996b; Stover, Neely, & Gorga, 1996; Bowman et al., 1997; Bowman et al., 1998).

the f_2 sweep technique. In general, latencies diminish as stimulus intensity increases (Figure 10–3). In addition, DPOAE latencies are shorter for higher f_2/f_1 ratios, and longer for lower f_2/f_1 ratios. There appears to be no gender effect for latency of the $2f_1-f_2$ DPOAE, but men do show longer latencies than females for the DP at $2f_2-f_1$ (Moulin & Kemp, 1996). Both f_1 and f_2 sweep techniques for measuring DPOAE latency or phase can be effectively used to investigate filter response properties of the cochlea which are, in turn, related to tuning curve or Q_{10}, characteristics (i.e., sharpness of tuning curves). Thus, DPOAE latency may offer even greater enhancement of sensitivity to cochlear dysfunction. A potential clinical disadvantage of DPOAE latency, however, is considerable intersubject variability which is, in part, due to individual variations in tympanic membrane and middle-ear status, such as middle ear pressure (e.g., Moulin & Kemp, 1996a).

The literature on latency in human subjects often addresses the topic of multicomponent DPOAEs, specifically the $2f_1-f_2$ and $2f_2-f_1$ DPOAEs (Frank & Kossl, 1996; Moulin, 1996a, 1996b; Wable, Collet, & Chery-Croze, 1996; Stover, Neely, & Gorga, 1996). Although the $2f_1-f_2$ DP is prominent in humans, the DP at $2f_2-f_1$ can be consistently record- *For a listing of the many* ed and is attracting considerable research interest because of its poten- *potential distortion* tial contribution to our understanding of cochlear processes. One very *products, see Chapter 4,* interesting line of research is the study of multicomponent DPOAEs to *and specifically Table 4–3.* explore the possibility that DPs are generated by multiple sources within the cochlea (e.g., Stover, Neely, & Gorga, 1996). The reader is encouraged to consult these studies for detailed discussion of the techniques used to measure multicomponent DPOAE, and thoughtful consideration of the differential influence of various stimulus and subject factors on the properties of multiple DP components.

SOPHISTICATED ANALYSIS STRATEGIES

There is ongoing interest in the development of a statistically based approach for identification of hearing loss with OAE data (Gorga et al., 1993; Prieve et al., 1993; Hatzopouos, Mazzoli, & Martini, 1995; Gorga, Neely, & Dorn, 1999). Examples of the statistical methods are spectral multivariate discriminant analysis, linear discriminant models, and quadradic (second-order) discriminant models (e.g., Hatzopouos, Mazzoli, & Martini, 1995). Other highly mathematical methods for signal analysis, such as wavelet analysis, time-frequency distributions (the Wigner Distribution and the Choi-Williams Distribution), Wiener kernel analysis, derived nonlinear response estimation, manipulation of OAE time-windowing, and linear/nonlinear system-identification techniques are also being applied to OAE data (e.g., Wit, van Dijk, & Avan, 1994; Whitehead et al., 1995; Ravazzani, Tognola, & Grandori, 1996; Blinowska & Durka, 1997; Ozdamar et al., 1997; van Dijk, Maat, & Wit, 1997; Krishnan & Chertoff, 1999). One ultimate goal of such work is to increase the overall accuracy of OAE detection and analysis, especially with specific OAE applications such as newborn hearing screening. In this respect, these studies are related in their overall objective to work on automated confirmation of the presence of OAEs versus just noise (Welzl-Muller & Stephan, 1994). Automated signal detection algorithms are now being incorporated into clinical OAE devices, as noted above.

CLOSING COMMENT

The rapidly expanding basic study of OAEs, and inseparably the cochlea as well, will continue to provide the knowledge base and technologic foundation essential for maximal exploitation of OAEs clinically. The goals and accomplishments of the basic scientist and clinician alike will be greatly enhanced by a regular exchange of ideas and experiences and mutual respect.

APPENDIX

Normative Data for
Otoacoustic Emissions

DPOAE NORMATIVE DATA

There are two general possibilities for accessing normative data for adult subjects. One is to rely on normative databases supplied by the manufacturer of the device you'll be using in the clinic. You will need to follow closely the test protocol that was employed during collection of these normative data, especially the stimulus intensity levels, the f_2/f_1 ratio, and the stimulus frequencies. If the persons responsible for collecting normative data used stimulus intensity levels of $L_1 = 65$ dB and $L_2 = 55$ dB, an f_2/f_1 ratio of 1.22, and three stimuli per octave from 500 to 4000 Hz, then you would need to use a similar protocol. Clearly, the flexibility of your clinical test protocol would be very limited. You would, for example, have no normative data for other intensity levels, or higher test frequencies, or for intermediate frequencies when more frequencies per octave were presented. If another database is used, it is also important to verify a variety of potential factors in DPOAE measurement outcome. What were the criteria for normal hearing used by the data collectors? That is, were normal subjects required to have hearing thresholds of 15 dB or better or 25 dB or better? Were subjects with a history of noise exposure, or reporting tinnitus, excluded from the database? Where were the data collected—a noisy room, a quiet room, or a sound booth? Nonetheless, some manufacturer's can supply extensive normative data, often installed on the OAE system you've purchased. Examples of normative databases from several manufacturers can be found in Chapter 7.

A second option is to collect your own database. This provides almost unlimited flexibility. The subject criteria (e.g., gender and age), the test conditions, and all test parameters can be tailor-made to your DPOAE applications, clinical setting, and patient population. However, careful subject selection and screening (for hearing thresholds, middle ear status, and otologic history) and actual OAE data collection for various stimulus and frequency combinations is time consuming (on the positive side, you will gain clinical experience in the process). And, normative statistics will need to be calculated (e.g., means, standard deviations, percentiles) for DPOAEs and noise floor values. How many normal subjects and/or ears are necessary for an adequate data base? The safest approach is to collect data from at least 20 ears, and then to calculate the normative statistics mentioned above for the next five subjects. If variability is stable, data collection can be terminated. If not, then it should continue until variability no longer decreases with additional subjects.

Adult normative data for five different DPOAE devices are summarized in Tables A–1 through A–5. Subjects were 30 young adults aged 21 to 28 years (15 male and 15 female) with hearing thresholds of 15 dB HL or better for audiometric frequencies of 500 through 8000 Hz. There were no gender differences in DPOAE amplitude. All had normal (type A) tympanograms. None reported tinnitus or exposure to excessive levels of sound. DPOAE data were collected in a quiet but not sound-treated room with an average ambient noise level of 56 dBC. Three testers collected all data. There were no significant differences in the data collected among the three testers. Important test parameters are summarized in the caption for each table. The test conditions and parameters, and these normative data, were published in an article by Ben Hornsby, Tim Kelly and Hall entitled "Normative data for five FDA-approved distortion product OAE systems" in *The Hearing Journal 49*(9): 1996.

Manufacturers of specific devices will probably be quite willing to refer new users to published or unpublished normative adult databases. One very carefully collected normative database for a clinical device (the Bio-Logic Scout) was published by Mike Gorga and colleagues at the Boys Town National Research Hospital in Omaha Nebraska (Gorga MP, Neely ST, Ohlrich B, Hoover B, Redner J, Peters J. From laboratory to clinic: A large scale study of distortion product otoacoustic emissions in ears with normal hearing and ears with hearing loss. *Ear and Hearing 18*:440–455, 1997).

Neonatal normative data for multiple clinical DPOAE devices are needed but lacking. Collecting such data is no easy task. The major logistical problem is verifying that the subjects are indeed normal hearing. There is no "gold standard" for hearing status period from prematurity (about 30 weeks) through age 3 to 4 years when valid frequency- and ear-specific audiometry might be consistently completed. Typically, infants in the well baby nursery are assumed to have normal hearing sensitivity, and this assumption is supported by the presence of a normal ABR at 20 or 30 dB nHL. However, even if normative data are carefully collected with a clinical OAE device from a large series of such infants with an adequate sample at different ages (in months), these data are really appropriate only for that device, and not the 9 or 10 other brands on the market. Developmental trends in OAEs, discussed in Chapter 5, provide some useful guidelines for interpreting infant DPOAE data in the context of adult norms. Despite the multiple technical and methodologic challenges, a large-scale and conscientious effort to amass an infant DPOAE database is clearly warranted, and is in the best interests of clinicians, manufacturers and, first and foremost, the children.

Soon, we will begin to see published normative DPOAE data for infants and older children as clinical devices are incorporated into routine pediatric audiology practice. As an example, you might review the following article:

Bowes M, Smith C, Tan AK, Varette-Cerre P. Screening of high-risk infants using the distortion product otoacoustic emissions. *Journal of Otolaryngology 28*: 181–184, 1999. [Faculty of Health Sciences, Queen's University, Kingston, Ontario, Canada]

TEOAE NORMATIVE DATA

Surprisingly scant published normative data exist for TEOAEs, even for adults. This is remarkable considering that a clinical device was first introduced over 10 years ago, and many hundreds of researchers and clinicians have studied or applied TEOAEs in thousands of normal subjects and diverse patient populations. The importance of developing TEOAE normative databases was recognized early on. For example, David Kemp in presenting some preliminary normative data for the ILO88 device at the end of a paper offering guidelines for clinical use of TEOAEs cautioned against its use for clinical interpretation "because of the lack of agreed-on calibration standards" (Kemp, 1990, p. 104). Instead, he suggested that the data "be used as a model with which to design local normative data pools" (Kemp, 1990, p. 104).

Adult normative data, collected with the current default parameters for the ILO88 device, are summarized in Table A1–A6. Because data collection was completed in 1994, current ILO88 devices differ in software and probe design. The suggestions made above for DPOAE normative data collection generally apply also to TEOAEs.

Normative data are equally important in pediatric populations. The following selected recent articles include normative TEOAE data for newborn infants. As noted above, the data are specific to the brand and model of equipment used by the authors. Normative data reported in years past may not be relevant due to advances in hardware, software, and probe design. Many other papers describing TEOAEs in infants and children are cited in the section on age in Chapter 5 .

■ Driscoll et al. Transient evoked otoacoustic emissions in two-month-old infants: A normative study. *Audiology 38*: 181–186, 1999. [Department of Speech Pathology & Audiology, The University of Queensland, St. Lucia, Australia]

■ Paludetti G et al. Transient evoked otoacoustic emissions (TEOAEs) in newborns: Normative data. *International Journal of Pediatric Otorhinolaryngology 47*: 235–241, 1999. [ENT Institute, Catholic University of the Sacred Heart, Rome, Italy]

Table A–1. Data for the **Bio-logic Scout** device for 40 ears collected from young audiometrically normal adults (hearing threshold levels 15 dB or better from 250 to 8000 Hz and type A tympanograms) in a quiet, non-sound-treated room. Test protocol includes: $f_2/f_1 = 1.2$; $L_1 = 65$; $L_2 = 55$ dB SPL. Frequency displayed is f_2 .

Frequency		Mean	SD	1%ile	5%ile	10%ile	99%ile	95%ile	90%ile
634	DP	9.25	5.97	6.69	7.34	7.66	11.81	11.16	10.84
	NF	5.63	6.68	−8.49	−7.77	−7.41	−2.77	−3.5	−3.85
805	DP	9.01	6.39	6.27	6.96	7.31	11.74	11.05	10.71
	NF	−7.43	8.65	−11.14	−10.2	−9.74	−3.73	−4.67	−5.13
1001	DP	10.18	6.56	7.38	8.09	8.44	12.99	12.28	11.93
	NF	−11.28	7.72	−14.58	−13.75	−13.33	−7.97	−8.81	−9.22
1586	DP	10.65	6.63	7.81	8.53	8.88	13.48	12.76	12.41
	NF	−16.45	7.56	−19.69	−18.87	−18.47	−13.21	−14.03	−14.44
2002	DP	6.85	6.4	4.11	4.81	5.15	9.6	8.9	8.56
	NF	−19.41	6.07	−22.01	−21.35	−21.03	−16.81	−17.46	−17.79
3174	DP	6.1	5.18	3.88	4.44	4.71	8.31	7.75	7.48
	NF	−21.16	6.04	−23.74	−23.09	−22.77	−18.57	−19.23	−19.55
4003	DP	6.1	5.68	3.66	4.28	4.58	8.53	7.91	7.61
	NF	−24.65	7.08	−27.68	−26.92	−26.54	−21.62	−22.39	−22.77
6347	DP	1.22	8.51	−2.42	−1.5	−1.04	4.87	3.95	3.49
	NF	−25.24	6.38	−27.97	−27.28	−26.93	−22.5	−23.19	−23.54

DP = amplitude of DP in dB SPL.

NF = amplitude of noise floor in dB SPL.

Table A–2. DPOAE data in dB SPL for the **Mimosa Acoustics/Starkey DP2000** device for 40 ears collected from young audiometrically normal adults (hearing levels 15 dB or better from 250 to 8000 Hz & type A tympanograms) in a quiet, non-sound-treated room. Test protocol includes: $f_2/f_1 = 1.2$; $L_1 = 65$; $L_2 = 55$ dB SPL. Frequency is geometric mean of f_1 and f_2 .

Frequency		Mean	SD	1%ile	5%ile	10%ile	99%ile	95%ile	90%ile
534	DP	6.78	5.74	4.17	4.84	5.16	9.39	8.72	8.40
	NF	6.29	6.69	3.25	4.02	4.40	9.32	8.55	8.17
704	DP	8.68	6.23	5.85	6.57	6.92	11.51	10.79	10.43
	NF	.31	6.27	−2.54	−1.82	−1.46	3.15	2.43	2.07
1070	DP	6.69	7.92	3.1	4.01	4.46	10.29	9.37	8.92
	NF	−4.34	8.63	−8.25	−7.26	—6.77	−.42	−1.42	−1.91
1408	DP	9.93	6.82	6.83	7.62	8.01	−7.09	−7.85	−8.22
	NF	−10.06	6.53	−13.02	−12.26	−11.89	−7.09	−7.85	−8.22
2113	DP	3.14	5.7	.55	1.21	1.53	5.73	5.07	4.74
	NF	−15.92	6.1	−18.69	−17.98	−17.63	−13.15	−13.85	−14.2
3084	DP	6.76	5.17	4.41	5.01	5.30	9.11	8.51	8.21
	NF	−19.65	10.05	−24.21	−23.05	−22.48	−15.08	−16.25	−16.82
3935	DP	7.48	4.67	5.36	5.9	6.16	9.59	9.05	8.79
	NF	−25.19	5.98	−27.9	−27.21	−26.87	−22.47	−23.17	−23.5
5710	DP	3.47	5.89	.79	1.47	1.81	6.14	5.46	5.12
	NF	−23.04	10.25	−27.7	−26.51	−25.93	−18.39	−19.58	−20.16

DP = amplitude of DP in dB SPL.

NF = amplitude of noise floor in dB SPL.

Table A–3. Data for **Grason Stadler 60** in dB SPL (N = 41 ears) collected from young audio-metrically normal adults (hearing threshold levels 15 dB or better from 250 to 8000 Hz and type A tympanograms) in a quiet, non-sound-treated room. Test protocol includes: f_2/f_1 = 1.2; L_1 = 65 / L_2 = 55 dB SPL. Frequency is f_2. DP = distortion product amplitude in dB SPL; NF = noise floor level in dB SPL. You can enter these normative data into your GSI 60.

Frequency		Mean	SD	1%ile	5%ile	10%ile	99%ile	95%ile	90%ile
562	DP	4.59	5.7	2.18	2.79	3.09	6.99	6.38	6.08
	NF	−5.88	3.11	−7.19	−6.86	−6.7	−4.57	−4.9	−5.06
781	DP	5.61	6.47	2.88	3.57	3.91	8.34	7.65	7.31
	NF	−7.73	2.29	−8.7	−8.46	−8.33	−6.76	−7.01	−7.13
1093	DP	7.2	7.74	3.92	4.75	5.16	10.47	9.64	9.23
	NF	−8.24	2.21	−9.18	−8.94	−8.83	−7.31	−7.55	−7.66
1562	DP	6.68	6.22	4.06	4.72	5.05	9.31	8.65	8.32
	NF	−8.95	2.59	−10.04	−9.77	−9.63	−7.86	−8.13	−8.27
1968	DP	3.15	7.48	−.01	.79	1.18	6.3	5.51	5.11
	NF	−10.63	3.09	−11.94	−11.61	−11.45	−9.33	−9.66	−9.82
3093	DP	3.63	4.92	1.55	2.08	2.34	5.71	5.19	4.93
	NF	−11.29	2.91	−12.52	−12.21	−12.06	−10.06	−10.37	−10.53
3937	DP	4.88	6.11	2.3	2.95	3.27	7.46	6.81	6.48
	NF	−10.24	2.67	−11.37	−11.09	−10.95	−9.12	−9.4	−9.54
6250	DP	−5.54	8.15	−8.98	−8.11	−7.68	−2.09	−2.96	−3.39
	NF	−10.1	3.28	−11.48	−11.13	−10.96	−8.71	−9.06	−9.24

Table A–4. Data in dB SPL for the **Madsen Celesta** for 30 ears collected from young audiometrically normal adults (hearing threshold levels 15 dB or better from 250 to 8000 Hz and type A tympanograms) in a quiet, non-sound-treated room. Test protocol includes: $f_2/f_1 = 1.2$; $L_1 = 65$; $L_2 = 55$ dB SPL. Frequency is geometric mean of f_1 and f_2.

Frequency		Mean	SD	1%ile	5%ile	10%ile	99%ile	95%ile	90%ile
500	DP	4.9	4.92	2.42	3.06	3.37	7.38	6.74	6.43
	NF	−9.97	4.33	−12.14	−11.58	−11.31	−7.79	−8.35	−8.62
753	DP	11.3	5.44	8.56	9.27	9.61	14.04	13.33	12.99
	NF	−5.63	6.08	−8.69	−7.9	−7.52	−2.57	−3.36	−3.75
1006	DP	11.9	6.98	8.39	9.29	9.73	15.41	14.51	14.07
	NF	−8.23	4.48	−10.49	−9.91	−9.62	−5.98	−6.56	−6.84
1512	DP	7.9	6.97	4.39	5.3	5.74	11.41	10.5	10.06
	NF	−11.43	6.59	−14.75	−13.89	−13.48	−8.12	−8.97	−9.39
2011	DP	4.8	5.39	2.09	2.79	3.13	7.51	6.81	6.47
	NF	−17.03	3.32	−18.7	−18.27	−18.06	−15.36	−15.79	−16
3023	DP	.6	4.5	-1.66	−1.08	−.8	2.86	2.28	2
	NF	−22.43	3.19	−24.04	−23.63	−23.42	−20.83	−21.24	−21.44
4036	DP	8.03	5.75	5.14	5.89	6.25	10.93	10.18	9.82
	NF	−19.3	3.72	−21.17	−20.69	−20.46	−17.43	−17.91	−18.14
6060	DP	14.17	8.03	10.12	11.17	11.67	18.21	17.17	16.66
	NF	−16.6	3.42	−18.32	−17.88	−17.66	−14.88	−15.32	−15.54

DP = amplitude of DP in dB SPL.

NF = amplitude of noise floor in dB SPL.

More extensive manufacturer's normative data are displayed in Tables 7–4 through 7–6 in Chapter 7.

Table A–5. Data for the **Virtual 330** device for 46 ears collected from young audiometrically normal adults (hearing threshold levels 15 dB or better from 250 to 8000 Hz and type A tympanograms) in a quiet, non-sound-treated room. Test protocol includes: $f_2/f_1 = 1.2$; $L_1 = 65$; $L_2 = 55$ dB SPL. Frequency is geometric mean of f_1 and f_2.

Frequency		Mean	SD	1%ile	5%ile	10%ile	99%ile	95%ile	90%ile
500	DP	4.12	8.38	.54	1.44	1.89	7.71	6.81	6.36
	NF	9.06	7.55	5.83	6.65	7.05	12.3	11.48	11.08
700	DP	7.97	6.75	5.08	5.82	6.18	10.87	10.13	9.77
	NF	.38	6.26	−2.3	−1.62	−1.29	3.06	2.38	2.05
1000	DP	.48	6.81	−2.43	−1.7	−1.33	3.39	2.66	2.29
	NF	−7.42	6.98	−10.41	−9.65	−9.28	−4.43	−5.19	−5.56
1580	DP	5.19	6.63	2.35	3.07	3.42	8.03	7.31	6.96
	NF	−14.82	7.04	−17.83	−17.07	−16.69	−11.81	−12.57	−12.94
2000	DP	2.27	6.92	−.69	.06	.43	5.24	4.49	4.12
	NF	−19.72	6.45	−22.48	−21.78	−21.44	−16.96	−17.65	−18
3180	DP	−7.7	8.48	−11.33	−10.41	−9.96	−4.07	−4.99	−5.44
	NF	−25.63	5.95	−28.18	−27.54	−27.22	−23.09	−23.73	−24.05
4000	DP	7.32	9.69	3.18	4.23	4.74	11.47	10.42	9.91
	NF	−16.61	4.89	−18.71	−18.18	−17.92	−14.52	−15.05	−15.31
6350	DP	−4.2	9.15	−8.12	−7.13	−6.64	−.28	−1.27	−1.76
	NF	−31.72	4.33	−33.57	−33.1	−32.87	−29.87	−30.33	−30.57

DP = amplitude of DP in dB SPL.

NF = amplitude of noise floor in dB SPL.

The Virtual Corporation is no longer in business (as of 1998).

Table A–6. Transient evoked otoacoustic emissions (TEOAE) normal findings recorded from 20 audiologically normal females and males at Vanderbilt University Medical Center by Jane E. Baer, Ph.D. TEOAE amplitude ("echo") and reproducibility data are reported for octave bands for each gender, and each ear. Data were collected with the ILO88 device (in 1993).

Parameter	Female (N = 20)				Male (N = 20)			
	Mean	SD	10%ile	90%ile	Mean	SD	10%ile	90%ile
Right Ear								
Echo (dB)								
overall (whole)	12.49	3.46	8.65	17.95	8.74	3.07	4.2	12.65
1000 Hz	10.55	4.26	6	16.5	4.95	4.81	0	11.6
2000 Hz	14.1	5.07	6.5	21.5	8.58	5.78	.4	14.6
3000 Hz	12.4	6.53	5.5	21	6.84	5	0	14
4000 Hz	10.6	6	2	19	6.63	4.34	2	11
5000 Hz	4.1	6.21	−1	12	−0.42	2.27	−3.6	2
Reproducibility (%)								
overall (whole)	92	4.67	85	98	75.85	17.65	53.5	93
1000 Hz	89	7.88	78	97	69.53	23.08	46.2	93.2
2000 Hz	93.35	6.75	82	99	80	24.62	47.6	96.6
3000 Hz	87.1	21.74	76.5	98.5	71.79	28.75	17.2	96
4000 Hz	80.3	29.12	31	98.5	66.26	36.07	0	92
5000 Hz	38.15	43.82	0.00	94	4	17.44	0	0
Low noise stimuli (%)	96.2	3.41	90.5	99.5	93.4	7	82.5	99
Noise level (dB)	33.81	1.23	32.0	35.45	35.36	1.7	33.1	37.1
Stimulus intensity (dB)	82.65	2.94	79.5	84.0	79.6	1.49	78	82
Stimulus stability (%)	94	4.58	88.5	99	88.1	12.48	79.5	100
Test time (sc)	0.46	1.0	44	48	47	4	44	53
Left Ear								
Echo (dB)								
overall (whole)	11.68	2.8	8.6	15.85	6.72	3.3	2.85	12.65
1000 Hz	9.26	4.6	4	15.2	2.15	4.08	−2	7
2000 Hz					5.4	5.82	−2	13.5
3000 Hz	12	5.08	5.4	18	4.55	5.37	−1	11
4000 Hz	9.63	6.18	0.4	16.2	3.5	5.71	−5	10
5000 Hz	3.26	6.01	−5	12.6	0.3	5.02	−5	7
Reproducibility (%)								
overall (whole)	90.2	5.36	81.5	96.5	62.95	22.61	32.5	91.5
1000 Hz	84.74	14.24	70.8	96.6	46.25	33.77	0	83
2000 Hz	91.74	7.19	81	98	62.65	35.44	0	95
3000 Hz	87	22.19	76.8	98	49.25	42.5	0	92.5
4000 Hz	79.53	29.76	23.2	97.6	48.2	41.02	0	90
5000 Hz	39.98	43.76	0	94	16.5	34.21	0	82.5
Low noise stimuli (%)	95.25	5.05	86.5	99	94.45	5.89	85.5	99
Noise level (dB)	34.23	1.41	32.4	36.1	35.68	1.96	32.9	38.5
Stimulus intensity (dB)	82.65	2.76	80	85.5	80.15	2.01	77.5	83
Stimulus stability (%)	93.8	4.94	85.5	100	92.65	4.8	85	98.5

APPENDIX

B

Otoacoustic Emissions Quiz

(Answers on page 572)

1. Potential applications of otoacoustic emissions include all of the following *except*:

   a. assessment of malingerers

   b. monitoring for ototoxicity

   c. confirmation of cochlear integrity in CAPD assessment

   d. estimation of conductive hearing loss

   e. differentiation of cochlear vs. retrocochlear auditory dysfunction

2. Otoacoustic emissions:

   a. require an airtight seal to obtain a reliable recording

   b. increase in strength as age increases

   c. are produced by the outer hair cells

   d. are only affected by pure sensory pathologies

3. Absence of detectable otoacoustic emissions could be due to:

   a. 60 dB hearing loss in infants

   b. excessive noise exposure and hearing loss of 20 dB at all frequencies

   c. otitis media

   d. outer hair cell damage secondary to ototoxicity

   e. all of the above

4. Which of the following are response parameters for transient evoked otoacoustic emissions?

   a. amplitude versus noise

   b. amplitude

   c. reproducibility

   d. spectrum

   e. none of the above

   f. all of the above

5. Which of the following have been used as a criterion for the *presence* of DPOAE?

   a. amplitude minus noise floor ≥ 5 dB

   b. amplitude reliability within ± 2 dB for at least two replications

   c. absolute DP amplitude ≥ 10 dB

   d. all of the above

6. Which best describes the relation between the efferent auditory system and OAEs?

   a. ipsilateral noise signals suppress OAE amplitude

   b. contralateral noise signals enhance OAE amplitude

   c. contralateral noise signals reduce the noise floor

   d. contralateral noise signals suppress OAE amplitude

   e. none of the above

7. Which of the following statements about outer hair cell motility is *not* accurate?

   a. influences tuning capabilities of cochlea

   b. depends on integrity of stria vascularis

   c. enhances auditory sensitivity

   d. occurs due to efferent system activation

   e. depends on blood supply to the cochlea

8. The term "auditory neuropathy" specifically refers to:

    a. disease of the auditory system

    b. hearing loss due to diabetes mellitus

    c. cochlear dysfunction

    d. evidence of auditory dysfunction but normal OAE findings

    e. evidence of auditory dysfunction with abnormal OAE findings

9. OAE findings are *not* likely to be influenced by which of the following auditory pathologies?

    a. Cytomegalovirus (inflammatory disease)

    b. extended Lasix and aminoglycoside administration

    c. inner hair cell damage

    d. excessive noise exposure

    e. large acoustic tumor within the internal auditory canal

10. A typical value for each of the following DPOAE f_2/f_1 ratio is:

    a. 65 dB SPL

    b. -3 dB

    c. 1.2

    d. 65/55

    e. 1.5

11. Which two of the following tend to have the largest TEOAE amplitudes?

    a. term neonates

    b. heterosexual men

    c. homosexual women

    d. heterosexual women

    e. bisexual men

12. DPOAE amplitude and sensitivity to cochlear dysfunction is greatest with which of the following stimulus paradigms?

    a. $L_1 = L_2$

    b. $L_2 - L_1 = -10$ dB

    c. $L_1 - L_2 = -10$ dB

    d. $L_1 = L_2 = 75$ dB

    e. $L_1 = L_2 = 45$ dB

13. OAE can be recorded in most patients with patent ventilation tubes:

    a. true

    b. false

14. The best explanation for why OAEs are not recorded in some patients with neoplastic retrocochlear pathology (i.e., a acoustic tumor) is:

    a. the tumor compromises efferent system function

    b. the tumor compresses outer hair cells

    c. the tumor compromises blood flow to the cochlea

    d. there is no loudness recruitment

    e. OAEs are recorded in all patients with acoustic tumors

15. Which two of the following possibilities are most likely in a patient with normal OAEs and an abnormal audiogram from 250 to 8000 Hz?

    a. malingerering (pseudohypacusis)

    b. collapsing ear canals

    c. sensorineural hearing loss

    d. retrocochlear auditory dysfunction

    e. this pattern is impossible

16. Which of the following is not and never will be a valuable application of OAEs?

    a. newborn hearing screening

    b. contributing to the diagnosis of auditory neuropathy

    c. monitoring ototoxicity

    d. documenting the degree of hearing loss

    e. early detection of noise-induced cochlear dysfunction

17. Among this list, who can be given credit with discovering OAEs?

    a. Georg von Békésy

    b. Hallowell Davis

    c. David Kemp

    d. James Jerger

    e. Michael Gorga

18. Among this group of distinguished audiologists/scientists, who discovered OHC motility?

    a. David Kemp

    b. Georg von Békésy

    c. Robert Galambos

    d. William Brownell

    c. Daniel Geisler

19. It would be a bad idea to monitor with OAEs for ototoxicity with a patient receiving which one of the following drugs?

    a. furosemide

    b. gentimicin

    c. vancomycin

    d. cisplatin

    e. carboplatin

20. Ambient (environmental) noise is usually greatest in OAE recordings for which of the following frequency regions?

    a. 500 to 4000 Hz

    b. 100 to 1000 Hz

    c. 500 to 1500 Hz

    d. 2000 to 4000 Hz

    e. >5000 Hz

21. Which one of the following factors does *not* usually reduce OAE newborn screening failure rate?

    a. delay screening until after 36 hours

    b. conduct screening within first 36 hours

    c. experienced tester

    d. quiet test environment

    e. manipulation of the ear canal

22. Which of the following factors has the greatest effect on TEOAEs?

    a. body temperature

    b. state of arousal (asleep versus awake)

    c. speech discrimination scores

    d. gender

    e. age

23. With appropriate manipulation of stimulus parameters (e.g., intensity), TEOAEs and DPOAEs have equivalent sensitivity to cochlear (outer hair cell) dysfunction:

    a. true

    b. false

24. OAEs have greater sensitivity than the audiogram to most cochlear pathology:

    a. true

    b. false

25. Which one of the following is a limitation of TEOAEs in comparison to DPOAEs?

    a. longer test time

    b. limited frequency specificity within the 1000 to 4000 Hz region

    c. less sensitivity to cochlear deficits

    d. upper frequency limit of 5000 Hz

    e. greater influence of middle ear pathology

ANSWERS TO QUIZ

1.	d		14.	c
2.	c		15.	a, d
3.	e		16.	d
4.	f		17.	c
5.	d		18.	d
6.	d		19.	e
7.	d		20.	c
8.	d		21.	b
9.	c		22.	d
10.	c		23.	a
11.	a, d		24.	a
12.	c		25.	d
13.	a			

REFERENCES

Abbas, P. J., & Sachs, M. B. (1976). Two-tone suppression in auditory nerve fibers: Extension of a stimulus-response relationship. *Journal of the Acoustical Society of America, 59,* 112–122.

Abdala, C. (1996). Distortion product otoacoustic emission (2f1–f2) amplitude as a function of f2/f1 frequency ratio and primary tone level separation in human adults and neonates. *Journal of the Acoustical Society of America, 100,* 3726–3740.

Abdala, C. (1998). A developmental study of distortion product otoacoustic emission (2f1–f2) suppression in humans. *Hearing Research, 121,* 125–138.

Abdala, C., Ma, E., & Sininger, Y. S. (1999). Maturation of medial efferent system function in humans. *Journal of the Acoustical Society of America, 105*(4), 2392–2402.

Abdala, C., Sininger, Y., Ekelid, M., & Zeng, F.-G. (1996). Distortion product otoacoustic emission suppression tuning curves in human adults and neonates. *Hearing Research, 98,* 38–53.

Abdala, C., & Sininger, Y. S. (1996). The development of cochlear frequency resolution in the human auditory system. *Ear & Hearing, 17,* 374–385.

Abdala, C., & Yoshinaga-Itano, C. (1997). Parent's reactions to newborn hearing screening. *Audiology Today, 9*(1), 24–25.

Abdo, M. H., Feghali, J. G., & Stapells, D. R. (1992). *Temporal and spectal analysis of click and tone transient-evoked otoacoustic emissions.* Paper presented at the Association for Research in Otolaryngology.

Abdul-Baqi, K. J. (1991). Chloral hydrate and middle ear pressure. *Journal of Laryngology and Otology, 105,* 421–423.

Aidan, D., Avan, P., & Bonfils, P. (1999). Auditory screening in neonates by means of transient evoked otoacoustic emissions: A report of 2842 recordings. *Annals of Otology, Rhinology, and Laryngology, 108*(6), 525–531.

Allen, G., Tiu, C., Koike, K., Ritchey, K., Kurs-Lasky, M., & Wax, M. (1998). Transient-evoked otoacoustic emissions in children after cisplatin chemotherapy. *Otolaryngology—Head and Neck Surgery, 118,* 584–588.

Allen, J. B., & Fahey, P. F. (1992). Using acoustic distortion products to measure the cochlear amplifier gain on the basilar membrane. *Journal of the Acoustical Society of America, 92,* 178–188.

Allen, J. B., & Lonsbury-Martin, B. L. (1993). Otoacoustic emissions. *Journal of the Acoustical Society of America, 93,* 568–569.

Amedee, R. G. (1995). The effects of chronic otitis media with effusion on the measurement of transiently evoked otoacoustic emissions. *Laryngoscope, 105,* 589–595.

American Academy of Pediatrics Joint Committee on Infant Hearing. (1995). Position statement. *Pediatrics, 95,* 1–5.

American Academy of Pediatrics Task Force on Newborn and Infant Hearing. (1999). Newborn and infant hearing: Diagnosis and intervention. *Pediatrics, 103,* 527–529.

American Speech-Language-Hearing Association. (1990). Guidelines for screening for hearing impairment and middle ear disorders. *Asha, 32*(Suppl. 2), 17–24.

Anderson, S. D. (1980). Some ECMR properties in relation to other signals from the auditory periphery. *Hearing Research, 2*, 273–296.

Anderson, S. D., & Kemp, D. T. (1979). The evoked cochlear mechanical response in laboratory primates: preliminary report. *Archives of Otorhinolaryngology, 224*, 47–54.

Anson, B. J., Bast, T. H., & Richany, S. F. (1955). The fetal and early postnatal development of the tympanic ring and related structures in man. *Annals of Otology, Rhinology, and Laryngology, 64*, 802–823.

Anteunis, L. J. C., Brienesse, P., & Schrander, J. J. P. (1998). Otoacoustic emissions in screening cleft lip and/or palate children for hearing loss—a feasibility study. *International Journal of Pediatric Otorhinolaryngology, 44*, 259–266.

Antonelli, A., & Grandori, F. (1996). Long term stability, influence of the head position and modelling considerations for evoked otoacoustic emissions. *Scandinavian Audiology, 25*(Suppl.), 97–108.

Apostolopoulos, N. K., Psarommatis, I. M., Tsakanikos, M. D., Dellagrammatikas, H. D., & Douniadakis, D. E. (1999). Otoacoustic emission-based hearing screening of a Greek NICU population. *International Journal of Pediatric Otorhinolaryngology, 47*, 41–48.

Aran, J.-M., Erre, J. P., & Avan, P. (1996). Contralateral suppression of transient otoacoustic emissions in guinea pigs: Effects of gentamicin. In L. Collet & F. Grandori (Eds.), *Suppression effects of otoacoustic emissions* (Vol. III, pp. 96–100). Milan, Italy: Casa Editrice G. Sefanoni-Lecco.

Aran, J. M., Rarey, K. E., & Hawkins, J. E. (1984). Functional and morphological changes in experimental endolympatic hydrops. *Acta Otolaryngologica (Stockholm), 97*, 547–557.

Arnold, D. J., Lonsbury-Martin, B. L., & Martin, G. K. (1999). High-frequency hearing influences lower-frequency distortion-product otoacoustic emissions. *Archives of Otolaryngology, 125*, 215–222.

Arnold, S., & Burkard, R. (1998). The auditory evoked potential difference tone and cubic difference tone measured from the inferior colliculus of the chinchilla. *Journal of the Acoustical Society of America, 104*, 1565–1574

Arthur, R. M., Pfeiffer, R. R., & Suga, N. (1971). Properties of "two-tone inhibition" in primary auditory neurons. *Journal of Physiology, 212*, 593–609.

Ashmore, J. F. (1987). A fast motile response in guinea-pig outer hair cells: The cellular basis for the cochlear amplifier. *Journal of Physiology (London), 388*, 323–347.

Ashmore, J. F., & Holley, M. C. (1988). Temperature-dependence of a fast motile response in isolated outer hair cells of the guinea pig cochlea. *Quarterly Journal of Experimental Physiology, 73*, 143–145.

Ashmore, J. R., & Russell, I. J. (1982). Effect of efferent nerve stimulation on hair cells in the frog sacculus. *Journal of Physiology, 329*, 26–27P.

Attias, J., Bresloff, I., & Furman, V. (1996). The influence of the efferent auditory system on otoacoustic emissions in noise induced tinnitus: clinical relevance. *Acta Otolaryngologica, 116*, 534–539.

Attias, J., Bresloff, I., Reshef, I., Horowitz, G., & Furman, V. (1998). Evaluating noise induced hearing loss with distortion product otoacoustic emissions. *British Journal of Audiology, 32*, 39–46.

Attias, J., Furst, M., Furman, V., Reshef, I., Horowitz, G., & Bresloff, I. (1995). Noise-induced otoacoustic emission loss with or without hearing loss. *Ear & Hearing, 16*, 612–618.

Avan, P., & Bonfils, P. (1991). Analysis of possible interactions of an attentional task with cochlear micromechanics. *Hearing Research, 57*, 269–275.

Avan, P., Elbez, M., & Bonfils, P. (1997). Click-evoked otoacoustic emissions and the influence of high-frequency hearing losses in humans. *Journal of the Acoustical Society of America, 101*, 2771–2777.

Axelsson, A., & Lindgren, F. (1977). Does pop music cause hearing damage? *Audiology, 16*, 432–437.

Axelsson, A., & Lindgren, F. (1981). Pop music and hearing. *Ear & Hearing, 2*, 64–69.

Baguley, D. M., & McFerran, D. J. (1999). Tinnitus in childhood. *International Journal of Pediatric Otolaryngology, 49*, 99–105.

Baldwin, M., & Watkin, P. (1992). The clinical application of otoacoustic emissions in paediatric audiological assessment. *Journal of Laryngology and Otology, 106*, 301–306.

Balfour, P. B., Pillion, J. P., & Gaskin, A. E. (1998). Distortion product otoacoustic emission and auditory brainstem response measures of pediatric sensorineural hearing loss. *Ear & Hearing, 19*, 463–472.

Balkany, T., Berman, S., Simmons, M., & Jafek, B. (1978). Middle ear effusion in neonates. *Laryngoscope, 88*, 398–405.

Bantock, H., & Croxson, S. (1998). Universal hearing screening using transient otoacoustic emissions in a community health clinic. *Archives of Diseases in Children, 78*, 249–252.

Bargones, J. Y., & Burns, E. M. (1988). Suppression tuning curves for spontaneous otoacoustic emissions infants and adults. *Journal of the Acoustical Society of America, 83*, 1809–1815.

Bartlett, J. (1980). *Familiar quotations* (15th ed.). Boston: Little, Brown & Company.

Beck, A., Maurer, J., Welkoborsky, H. J., & Mann, W. (1992). Changes in transitory evoked otoacoustic emissions in chemotherapy with cisplatin and 5 FU. *Hals-Nasen-Ohren (HNO)*, 40, 123–127.

Behroozi, K. B. (1997). Noise-related ailments of performing musicians: A review. *Medical Problems of Performing Artists*, 12, 19–22.

Bell, A. (1992). Circadian and menstrual rhythms in frequency variations of spontaneous otoacoustic emissions from human ears. *Hearing Research*, 58, 91–100.

Bennett, M. J. (1980). Trials with the auditory response cradle II—the neonatal respiratory response to an auditory stimulus. *Audiology*, 14, 1–6.

Bergman, B., Gorga, M., Neely, S., Kaminski, J., Beauchaine, K., & Peters, J. (1995). Preliminary descriptions of transient-evoked and distortion-product otoacoustic emissions from graduates of an intensive care unit. *Journal of the American Academy of Audiology*, 6, 150–162.

Berlin, C., Bordelon, J., St.John, P., Wilensky, D., Hurley, A., Kluka, E., & Hood, L. (1998). Reversing click polarity may uncover auditory neuropathy in infants. *Ear & Hearing*, 19, 37–47.

Berlin, C., Hood, L., Cecola, P., Jackson, D., & Szabo, P. (1993). Does Type I afferent neuron dysfunction reveal itself through lack of efferent suppression? *Hearing Research*, 65, 40–50.

Berlin, C. I., Hood, L. J., Hurley, A., & Wen, H. (1994). Contralateral suppression of otoacoustic emissions: An index of the function of the medial olivocochlear system. *Otolaryngology—Head and Neck Surgery*, 110, 3–21.

Berlin, C., Hood, L., Hurley, A., Wen, H., & Kemp, D. (1995). Binaural noise suppresses linear click-evoked otoacoustic emissions more than ipsilateral or contralateral noise. *Hearing Research*, 87, 96–103.

Berlin, C., Hood, L., Wen, H., Szabo, P., Cecola, R., Rigby, P., & Jackson, D. (1993). Contralateral suppression of non-linear click-evoked otoacoustic emissions. *Hearing Research*, 71, 1–11.

Berman, S. A., Balkany, T. J., & Simmons, M. A. (1978). Otitis media in the neonatal intensive care unit. *Pediatrics*, 62, 198–201.

Berndt, H., & Wagner, H. (1981). Influence of body temperature on the set-up and recovery of noise-induced cochlea damage. *Archives of Otorhinolaryngology*, 232, 199–202.

Berninger, E., Karlsson, K. K., & Alvan, G. (1998). Quinine reduces the dynamic range of the auditory system. *Acta Otolaryngologica (Stockholm)*, 118, 46–51.

Berninger, E., Karlsson, K. K., Hellgren, U., & Eskilsson, G. (1995). Magnitude changes in transient evoked otoacoustic emissions and high-level 2f1–f2 distortion products in man during quinine administration. *Scandinavian Audiology*, 24, 27–32.

Bertoli, S., & Probst, R. (1997). The role of transient-evoked otoacoustic emission testing in the evaluation of elderly persons. *Ear & Hearing*, 18, 286–293.

Bess, F. H. (1993, November). *Universal hearing screening of newborns and infants: A critical review of the evidence.* Paper presented at the Newborn Hearing Screening Symposium, Nashville, TN.

Bess, F. H., & Paradise, J. L. (1994). Universal screening for infant hearing impairment: not simple, not risk-free, not necessarily beneficial, and not presently justified. *Pediatrics*, 93, 330–334.

Bilger, R., Matthies, M., Hammel, D., & Demorest, M. (1990). Genetic implications of gender differences in the prevalence of spontaneous otoacoustic emissions. *Journal of Speech and Hearing Research*, 33, 418–432.

Blinowska, K. J., & Durka, P. J. (1997). Introduction to wavelet analysis. *British Journal of Audiology*, 31, 449–459.

Blinowska, K. J., Durka, P. J., Skierski, A., Grandori, F., & Tognola, G. (1997). High resolution time-frequency analysis of otoacoustic emissions. *Technological Health Care*, 5, 407–418.

Bluestone, C. D., & Klein, J. O. (1990). Methods of examination: Clinical examination in pediatric otolaryngology. In C. D. Bluestone & S. E. Stool (Eds.), *Pediatric otolaryngology* (2nd ed., pp. 119–121). Philadelphia: W.B. Saunders.

Bobbin, R. P., & Konishi, T. (1971). Acetylcholine mimics crossed olivocochlear bundle stimulation. *Nature*, 231, 222–223.

Bonfils, P. (1989). Spontaneous otoacoustic emissions: Clinical interest. *Laryngoscope*, 99, 752–756.

Bonfils, P., Avan, P., Francois, M., Trotoux, J., & Narcy, P. (1992). Distortion-product otoacoustic emissions in neonates: Normative data. *Acta Otolaryngologica (Stockholm)*, 112, 739–744.

Bonfils, P., Avan, P., Londero, A., Trotoux, J., & Narcy, P. (1991). Objective low-frequency audiometry by distortion-product acoustic emissions. *Archives of Otolaryngology—Head and Neck Surgery*, 117, 1167–1171.

Bonfils, P., Bertrand, Y., & Uziel, A. (1988). Evoked otoacoustic emissions: Normative data and presbycusis. *Audiology*, 27, 27–35.

Bonfils, P., Dumont, A., Marie, P., Francois, M., & Narcy, P. (1990). Evoked otoacoustic emissions in newborn hearing screening. *Laryngoscope*, 100, 186–189.

Bonfils, P., Francois, M., Avan, P., Londero, A., Trotoux, J., & Narcy, P. (1992). Spontaneous and evoked otoacoustic emissions in preterm neonates. *Laryngoscope, 102*, 182–186.

Bonfils, P., Piron, J. P., Uziel, A., & Pujol, R. (1988). A correlative study of evoked otoacoustic emission properties and audiometric thresholds. *Archives of Otorhinolaryngology, 245*, 53–56.

Bonfils, P., & Uziel, A. (1988). Evoked otoacoustic emissions in patients with acoustic neuromas. *American Journal of Otology, 9*, 412–441.

Bonfils, P., & Uziel, A. (1989). Clinical applications of evoked acoustic emissions: Results in normally hearing and hearing-impaired subjects. *Annals of Otology, Rhinology, and Laryngology, 98*, 326–332.

Bonfils, P., Uziel, A., & Narcy, P. (1989). The properties of spontaneous and evoked acoustic emissions in neonates and children: A preliminary report. *Archives of Otorhinolaryngology, 246*, 249–251.

Bonfils, P., Uziel, A., & Pujol, R. (1988a). Evoked otoacoustic emissions: A fundamental and clinical survey. *Otology, Rhinology, and Laryngology, 50*, 212–218.

Bonfils, P., Uziel, A., & Pujol, R. (1988b). Screening for auditory dysfunction in infants by evoked otoacoustic emissions. *Archives of Otolaryngology—Head and Neck Surgery, 114*, 887–890.

Borg, E. (1997). Perinatal asphyxia, hypoxia, ischemia, and hearing loss. An overview. *Scandinavian Audiology, 26*, 77–91.

Bowes, M., Smith, C., Tan, A. K., & Varette-Cerre, P. (1999). Screening of high-risk infants using distortion product otoacoustic emissions. *Journal of Otolaryngology, 28*(4), 181–184.

Bowman, D. M., Eggermont, J. J., Brown, D. K., & Kimberley, B. P. (1998). Estimating cochlear filter response properties from distortion product otoacoustic emission (DPOAE) phase delay measurements in normal hearing human adults. *Hearing Research, 119*(3), 14–26.

Bowman, D. M., Brown, D. K., Eggermont, J. J., & Kimberley, B. P. (1997). The effect of sound intensity on f1-sweep and f2-sweep distortion product otoacoustic emissions phase delay estimates in human subjects. *Journal of the Acoustical Society of America, 101*, 1550–1559.

Bray, P. (1989). *Click evoked otoacoustic emissions and the development of clinical otoacoustic hearing test instrument.* Unpublished Ph.D. dissertation, London University, London.

Bray, P., & Kemp, D. T. (1987). An advanced cochlear echo technique suitable for infant screening. *British Journal of Audiology, 21*, 191–204.

Brienesse, P., Anteunis, L., Wit, H., Gavilanes, D., & Maertzdorf, W. (1996). Otoacoustic emissions in preterm infants: Indications for cochlear development? *Audiology, 35*, 296–306.

Brienesse, P., Anteunis, L. J. C., Maertzdorf, W. J., Blanco, C. E., & Manni, J. J. (1997). Frequency shift of individual spontaneous emissions in preterm infants. *Pediatric Research, 42*, 478–483.

Brienesse, P., & Debyelaan, P. (1997). Maturation of otoacoustic emissions: Longitudinal versus cross-sectional study. *International Journal of Pediatric Otorhinolaryngology, 40*, 73–74.

Brienesse, P., Maertzdorf, W., Anteunis, L., Mannis, J., & Blanco, C. (1998a). Long-term and short-term variations in amplitude and frequency of spontaneous otoacoustic emissions in pre-term infants. *Audiology, 37*(5), 278–284.

Brienesse, P., Maertzdorf, W. J., Anteunis, L. J., Mannis, J. J., & Blanco, C. E. (1998b). Click-evoked otoacoustic emission measurement in preterm infants. *European Journal of Pediatrics, 157*, 999–1003.

Bright, K. E., & Glattke, T. J. (1984, November). *Spontaneous otoacoustic emissions in normal listeners.* Paper presented at the American Speech-Language-Hearing Association Convention.

Brown, A., McDowell, B., & Forge, A. (1989). Acoustic distortion products can be used to monitor the effects of chronic gentamicin treatment. *Hearing Research, 42*, 143–156.

Brown, A., Williams, D., & Gaskill, S. (1993). The effect of aspirin on cochlear mechanical tuning. *Journal of the Acoustical Society of America, 93*, 3298–3307.

Brown, A. M. (1993). Distortion in the cochlea: Acoustic f2–f1 at low stimulus levels. *Hearing Research, 70*, 160–166.

Brown, A. M. (1987). Acoustic distortion from rodent ears: A comparison of responses from rats, guinea pigs and gerbils. *Hearing Research, 31*, 25–38.

Brown, A. M. (1988). Continuous low level sound alters cochlear mechanics: An efferent effect? *Hearing Research, 34*, 27–38.

Brown, A. M., & Gaskill, S. A. (1990). Measurement of acoustic distortion reveals underlying similarities between human and rodent mechanical responses. *Journal of the Acoustical Society of America, 88*, 840–849.

Brown, A. M., & Kemp, D. T. (1984). Suppressibility of the 2f1–f2 stimulated acoustic emissions in gerbil and man. *Hearing Research, 13*, 29–37.

Brown, A. M., & Kemp, D. T. (1985). Intermodulation distortion in the cochlea: Could basal vibration be the major cause of round window CM distortion? *Hearing Research, 19*, 191–198.

Brown, D. R., Watchko, J. F., & Sabo, D. (1991). Neonatal sensorineural hearing loss associated with furosemide: A case-control study. *Developmental Medicine and Child Neurology, 33*, 816–823.

Brown, M. C., Smith, D. I., & Nutall, A. L. (1983). The temperature dependency of neural and hair cell responses evoked by high frequencies. *Journal of the Acoustical Society of America, 73*, 1662–1670.

Brown, R. D., & McElwee, T. W. (1972). Effects of intra-arterially and intravenously administered ethacrynic acid and furosemide on cochlear N2 in cats. *Toxicology and Applied Pharmacology, 22*, 589–594.

Brownell, W. E. (1983). Observations on a motile response in isolated outer hair cells. In W. R. Webster & L. M. Aitken (Eds.), *Mechanisms of hearing* (pp. 5–10). Monash, Australia: Monash University Press.

Brownell, W. E. (1984). Microscopic observation of cochlear hair cell motility. *Scanning Electron Microscopy, 3*, 1401–1406.

Brownell, W. E. (1990). Outer hair cell electromotility and otoacoustic emissions. *Ear & Hearing, 11*, 89–92.

Brownell, W. E., Bader, C. R., Bertrand, D., & Ribaupierre, Y. (1985). Evoked mechanical responses of isolated cochlear outer hair cells. *Science, 227*, 194–196.

Brownell, W. E., Manis, P. B., Zidanic, M., & Spirou, G. A. (1983). Acoustically evoked radial current densities in scala tympani. *Journal of the Acoustical Society of America, 74*, 792–800.

Buki, B., Katona, G., Noszek, L., Jancso, G., & Ribari, O. (1993). Otoacoustic emission audiometry in adults and neonates (in Hungarian). *Orvosi Hetilap, 133*, 2067–2969.

Bulla, W. A., & Hall, J. W., III. (1998). Daily noise-level exposures of professional music recording engineers. *Journal of the Audio Engineering Society.*

Buller, G., & Lutman, M. E. (1998). Automatic classification of transiently evoked otoacoustic emissions using an artificial neural network. *British Journal of Audiology, 32*, 235–247.

Bunch, C. C. (1943). *Clinical audiometry.* St. Louis: C.V. Mosby.

Buno, W. (1978). Auditory nerve activity influenced by contralateral ear sound stimulation. *Experimental Neurology, 59*, 62–74.

Burkhard, R., Shi, Y., & Hecox, K. (1990). A comparison of maximum length and Legendre sequences for the derivation of brain-stem auditory-evoked responses at rapid rates of stimulation. *Journal of the Acoustical Society of America, 87*, 1656–1664.

Burns, E., Campbell, S., & Arehart, K. (1994). Longitudinal measurements of spontaneous otoacoustic emissions infants. *Journal of the Acoustic Society of America, 95*, 385–394.

Burns, E. M., Arehart, K. H., & Campbell, S. L. (1992). Prevalence of spontaneous otoacoustic emissions in neonates. *Journal of the Acoustical Society of America, 91*, 1571–1575.

Burns, E. M., Harrison, W. A., Bulen, J. C., & Keefe, D. H. M. (1993). Voluntary contraction of middle ear muscles: Effects on input impedance, energy reflectance and spontaneous otoacoustic emissions. *Hearing Research, 67*, 117–127.

Burns, E. M., & Keefe, D. H. (1991). *Intermittent tinnitus resulting from unstable otoacoustic emissions.* Presented at Tinnitus 91: 4th International Tinnitus Symposium.

Burns, E. M., Keefe, D. H., & Ling, R. (1998). Energy reflectance in the ear canal can exceed unity near spontaneous otoacoustic emission frequencies. *Journal of the Acoustical Society of America, 103*, 462–474.

Burns, E. M., Strickland, E. A., Tubis, A., & Jones, K. (1984). Interaction among spontaneous otoacoustic emissions. I. Distortion products and linked emissions. *Hearing Research, 16*, 271–278.

Butinar D., Zidar, J., Leonardis, L., Popovic, M., Kalaydijieva, L., Angelicheva, D., Sinninger, Y., Keats, B., & Starr, A. (1999). Hereditary auditory, vestibular, motor, and sensory neuropathy in a Slovenian Roma (Gypsy) kindred. *Annals of Neurology, 46*, 36–44.

Cacace, A., McClelland, W., Weiner, J., & McFarland, D. (1996). Individual differences and the reliability of 2f1–f2 distortion-product otoacoustic emissions: Effects of time-of-day, stimulus variables, and gender. *Journal of Speech and Hearing Research, 39*, 1138–1148.

Campbell, K. C., & Durrant, J. (1993). Audiologic monitoring for ototoxicity. *Otolaryngology Clinics of North America, 26*, 903–914.

Cane, M., O'Donoghue, G., & Lutman, M. (1992). The feasibility of using oto-acoustic emissions to monitor cochlear function during acoustic neuroma surgery. *Scandinavian Audiology, 21*, 173–176.

Cane, M. A., Lutman, M. E., & O'Donoghue, G. M. (1994). Transiently evoked otoacoustic emissions in patients with cerebellopontine angle tumors. *American Journal of Otology, 15*(2), 207–216.

Canlon, B., & Fransson, A. (1995). Morphological and functional preservation of the outer hair cells from noise trauma by sound conditioning. *Hearing Research, 84*, 112–124.

Capps, M. J., & Ades, H. W. (1968). Auditory frequency discrimination after transection of the olivocochlear bundle in squirrel monkeys. *Experimental Neurology, 21*, 147–158.

Carhart, R. (1946). Monitored live voice as a test of auditory acuity. *Journal of the Acoustical Society of America, 17*, 339–349.

Carhart, R. (1965). Problems in the measurement of speech discrimination. *Archives of Otolaryngology, 82*, 253–260.

Castello, E. (1997). Distortion products in normal hearing patients with tinnitus. *Boll Soc Ital Biol Sper, 73*, 93–100.

Castor, X., Veuillet, E., Morgon, A., & Collet, L. (1994). Influence of aging on active cochlear micromechanical properties and on the medial olivocochlear system in humans. *Hearing Research, 77*, 1–8.

Cavanaugh, R., Jr. (1987). Pneumatic otoscopy in healthy full-term infants. *Pediatrics, 79*(4), 520–523.

Ceranic, J. B., Prasher, D. K., & Luxon, L. M. (1995). Tinnitus and otoacoustic emissions. *Clinical Otolaryngology, 20*, 192–200.

Ceranic, B. J., Prasher, D. K., & Luxon, L. M. (1998). Presence of tinnitus indicated by variable spontaneous otoacoustic emissions. *Audiology and Neuro-Otology, 3*, 332–344.

Ceranic, B. J., Prasher, D. K., Raglan, E., & Luxon, L. M. (1998). Tinnitus after head injury: Evidence from otoacoustic emissions. *Journal of Neurology, Neurosurgery and Psychiatry, 65*, 523–529.

Cevette, M. J. (1984). Auditory brainstem response testing in the intensive care unit. *Seminars in Hearing, 5*, 57–69.

Chang, K. W., Vohr, B. R., Norton, S. J., & Lekas, M. D. (1993). External and middle ear status related to evoked otoacoustic emission in neonates. *Archives of Otolaryngology—Head and Neck Surgery, 119*, 276–282.

Chang, S. O., Jang, Y. J., & Rhee, C. K. (1998). Effects of middle ear effusion on transient evoked otoacoustic emissions in children. *Auris Nasus Larynx, 25*(3), 243–247.

Chapman, P. (1982). Rapid onset of hearing loss after cisplatin therapy: Case reports and a literature review. *Journal of Laryngology and Otology, 96*, 159–162.

Chase, P., & Hall, J., III. (1998). *Test/retest reliability of distortion product otoacoustic emissions in newborns.* Paper presented at the European Consensus Conference on Neonatal Hearing Screening, Milan, Italy.

Cheatham, M. A., & Dallos, P. (1989). Two-tone suppression in inner ear responses. *Hearing Research, 40*, 187–196.

Cheatham, M. A., & Dallos, P. (1990). Comparison of low- and high-side two-tone suppression in inner ear cell and organ of Corti responses. *Hearing Research, 50*, 193–210.

Cheatham, M. A., & Dallos, P. (1992). Two-tone suppression in inner hair cell responses: Correlates of rate suppression in the auditory nerve. *Hearing Research, 60*, 1–12.

Chen, A. Y., & Brownell, W. E. (1999). Effect of temperature on lateral wall mechanics of the guinea pig outer hair cell. *Otolaryngology—Head and Neck Surgery, 120*, 46–50.

Chertoff, M. E., & Guruprasad, S. N. (1997). Application of a stimulus spectral calibration routine to click evoked otoacoustic emissions. *Journal of the American Academy of Audiology, 8*, 333–341.

Chery-Croze, S., Collet, L., & Morgon, A. (1993). Medial olivocochlear system and tinnitus. *Acta Otolaryngologica, 113*, 285–290.

Chery-Croze, S., Moulin, A., & Collet, L. (1993). Effect of contralateral sound stimulation on the distortion product 2F1–F2 in humans: Evidence of a frequency specificity. *Hearing Research, 68*, 53–58.

Chery-Croze, S., Moulin, A., Collet, L., & Morgon, A. (1994). Is the test of medial efferent system function a relevant investigation of tinnitus? *British Journal of Audiology, 28*, 13–25.

Chery-Croze, S., Truy, E., & Morgon, A. (1994). Contralateral suppression of transient otoacoustic emissions and tinnitus. In L. Collet & F. Grandori (Eds.), *Suppression effects of otoacoustic emissions* (Vol. III, pp. 82–95). Milan, Italy: Casa Editrice G. Sefanoni-Lecco.

Chida, E. (1998). Distortion product otoacoustic emissions for the assessment of auditory sensitivity. *Nippon Jibiinkoka Gakkai Kaiho, 101*, 1335–1347.

Chisin, R., Perlman, M. D., & Sohmer, H. (1979). Cochlear and brain stem responses in hearing loss following neonatal hyperbilirubinemia. *Annals of Otology, Rhinology, and Laryngology, 88*, 352–357.

Choi, S. S., Pafitis, I. A., Zalzal, G. H., Herer, G. R., & Patel, K. M. (1999). Clinical applications of transiently evoked otoacoustic emissions in the pediatric population. *Annals of Otology, Rhinology, and Laryngology, 198*, 132–138.

Church, M. W., Kaltenbach, J. A., Blakely, B. W., & Burgio, D. L. (1995). The comparative effects of sodium thiosulphate, diethyldithiocarbamate, fosfomycin, and WR-2721 on ameliorating cisplatin-induced ototoxicity. *Hearing Research, 86*, 195–203.

Chuang, S. W., Gerber, S. E., & Thornton, A. R. D. (1993). Evoked otoacoustic emissions in preterm infants. *International Journal of Pediatric Otorhinolaryngology, 26,* 39–45.

Church, M. W., Kaltenbach, J. A., Blakely, B. W., & Burgio, D. L. (1995). The comparative effects of sodium thiosulphate, diethyldithiocarbamate, fosfomycin, and WR-2721 on ameliorating cisplatin-induced ototoxicity. *Hearing Research, 86,* 195–203.

Cianfrone, G., Mattia, M., Cervellini, M., & Musacchio, A. A. (1993). Some effects of tonal fatiguing on spontaneous and distortion product otoacoustic emissions. *British Journal of Audiology, 27,* 123–130.

Cianfrone, M., Mattia, M., Altissimi, G., & Turchetta, R. (1990). Distortion product otoacoustic emissions and spontaneous otoacoustic emission suppression in humans. In G. F. Grandori, G. Cianfrone, & D. T. Kemp (Eds.), *Cochlear mechanisms and otoacoustic emissions* (Vol. 7, pp. 126–138). Basel: Karger.

Clark, W. W., Kim, D. O., Zurek, P. M., & Bohne, B. A. (1984). Spontaneous otoacoustic emissions in chinchilla ear canals: Correlation with histopathology and suppression by external tones. *Hearing Research, 16,* 299–314.

Clemens, C., & Neumann, R. S. J. (1989). Psychological adjustment to the results of neonatal hypothyroid screening. *Acta Paediatrica Scandinavia, 78,* 447–448.

Cohn, E. S., Kelley, P. M., Fowler, T. W., Gorga, M. P., Lefkowitz, D. M., Kuehn, H. J., Schaefer, G. B., Gobar, L. S., Hahn, F. J., Harris, D. J., & Kimberling, W. J. (1999). Clinical studies of families with hearing loss attributable to mutations in the connexin 26 gene (GJB2/DFNB1). *Pediatrics, 103,* 546–550.

Coleman, G. B., Kaltenbach, J. A., & Falzarano, P. R. (1995). Postnatal development of the mammalian tectorial membrane. *American Journal of Otology, 16,* 620–627.

Coles, R. R. A., Snashell, S. E., & Stephens, S. D. G. (1975). Some varieties of objective tinnitus. *British Journal of Audiology, 9,* 1–6.

Collet, L. (1993). Use of otoacoustic emissions to explore the medial olivocochlear system in humans. *British Journal of Audiology, 27,* 155–159.

Collet, L., Chanal, J. M., Hellal, H., Gartner, M., & Morgon, A. (1989). Validity of bone conduction stimulated ABR, MLR and otoacoustic emissions. *Scandinavian Audiology, 18,* 43–46.

Collet, L., Gartner, M., Moulin, A., Fauffman, I., Disant, F., & Morgon, A. (1989). Evoked otoacoustic emissions and sensorineural hearing loss. *Archives of Otolaryngology—Head and Neck Surgery, 115,* 1060–1062.

Collet, L., Gartner, M., Veuillet, E., Moulin, A., & Morgon, A. (1993). Evoked and spontaneous otoa-

coustic emissions: A comparison of neonates and adults. *Brain Development, 15,* 249–252.

Collet, L., & Grandori, F. (1994). *Suppression effects of otoacoustic emissions.* (Vol. III). Milan, Italy: Casa Editrice G. Sefanoni-Lecco.

Collet, L., Kemp, D. T., Veullet, E., Duclaux, R., Mouline, A., & Morgan, A. (1990). Effect of contralateral auditory stimuli on active cochlear-micromechanical properties in human subjects. *Hearing Research, 43,* 251–262.

Collet, L., Moulin, A., Gartner, M., & Morgon, A. (1990). Age-related changes in evoked otoacoustic emissions. *Annals of Otology, Rhinology, and Laryngology, 99,* 993–997.

Collet, L., Veuillet, E., Bene, J., & Morgon, A. (1992). Effects of contralateral white noise on click-evoked emissions in normal and sensorineural ears: Towards an exploration of the medial olivocochlear system. *Audiology, 31,* 1–7.

Collet, L., Veuillet, E., Chanal, J. M., & Morgon, A. (1991). Evoked otoacoustic emissions and sensorineural hearing loss. *Audiology, 30,* 164–171.

Coletti, V., Fiorino, F. G., Bruni, L., & Biasi, D. (1997). Middle ear mechanics in subjects with rheumatoid arthritis. *Audiology, 36,* 136–146.

Comis, S. D., Osborne, M. P., & Jeffries, J. R. (1990). Effect of furosemide upon morphology of hair bundles in guinea pig cochlear hair cells. *Acta Otolaryngologica, 109,* 49–56.

Committee on Conservation of Hearing. (1959). Guide for the evaluation of hearing impairment. *Transactions of the American Academy of Ophthalmology and Otolaryngology, 63,* 238.

Committee on Hearing and Equilibrium, American Academy of Otolaryngology—Head and Neck Surgery. (1979). Guides to the evaluation of permanent impairment. *Journal of the American Medical Association, 133,* 396–397.

Conlee, J. W., & Shapiro, S. M. (1991). Morphological changes in the cochlear nucleus and nucleus of the trapezoid body in Gunn rat pups. *Hearing Research, 57,* 23–30.

Cooper, N. P. (1996). Two-tone suppression in cochlear mechanics. *Journal of the Acoustical Society of America, 99,* 3087–3098.

Cooper, N. P., & Rhode, W. S. (1996). Two-tone suppression in apical cochlear mechanics. *Auditory Neuroscience, 3,* 123–134.

Corso, J. F. (1958). Proposed laboratory standards of normal hearing. *Journal of the Acoustical Society of America, 30,* 14–23.

Corso, J. F. (1962). Body position and auditory thresholds. *Perceptual Motor Skills, 14,* 499–507.

Cullington, H., Kumar, B., & Flood, L. (1998). Feasibility of otoacoustic emissions as a hearing screen following grommet insertion. *British Journal of Audiology, 32*, 57–62.

Dallmayr, C. (1985). Spontane oto-akustische emissionen: Statistik und reaktion auf akustische stortone. *Acustica, 59*, 67–75.

Dallos, P., Billone, M. C., Durrant, J. D., Wang, C.-Y., & Raynor, S. (1972). Cochlear inner and outer hair cells: functional differences. *Science, 177*, 356–358.

Dallos, P., Geisler, C. D., Matthews, J. W., Ruggero, M. A., & Steele, C. R. (Eds.). (1990). *The mechanics and biophysics of hearing.* New York: Springer-Verlag.

Dallos, P., Popper, A., & Fay, R. (Eds.). (1996). *The cochlea.* New York: Springer.

Dallos, P., & Sweetman, R. H. (1969). Distribution pattern of cochlear harmonics. *Journal of the Acoustical Society of America, 45*, 37–46.

Daniel, H. J., Hume, W. G., Givens, G. D., & Jordan, J. H. (1985). Body position and acoustic admittance. *Ear & Hearing, 6*, 76–79.

Davis, A., & Wood, S. (1992). The epidemiology of childhood hearing impairment: Factors relevant to planning of services. *British Journal of Audiology, 26*, 77–90.

Davis, A., Wood, S., Healy, R., Webb, H., & Rowe, S. (1995). Risk factors for hearing disorders: Epidemiologic evidence of change over time in the UK. *Journal of the American Academy of Audiology, 6*, 365–370.

Davis, H. (1983). An active process in cochlear mechanics. *Hearing Research, 9*, 79–90.

Davis, H., Morgan, C. T., Hawkins, J. E., Galambos, R., & Smith, F. W. (1950). Temporary deafness following exposure to loud noises and tone. *Acta Otolaryngologica*, Suppl. 88.

Daya, H., Hinton, A. E., Radomskiej, P., & Huchzermeyer, P. (1996). Otoacoustic emissions: Assessment of hearing after tympanostomy tube insertion. *Clinical Otolaryngology, 21*, 492–494.

Decker, T. N. (Ed.). (1992). *Otoacoustic emissions* (Vol. 13). New York: Thieme.

Decreton, S. J. R. C., Hanssens, K., & DeSloovere, M. (1991). Evoked otoacoustic emissions in infant hearing screening. *International Journal of Pediatric Otorhinolaryngology, 21*, 235–247.

Delb, W., Hoppe, W., Liebel, J., & Iro, H. (1999). Determination of acute noise effects using distortion product otoacoustic emissions. *Scandinavian Audiology, 28*(2), 67–76.

Delgutte, B. (1990). Two-tone rate suppression in auditory-nerve fibers: Dependence on suppressor frequency and level. *Hearing Research, 49*, 225–246.

Deliac, P., Demarquez, J. P., Barberot, J. P., Sandler, B., & Paty, J. (1990). Brainstem auditory evoked potentials in icteric fullterm newborns: Alterations with exchange transfusions. *Neuropaediatrics, 21*, 115–118.

Deltenre, P., Mansbach, A. L., Bozet, C., Christiaens, F., Barthelemy, P., Paulissen, D., & Renglet, T. (1999). Auditory neuropathy with preserved cochlear microphonics and secondary loss of otoacoustic emissions. *Audiology, 38*(4), 187–195.

Deltenre, P., Mansbach, A. L., Bozet, C., Clerex, A., & Hecox, K. E. (1997). Auditory neuropathy: A report on three cases with early onsets and major neonatal illnesses. *Electroencephalography and Clinical Neurophysiology, 104*, 17–22.

Dempster, J. H., & Mackensie, K. (1990). The resonance frequency of the external auditory canal in children. *Ear & Hearing, 11*, 296–298.

den Hartigh, J., Hilders, C. G. J. M., Schoemaker, R., Hulshof, J. H., Cohen, A., & Vermeij, P. (1994). Tinnitus suppression by intravenous lidocaine in relation to plasma concentration. *Clinical Pharmacology and Therapeutics, 54*, 415–420.

Dennis, J. M., Sheldon, R., Toubas, P., & McCaffee, M. (1984). Identification of hearing loss in the neonatal intensive care unit population. *American Journal of Otology, 5*, 201–205.

Deol, M. (1981). The inner ear in Bronx Waltzer mice. *Acta Otolaryngologica (Stockholm), 92*, 331–336.

Desa, D. J. (1973). Infection and amniotic aspiration of middle ear in stillbirths and neonatal deaths. *Archives of Disease in Childhood, 48*, 872–880.

Desai, A., Reed, D., Cheyne, A., Richards, S., & Prasher, D. (1999). Absence of otoacoustic emissions in subjects with normal audiometric thresholds implies exposure to noise. *Noise and Health, 2*, 58–65.

Desmedt, J. E., & Monaco, P. (1961). Mode of action of the efferent olivo-cochlear bundle on the inner ear. *Nature, 192*, 1263–1265.

Dewson, J. H. (1968). Efferent olivocochlear bundle: some relationships to stimulus discrimination in noise. *Journal of Neurophysiology, 31*, 122–130.

Dhar, S., Long, G. R., & Culpepper, N. B. (1998). The dependence of the distortion product 2f1–f2 on primary levels in non-impaired human ears. *Journal of Speech Language Hearing Research, 41*(6), 1307–1318.

Dibble, K. (1995). Hearing loss & music. *Journal of the Audio Engineering Society, 43*, 251–266.

DiNardo, W., Ghirlanda, G., Paludetti, G., Cercone, S., Saponara, C., DelNinno, M., DiGirolamo, S., Magnani, P., & DiLeo, M. A. (1998). Distortion-product otoacoustic emissions and selective sensorineural loss in IDDM. *Diabetes Care, 21*(8), 1317–1321.

Dirckx, J. J. J., Daemers, K., Somers, T., Offeciers, F. E., & Govaerts, P. J. (1996). Numerical assessment of TOAE screening results: Currently used criteria and their effect on TOAE prevalence figures. *Acta Otolaryngologica (Stockholm), 116*, 672–679.

Dohlen, P., Hennaux, C., Chantry, P., & Hennebert, D. (1991a). Evoked oto-acoustic emissions: Normative results in newborns and adults (in French). *Acta Oto-rhino-laryngologica Belgium, 45*, 381–385.

Dohlen, P., Hennaux, C., Chantry, P., & Hennebert, D. (1991b). The occurrence of oto-acoustic emissions in a normal adult population and neonates. *Scandinavian Audiology, 20*, 203–204.

Dohlen, P., Hennaux, C., Chantry, P., & Hennebert, D. (1992). Evoked oto-acoustic emissions: Normative results in high-risk infants (in French). *Acta Oto-rhino-laryngologica Belgium, 46*, 391–395.

Don, M., & Eggermont, J. J. (1978). Analysis of click evoked brainstem potentials in man using high pass noise masking. *Journal of the Acoustical Society of America, 63*, 1084–1092.

Don, M., Ponton, C. W., Eggermont, J. J., & Masuda, A. (1993). Gender differences in cochlear response time: An explanation for gender amplitude differences in the unmasked auditory brain-stem response. *Journal of the Acoustical Society of America, 94*, 2135–2148.

Dorn, P. A., Piskorski, P., Keefe, D. H., Neely, S. T., & Gorga, M. P. (1998). On the existence of an age/threshold/frequency interaction in distortion product otoacoustic emissions. *Journal of the Acoustical Society of America, 104*, 964–971.

Downs, M. P. (1970). The identification of congenital deafness. *Transactions of the American Academy of Ophthalmology and Otolaryngology, 74*, 1208–1214.

Downs, M. P. (1994). Pediatric audiology—perspective. *Seminars in Hearing, 15*, 1–15.

Downs, M. P., & Hemenway, W. G. (1969). Report on the hearing screening of 17,000 neonates. *International Audiology, 8*, 72–76.

Downs, M. P., & Sterritt, G. M. (1964). Identification audiometry for neonates: A preliminary report. *Journal of Auditory Research, 4*, 69–80.

Doyle, K., Burggraaf, B., Fujikawa, S., & Kim, J. (1997). Newborn hearing screening by otoacoustic emissions and automated auditory brainstem response. *International Journal of Pediatric Otorhinolaryngology, 41*, 111–119.

Doyle, W. J., & Fria, T. J. (1985). The effects of hypothermia on the latencies of the auditory brain stem response (ABR) in the rhesus monkey. *Electroencephalography and Clinical Neurophysiology, 60*, 258–266.

Driscoll, C., Kei, J., Murdoch, B., McPherson, B., Smyth, V., Latham, S., & Loscher, J. (1999). Transient evoked otoacoustic emissions in two-month-old infants: A normative study. *Audiology, 38*(4), 181–186.

Dulon, D., Zajic, G., Aran, J.-M., & Schacht, J. (1989). Aminoglycoside antibiotics impair calcium entry but not viability and motility in isolated cochlear outer hair cells. *Journal of Neuroscience Research, 24*, 338–346.

Eatock, R. A., & Manley, G. A. (1981). Auditory nerve fibre activity in the Tokay Gecko. II. Temperature effect on tuning. *Journal of Comparative Physiology, 142*, 219–226.

Eavey, R. D. (1993). Abnormalities of the neonatal ear: Otoscopic observations, histologic observations, and a model for contamination of the middle ear by cellular contents of amniotic fluid. *Laryngoscope, 103*(Suppl. 58), 1–31.

Eddins, A. C., Zuskov, M., & Salvi, R. J. (1999). Changes in distortion product otoacoustic emissions during prolonged noise exposure. *Hearing Research, 127*, 119–128.

Edwards, C. G., Durieux-Smith, A., & Picton, T. W. (1985). Auditory brainstem response audiometry in neonatal hydrocephalus. *Journal of Otolaryngology, 14*, 40–46.

Egan, J. (1948). Articulation testing methods. *Laryngoscope, 58*, 955–991.

Eggermont, J. J., & Odenthal, D. W. (1974). Action potentials and summating potentials in the normal human cochlea. *Acta Otolaryngologica, Suppl. 316*, 39–61.

El Barbary, A. (1991). Auditory nerve of the normal and jaundiced rat. I. Spontaneous discharge rate and cochlear nerve histology. *Hearing Research, 54*, 75–90.

El-Refaie, A., Parker, D. J., & Bamford, J. M. (1996). Otoacoustic emission versus ABR screening: the effect of external and middle ear abnormalities in a group of SCBU neonates. *British Journal of Audiology, 30*, 3–8.

Elberling, C., Parbo, J., Johnsen, N. J., & Bagi, P. (1985). Evoked acoustic emission: Clinical application. *Acta Otolaryngologica, 421*, 77–85.

Elliott, E. (1958). A ripple effect in the audiogram. *Nature, 181*, 1076.

Elssmann, S., Matkin, N., & Sabo, M. (1987). Early identification of congenital sensorineural hearing impairment. *Hearing Journal, 40*(9), 13–17.

Engdahl, B. (1996). Effects of noise and exercise on distortion product otoacoustic emissions. *Hearing Research, 93*, 72–82.

Engdahl, B., Arnesen, A. R., & Mair, I. W. S. (1991). Otoacoustic emissions (Norwegian language). *Tidsskr Nor Loegeforen, 111*, 2655–2666.

Engdahl, B., Arnesen, A. R., & Mair, I. W. S. (1994). Reproducibility and short-term variability of transient evoked otoacoustic emissions. *Scandinavian Audiology, 23*, 99–104.

Engdahl, B., & Kemp, D. T. (1996). The effect of noise exposure on the details of distortion product otoacoustic emissions in humans. *Journal of the Acoustical Society of America, 99*, 1573–1587.

Eshraghi, A., Francois, M., & Narcy, P. (1996). Evolution of transient evoked otoacoustic emissions in preterm newborns: A preliminary study. *International Journal of Pediatric Otolaryngology, 37*, 121–127.

Evans, B. N. (1990). Fatal contractions: Ultrastructural and electromechanical changes in outer hair cells following transmembranous electrical stimulation. *Hearing Research, 45*, 265–282.

Evans, B. N., & Dallos, P. (1993). Stereocilia induced somatic motility of cochlear outer hair cells. *Proceedings of the New York Academy of Science, 90*, 8347–8351.

Eysholdt, U., & Schreiner, C. (1982). Maximum length sequences: A fast method for measuring brainstem-evoked responses. *Audiology, 21*, 242–250.

Fabiani, M. (1993). Evoked otoacoustic emissions in the study of adult sensorineural hearing loss. *British Journal of Audiology, 27*, 131–137.

Fabiani, M., Petrolito, G., Anastasi, S., Pascarella, M. A., Sciarretta, G., Saponara, M., D'Ambrosio, L., Jagher, P. M., & Munarin, F. (1992). Lesioni uditive negli atleti praticanti attivita sportive con armi da fuoco. *Medicine Sport, 45*, 369–379.

Fahey, P. F., & Allen, J. B. (1985). Nonlinear phenomena as observed in the ear canal and at the auditory nerve. *Journal of the Acoustical Society of America, 77*, 599–612.

Feinmesser, M., & Tell, L. (1976). Neonatal screening for detection of hearing loss. *Archives of Otolaryngology, 102*, 297–299.

Ferber-Viart, C., Colleaux, B., Laoust, L., Dubreuil, C., & Duclaux, R. (1998). Is the presence of transient evoked otoacoustic emissions in ears with acoustic neuroma significant? *Laryngoscope, 108*, 605–609.

Ferber-Viart, C., Savourey, G., Garcia, C., Duclaux, R., Bittel, J., & Collet, L. (1995). Influence of hyperthermia on cochlear micromechanical properties in humans. *Hearing Research, 91*, 202–207.

Fex, J. (1959). Augmentation of the cochlear microphonics by stimulation of efferent fibers to cochlea. *Acta Otolaryngologica, 50*, 540.

Finitzo, T., Albright, K., & O'Neal, J. (1998). The newborn with hearing loss: Detection in the nursery. *Pediatrics, 102*(6), 1452–1460.

Fitzgerald, J. J., Robertson, D., & Johnstone, B. M. (1993). Effects of intra-cochlear perfusion of salicylates on cochlear microphonic and other auditory responses in guinea pig. *Hearing Research, 67*, 147–156.

Fleischman, R. W., Standnicki, S. W., Ethieu, M. F., & Schaeppi, U. (1975). Ototoxicity of cis-dichlorodiamine platinum (II) in the guinea pig. *Toxicology and Applied Pharmacology, 33*, 320–332.

Flock, A. (1980). Contractile proteins in hair cells. *Hearing Research, 2*, 411–412.

Folsom, R., Burns, E., Morrison, R., & Zettner, E. (1995). Comparison of peripheral vs. central tuning in human adults and infants. *Association for Research in Otolaryngology, 18*, 120.

Folsom, R., & Wynne, M. (1987). Auditory brainstem responses from human adults and infants: Wave-V tuning curves. *Journal of the Acoustical Society of America, 81*, 412–417.

Folsom, R. L., & Owsley, R. M. (1985). N1 action potentials in humans: influence of stimultaneous contralateral stimulation. *Acta Otolaryngologica, Suppl. 421*, 77–85.

Fortnum, H., & Davis, A. (1997). Epidemiology of permanent childhood hearing impairment in the Trent region, 1985–1993. *British Journal of Audiology, 31*, 409–446.

Fortnum, H., Farnsworth, A., & Davis, A. (1993). The feasibility of evoked otoacoustic emissions as an in-patient hearing check after meningitis. *British Journal of Audiology, 27*, 227–231.

Fradis, M., Podoshin, L., Ben-David, J., & Reiner, B. (1985). Treament of Meniere's disease by intratympanic injection with lidocaine. *Archives of Otolaryngology—Head and Neck Surgery, 111*, 491–493.

Francois, M. (1999). Les otoemissions provoquees chez le nouveau-ne. *Archives of Pediatrics, 6*(Suppl. 6), 351–352.

Francois, M., Laccourreye, L., Tran Ba Huy, E., & Narcy, P. (1997). Hearing impairment in infants after meningitis: detection by transient evoked otoacoustic emissions. *Journal of Pediatrics, 130*, 712–717.

Frank, G., & Kossl, M. (1995). The shape of 2f1–f2 suppression tuning curves reflects basilar membrane specializations in the mustached bat *Pteronotus parnellii*. *Hearing Research, 83*, 150–160.

Franklin, D. J., Lonsbury-Martin, B. L., Stagner, B. B., & Martin, G. K. (1991). Altered susceptibility of 2f1-f2 acoustic distortion products to the effects of repeated noise exposure in rabbits. *Hearing Research, 53*, 185–208.

Franklin, D. J., McCoy, M. J., Martin, G. K., & Lonsbury-Martin, B. L. (1992). Test-retest reliability of distortion-product and transiently evoked otoacoustic emissions. *Ear & Hearing, 13*, 417–429.

Freeman, S., Plotnik, M., Elidan, J., & Sohmer, H. (1999). Differential effect of the loop diuretic furosemide on short latency auditory and vestibular-evoked potentials. *American Journal of Otology, 20*, 41–45.

Frick, L. R., & Matthies, M. L. (1988). Effects of external stimuli on spontaneous otoacoustic emissions. *Ear & Hearing, 9*, 190–197.

Fritze, W. (1983). Registration of spontaneous cochlear emissions by means of Fourier transformation. *Archives of Otorhinolaryngology, 238*, 189–196.

Froehlich, P., Collet, L., Chanal, J. M., & Morgon, A. (1990). Variability of the influence of a visual task on the active micromechanical properties of the cochlea. *Brain Research, 508*, 286–288.

Froehlich, P., Collet, L., & Morgon, A. (1993). Transiently evoked otoacoustic emissions amplitudes change with changes of directed attention. *Physiologic Behavior, 53*, 679–682.

Froehlich, P., Collet, L., Valatx, J., & Morgon, A. (1993). Sleep and active cochlear micromechanical properties in human subjects. *Hearing Research, 66*, 1–7.

Froehlich, P., Ferber, C., Remond, J., Jaboulay, J. M., Morgon, A., Duclaux, R., & Collet, L. (1994). Lack of association between transiently evoked emission amplitude and experimentation linked-factors (repeated acoustic stimulation, cerebrospinal fluid pressure, supine and sitting positions, and alertness levels). *Hearing Research, 75*, 184–190.

Frolenkov, G. I., Belyantseva, I. A., Kurc, M., Mastroianni, M. A., & Kachar, B. (1998). Cochlear outer hair cell electromotility can provide force for both low and high intensity distortion product otoacoustic emissions. *Hearing Research, 126*, 67–74.

Furst, M., Rabinowitz, W. M., & Zurek, P. M. (1988). Ear canal acoustic distortion at 2f1–f2 from human ears: Relation to other emissions and perceived combination tones. *Journal of the Acoustical Society of America, 84*, 215–221.

Fyro, K., & Bodegard, G. (1987). Four year follow-up of psychological reactions to false positive screening tests for congenital hypothyroidism. *Acta Paediatrica Scandinavia, 76*, 107–114.

Fyro, K., & Bodegard, G. (1988). Difficulties in psychological adjustment to a new neonatal screening programme. *Acta Paediatrica Scandinavia, 77*, 226–231.

Galambos, R. (1956). Suppression of auditory-nerve activity by stimulation of efferent fibers to the cochlea. *Journal of Neurophysiology, 19*, 424–437.

Gaskill, S., & Brown, A. (1993). Comparing the level of the acoustic distortion product 2f1–f2 with behavioral threshold audiograms from normal-hearing and hearing-impaired ears. *British Journal of Audiology, 27*, 397–407.

Gaskill, S. A., & Brown, A. M. (1990). The behavior of the acoustic distortion product, 2f1–f2, from the human ear and its relation to auditory sensitivity. *Journal of the Acoustical Society of America, 88*, 821–839.

Giard, M. H., Collet, L., Bouchet, P., & Pernier, J. (1994). Auditory selective attention in the human cochlea. *Brain Research, 633*, 353–356.

Gifford, M. L., & Guinan, J. J. (1987). Effects of electrical stimulation of medial olivocochlear neurons on ipsilateral and contralateral cochlear responses. *Hearing Research, 29*, 179–194.

Gill, A. W., Gosling, D., Kelly, C., Walker, P., & Wooderson, S. (1998). Predischarge screening of very low birthweight infants by click evoked otoacoustic emissions. *Journal of Paediatric Child Health, 34*(5), 456–459.

Giraud, A. L., Collet, L., Chery-Croze, S., Magnan, J., & Chays, A. (1995). Evidence of a medial olivocochlear involvement in contralateral suppression of otoacoustic emissions in humans. *Brain Research, 705*, 15–23.

Gitter, A. H. (1992). The length of isolated outer hair cells is temperature dependent. *Journal of Otorhinolaryngology, 54*, 121–123.

Glanville, J. D., Coles, R. R. A., & Sullivan, B. M. (1971). A family with high-tonal objective tinnitus. *Journal of Laryngology and Otology, 85*, 1–10.

Glattke, T., & Kujawa, S. (1991). Otoacoustic emissions. *American Journal of Audiology, 1*, 29–40.

Glattke, T. J., Pafitis, I. A., Cummiskey, C., & Herer, G. R. (1995). Identification of hearing loss in children using measures of transient otoacoustic emission reproducibility. *American Journal of Audiology, 4*, 71–86.

Gobsch, H., Kevanishvili, Z., Gamgegeli, Z., & Gvelesiani, T. (1992). Behaviour of delayed evoked otoacoustic emission under forward masking paradigm. *Scandinavian Audiology, 21*, 143–148.

Gobsch, H., & Tietze, G. (1993). Interrelation of spontaneous and evoked otoacoustic emissions. *Hearing Research, 69*, 176–181.

Goforth, L., Hood, L. J., & Berlin, C. I. (1998). Development of efferent function in neonates. *Association for Research in Otolaryngology, 21*.

Gold, T. (1948). Hearing. II. The physical basis of the action of the cochlea. *Proceedings of the Royal Society of Britain, 135*, 492–498.

Gold, T. (1989). Historical background to the proposal, 40 years ago, of an active model for cochlear frequency analysis. In J. Wilson & D. Kemp (Eds.), *Cochlear mechanics* (pp. 299–305). New York: Plenum.

Gold, T., & Pumphrey, R. (1948). Hearing. I. The cochlea as a frequency analyzer. *Proceedings of the Royal Society of Britain, 135,* 462–491.

Goldstein, A. J., & Mizukoshi, O. (1967). Separation of the organ of Corti into its component cells. *Annals of Otology, Rhinology, and Laryngology, 76,* 414–426.

Goldstein, J. L. (1967). Auditory nonlinearity. *Journal of the Acoustical Society of America, 41,* 676–689.

Goldstein, J. L., & Kiang, N. Y. S. (1968). Neural correlates of the aural combination tone 2f1–f2. *Proceedings of the IEEE, 56*(6), 981–992.

Goodhill, V. (1950). Nuclear deafness and the nerve deaf child: the importance of the Rh factor. *Transactions of the American Academy of Ophthalmology and Otolaryngology, 44,* 671–686.

Gorga, M., Neely, S., Bergman, B., Beauchaine, K., Kaminski, J., Peters, J., Schulte, L., & Jesteadt, W. (1993). A comparison of transient-evoked and distortion product otoacoustic emissions in normal-hearing and hearing-impaired subjects. *Journal of the Acoustical Society of America, 94*(5), 2639–2648.

Gorga, M., Neely, S., Ohlrich, B., Hoover, B., Redner, J., & Peters, J. (1997). From laboratory to clinic: A large scale study of distortion product otoacoustic emissions in ears with normal hearing and ears with hearing loss. *Ear & Hearing, 18,* 440–455.

Gorga, M., Stelmachowicz, P., Barlow, S., & Brookhauser, P. (1995). Case of recurrent, reversible, sudden sensorineural hearing loss in a child. *Journal of the American Academy of Audiology, 6,* 163–172.

Gorga, M. P. (1994). *Otoacoustic emissions and infant screening.* Paper presented at the Winter Meeting of the Illinois Chapter of the American Academy of Audiology, Chicago.

Gorga, M. P., Kaminski, J. R., & Beauchaine, K. A. (1988). Auditory brainstem responses from graduates of an intensive care nursery using an insert earphone. *Ear & Hearing, 9,* 144–147.

Gorga, M. P., Neely, S. T., Bergman, B., Beauchaine, K. L., Kaminski, J. R., Peters, J., & Jesteadt, W. (1993). Otoacoustic emissions from normal-hearing and hearing-impaired subjects: Distortion product responses. *Journal of the Acoustical Society of America, 93,* 2050–2060.

Gorga, M. P., Neely, S. T., Bergman, B. M., Beauchaine, K. L., Kaminski, J. R., & Liu, Z. (1994). Towards understanding the limits of distortion product otoacoustic emission measurements. *Journal of the Acoustical Society of America, 96,* 1494–1500.

Gorga, M. P., Neely, S. T., & Dorn, P. A. (1999). DPOAE test performance for a priori criteria and for multifrequency gold standards. *Ear & Hearing, 20,* 345–362.

Gorga, M. P., Reiland, J. K., Beauchaine, K. A., Worthington, D. W., & Jesteadt, W. (1987). Auditory brainstem responses from graduates of an intensive care nursery: Normal patterns of response. *Journal of Speech and Hearing Research, 30,* 311–318.

Gorga, M. P., Stover, L., Neely, S. T., & Montoya, D. (1996). The use of cumulative distributions to determine critical values and levels of confidence for clinical distortion product otoacoustic emissions measurements. *Journal of the Acoustical Society of America, 100,* 968–977.

Graham, J. M., Drenovak, M., Akhtar, S., & Bantock, H. (1997). *Case report of a child who developed severe hyperbilirubinemia with preserved otoacoustic emissions but absent auditory brainstem responses and in whom normal hearing thresholds developed by 14 months of age.* Paper presented at the British Cochlear Implant Group, England.

Graham, R. L., & Hazell, J. W. P. (1996). Contralateral suppression of transient otoacoustic emissions: Intraindividual variability in tinnitus and normal subjects. In L. Collet & F. Grandori (Eds.), *Suppression effects of otoacoustic emissions* (Vol. III, pp. 56–70). Milan, Italy: Casa Editrice G. Sefanoni-Lecco.

Grandori, F. (1985). Nonlinear phenomena in click- and toneburst evoked otoacoustic emissions from human ears. *Audiology, 25,* 71–80.

Grandori, F., Cianfrone, G., & Kemp, D. T. (Eds.). (1990). *Cochlear mechanisms and otoacoustic emissions.* Basel: Kruger.

Grandori, F., Collet, L., Kemp, D., Salomen, G., Schorn, K., & Thornton, R. (Eds.). (1994). *Advances in otoacoustic emissions. I. Fundamentals and clinical applications.*

Grandori, F., & Ravazzani, P. (1993). Non-linearities of click-evoked otoacoustic emissions and the derived non-linear technique. *British Journal of Audiology, 27,* 97–102.

Gratton, M. A. (1990). The interaction of cisplatin and noise on the peripheral auditory system. *Hearing Research, 50,* 211–224.

Gray, L. (1990). Development of temporal integration in newborn chicks. *Hearing Research, 45,* 169–177.

Greville, A. (1996). Identification of hearing loss in infants. *The New Zealand Medical Journal, 109,* 21–22.

Grewe, T., Danhauer, J., Danhauer, K., & Thornton, A. (1994). Clinical use of otoacoustic emissions in children with autism. *International Journal of Pediatric Otorhinolaryngology, 30,* 123–132.

Grose, J. H. (1983). The effect of contralateral stimulation on spontaneous otoacoustic emissions. *Journal of the Acoustical Society of America, 74*, S38.

Guggenheim, P. (1971). Mesenchyme in the middle ear. *Laryngoscope, 81*, 1665–1670.

Guinan, J. J., Jr. (1986). Effect of efferent neural activity on cochlear mechanics. *Scandinavian Audiology,* Suppl. 25, 53–62.

Guinan, J. J., Jr. (1996). Physiology of olivocochlear efferents. In P. Dallos, A. N. Popper, & R. R. Fay (Eds.), *The cochlea* (pp. 435–502). New York: Springer.

Guinan, J. J., Jr., Warr, W. B., & Norris, B. E. (1983). Differential olivocochlear projections from lateral versus medial zones of superior olivary complex. *Journal of Comparative Neurology, 221*, 358–370.

Gvelesiani, T. G., Gunenkov, A. V., & Tavartkiladze, G. A. (1998). Relationship between otoacoustic emissions and ear resonance. *Association for Research in Otolaryngology, 21*.

Haggard, M. (1992). Screening children's hearing. *British Journal of Audiology, 26*, 209–215.

Haggerty, H. S., Lusted, H. S., & Morton, S. C. (1993). Statistical quantification of 24 hour and monthly variabilities of spontaneous otoacoustic emission frequency in humans. *Hearing Research, 70*, 31–49.

Haginomori, S. I. (1998). Spontaneous otoacoustic emissions in patients with endolymphatic hydrops. *Association for Research in Otolaryngology, 21*.

Haginomori, S. I., Makimoto, K., Araki, M., Kawakami, M., & Takahashi, H. (1995). Effect of lidocaine injection on evoked otoacoustic emissions with tinnitus. *Acta Otolaryngologica (Stockholm), 115*, 488–492.

Hall, D. M., & Garner, J. (1988). Feasibility of screening all neonates for hearing loss. *Archives of Diseases of Childhood, 63*, 652–653.

Hall, J. L. (1972). Auditory distortion products f2–f1 and 2f1–f2. *Journal of the Acoustical Society of America, 51*, 1863–1871.

Hall, J. L. (1974). Two-tone distortion products in a nonlinear model of the basilar membrane. *Journal of the Acoustical Society of America, 56*, 1818–1828.

Hall, J. W., III. (1986). Auditory brainstem response spectral content in comatose head-injured patients. *Ear & Hearing, 7*, 383–387.

Hall, J. W., III. (1992). *Handbook of auditory evoked responses*. Needham Heights, MA: Allyn & Bacon.

Hall, J. W., III. (1992). Otoacoustic emissions: Facts and fantasies. *The Hearing Journal, 45*(11), 7–52.

Hall, J. W., III. (1994). Clinical application of otoacoustic emissions: What do we know about factors influencing measurement and analysis? *Otolaryngology—Head and Neck Surgery, 110*, 22–38.

Hall, J. W., III., Baer, J. E., Chase, P. A., & Rupp, K. A. (1994, April 29, 1994). *Transient and distortion product otoacoustic emissions in infant hearing screening*. Paper presented at the American Academy of Audiology, Richmond, VA.

Hall, J. W., III, Berry, G. A., & Olson, K. (1982). Identification of serious hearing loss with acoustic reflex data: Clinical experience with some new guidelines. *Scandinavian Audiology, 11*, 251–255.

Hall, J. W., III, Brown, D. P., & Mackey-Hargadine, J. R. (1985). Pediatric applications of serial ABR and middle-latency evoked response recordings. *International Journal of Pediatric Otorhinolaryngology, 9*, 201–218.

Hall, J. W., III, Bull, J., & Cronau, L. (1988). The effect of hypo- versus hyperthermia on auditory brainstem response: Two case reports. *Ear & Hearing, 9*, 137–143.

Hall, J. W., III, & Bulla, W. A. (1999). Assessment of music-induced auditory dysfunction. *The Hearing Review, 6*(2), 20–27.

Hall, J. W., III, & Chase, P. A. (1993). Answers to 10 common clinical questions about otoacoustic emissions. *The Hearing Journal, 46*(10), 29–32.

Hall, J. W., III, Herndon, D. N., Gary, L. B., & Winkler, J. B. (1986). Auditory brainstem response in young burn-wound patients treated with ototoxic drugs. *International Journal of Pediatric Otorhinolaryngology, 12*, 187–203.

Hall, J. W., III, Kileny, P. R., & Ruth, R. A. (1987, August). *Clinical validation study of the ALGO-1 automated hearing screener*. Paper presented at the 10th International Evoked Response Audiometry Study Group Meeting, Charlottesville, Virginia.

Hall, J. W., III, Kripal, J. P., & Hepp, T. (1988). Newborn hearing screening with auditory brainstem response: measurement problems and solutions. *Seminars in Hearing, 9*(1), 15–33.

Hall, J. W., III, & Mueller, H. G., III. (1997). *Audiologists' Desk Reference. Volume I*. San Diego: Singular Publishing Group.

Hall, J. W., III, & Santucci, M. (1995). Protecting the professional ear: Conservation strategies and devices. *The Hearing Journal, 48*, 37–45.

Hall, J. W., III, Winkler, J. B., Herndon, D. N., & Gary, L. B. (1987). Auditory brainstem response in auditory assessment of acute severely burned children. *Journal of Burn Care and Rehabilitation, 8*, 195–198.

Halpern, J., Hosford-Dunn, H., & Malachowski, N. (1987). Four factors that accurately predict hearing loss in "high risk" neonates. *Ear & Hearing, 8*, 21–25.

Hamernik, R. P., Ahroon, W. A., Jock, B. M., & Bennett, J. A. (1998). Noise-induced threshold shift dynamics measured with distortion-product otoacoustic emissions and auditory evoked potentials in chinchillas with inner hair cell deficient cochleas. *Hearing Research, 118*, 73–82.

Hamernik, R. P., Ahroon, W. A., & Lei, S. F. (1996). The cubic distortion product otoacoustic emissions from the normal and noise-damaged chinchilla cochlea. *Journal of the Acoustical Society of America, 100*, 1003–1012.

Hamernik, R. P., Henderson, D., & Salvi, R. J. (Eds.). (1982). *New perspectives on noise-induced hearing loss.* New York: Raven Press.

Hamill-Ruth, R. J., Ruth, R. A., Googer, K., Volles, D., Deivert, M., & Turrentine, B. (1998). Use of otoacoustic emissions to screen for hearing loss in critically ill patients. *Audiology, 37*, 344–352.

Harel, N., Kakigi, A., Hirakawa, H., Mount, R. J., & Harrison, R. V. (1997). The effects of anesthesia on otoacoustic emissions. *Hearing Research, 110*, 25–33.

Harris, F. (1990). Distortion-product otoacoustic emissions in humans with high frequency sensorineural hearing loss. *Journal of Speech and Hearing Research, 33*, 594–600.

Harris, F., & Glattke, T. (1992). The use of suppression to determine the characteristics of otoacoustic emissions. *Seminars in Hearing, 13*, 67–80.

Harris, F., & Probst, R. (1992). Transiently evoked otoacoustic emissions in patients with Meniere's disease. *Acta Otolaryngologica (Stockholm), 112*, 36–44.

Harris, F., Probst, R., & Wenger, R. (1991). Repeatability of transiently evoked otoacoustic emissions in normally hearing humans. *Audiology, 30*, 135–141.

Harris, F., Probst, R., & Xu, L. (1992). Suppression of the 2f1–f2 otoacoustic emission in humans. *Hearing Research, 64*, 133–141.

Harris, F. P., Lonsbury-Martin, B. L., Stagner, B. B., Coats, A. C., & Martin, G. K. (1989). Acoustic distortion products in humans: Systematic changes in amplitude as a function of f2/f1 ratio. *Journal of the Acoustical Society of America, 85*, 220–229.

Harris, F. P., & Probst, R. (Eds.). (1994). *Technical issues related to the clinical measurement of transiently evoked and distortion-product otoacoustic emissions.* (Vol. II). Milan, Italy: Commission of the European Communities.

Harrison, M., & Roush, J. (1996). Age of suspicion, identification, and intervention for infants and young children with hearing loss: A national study. *Ear & Hearing, 17*, 55–62.

Harrison, R. V. (1998). An animal model of auditory neuropathy. *Ear & Hearing, 19*, 355–361.

Harrison, W. A., & Burns, E. M. (1993). Effects of contralateral acoustic stimulation on spontaneous otoacoustic emissions. *Journal of the Acoustical Society of America, 94*, 2649–2658.

Hassmann, E., Skotnicka, B., Midro, A. T., & Musiatowicz, M. (1998). Distortion products otoacoustic emissions in diagnosis of hearing loss in Down syndrome. *International Journal of Pediatric Otorhinolaryngology, 45*, 199–206.

Hatzopoulos, S., Mazzoli, M., & Martini, A. (1995). Identification of hearing loss using TEOAE descriptors: Theoretical foundations and preliminary results. *Audiology, 34*, 248–259.

Haughton, P. M. (1998). Random noise in the spectra of evoked otoacoustic emissions. *British Journal of Audiology, 32*, 337–349.

Hauser, R., & Probst, R. (1991). The influence of systematic primary-tone level variation L2–L1 on the acoustic distortion product emission 2f1–f2 in normal human ears. *Journal of the Acoustical Society of America, 89*, 280–286.

Hauser, R., Probst, R., Harris, F., & Frei, F. (1992). Influence of general anesthesia on transiently evoked otoacoustic emissions in humans. *Annals of Otology, Rhinology, and Laryngology, 101*, 994–999.

Hauser, R., Probst, R., & Harris, F. P. (1993). Effects of atmospheric pressure variation on spontaneous, transiently evoked, and distortion product otoacoustic emissions in normal human ears. *Hearing Research, 69*, 133–145.

He, D. Z. Z., Evans, B. N., & Dallos, P. (1994). First appearance and development of electromotility in neonatal gerbil outer hair cells. *Hearing Research, 78*, 77–90.

He, N.-J., & Schmiedt, R. A. (1993). Fine structure of the 2f1–f2 acoustic distortion product: Changes with primary level. *Journal of the Acoustical Society of America, 94*, 2659–2669.

He, N.-J., & Schmiedt, R. A. (1997). Fine structure of the 2f1–f2 acoustic distortion product: Effects of primary level and frequency ratios. *Journal of the Acoustical Society of America, 101*, 3554–3565.

Heil, H., Erre, J. P., Aurousseau, C., Bouali, R., Dulon, D., & Aran, J. M. (1993). Gentamicin uptake by cochlear hair cells precedes hearing impairment during chronic treatment. *Audiology, 32*, 78–87.

Heitmann, J., Waldmann, B., Schnitzier, H. U., Plinkert, P. K., & Zenner, H. P. (1998). Suppression of distortion product otoacoustic emissions (DPOAE) near 2f1–f2 removes DP-gram fine structure—evidence for a second generator. *Journal of the Acoustical Society of America, 103*, 1527–1531.

Henderson, D., Hamernik, R. P., Mills, J., & Dosanjh, D. (Eds.). (1976). *Effects of noise on hearing.* New York: Raven.

Henderson, D., Subramaniam, M., & Boettcher, F. A. (1993). Individual susceptibility to noise-induced hearing loss: An old topic revisited. *Ear & Hearing, 14,* 152–168.

Henley, C., Weatherly, R., Martin, G., & Lonsbury-Martin, B. (1996). Sensitive developmental periods for kanamycin ototoxic effects on distortion-product otoacoustic emissions. *Hearing Research, 98,* 93–103.

Henley, C. M., & Rybak, L. P. (1995). Ototoxicity in developing mammals. *Brain Research Reviews, 20,* 68–90.

Henry, K. R., & Chole, R. A. (1984). Hypothermia protects the cochlea from noise damage. *Hearing Research, 16,* 225–230.

Herer, G. R., Glattke, T. J., Pafitis, I. A., & Cummiskey, C. (1996). Detection of hearing loss in young children and adults using otoacoustic emissions. *Folia Phoniatrica et Logopaedica, 48,* 17–121.

Hess, M., Finckh-Kramer, U., Bartsch, M., Kewitz, G., Versmold, H., & Gross, M. (1998). Hearing screening in at-risk neonate cohort. *International Journal of Pediatric Otorhinolaryngology, 46,* 81–89.

Hess, M. M., Lamprecht, A., Kirkopoulos, S., & Fournell, A. (1991). Messung evozierter otoakustischer Emissionen zu verschiedenen Zeitpunkten einer Intubationsarkose. *Folia Phoniatrica, 43,* 68–73.

Hicks, M. L., & Bacon, S. P. (1999). Psychophysical measures of auditory nonlinearities as a function of frequency in individuals with normal hearing. *Journal of the Acoustical Society of America, 105,* 326–341.

Hine, J. E., & Thornton, A. R. D. (1997). Transient evoked otoacoustic emissions recorded using maximum length sequences as a function of stimulus rate and level. *Ear & Hearing, 18,* 121–128.

Hine, J. E., Thornton, A. R. D., & Brookes, G. B. (1997). Effect of olivocochlear bundle section on evoked otoacoustic emissions recorded using maximum length sequences. *Hearing Research, 108,* 28–36.

Hinz, M., & von Wedel, H. (1984). Otoacoustische Emissionnen bei Patienten mit Hörsturzt. *Archives of Otolaryngology,* Suppl. 11, 128–130.

Hirsh, I. J., Davis, H., Silverman, S. R., Reynolds, E. G., Eldert, E., & Benson, R. W. (1952). Development of materials for speech audiometry. *Journal of Speech and Hearing Disorders, 17,* 321–337.

Hofstetter, P., Ding, D., Powers, N., & Salvi, R. (1997). Quantitative relationship of carboplatin dose to magnitude of inner and outer hair cell loss and the reduction in distortion product otoacoustic emission amplitude in chinchillas. *Hearing Research, 112,* 199–215.

Holte, L., Margolis, R. H., & Cavanaugh, J. (1991). Developmental changes in multifrequency tympanometry. *Audiology, 30,* 1–24.

Holtz, M., Harris, F., & Probst, R. (1994). Otoacoustic emissions: An approach for monitoring aminoglycoside-induced ototoxicity. *Laryngoscope, 104,* 1130–1134.

Holtz, M. A., Probst, R., Harris, F. P., & Hauser, R. (1993). Monitoring the effects of noise exposure using transiently evoked otoacoustic emissions. *Acta Otolaryngologica, 113,* 478–482.

Hood, L. J. (1998). Auditory neuropathy: What is it and what can we do with it? *The Hearing Journal, 51,* 10, 12, 13,16–18.

Hood, L. J., Hurley, A. E., Goforth, L., Bordelon, J., & Berlin, C. I. (1997). Aging and efferent suppression of otoacoustic emissions. *Association for Research in Otolaryngology.*

Horner, K., & Cazals, Y. (1989). Distortion products in early stage experimental hydrops in the guinea pig. *Hearing Research, 43,* 71–80.

Horner, K. C., Guilhaume, A., & Cazals, Y. (1988). Atrophy of middle and short stereocilia on the outer hair cells of guinea pig cochleas with experimentally induced hydrops. *Hearing Research, 32,* 41–48.

Hornsby, B., Kelly, T., & Hall, J., III. (1996). Normative data for five FDA-approved distortion product OAE systems. *Hearing Journal, 49*(9), 39–46.

Hotaling, A., Blank, C., Park, A., Matz, G., Yost, W., & Raffin, M. (1994). *Distortion-product otoacoustic non-emissions.* Paper presented at the American Auditory Society 20th Annual Meeting, Halifax, Nova Scotia.

Houtgast, T. (1972). Psychophysical evidence for lateral inhibition in hearing. *Journal of the Acoustical Society of America, 5,* 1885–1894.

Huang, J.-M., Berlin, C. I., Cullen, J. K., Jr., & Wickremasinghe, A. R. (1994). Development of contralateral suppression of the VIIIth nerve compound action potential (CAP) in the Mongolian gerbil. *Hearing Research, 78,* 243–248.

Hubbard, A. E., & Geisler, C. D. (1972). A hybrid-computer model of the cochlear partition. *Journal of the Acoustical Society of America, 51,* 1895–1903.

Huizing, E. H., & Spoor, A. (1973). An unusual type of tinnitus. *Archives of Otolaryngology, 98,* 134–136.

Hudgins, C. V., Hawkins, J. E., Jr., Karlin, J. E., & Stevens, S. S. (1947). The development of recorded auditory tests for measuring hearing loss for speech. *Laryngoscope, 57,* 57–89.

Humes, L. E. (1980). Growth of L(f2–f1) and L(2f1–f2) with input level: Influence of f2/f1. *Hearing Research, 2*, 115–122.

Hung, K. L. (1989). Auditory brainstem responses in patients with neonatal hyperbilirubinemia. *Brain and Development, 11*, 297–301.

Hunter, L. L., & Margolis, R. H. (1992). Multifrequency tympanometry: Current clinical applications. *American Journal of Audiology, 1*, 33–43.

Hunter, M. F., Kimm, L., Cafarelli Dees, D., Kennedy, C. R., & Thornton, A. R. D. (1994). Feasibility of otoacoustic emission detection followed by ABR as a universal infant screening test for hearing impairment. *British Journal of Audiology, 28*, 235–248.

Hurley, R. M., & Musiek, F. M. (1994). Effectiveness of transient-evoked otoacoustic emissions (TEOAE) in predicting hearing level. *Journal of the American Academy of Audiology, 5*, 195–203.

Hussain, D. M., Gorga, M. P., Neely, S. T., Keefe, D. H., & Peters, J. (1998). Transient evoked otoacoustic emissions in patients with normal hearing and patients with hearing loss. *Ear & Hearing, 19*, 434–449.

Igarashi, M., Cranford, J. L., Allen, E. A., & Alford, B. R. (1979). Behavioral auditory function after transection of crossed olivocochlear bundle in the cat. I. Pure-tone intensity discrimination. *Acta Otolaryngologica, 87*, 429–433.

Inamura, N., Kusakari, J., & Takasaka, T. (1987). Effect of hypothermia on the cochlear potentials. *Acta Otolaryngologica, Suppl. 435*, 33–39.

Ito, H. (1984). Auditory brainstem response in NICU infants. *International Journal of Pediatric Otorhinolaryngology, 8*, 155–162.

Iwasaki, S., Mizuta, K., & Hoshino, T. (1998). Tone burst-evoked otoacoustic emissions in cats with acoustic overstimulation and anoxia. *Hearing Research, 118*, 83-89.

Jacobson, J., & Jacobson, C. (1994). The effects of noise in transient EOAE newborn hearing screening. *International Journal of Pediatric Otorhinolaryngology, 29*, 235–248.

Jacobson, J. T., & Mencher, G. T. (1981). Intensive care nursery noise and its influence on newborn hearing screening. *International Journal of Pediatric Otorhinolaryngology, 3*, 45–54.

Jacobson, J. T., & Morehouse, C. R. (1984). A comparison of auditory brainstem response and behavioral screening in high risk and normal newborn infants. *Ear & Hearing, 5*, 247–253.

Jaffe, B., Hurtado, F., & Hurtado, E. (1967). Tympanic membrane mobility in the newborn (with seven months follow-up). *Laryngoscope, 80*, 36–47.

Jaffe, B. F. (1980). Amniotic fluid microviscosity and middle ear effusion. *Pediatrics, 65*, 362–363.

Janssen, T., Kummer, P., Boege, P., & Arnold, W. (1998). Growth behavior of the 2f1–f2 distortion product otoacoustic emissions in sensorineural hearing loss with and without tinnitus. *Association for Research in Otolaryngology.*

Jerger, J. (1970). Clinical experience with impedance audiometry. *Archives of Otolaryngology, 92*, 311–324.

Jerger, J. (1997). Universal hearing screening and human rights. *Audiology Today, 9*(1), 9.

Jerger, J., & Jerger, S. (1971). Diagnostic significance of PB word functions. *Archives of Otolaryngology, 93*, 573–580.

Jerger, J., & Keith, W. (1980). Inter- versus intrasubject variability in acoustic immittance. *Ear and Hearing, 1*, 338–340.

Jerger, J. F., & Hayes, D. (1976). The cross-check principle in pediatric audiology. *Archives of Otolaryngology, 102*, 614–620.

Jewett, D. L., & Williston, J. S. (1971). Auditory evoked far fields averaged from the scalp of humans. *Brain, 4*, 681–696.

Jock, B., Hamernik, R., Aldrich, L., Ahroon, W., Petriello, K.-L., & Johnson, A. (1996). Evoked-potential thresholds and cubic distortion product otoacoustic emissions in the chinchilla following carboplatin treatment and noise exposure. *Hearing Research, 96*, 179–190.

Joglekar, V. (1980). Barrier properties of vernix caseosa. *Archives of Diseases of Childhood, 55*(10), 817–819.

Johannesen, P. T., Rasmussen, A. N., & Osterhammel, P. A. (1998a). Instrumentation for transient evoked otoacoustic emissions elicited by maximum length sequences. *Scandinavian Audiology, 27*, 37–42.

Johannesen, P. T., Rasmussen, A. N., & Osterhammel, P. A. (1998b). Neonatal hearing screening using transient evoked otoacoustic emissions elicited by maximum length sequences. *Revista Brasiliera de Otorrinolaringologia, 64*(5), 485–492.

Johnsen, N., Bagi, P., Parbo, J., & Elberling, C. (1988). Evoked acoustic emissions from the human ear. IV. Final results in 100 neonates. *Scandinavian Audiology, 17*, 27–34.

Johnsen, N., Parbo, J., & Elberling, C. (1993). Evoked acoustic emissions from the human ear. *Scandinavian Audiology, 22*, 87–95.

Johnsen, N. J., Bagi, P., & Elberling, C. (1983). Evoked acoustic emissions from the human ear. III. Findings in neonates. *Scandinavian Audiology, 12*, 17–24.

Johnsen, N. J., & Elberling, C. (1982). Evoked acoustic emissions from the human ear. II. Normative data in young adults and influence of posture. *Scandinavian Audiology, 11*, 68–77.

Johnsen, N. J., & Elberling, C. (1982). Evoked acoustic emissions from the human ear: I. Equipment and response parameters. *Scandinavian Audiology, 11*, 3–12.

Johnson, E. (1965). Auditory test results in 110 surgically confirmed retrocochlear lesions. *Journal of Speech and Hearing Disorders, 30*, 307–317.

Johnstone, B. M., Patuzzi, R., & Yates, G. K. (1986). Basilar membrane measurements and the travelling wave. *Hearing Research, 22*, 147–153.

Johnstone, B. M., & Sellick, P. M. (1972). The peripheral auditory apparatus. *Quarterly Review in Biophysics, 5*, 1-57.

Joint Committee on Infant Hearing. (1982, November) .1982 position statement. *Ear & Hearing, 4*, 3–4.

Joint Committee on Infant Hearing. (1994). 1994 position statement. *Audiology Today, 6*(6), 6–9.

Jones, A. T. (1935). The discovery of difference tones. *American Physics Teacher, 3*, 49–51.

Jones, K., Tubis, A., Long, G. R., Burns, E. M., & Strickland, E. A. (1986). Interactions among multiple spontaneous otoacoustic emissions. In J. B. Allen, J. L. Hall, A. Hubbard, S. T. Neely, & A. Tubis (Eds.), *Peripheral auditory mechanisms* (pp. 266–273). Berlin: Springer-Verlag.

Kaga, K., Kitazumi, E., & Kodama, K. (1979). Auditory brainstem responses of kernicterus infants. *International Journal of Pediatric Otorhinolaryngology, 1*, 255–264.

Kaga, K., Nakamura, M., Shinogami, M., Tsuzuku, T., Yamdad, B., & Shindo, M. (1996). Auditory nerve disease of both ears revealed by auditory brainstem responses, electrocochleography, and otoacoustic emissions. *Scandinavian Audiology, 25*, 233–238.

Kakigi, A., Hirakawa, H., Harel, N., Mount, R. J., & Harrison, R. V. (1998a). Basal cochlear lesions result in increased amplitude of otoacoustic emissions. *Audiology & Neuro-Otology, 3*, 361–372.

Kakigi, A., Hirakawa, H., Harel, N., Mount, R. J., & Harrison, R. V. (1998b). Comparison of distortion-product and transient evoked otoacoustic emissions with ABR threshold shift in chinchillas with ototoxic damage. *Auris Nasus Larynx, 25*(3), 223–232.

Kalinec, F., & Kachar, B. (1993). Inhibition of outer hair cell electromotility by sulfhydryl specific reagents. *Neuroscience Letters, 157*, 231–234.

Kaltenbach, J. A., Church, M. W., Blakley, B. W., McCaslin, D. L., & Burgio, D. L. (1997). Comparison of five agents in protecting the cochlea against the ototoxic effects of cisplatin in the hamster. *Otolaryngology—Head and Neck Surgery, 117*, 493–500.

Kanne, T. J., Schaefer, L., & Perkins, J. A. (1999). Potential pitfalls of initiating a newborn hearing screening program. *Archives of Otolaryngology—Head and Neck Surgery, 125*, 28–32.

Kapadia, S., & Lutman, M. E. (1997). Are normal hearing thresholds a sufficient condition for click-evoked otoacoustic emissions? *Journal of the Acoustical Society of America, 101*, 3566–.

Karlsson, K. K., Berninger, E., & Alvan, G. (1991). The effect of quinine on psychoacoustic tuning curves, stapedius reflexes and evoked otoacoustic emissions in healthy volunteers. *Scandinavian Audiology, 20*, 83–90.

Karlsson, K. K., Berninger, E., Gustafsson, L. L., & Alvan, G. (1995). Pronounced quinine-induced cochlear hearing loss. Mechanistic study in one volunteer at multiple stable plasma concentrations. *Journal of Audiological Medicine, 4*, 12–24.

Karlsson, K. K., & Flock, A. (1990). Quinine causes isolated outer hair cells to change length. *Neuroscience Letters, 116*, 101–105.

Karzon, R. K., Garcia, P., Peterein, J. L., & Gates, G. A. (1994). Distortion product otoacoustic emissions in the elderly. *American Journal of Audiology, 5*, 596–605.

Katona, G., Buki, B., Farkas, Z., Pytel, J., Simon-Nagy, E., & Hirschberg, J. (1993). Transitory evoked otoacoustic emissions in a child with profound hearing loss. *International Journal of Pediatric Otorhinolaryngology, 26*, 263–267.

Katona, G., & Czinner, A. (1999). Objective audiologic assessment of children treated with amikacin. *Orv Hetil, 140*, 1305–1307.

Kawase, T., & Liberman, M. C. (1993). Antimasking effects of the olivocochlear reflex. I. Enhancement of compound action potentials to masked tones. *Journal of Neurophysiology, 70*, 2519–2532.

Keefe, D. H., & Levi, E. (1996). Maturation of the middle and external ears: Acoustic power-based responses and reflectance tympanometry. *Ear & Hearing, 17*, 361–373.

Keefe, D. H., Ling, R., & Bulen, J. C. (1992). Method to measure acoustic impedance and reflection coefficient. *Journal of the Acoustical Society of America, 91*, 470–485.

Kei, J., McPherson, B., Smyth, V., Latham, S., & Loscher, J. (1997). Transient evoked otoacoustic emissions in infants: Effects of gender, ear asymmetry, and activity status. *Audiology, 36*, 61–71.

Keith, R. W. (1975). Middle ear function in neonates. *Archives of Otolaryngology, 101*, 376–379.

Kemp, D. T. (1978). Stimulated acoustic emissions from within the human auditory system. *Journal of the Acoustical Society of America, 64*, 1386–1391.

Kemp, D. T. (1979a). Evidence for a new element in cochlear mechanics. *Scandinavian Audiology,* Suppl. 9, 35–47.

Kemp, D. T. (1979b). Evidence of mechanical nonlinearity and frequency selective wave amplification in the cochlea. *Archives of Otorhinolaryngology, 224,* 37–45.

Kemp, D. T. (1979c). The evoked cochlear mechanical response of the auditory microstructure in models of the auditory system and related signal processing techniques. *Scandinavian Audiology, 9,* 35–47.

Kemp, D. T. (1980). Towards a model for the origin of cochlear echoes. *Hearing Research, 2,* 533–548.

Kemp, D. T. (1986). Otoacoustic emissions, travelling waves, and cochlear mechanisms. *Hearing Research, 22,* 95–113.

Kemp, D. T. (1988). Developments in cochlear mechanics and techniques for noninvasive evaluation. *Advances in Audiology, 5,* 27-45.

Kemp, D. T. (1990). A guide to the effective use of otoacoustic emissions. *Ear & Hearing, 11*(2), 93–105.

Kemp, D. T., Bray, P., Alexander, L., & Brown, A. M. (1986). Acoustic emission cochleography—practical aspects. *Scandinavian Audiology,* Suppl. 25, 71–94.

Kemp, D. T., & Brown, A. M. (1984). Ear canal acoustic and round window electrical correlates of 2f1–f2 distortion generated in the cochlea. *Hearing Research, 13,* 39–46.

Kemp, D. T., & Chum, R. A. (1980). Properties of the generator of stimulated acoustic emissions. *Hearing Research, 2,* 213–232.

Kemp, D. T., & Martin, J. A. (1976). Active resonant systems in audition. *13th International Congress of Audiology,* 64–65.

Kemp, D. T., & Ryan, S. (1991). Otoacoustic emission tests in neonatal screening programmes. *Acta Otolaryngologica (Stockholm),* Suppl. 482, 73–84.

Kemp, D. T., Ryan, S., & Bray, P. (1990). A guide to the effective use of otoacoustic emissions. *Ear & Hearing, 11,* 93-105.

Kennedy, C., Kimm, L., Cafarelli Dees, D., Evans, P., Hunter, M., Lenton, S., & Thornton, R. (1991). Otoacoustic emissions and auditory brainstem responses in the newborn. *Archives of Diseases in Childhood, 66,* 1124–1129.

Kettembeil, S., Manley, G. A., & Siegl, E. (1995). Distortion-product otoacoustic emissions and their anesthesia sensitivity in European starling and the chicken. *Hearing Research, 86,* 47–62.

Kevanishvili, Z., Gobsch, H., Gvelesiani, T., & Gamgebeli, Z. (1992). Evoked otoacoustic emission behavior under forward masking paradigm. *Otorhinolaryngology, 54,* 229–234.

Khalfa, S., & Collet, L. (1996). Functional asymmetry of medial olivocochlear system in humans: Towards a peripheral auditory lateralization. *Neuroreport, 7,* 993–996.

Khalfa, S., Morlet, T., Micheyl, C., Morgon, A., & Collet, L. (1997). Evidence for peripheral hearing asymmetry in humans: Clinical implications. *Acta Otolaryngologica, 117,* 192–196.

Khalfa, S., Veuillet, E., & Collet, L. (1998). Infuence of handedness on peripheral auditory asymmetry. *European Journal of Neuroscience, 10*(8), 2731–2737.

Khanna, S. M., & Leonard, D. G. B. (1982). Basilar membrane tuning in the cat cochlea. *Science, 215,* 305–306.

Khvoles, R., Freeman, S., & Sohmer, H. (1998). Effect of temperature on the transient and distortion product otoacoustic emissions in rats. *Audiology and Neuro-Otology, 3,* 349–360.

Kileny, P. R., Connelly, C., & Robertson, C. M. T. (1980). Auditory brainstem responses in perinatal asphyxia. *International Journal of Pediatric Otorhinolaryngology, 2,* 147–159.

Kileny, P. R., Edwards, B. M., Disher, M. J., & Telian, S. A. (1998). Hearing improvement after resection of cerebellopontine angle meningioma: Case study of the preoperative role of transient evoked otoacoustic emissions. *Journal of the American Academy of Audiology, 9,* 251–256.

Kileny, P. R., & Robertson, C. M. T. (1985). Neurological aspects of infant hearing assessment. *Journal of Otolaryngology, 14,* 34–39.

Kim, D., Paparello, J., Jung, M., Smurzynski, J., & Sun, X. (1996). Distortion product otoacoustic emission test of sensorineural hearing loss: Performance regarding sensitivity, specificity, and receiver operating characteristics. *Acta Otolaryngologica (Stockholm), 116,* 3–11.

Kim, D. O. (1980). Cochlear mechanics: Implications of electrophysiological and acoustical observations. *Hearing Research, 2,* 297–317.

Kim, D. O. (1986). Active and nonlinear cochlear biomechanics and the role of the outer-hair-cell subsystem in the mammalian auditory system. *Hearing Research, 22,* 105–114.

Kim, D. O., Leonard, G., Smurzynski, J., & Jung, M. D. (1992). Otoacoustic emissions and noise-induced hearing loss: Hearing studies. In A. L. Dancer, D. Henderson, R. J. Salvi, & R. P. Hamernik (Eds.), *Noise-induced hearing loss* (pp. 98-105). St. Louis, MO: Mosby Year Book Press.

Kim, D. O., Molnar, C. E., & Matthews, J. W. (1979). Cochlear mechanics: physiologically vulnerable nonlinear behavior as reflected in ear-canal pressure and cochlear-nerve-fiber responses. *Journal of the Acoustical Society of America, 65,* S28.

Kim, D. O., Molnar, C. E., & Matthews, J. W. (1980). Cochlear mechanics: Nonlinear behavior in two-tone responses as reflected in cochlear-nerve-fiber responses and in ear-canal sound pressure. *Journal of the Acoustical Society of America, 67,* 1704–1721.

Kim, D. O., Siegel, J., & Molnar, C. E. (1979). Cochlear non-linear phenomena in two-tone responses. *Scandinavian Audiology,* (Suppl. 9), 63–81.

Kim, D. O., Sun, X.-M., Jung, M. D., & Leonard, G. (1997). A new method of measuring distortion product otoacoustic emissions using multiple tone pairs: Study of human adults. *Ear & Hearing, 18,* 277–285.

Kimberley, B. P., Brown, D. K., & Eggermont, J. J. (1993). Measuring human cochlear traveling wave delay using distortion product emissions phase responses. *Journal of the Acoustical Society of America, 94,* 1343–1350.

Kimberley, B. P., Hernadi, I., Lee, A. M., & Brown, D. K. (1994). Predicting pure tone thresholds in normal and hearing-impaired ears with distortion product emission and age. *Ear & Hearing, 15,* 199–209.

Kimberley, B. P., Kimberley, B. M., & Roth, L. (1994). A neural network approach to the prediction of pure tone thresholds with distortion product emissions. *ENT Journal, 73*(11), 812–823.

Kimberley, B. P., & Nelson, D. A. (1989). Distortion product emissions and sensorineural hearing loss. *Journal of Otolaryngology, 18,* 365-369.

Kimura, R., & Wersall, J. (1962). Termination of the olivocochlear bundle in relation to the outer hair cells of the organ of Corti in guinea pig. *Acta Otolaryngologica (Stockholm), 55,* 11–32.

Kirk, D. L., & Johnstone, B. M. (1993). Modulation of f2–f1: Evidence for a GABA-ergic efferent system in apical cochlea of the guinea pig. *Hearing Research, 67,* 20–34.

Kirk, D. L., & Yates, G. K. (1998). 4-aminopyridine in scala media reversibly alters the cochlear potentials and suppresses electrically evoked otoacoustic emissions. *Audiology and Neuro-Otology, 3,* 21–39.

Kochs, E. (1995). Electrophysiological monitoring and mild hypothermia. *Journal of Neurosurgery and Anesthesiology, 7,* 222–228.

Koike, K. J., & Wetmore, S. J. (1999). Interactive effects of the middle ear pathology and the associated hearing loss on transient-evoked otoacoustic emission measures. *Otolaryngology—Head and Neck Surgery, 121,* 238–244.

Kok, M. R., van Zanten, G. A., & Brocaar, M. P. (1992). Growth of evoked otoacoustic emissions during the first days postpartum. *Audiology, 31,* 140–149.

Kok, M., van Zanten, G., & Brocaar, M. (1993). Aspects of spontaneous otoacoustic emissions in healthy newborns. *Hearing Research, 69,* 115–123.

Kok, M., van Zanten, G., Brocaar, M., & Jongejan, H. (1994). Click-evoked oto-acoustic emissions in very-low-birth-weight infants: A cross-sectional data analysis. *Audiology, 33,* 152–164.

Kok, M., van Zanten, G., Brocaar, M., & Wallenburg, H. (1993). Click-evoked oto-acoustic emissions in 1036 ears of healthy newborns. *Audiology, 32,* 213–224.

Kok, R. (1994). *Oto-acoustic emissions in healthy newborns and very-low-birth-weight infants.* Rotterdam, The Netherlands: Erasmus.

Kokesh, J., Norton, S., & Duckert, L. (1994). Effect of perilymphatic fistulas on evoked otoacoustic emissions in the guinea pig. *American Journal of Otology, 15*(4), 466–473.

Konishi, T., Salt, A. N., & Hamrick, P. E. (1981). Effects of hyperthermia on ionic movement in the guinea pig cochlea. *Hearing Research, 4,* 265–278.

Konradsson, K. (1996). Bilaterally preserved otoacoustic emissions in four children with profound idiopathic unilateral sensorineural hearing loss. *Audiology, 35,* 217–227.

Kopke, R. D., Liu, W., Gabaizadeh, R., Jacono, A., Feghali, J., Spray, D., Garcia, P., Steinman, H., Malgrange, B., Ruben, R. J., Rybak, L., & Van de Water, T. R. (1997). Use of organotypic cultures of Corti's organ to study the protective effects of antioxidant molecules on cisplatin-induced damage of auditory hair cells. *American Journal of Otology, 18,* 559–571.

Koppl, C., & Manley, G. (1993). Distortion-product otoacoustic emissions in the bobtail lizard. II. Suppression tuning characteristics. *Journal of the Acoustical Society of America, 93,* 2834–2843.

Kraus, N., Ozdamar, O., Stein, L., & Reed, N. (1984). Absent auditory brainstem response: Peripheral hearing loss or brain stem dysfunction. *Laryngoscope, 94,* 400–406.

Krishnan, G., & Chertoff, M. E. (1999). Insights into linear and nonlinear cochlear transduction: Application of a new system-identification procedure on transient-evoked otoacoustic emissions data. *Journal of the Acoustical Society of America, 105,* 770–781.

Kruger, B. (1987). An update on the external ear canal resonance in infants and young children. *Ear & Hearing, 8,* 333–336.

Kruger, B., & Ruben, R. J. (1987). The acoustic properties of the infant ear. *Acta Otolaryngolgica, 103,* 578–585.

Kruglov, A.V., Artamasov, S. V., Frolenkov, G. I., & Tavartkiladze, G. A. (1997). Transient evoked otoacoustic emission with unexpectedly short latency. *Scandinavian Audiology, 117,* 234–255.

Krumholtz, A., Felix, J. K., Goldstein, P. J., & McKenzie, E. (1985). Maturation of the brain stem auditory evoked potential in premature infants. *Electroencephalograpy and Clinical Neurophysiology, 62,* 124–134.

Kujawa, S. G., Fallon, M., & Bobbin, R. P. (1992). Intracochlear salicylate reduces low-intensity acoustic and cochlear microphonic distortion products. *Hearing Research, 64,* 73–80.

Kujawa, S. G., Glattke, T. J., Fallon, M., & Bobbin, R. P. (1992). Intracochlear application of acetylcholine alters sound-induced mechanical events within the cochlear partition. *Hearing Research, 61,* 106–116.

Kukawa, S. G., Glattke, T. J., Fallon, M., & Bobbin, R. P. (1993). Contralateral sound suppresses distortion product otoacoustic emissions through cholinergic mechanisms. *Hearing Research, 68,* 97–106.

Kujawa, S. G., Glattke, T. J., Fallon, M., & Bobbin, R. P. (1994). A nicotinic-like receptor mediates suppression of distortion product otoacoustic emissions by contralateral sound. *Hearing Research, 74,* 122–134.

Kulawiec, J. T., & Orlando, M. S. (1995). The contribution of spontaneous otoacoustic emissions to the click evoked otoacoustic emissions. *Ear & Hearing, 16,* 515–520.

Kumagai, S. (1995). Distortion-product otoacoustic emissions in kanamycin treated guinea pig cochlea. *Nippon Jibiinkoko Gakkai Kaiho, 98,* 368–379.

Kummer, P., Janssen, T., & Arnold, W. (1995). Suppression tuning characteristics of the 2f1–f2 distortion product otoacoustic emission in humans. *Journal of the Acoustical Society of America, 98,* 197–210.

Kumpf, W., & Hoke, M. (1970). Ein konstantes Ohrgerausch bei 4000 Hz. *Archives Klinikum Experimental Ohren-Nasen-Kehlkopfheikd, 196,* 243–247.

Kusakari, J., Ise, I., Comegys, T. H., Thalmann, T., & Thalmann, R. (1978). Effect of ethacrynic acid, furosemide, and ouabain upon the endolymphatic potential and upon high energy phosphates of the stria vascularis. *Laryngoscope, 88,* 12–37.

Kusuki, M., Sakashita, T., Kubo, T., Kyunai, K., Ueno, K., Hikawa, C., Wada, T., & Nakai, Y. (1998). Changes in distortion product otoacoustic emissions from ears with Meniere's disease. *Acta Otolaryngologica (Stockholm), 538,* 78–89.

Laccourreye, L., Francois, M., Tran Ba Huy, E., & Narcy, P. (1996). Bilateral evoked emissions in a child with profound hearing loss. *Annals of Otology, Rhinology, and Laryngology, 105,* 286–288.

Lafreniere, D., Jung, M., Smurzynski, J., Leonard, G., Kim, D., & Sasek, J. (1991). Distortion-product and click-evoked otoacoustic emissions in healthy newborns. *Archives of Otolaryngology—Head and Neck Surgery, 117,* 1382–1389.

Lamprecht, A. (1991). Click-evoked oto-acoustic emissions in normal and hearing-impaired adults and children (in German). *Laryngo-Rhino-Otologogy, 70,* 1–4.

Lamprecht-Dinnesin, A., Pohl, M., Hartmann, S., Heinecke, A., Ahrens, S., Muller, E., & Riebandt, M. (1998). Effects of age, gender, and ear side on SOAE parameters in infancy and childhood. *Audiology and Neuro Otology, 3,* 386–401.

Lasky, R., Perlman, J., & Hecox, K. (1993). Distortion-product otoacoustic emissions in human newborns and adults. *Ear & Hearing, 13,* 430–441.

Lasky, R. E. (1998a). Distortion product otoacoustic emissions in human newborns and adults. I. Frequency effects. *Journal of the Acoustical Society of America, 103,* 981–991.

Lasky, R. E. (1998b). Distortion product otoacoustic emissions in human newborns and adults. II. Level effects. *Journal of the Acoustical Society of America, 103,* 992–1000.

Laurikainen, E. A., Johansson, R. K., & Kileny, P. R. (1996). Effects of intratympanically delivered lidocaine on the auditory system of humans. *Ear & Hearing, 17,* 49–54.

Laurikainen, E. A., Kim, D., Didier, A., Ren, T., Miller, J. M., Quirk, W. S., & Nutall, A. L. (1993). Stellate ganglion drives sympathetic regulation of cochlear blood flow. *Hearing Research, 64,* 199–204.

Lavigne-Rebillard, M., & Pujol, R. (1986). Development of the auditory hair cell surface in human fetuses: A scanning electron microscopy study. *Anatomic Embryology, 174,* 369–377.

Lavigne-Rebillard, M., & Pujol, R. (1988). Hair cell innervation in the fetal human cochlea. *Acta Otolaryngologica (Stockholm), 105,* 398–402.

Lavigne-Rebillard, M., & Pujol, R. (1990). Auditory hair-cells in human fetuses: Synaptogenesis and ciliogenesis. *Journal of Electron Microscopy Technique, 15,* 115–122.

Leake, P. A., Kuntz, A. L., Moore, C. M., & Chambers, P. L. (1997). Cochlear pathology induced by aminoglycoside ototoxicity during postnatal maturation in cats. *Hearing Research, 113,* 117–132.

LeCates, W. W., Kuo, S. C., & Brownell, W. E. (1995). Temperature dependent length changes of the outer hair cell. *Association for Research in Otolaryngology, 18*, 156.

Lecusay, R. A., Fletcher, C. A., Lonsbury-Martin, B. L., Stagner, B. B., Waxman, G. M., & Martin, G. K. (1996). Otoacoustic emissions in normal-hearing humans: Musicians vs. non-musicians. *Association for Research in Otolaryngology, 19*, 25.

Lee, J., & Kim, J. (1999). The maximum permissable ambient noise and frequency-specific averaging time on the measurement of distortion product otoacoustic emissions. *Audiology, 38*, 19–23.

Lenhardt, M. L., McArtor, R., & Bryant, B. (1984). Effects of neonatal hyperbilirubinemia on the brainstem electric response. *Journal of Pediatrics, 104*, 281–284.

Lenneberg, E. H. (1967). *Biological foundations of language.* New York: John Wiley & Sons.

Lenoir, M., & Puel, J.-L. (1987). Development of 2f1–f2 otoacoustic emissions in the rat. *Hearing Research, 29*, 265–271.

LePage, E., & Johnstone, B. (1980). Nonlinear mechanical behavior of the basilar membrane in the basal turn of the guinea pig cochlea. *Hearing Research, 2*, 183–189.

Lerner, S. A., & Matz, G. J. (1979). Suggestions for monitoring patients during treatment with aminoglycoside antibiotics. *Otolaryngology—Head and Neck Surgery, 87*, 222-228.

LePage, E. L. (1989). Functional role of the olivocochlear bundle: A motor unit control system in the mammalian cochlea. *Hearing Research, 38*, 177–198.

LePage, E. L., & Murray, N. M. (1998). Latent cochlear damage in personal stereo users: A study based on click-evoked otoacoustic emissions. *Medical Journal of Australia, 169*, 588–592.

Lerner, S. A., & Matz, G. J. (1979). Suggestions for monitoring patients during treatment with aminoglycoside antibiotics. *Otolaryngology—Head and Neck Surgery, 87*, 222–228.

Levi, G., Sohmer, H., & Kapitulnik, J. (1981). Auditory nerve and brain stem responses in homozygous jaundiced Gunn rats. *Archives of Otolaryngology, 232*, 139–143.

Levi, H., Adelman, C., Geal-Dor, M., Elidan, J., Eliashar, R., Sichel, J.-Y., Bar-Oz, B., Weinstein, D., Freeman, S., & Sohmer, H. (1997). Transient evoked otoacoustic emissions in newborns in the first 48 hours after birth. *Audiology, 36*, 181–186.

Liberman, M. C. (1980). Efferent synapses in the inner hair cell area of the cat cochlea: An electron-microscopic study of serial sections. *Hearing Research, 3*, 189–204.

Liberman, M. C. (1988). Response properties of cochlear efferent neurons: monoaural versus binaural stimulation and the effects of noise. *Journal of Neurophysiology, 60*, 1799–1798.

Liberman, M. C. (1989). Rapid assessment of sound-evoked olivocochlear feedback: Suppression of compound action potential by contralateral sound. *Hearing Research, 38*, 1779–1798.

Liberman, M. C., & Brown, M. C. (1986). Physiology and anatomy of single olivocochlear neurons in the cat. *Hearing Research, 24*, 17–36.

Lichtenstein, V., & Stapells, D. R. (1996). Frequency-specific identification of hearing loss using transient-evoked otoacoustic emissions to clicks and tones. *Hearing Research, 98*, 125–136.

Lina-Granade, G., & Collet, L. (1995). Effect of interstimulus interval on evoked otoacoustic emissions. *Hearing Research, 87*, 55–61.

Lina Granade, G., Collet, L., & Morgon, A. (1994). Auditory-evoked brainstem responses elicited by Maximum Length Sequences in normal and sensorineural ears. *Audiology, 33*, 218–236.

Lina-Granade, G., Liogier, X., & Collet, L. (1997). Contralateral suppression and stimulus rate effects on evoked otoacoustic emissions. *Hearing Research, 197*, 83–92.

Lind, O. (1994). Contralateral suppression of TEOAE. Attempts to find a latency. *British Journal of Audiology, 28*, 219–225.

Lind, O. (1995). Transient-evoked otoacoustic emissions and contralateral suppression in patients with unilateral tinnitus. *Scandinavian Audiology, 25*, 167–172.

Lind, O. (1998). A clinical study on the growth of distortion product otoacoustic emissions and hearing loss at 2 KHz in humans. *Scandinavian Audiology, 27*, 207–212.

Littman, T. A., Cullen, J. K., Jr., & Bobbin, R. P. (1992). The effect of olivocochlear bundle transection on tuning curves and acoustic distortion products. *Journal of the Acoustical Society of America, 92*, 1945–1952.

Littman, T. A., Magruder, A., & Strother, D. R. (1998). Monitoring and predicting ototoxic damage using distortion-product otoacoustic emissions: A pediatric case study. *Journal of the American Academy of Audiology, 9*, 257–262.

Liu, B., Liu, C., & Song, B. (1996). Otoacoustic emissions and tinnitus. *Chung Hua Erh Pi Yen Hou Yo Tsa Chih, 31*, 231–233.

Liu, X. Z., & Newton, V. (1997). Distortion product emissions in normal-hearing and low-frequency hearing loss carriers of gene for Waardenburg's syndrome. *Annals of Otology, Rhinology, and Laryngology, 106,* 220–225.

Long, G. R. (1984). The microstructure of quiet and masked thresholds. *Hearing Research, 15,* 73–87.

Long, G. R., & Tubis, A. (1988). Modification of spontaneous and evoked otoacoustic emissions and associated psychoacoustic microstructure by aspirin consumption. *Journal of the Acoustical Society of America, 84,* 1343–1353.

Long, G. R., Tubis, A., & Jones, K. (1986). Synchronization of spontaneous otoacoustic emissions and driven limit cycle oscillators. *Journal of the Acoustical Society of America, 81,* S120.

Long, G. R., Tubis, A., & Jones, K. (1991). Modeling synchronization and suppression of spontaneous otoacoustic emissions using Van der Pol oscillators: Effects of aspirin administration. *Journal of the Acoustical Society of America, 89,* 1201-1212.

Lonsbury-Martin, B. (1994). Introduction to otoacoustic emissions. *American Journal of Otology, 15*(Suppl. 1), 1–12.

Lonsbury-Martin, B., Cutler, W., & Martin, G. (1991). Evidence for the influence of aging on distortion-product otoacoustic emissions in humans. *Journal of the Acoustical Society of America, 89,* 1749–1759.

Lonsbury-Martin, B., McCoy, M., Whitehead, M., & Martin, G. (1993). Clinical testing of distortion-product otoacoustic emissions. *Ear & Hearing, 1,* 11–22.

Lonsbury-Martin, B., Whitehead, M. L., Henley, C. M., & Martin, G. K. (1991). Differential effects of sodium salicylate on the distinct classes of otoacoustic emissions. [Abstract]. *Association for Research in Otolaryngology, 14,* 67.

Lonsbury-Martin, B. L., Harris, F. P., Stagner, B. B., Hawkins, M. D., & Martin, G. K. (1990). Distortion product emissions in humans. I. Basic properties in normally hearing subjects. *Annals of Otology, Rhinology, and Laryngology,* Suppl. 99, 3–14.

Lonsbury-Martin, B. L., Harris, F. P., Stagner, B., Hawkins, M. D., & Martin, G. K. (1990). Distortion-product emissions in humans: II. Relations to acoustic immittance and stimulus-frequency and spontaneous otoacoustic emissions in normally hearing subjects. *Annals of Otology, Rhinology, and Laryngology,* Suppl. 147, 15–29.

Lonsbury-Martin, B. L., & Martin, G. K. (1990). The clinical utility of distortion-product otoacoustic emissions. *Ear & Hearing, 11*(2), 144–154.

Lonsbury-Martin, B. L., Martin, G. K., McCoy, M. J., & Whitehead, M. L. (1994). Otoacoustic emission testing in young children: Middle ear influences. *American Journal of Otology, 15,* 13–20.

Lonsbury-Martin, B. L., Martin, G. K., Probst, R., & Coats, A. C. (1988). Spontaneous otoacoustic emissions in a nonhuman primate: II. Cochlear anatomy. *Hearing Research, 33,* 69–94.

Lonsbury-Martin, B. L., Whitehead, M. L., & Martin, G. K. (1991). Clinical applications of otoacoustic emissions. *Journal of Speech and Hearing Research, 34,* 964-981.

Low, R., Brown, A. N., & Sheppard, S. L. (1995). Delay in the development of neural responses in a human infant with normal cochlear responses. *British Journal of Audiology, 29,* 31.

Lucertini, M., Bergamaschi, A., & Urbani, L. (1996). Transient evoked otoacoustic emissions in occupational medicine as an auditory screening test for employment. *British Journal of Audiology, 30,* 79–88.

Lucertini, M., Tufarelli, D., & Urbani, L. (1998). Influence of a 6–8 kHz audiometric notch on transient evoked otoacoustic emissions. *European Archives of Otorhinolaryngology, 208.*

Luterman, D., & Chasin, J. (1970). The pediatrician and the parent of the deaf child. *Pediatrics, 45,* 115–116.

Lutman, M. E. (1989). Evoked otoacoustic emissions in adults: Implications for screening. *Audiology in Practice, 6*(3), 6–8.

Lutman, M. E. (1993). Reliable identification of click-evoked otoacoustic emissions using signal-processing techniques. *British Journal of Audiology, 27,* 102–108.

Lutman, M. E., Mason, S. M., Sheppard, S., & Gibbin, K. P. (1989). Differential diagnostic potential of otoacoustic emissions: A case study. *Audiology, 28,* 205–210.

Lutman, M. E. et al. (1994). The distribution of hearing threshold levels in the general population aged 18-30 years. *Audiology, 33,* 327-350.

Maat, B., van Dijk, P., & Wit, H. P. (1994). Noise evoked otoacoustic emissions: Just another way of measuring? In F. Grandori (Ed.), *Advances in otoacoustic emissions: Fundamentals and clinical applications* (Vol. II, pp. 21–31). Milan: Stefanoni Lecco.

Macdonald, M. R., Harrison, R. V., Wake, M., Bliss, B., & Macdonald, R. E. (1994). Ototoxicity of carboplatin: Comparing animal and clinical models at the Hospital for Sick Children. *Journal of Otolaryngology, 23,* 151–159.

Macrae, J. H. (1972). Effects of body position on the auditory system. *Journal of Speech and Hearing Research, 15,* 330–339.

Madeira da Silva, J. F. H., Reis, J. L., & Penha, R. (1994). Distortion product otoacoustic emissions: a latency study. In F. Grandori (Ed.), *Advances in otoacoustic emissions. I. Fundamentals and clinical applications* (pp. 48–64). Milan: Stefanoni Lecco.

Magnuson, M., & Hergils, L. (1999). The parents' view on hearing screening in newborns. Feelings, thoughts and opinions on otoacoustic emissions. *Scandinavian Audiology, 28*(1), 47–56.

Maison, S., Micheyl, C., Chays, A., & Collet, L. (1997). Medial olivocochlear system stabilizes active cochlear micromechanical properties. *Hearing Research, 113*, 89–98.

Maison, S., Micheyl, C., & Collet, L. (1997). Medial olivocochlear efferent system in humans studied with amplitude-modulated tones. *Journal of Neurophysiology, 77*, 1759–1768.

Maison, S., Micheyl, C., & Collet, L. (1998). Contralateral frequency-modulated tones suppress transient-evoked otoacoustic emissions in humans. *Hearing Research, 117*, 114–118.

Maison, S., Micheyl, C., & Collet, L. (1999). Sinusoidal amplitude modulation alters contralateral noise suppression of evoked otoacoustic emissions in humans. *Neuroscience, 91*, 133–138.

Manley, G. A., & Koppel, C. (1994). Spontaneous otoacoustic emissions in the bobtail lizard. III. Temperature effects. *Hearing Research, 72*, 171–180.

Margolis, R. H., & Trine, M. B. (1997). Influence of middle-ear disease on otoacoustic emissions. In M. S. Robinette & T. J. Glattke (Eds.), *Otoacoustic emissions: Clinical applications* (pp. 130–150). New York: Thieme.

Marshall, L., & Heller, L. (1996). Reliability of transient-evoked otoacoustic emissions. *Ear & Hearing, 17*, 237–254.

Marshall, L., & Heller, L. M. (1998). Transient-evoked otoacoustic emissions as a measure of noise-induced threshold shift. *Journal of Speech Language Hearing Research, 41*, 1319–1334.

Marshall, L., Heller, L. M., & Westhusin, L. J. (1997). Effect of negative middle-ear pressure on transient-evoked otoacoustic emissions. *Ear & Hearing, 18*, 218–226.

Marshall, R. E., Reichert, T. J., Kerley, S. M., & Davis, H. (1980). Auditory function in newborn intensive care unit patients revealed by auditory brainstem potentials. *Journal of Pediatrics, 96*, 731–735.

Martin, G. K., Jassir, D., Stagner, B. B., & Lonsbury-Martin, B. L. (1998). Effects of loop diuretics on the suppression tuning of distortion-product otoacoustic emissions in rabbits. *Journal of the Acoustical Society of America, 104*, 972–983.

Martin, G. K., Lonsbury-Martin, B. L., Probst, R., Sheinin, S. A., & Coats, A. C. (1987). Acoustic distortion products in rabbits. II. Sites of origin revealed by suppression contours and pure-tone exposures. *Hearing Research, 28*, 191–208.

Martin, G. K., Ohlms, L. A., Franklin, D. J., Harris, F. P., & Lonsbury-Martin, B. L. (1990). Distortion-product emissions in humans. III. Influence of sensorineural hearing loss. *Annals of Otology, Rhinology, and Laryngology, 99*(Suppl. 147), 30–42.

Martinez Ibarguen, A., Santaolalla Montoya, F., & Sanchez Del Rey, A. (1995). Normality parameters of the spontaneous otoacoustic emissions. *Acta Otorinolaringologica Espanol, 46*, 175–181.

Mason, J. A., & Herrmann, K. R. (1998). Universal infant hearing screening by automated auditory brainstem response measurement. *Pediatrics, 101*, 221–228.

Mathis, A., Probst, R., DeMin, N., & Hauser, R. (1991). A child with unusually high level spontaneous otoacoustic emission. *Archives of Otolaryngology—Head and Neck Surgery, 117*, 674–676.

Matkin, N. D., & Carhart, R. (1966). Auditory profiles associated with Rh incompatibility. *Archives of Otolaryngology, 64*, 502–513.

Matthews, J. W. (1983). Modeling reverse middle ear transmission of acoustic distortion products. In J. B. Allen, J. L. Hall, A. Hubbard, S. T. Neely, & A. Tubis (Eds.), *Peripheral auditory mechanisms* (pp. 258–265). New York: Springer-Verlag.

Matthews, J. W., Kim, D. O., Molnar, C. E., & Neely, S. T. (1981). Modeling reverse middle ear transmission: Aural acoustic distortion products, "echoes," and spontaneous emissions. *Journal of the Acoustical Society of America, 69*, 43.

Mauermann, M., Uppenkamp, S., & Kollmeier, B. (1998). DPOAE fine structure for different shapes of cochlear hearing loss-evidence for the distortion product frequency place as a source of DPOAE fine structure. *Association for Research in Otolaryngology, 21*.

Mauk, G., White, K., Mortensen, L., & Behrens, T. (1991). The effectiveness of screening programs based on high-risk characteristics in early identification of hearing impairment. *Ear & Hearing, 12*, 312–319.

Maurer, J., Beck, A., Mann, V., & Mintert, R. (1992). Changes in otoacoustic emissions with simultaneous acoustic stimulation of the contralateral ear in normal probands and patients with unilateral acoustic neurinoma. *Laryngorhinootologie, 71*, 69–73.

Maxon, A., White, K., Behrens, T., & Vohr, B. (1995). Referral rates and cost efficiency in a universal newborn hearing screening program using transient evoked otoacoustic emissions. *Journal of the American Academy of Audiology, 6*, 271–277.

Maxon, A. B., White, K. R., Vohr, B. R., & Behrens, T. R. (1993). Using transient evoked otoacoustic emissions for neonatal hearing screening. *British Journal of Audiology, 27*, 149–153.

May, B. J., & McQuone, S. J. (1995). Effects of bilateral olivocochlear lesions on pure-tone intensity discrimination in noise. *Auditory Neuroscience, 1*, 385–400.

McAlpine, D., & Johnstone, B. (1990). The ototoxic mechanism of cisplatinum. *Hearing Research, 47*, 191–204.

McFadden, D. (1993). A speculation about the parallel ear asymmetries and sex differences in hearing sensitivity and otoacoustic emissions. *Hearing Research, 68*, 143–151.

McFadden, D. (1998). Sex differences in the auditory system. *Developmental Neuropsychology, 14*(2/3), 261–298.

McFadden, D., & Loehlin, J. C. (1995). On the heritability of spontaneous otoacoustic emissions: A twins study. *Hearing Research, 85*, 181–198.

McFadden, D., Loehlin, J. C., & Pasanen, E. G. (1996). Additional findings on heritability and prenatal masculinization of cochlear mechanisms: Click-evoked otoacoustic emissions. *Hearing Research, 97*, 102–119.

McFadden, D., & Mishra, R. (1993). On the relation between hearing sensitivity and otoacoustic emissions. *Hearing Research, 71*, 208–213.

McFadden, D., & Pasanen, E. G. (1994). Otoacoustic emissions and quinine sulfate. *Journal of the Acoustical Society of America, 95*(6), 3460–3474.

McFadden, D., & Pasanen, E. G. (1998). Comparison of the auditory systems of heterosexuals and homosexuals: Click-evoked otoacoustic emissions. *Proceedings of the National Academy of Sciences, 95*, 2709–2713.

McFadden, D., Pasagen, E. G., & Callaway, N. L. (1998). Changes in otoacoustic emissions in a transsexual male during treatment with estrogen. *Journal of the Acoustical Society of America, 104*, 1555–1558.

McFadden, D., Pasanen, E. G., & Callaway, N. L. (1999). Spontaneous otoacoustic emissions in heterosexuals, homosexuals, and bisexuals. *Journal of the Acoustical Society of America, 105*, 2403–2413.

McFadden, D., Plattsmier, H. S., & Pasanen, E. G. (1984). Aspirin-induced hearing loss as a model of sensorineural hearing loss. *Hearing Research, 16*, 251–260.

McFadden, S. L., & Campo, P. (1998). Cubic distortion product otoacoustic emissions in young and aged chinchillas exposed to low-frequency noise. *Journal of the Acoustical Society of America, 104*, 2290–2297.

McHaney, V. A., Thibadoux, G., & Hayes, F. A. (1983). Hearing loss in children receiving cisplatin chemotherapy. *Journal of Pediatrics, 102*, 314–317.

McLellan, M., & Webb, C. (1957). Ear studies in the newborn infant. *Journal of Pediatrics, 51*, 672–677.

McLellan, M. S., Strong, J. P., Vautier, T., & Blatt, I. M. (1967). Otitis media in the newborn: Relationship to duration of rupture of amniotic membrane. *Archives of Otolaryngology, 85*, 54–56.

McNellis, E., & Klein, A. (1997). Pass/fail rates for repeated click-evoked otoacoustic emission and auditory brain stem response screenings in newborns. *International Journal of Pediatric Otorhinolaryngology, 116*, 431–437.

McPherson, B., Kei, J., Smyth, V., Latham, S., & Loscher, J. (1998). Feasibility of community-based hearing screening using transient evoked otoacoustic emissions. *Public Health, 112*, 147–152.

Meech, R. P., Campbell, K. C. M., Hughes, L. P., & Rybak, L. P. (1998). A semiquantitative analysis of the effects of cisplatin on the rat stria vascularis. *Hearing Research, 124*, 44–59.

Mehl, A. L., & Thomson, V. (1998). Newborn hearing screening: The great omission. *Pediatrics, 101*(1), 1.

Melding, P. S., Goodey, R. J., & Thorne, P. R. (1978). The use of intravenous lidocaine in the diagnosis and treatment of tinnitus. *Journal of Laryngology and Otology, 92*, 115–121.

Meredith, R., Stephens, D., Hogan, S., Cartlidge, P. H. T., & Drayton, M. (1994). Screening for hearing loss in an at-risk neonatal population using evoked otoacoustic emissions. *Scandinavian Audiology, 23*, 187–193.

Meric, C., & Collet, L. (1993). Comparative influence of repeated measurement and of attention on evoked otoacoustic emissions. *Acta Otolaryngologica, 113*, 471–477.

Meric, C., & Collet, L. (1994). Attention and otoacoustic emissions: A review. *Neuroscience Behavioral Review, 18*, 215–222.

Meyer, S. E., Jardine, C. A., & Deverson, W. (1997). Developmental changes in tympanometry: A case study. *British Journal of Audiology, 31*, 189–195.

Micheyl, C., & Collet, L. (1996). Involvement of the olivocochlear bundle in the detection of tones in noise. *Journal of the Acoustical Society of America, 99*, 1604–1610.

Micheyl, C., Maison, S., Carlyon, R. P., Andeol, G., & Collet, L. (1999). Contralateral suppression of transiently evoked otoacoustic emissions by harmonic complex tones in humans. *Journal of the Acoustical Society of America, 105*, 293–305.

Micheyl, C., Perrot, X., & Collet, L. (1997). Relationship between auditory intensity discrimination in noise and olivocochlear efferent system activity in humans. *Behavioral Neuroscience, 111*, 801–807.

Michie, P., LePage, E., Solowij, N., Haller, M., & Terry, L. (1996). Evoked otoacoustic emissions and auditory selective attention. *Hearing Research, 98*, 54–67.

Mills, D. M., Norton, S. J., & Rubel, E. W. (1993). Vulnerability and adaptation of distortion product otoacoustic emissions to endocochlear potential variation. *Journal of the Acoustical Society of America, 94*, 2108–2122.

Mills, D. M., & Rubel, E. W. (1994). Variation of distortion product otoacoustic emissions with furosemide injection. *Hearing Research, 77*, 183–199.

Mills, D. M., & Rubel, E. W. (1996). Development of the cochlear amplifier. *Journal of the Acoustical Society of America, 100*, 428–441.

Mills J. H., et al. (1998). Interaction of noise-induced hearing loss and presbyacusis. *Scandinavian Audioliogy, Suppl. 48*, 117-122.

Miltich, A. J. (1968). Human auditory threshold shifts following changes between upright, supine and inverted bodily positions. *Journal of Auditory Research, 8*, 367–377.

Miyamoto, R. T., Kirk, K. I., Renshaw, J., & Hussain, D. (1999). Cochlear implantation in auditory neuropathy. *Laryngoscope, 109*, 181–185.

Molini, E., Ricci, G., Alunnni, N., & Simoncelli, C. (1998). Otoacoustic distortion products in infants and adults: A comparative study. *Acta Otorhinolaryngology Italia, 18*, 74–82.

Molini, E., Simoncelli, C., Ricci, G., Capolunghi, B., Alunni, N., & von Garrel, C. (1991). Evoked otoacoustic emissions in newborn hearing screening (in German). *Laryngo-Rhino-Otologie, 70*, 412–416.

Moller, A. R., Jannetta, P. J., & Moller, M. B. (1981). Neural generators of brainstem potentials: Results from human intracranial recordings. *Annals of Otology, Rhinology, and Laryngology, 90*, 591–596.

Morell, R. J., Kim, H. J., Hood, L. J., Goforth, L., Friderici, K., Fisher, R., Van Camp, G., Berlin, C. I., Oddoux, C., Ostrer, H., Keats, B., & Friedman, T. B. (1998). Mutations in the connexin 26 gene (GJB2) among Ashkenazi Jews with nonsyndromic recessive deafness. *New England Journal of Medicine, 339*, 1500–1505.

Morlet, T., Collet, L., Duclaux, R., Lapillonne, A., B, S., Putet, G., & Morgon, A. (1995). Spontaneous and evoked otoacoustic emissions in pre-term and full-term neonates: Is there a clinical application? *International Journal of Pediatric Otorhinolaryngology, 33*, 207–211.

Morlet, T., Collet, L., Salle, B., & Morgon, A. (1993). Functional maturation of cochlear active mechanisms and of the medial olivocochlear system in humans. *Acta Otolaryngologica, 113*, 271–277.

Morlet, T., Ferber, C., Duclaux, R., Challamel, M.-J., & Collet, L. (1994). Effect of sleep stages on transiently evoked oto-acoustic emissions in infants. *Brain and Development, 16*, 115–120.

Morlet, T., Goforth, L., Hood, L. J., Ferber, C., Duclaux, R., & Berlin, C. I. (1999). Development of human cochlear active mechanism asymmetry: Involvement of the medial olivocochlear system. *Hearing Research, 134*, 153–162.

Morlet, T., Lapillonne, A., Ferbe, C., Duclaux, R., Sann, L., Putet, G., Salle, B., & Collet, L. (1995). Spontaneous otoacoustic emissions in preterm neonates: Prevalence and gender effects. *Hearing Research, 90*, 44–54.

Mott, J. B., Norton, S. J., Neely, S. T., & Warr, W. B. (1989). Changes in spontaneous otocoustic emissions produced by acoustic stimulation of the contralateral ear. *Hearing Research, 38*, 229–242.

Moulin, A., Bera, J.-C., & Collet, L. (1994). Distortion product otoacoustic emissions and sensorineural hearing loss. *Audiology, 33*, 305–326.

Moulin, A., & Carrier, S. (1998). Time course of the medial olivocochlear efferent effect on otoacoustic emissions in humans. *Neuroreport, 9*(16), 3741–3744.

Moulin, A., Collet, L., & Duclaux, R. (1993). Contralateral auditory stimulation alters acoustic distortion products in humans. *Hearing Research, 65*, 193–210.

Moulin, A., Collet, L., & Morgon, A. (1992). Influence of spontaneous otoacoustic emissions (SOAE) on acoustic distortion product input/output functions: Does the medial efferent system act differently in the vicinity of an SOAE? *Acta Otolaryngologica, 112*, 210-214.

Moulin, A., Collet, L., Veuillet, E., & Morgon, A. (1993). Interrelations between transiently evoked otoacoustic emissions and acoustic distortion products in normally hearing subjects. *Hearing Research, 65*, 216–233.

Moulin, A., & Kemp, D. T. (1996). Multicomponent acoustic distortion product otoacoustic emission phase in humans. II. Implications for distortion product otoacoustic emissions generation. *Journal of the Acoustical Society of America, 100*, 1640–1662.

Mountain, D. C. (1980). Changes in the endolymphatic potential and crossed bundle stimulation alter cochlear mechanics. *Science, 210*, 71–72.

Mountain, D. C., Geisler, C. D., & Hubbard, A. E. (1980). Stimulation of efferents alters the cochlear microphonic and the sound-induced resistance changes measured in scala media of the guinea pig. *Hearing Research, 3*, 231–240.

Mra, Z., & Wax, M. K. (1999). Effects of acute thyroxin depletion on hearing in humans. *Laryngoscope, 109*, 343–350.

Mueller, H. G. III., & Hall, J. W., III. (1998). *Audiologists' Desk Reference. Volume II.* San Diego: Singular Publishing Group.

Mulheran, M., & Degg, C. (1997). Comparison of distortion product OAE generation between a patient group requiring frequent gentamicin therapy and control subject. *British Journal of Audiology, 31*, 5–9.

Mulheran, M., & Harpur, E. (1998). The effect of gentamicin and furosemide given in combination on cochlear potentials in the guinea pig. *British Journal of Audiology, 32*, 47–56.

Murai, K., Tyler, R. S., Harker, L. A., & Stouffer, J. L. (1992). Review of pharmacological treatment of tinnitus. *American Journal of Otology, 13*, 454–464.

Musiek, F., Bornstein, S., & Rintelmann, W. (1995). Transient evoked otoacoustic emisions and pseudohypacusis. *Journal of the American Academy of Audiology, 6*, 293–301.

Musiek, F. E. (Ed.). (1992). Otoacoustic emissions and the olivocochlear bundle. *Hearing Journal, 45*,

Musiek, F. E., & Baran, J. A. (1996). Comparison of standard and abbreviated distortion product otoacoustic emissions procedures. *Journal of the American Academy of Audiology, 7*, 370–374.

Naeve, S. L., Margolis, R. H., Levine, S. C., & Fournier, E. M. (1992). Effect of ear-canal air pressure on otoacoustic emissions. *Journal of the Acoustical Society of America, 91*, 2091–2095.

Nakamura, H., Takada, S., Shimbuku, R., Matsuo, M., & Hirokuni, N. (1985). Auditory nerve and brainstem responses in newborn infants with hyperbilirubinemia. *Pediatrics, 75*, 703–708.

Nakamura, M., Yamasoba, T., & Kaga, K. (1997). Changes in otoacoustic emissions in patients with idiopathic sudden deafness. *Audiology, 36*, 121–135.

Neely, S. T., & Gorga, M. P. (1998). Comparison between intensity and pressure as measures of sound level in the ear canal. *Journal of the Acoustical Society of America, 104*, 2925–2934.

Neely, S. T., & Kim, D. O. (1983). An active cochlear model showing sharp tuning and high sensitivity. *Hearing Research, 9*, 123–130.

Neely, S. T., & Kim, D. O. (1986). An active model of cochlear biomechanics. *Journal of the Acoustical Society of America, 79*, 1472–1480.

Neely, S. T., Norton, S. J., Gorga, M. P., & Jesteadt, W. (1988). Latency of auditory brainstem responses and otoacoustic emissions using tone-burst stimuli. *Journal of the Acoustical Society of America, 83*, 652–656.

Nelson, D., & Kimberley, B. (1992). Distortion-product emissions and auditory sensitivity in human ears with normal hearing and cochlear hearing loss. *Journal of Speech and Hearing Research, 35*, 1142–1159.

Nelson, D. A. et al. (1996). Slopes of distortion-product otoacoustic emission growth curves corrected for noise-floor levels. *Journal of the Acoustical Society of America, 99*, 468-474.

Nemes, J. (1998). Universal newborn hearing screening: The question is, not if, but when? *The Hearing Journal, 51*(7), 21–69.

Neumann, J. (1997). *Recording techniques, theory, and audiological applications of otoacoustic emissions.* Oldenburg, Germany: Bibliotheks- und Informationssystem der Universität Oldenburg.

Neumann, J., Uppenkamp, S., & Killmeier, B. (1994). Suppression of transiently evoked otoacoustic emissions. *Journal of the Acoustical Society of America, 95*, 2844A.

Neumann, J., Uppenkamp, S., & Kollmeier, B. (1997). Interaction of otoacoustic emissions with additional tones: suppression or synchronization? *Hearing Research, 103*, 19–27.

Ng, J., & Yun, H. L. (1992). Otoacoustic emissions (OAE) in paediatric hearing screening—the Singapore experience. *The Journal of the Singapore Paediatric Society, 34*(1/2), 1–5.

Nieder, P. C., & Nieder, I. (1970). Crossed olivocochlear bundle: Electrical stimulation enhances masked neural responses to loud clicks. *Brain Research, 21*, 135–137.

Nieder, P., & Nieder, I. (1979). Stimulation of efferent olivocochlear bundle causes release from low level masking. *Nature, 227*, 184–185.

Nielsen, L. H., Popelka, G. R., Rasmussen, A. N., & Osterhammel, P. A. (1993). Clinical significance of probe-tone frequency ratio on distortion product otoacoustic emissions. *Scandinavian Audiology, 22*, 159–164.

National Institutes of Health. (1993, March 1–3). Identification of hearing impairment in infants and young children. *NIH Consensus Statement, 11.*

Niskar, A. S., Kieszak, S. M., Holmes, A., Esteban, E., Rubin, C., & Brody, D. J. (1998). Prevalence of hearing loss among children 6 to 19 years of age: The Third National Health and Nutrition Examination Study. *Journal of the American Medical Society, 279*(14), 1071–1075.

Norcia, A. M., Sato, T., Shinn, P., & Mertus, J. (1986). Methods for the identification of evoked response components in the frequency and combined frequency/time domains. *Electroencephalography and Clinical Neurophysiology, 65,* 212–226.

Norman, M., & Thornton, A. R. D. (1993). Frequency analysis of the contralateral suppression of evoked otoacoustic emissions by narrow-band noise. *British Journal of Audiology, 27,* 281–289.

Norrix, L. W., & Glattke, T. J. (1996). Distortion product otoacoustic emissions created through the interaction of spontaneous otoacoustic emissions and externally generated tones. *Journal of the Acoustical Society of America, 100,* 945–955.

Northern, J. L., & Hayes, D. H. (1994). Universal screening for infant hearing impairment: Necessary, beneficial and justifiable. *Audiology Today, 6,* 10–13.

Norton, S., Tucci, D., & Rubel, E. W. (1990). Comparison of acoustic and neural responses from avian ears following gentamicin [Abstract]. *Association for Research in Otolaryngology, 13,* 62.

Norton, S. J. (1993). Applications of transient evoked otoacoustic emissions to pediatric populations. *Ear & Hearing, 14,* 64–73.

Norton, S. J. (1994). Emerging role of evoked otoacoustic emissions in neonatal hearing screening. *American Jouranl of Audiology, 15*(Suppl. 1), 4–12.

Norton, S. J., Bargones, J. Y., & Rubel, E. W. (1991). Development of otoacoustic emissions in gerbil: Evidence for micromechanical changes underlying development of the place code. *Hearing Research, 51,* 73–92.

Norton, S. J., Mott, J. B., & Champlin, C. A. (1989). Behavior of spontaneous otoacoustic emissions following intense ipsilateral acoustic stimulation. *Hearing Research, 38,* 234–258.

Norton, S. J., & Neely, S. T. (1987). Tone burst evoked otoacoustic emissions from normal-hearing subjects. *Journal of the Acoustical Society of America, 81,* 1860–1872.

Norton, S. J., & Rubel, E. W. (1990). Active and passive ADP components in mammalian and avian ears. In P. Dallos, C. D. Geisler, J. W. Matthews, M. A. Ruggero, & C. R. Steele (Eds.), *Mechanics and biophysics of hearing* (pp. 219–226). New York: Springer-Verlag.

Norton, S. J. et al. (1990). Evoked otoacoustic emissions in normal-hearing infants and children:

Emerging data and issues. *Ear & Hearing, 11,* 121-127.

Noyes, W. S., McCaffrey, T. V., Fabry, D. A., Robinette, M. S., & Suman, V. J. (1996). Effect of temperature elevation on rabbit cochlear function as measured by distortion-product otoacoustic emissions. *Otolaryngology—Head and Neck Surgery, 115,* 548–552.

Nozza, R., Sabo, D., & Mandel, E. (1997). A role for otoacoustic emissions in screening for hearing impairment and middle ear disorders in school-age children. *Ear & Hearing, 18,* 227–239.

Nuttall, A. L., & Dolan, D. F. (1993). Two-tone suppression of inner hair cell and basilar membrane responses in the guinea pig. *Journal of the Acoustical Society of America, 93,* 390–400.

Nwaesi, C. G., Van Aerde, J. B. S., Boyden, M., & Perlman, M. (1994). Changes in auditory brainstem responses in hyperbilirubinemic infants before and after exchange transfusion. *Pediatrics, 74,* 800–803.

O'Brien, A. J. (1994). Temperature dependency of the frequency and level of a spontaneous otoacoustic emission during fever. *British Journal of Audiology, 28,* 281–290.

O'Mahoney, C. F., & Kemp, D. T. (1995). Distortion product otoacoustic emission delay measurement in human ears. *Journal of the Acoustical Society of America, 97,* 3721–3735.

Ochi, A., Yasuhara, A., & Kobayashi, Y. (1998). Comparison of distortion product otoacoustic emissions with auditory brain-stem response for clinical use in neonatal intensive care unit. *Electroencephalography and Clinical Neurophysiology, 108,* 577–583.

Oeken, J. (1998). Distortion product otoacoustic emissions in acute acoustic trauma. *Noise and Health, 1,* 56–66.

Ohlemiller, K. K., & Siegel, J. H. (1992). The effects of moderate cooling on gross cochlear potentials in the gerbil: Basal and apical differences. *Hearing Research, 63,* 79–89.

Ohlemiller, K. K., & Siegel, J. H. (1994). Cochlear basal and apical differences reflected in the effects of cooling on responses of single auditory nerve fibers. *Hearing Research, 80,* 174–190.

Ohlms, L. A., Chen, A. Y., Stewart, M. G., & Franklin, D. J. (1999). Establishing the etiology of childhood hearing loss. *Otolaryngology—Head and Neck Surgery, 120,* 159–163.

Ohlms, L. A., Lonsbury-Martin, B. L., & Martin, G. K. (1990a). Acoustic-distortion products: Separation of sensory from neural dysfunction in sensorineural hearing loss in humans and rabbits. *Otolaryngology—Head and Neck Surgery, 104,* 159–174.

Ohlms, L. A., Lonsbury-Martin, B. L., & Martin, G. K. (1990b). The clinical application of acoustic distortion products. *Otolaryngology—Head and Neck Surgery, 103*, 52–59.

Ohmura, M., & Yamamoto, E. (1990). Differences in endocochlear potentials in response to anoxia in maturing and mature guinea pigs. *European Archives of Otorhinolaryngology, 248*, 8–10.

Ohyama, K., Wada, H., & Takasaka, T. (1992). Effect of alteration of middle ear environment on distortion-product emissions, *Biophysics of hair cell sensory systems* (pp. 78–86).

Osterhammel, D., & Osterhammel, P. (1979). High frequency audiometry: Age and sex variations. *Scandinavian Audiology, 8*, 73–81.

Osterhammel, P., Nielsen, L., & Rasmussen, A. (1993). Distortion product otoacoustic emissions: The influence of the middle ear transmission. *Scandinavian Audiology, 22*, 111–116.

Osterhammel, P. A., Rasmussen, A. N., Olsen, S. T., & Nielsen, L. H. (1996). The influence of spontaneous otoacoustic emissions on the amplitude of transient-evoked emissions. *Scandinavian Audiology, 25*, 187–192.

Oudesluys-Murphy, A., van Straaten, H., Bholasingh, R., & van Zanten, G. (1996). Neonatal hearing screening. *European Journal of Pediatrics, 155*, 429–435.

Owens, J. J., McCoy, M. J., Lonsbury-Martin, B. L., & Martin, G. K. (1992). Influence of otitis media on evoked otoacoustic emissions in children. *Seminars in Hearing, 13*(1), 53–66.

Owens, J. J., McCoy, M. J., Lonsbury-Martin, B. L., & Martin, G. K. (1993). Otoacoustic emissions in children with normal ears, middle ear dysfunction, and ventilating tubes. *American Journal of Otology, 14*(1), 34–40.

Ozdamar, O., Delgado, R. E., Rahman, S., & Lopez, C. (1998). Adaptive Wiener filtering for improved acquisition of distortion product otoacoustic emissions. *Annals of Biomedical Engineering, 26*, 883–891.

Ozdamar, O., Zhang, J., Kalayci, T., & Ulgen, Y. (1997). Time-frequency distribution of evoked otoacoustic emissions. *British Journal of Audiology, 31*, 461–471.

Ozturan, O., & Oysu, C. (1999). Influence of spontaneous otoacoustic emissions on distortion product otoacoustic emissions amplitudes. *Hearing Research, 127*, 129–136.

Paintaud, G., Alvan, G., Berninger, E., Gustafsson, L. L., Idrizbegovic, E., Karlsson, K. K., & Wakelkamp, M. (1994). The concentration-effect relationship of quinine-induced hearing impairment. *Clinical Pharmacologic Therapy, 5*, 317–323.

Paludetti, G., Ottaviani, F., Fetoni, A. R., Zuppa, A. A., & Tortorola, G. (1999). Transient evoked otoacoustic emissions (TEOAEs) in newborns: Normative data. *International Journal of Pediatric Otolaryngology, 47*(3), 235–241.

Panosetti, E., Shi, B. X., Eloy, J. P., Orband, D., & Rasque, E. (1999). Oto-emissions provoquees a la naissance: l'experience luxembourgeoise (in French). *Archives of Pediatrics, 6*(Suppl. 2), 353–355.

Paparella, M. M., Shea, D., Meyerhoff, W. L., & Goycoolea, M. V. (1980). Silent otitis media. *Laryngoscope, 90*, 1089–1098.

Pappas, D. (1983). A study of the high-risk registry for sensorineural hearing impairment. *Archives of Otolaryngology—Head and Neck Surgery, 91*, 41–44.

Paradise, J. L. (1999). Universal newborn hearing screening: Should we leap before we look? *Pediatrics, 102*, 670–664.

Paradise, J. L., Smith, C. G., & Bluestone, C. D. (1976). Tympanometric detection of middle ear effusion infants and young children. *Pediatrics, 58*, 198–210.

Parham, K., Sun, X. M., & Kim, D. O. (1999). Distortion product otoacoustic emissions in the CBA/J mouse model of presbycusis. *Hearing Research, 134*, 29–38.

Parker, D. J., & Thornton, R. D. (1978). Cochlear traveling wave velocities calculated from the derived components of the cochlear nerve and brainstem evoked responses of the human auditory system. *Scandinavian Audiology, 7*, 67–70.

Parker, G., Webb, H., & Stevens, J. (1997,). *Outcome of infants with transient otoacoustic emissions present and high ABR threshold at birth.* Paper presented at the British Society of Audiology Annual Conference.

Pascal, J., Bourgeade, A., Lagier, M., & Legros, C. (1998). Linear and nonlinear model of the human middle ear. *Journal of the Acoustical Society of America, 104*, 1509–1516.

Patuzzi, R. (1993). Otoacoustic emissions and the categorization of cochlear and retro-cochlear lesions. *British Journal of Audiology, 27*, 91–95.

Patuzzi, R. (1996). Cochlear micromechanics and macromechanics. In P. Dallos, A. N. Popper, & R. R. Fay (Eds.), *The cochlea* (pp. 186–257). New York: Springer.

Peck, J. E. (1994a). Development of hearing. Part I. Phylogeny. *Journal of the American Academy of Audiology, 5*, 291–299.

Peck, J. E. (1994b). Development of hearing. Part II. Embryology. *Journal of the American Academy of Audiology, 5*, 359–365.

Peck, J. E. (1995). Development of hearing. Part III. Postnatal development. *Journal of the American Academy of Audiology, 6*(2), 113–123.

Penner, M. (1990). An estimate of the prevalence of tinnitus caused by spontaneous otoacoustic emissions. *Archives of Otolaryngology—Head and Neck Surgery, 116,* 418–423.

Penner, M., & Zhang, T. (1997). Prevalence of spontaneous otoacoustic emissions in adults revisited. *Hearing Research, 103,* 28–34.

Penner, M. J. (1989). Aspirin abolishes tinnitus caused by spontaneous otoacoustic emissions: A case study. *Archives of Otolaryngology—Head and Neck Surgery, 115,* 871–875.

Penner, M. J. (1994). Covariation of tinnitus pitch and the associated emission: A case study. *Otolaryngology—Head and Neck Surgery, 100,* 304–309.

Penner, M. J. (1995). Frequency variation of spontaneous otoacoustic emissions during a naturally occurring menstrual cycle, amenorrhea, and oral contraception: A brief report. *Ear & Hearing, 16,* 428–432.

Penner, M. J. (1996). The emergence and disappearance of one subject's spontaneous otoacoustic emissions. *Ear and Hearing, 17,* 116–119.

Penner, M. J., Brauth, S. E., & Jastreboff, P. (1994). Covariation of binaural, concurrently-measured spontaneous otoacoustic emissions. *Hearing Research, 73,* 190–194.

Penner, M. J., & Burns, E. M. (1987). The dissociation of SOAEs and tinnitus. *Journal of Speech and Hearing Research, 30,* 396–403.

Penner, M. J., & Coles, R. R. A. (1992). Indications for aspirin as a palliative for tinnitus caused by SOAEs: A case study. *British Journal of Audiology, 26,* 91–96.

Penner, M. J., & Glotzbach, L. (1994). Covariation of tinnitus pitch and the associated emission: A case study. *Otolaryngology—Head and Neck Surgery, 100,* 304–309.

Penner, M. J., Glotzbach, L., & Huang, T. (1993). Spontaneous otoacoustic emissions: Measurement and data. *Hearing Research, 68,* 229–237.

Penner, M. J. et al. (1997). Prevalence of spontaneous otoacoustic emissions in adults revisited. *Hearing Research, 103,* 28–34.

Perlman, M., Fainmesser, P., Sohmer, H., Tamari, H., Yohanen, W., & Pevsmer, B. (1983). Auditory nerve brainstem evoked responses in hyperbilirubinemic neonates. *Pediatrics, 72,* 658–664.

Perlstein, M. A. (1960). The late clinical syndrome of posticteric encephalopathy. *Pediatric Clinics of North America, 7,* 665–687.

Perrot, X., Micheyl, C., Khalfa, S., & Collet, L. (1999). Stronger bilateral efferent influences on cochlear biomechanical activity in musicians than in non-musicians. *Neuroscience Letters, 262*(3), 167–170.

Pestalozza, G., Romagnoli, M., & Tessitore, E. (1988). Incidence and risk factors of acute otitis media with effusion in children of different age groups. *Advances in Otorhinolaryngology, 40,* 47–56.

Pfeiffer, R. R., & Molnar, C. E. (1974). Characteristics of the (f2–f1) component in response patterns of single cochlear nerve fibers. *Journal of the Acoustical Society of America, 56,* S21.

Phillips, A. J., & Farrell, G. (1992). The effect of posture on three objective audiological measures. *British Journal of Audiology, 26,* 339–345.

Phillips, A. J., & Marchbanks, R. J. (1989). Effects of posture and age on tympanic membrane displacement measurements. *British Journal of Audiology, 23,* 279–284.

Picton, T., Kellett, A. J. C., Vezenyi, M., & Rabinovitch, D. E. (1993). Otoacoustic emissions recorded at rapid stimulus rates. *Ear & Hearing, 14,* 299–314.

Pike, D. A., & Bosher, S. K. (1980). The time course of the strial changes produced by intravenous furosemide. *Hearing Research, 3,* 79–89.

Pirila, T., Jounio-Ervasti, K., & Sorri, M. (1991). Hearing asymmetry among left-handed and right-handed persons in a random population. *Scandinavian Audiology, 20,* 223–226.

Plinkert, P. K., Arold, R., & Zenner, H. P. (1990). Evoked otoacoustic emissions—A screening method to detect hearing disorders in high-risk infants (in German). *Laryngo-Rhino-Otology, 69,* 108–110.

Plinkert, P. K., Gitter, A. H., & Zenner, H. P. (1990). Tinnitus associated spontaneous otoacoustic emissions. Active outer hair cell movements as a common origin? *Acta Otolaryngologica (Stockholm), 110,* 342–347.

Plinkert, P. K., & Krober, S. (1991). Früherkennung einer Cisplatin-Ototoxizitat durch evozierte otoakustische Emissionen. *Laryngo-Rhino-Otologie, 70,* 457–462.

Plinkert, P. K., Sesterhenn, G., Arold, R., & Zenner, H. P. (1990). Evaluation of otoacoustic emissions in high-risk infants by using an easy and rapid objective auditory screening method. *European Archives of Otorhinolaryngology, 247,* 356–360.

Plomp, R. (1965). Detectability thresholds for combination tones. *Journal of the Acoustical Society of America, 37,* 1110–1123.

Popelka, G. R., Karzon, R. K., & Arjmand, E. M. (1995). Growth of the 2f1–f2 distortion product otoacoustic emission for low-level stimuli in human neonates. *Ear & Hearing, 16,* 159–165.

Popelka, G. R., Karzon, R. K., & Clary, R. A. (1998). Identification of noise sources that influence distortion product otoacoustic emission measurements in human neonates. *Ear & Hearing, 19,* 319–328.

Popelka, G. R., Osterhammel, P. A., Nielsen, L. H., & Rasmussen, A. (1993). Growth of distortion product otoacoustic emissions with primary-tone level in humans. *Hearing Research, 71,* 12–22.

Prasher, D., Ryan, S., & Luxon, L. (1994). Contralateral suppression of transient otoacoustic emissionsand neuro-otology. In L. Collet & F. Grandori (Eds.), *Suppression effects of otoacoustic emissions* (Vol. III, pp. 71–81). Milan, Italy: Casa Editrice G. Sefanoni-Lecco.

Prasher, D., & Sulkowski, W. (1999). The role of otoacoustic emissions in screening and evaluation of noise damage. *International Journal of Medicine and Environmental Health, 12*(2), 183–192.

Pratt, H., Shi, Y., & Polyakov, A. (1998). Contralaterally evoked transient otoacoustic emissions. *Hearing Research, 115,* 39–44.

Preckel, M. P., Ferber-Viart, C., Leftheriotis, G., Dubreuil, C., Duclaux, R., Saumet, J. L., Banssillon, V., & Granry, J. C. (1998). Autoregulation of human inner ear blood flow during middle ear surgery with propofol or isoflurane anesthesia during controlled hypotension. *Anesthesiology and Analgesia, 87,* 1002–1008.

Prieve, B., & Falter, S. R. (1995). COAEs and SOAEs in adults with increasing age. *Ear & Hearing, 16,* 521–528.

Prieve, B., Gorga, M., & Neely, S. (1991). Otoacoustic emissions in an adult with severe hearing loss. *Journal of Speech and Hearing Research, 34,* 379–385.

Prieve, B., Gorga, M., Schmidt, A., Neely, S., Peters, J., Schultes, L., & Jesteadt, W. (1993). Analysis of transient-evoked otoacoustic emissions in normal-hearing and hearing-impaired ears. *Journal of the Acoustical Society of America, 93,* 3308–3319.

Prieve, B. A. (1992). Otoacoustic emissions in infants and children: Basic characteristics and clinical application. *Seminars in Hearing, 13*(1), 37–52.

Prieve, B. A., & Fitzgerald, T. S. (1998). Preliminary results from a longitudinal study of distortion product otoacoustic emissions in infants. *Association for Research in Otolaryngology, 21.*

Prieve, B. A., Fitzgerald, T. S., & Schulte, L. E. (1997). Basic characteristics of click-evoked otoacoustic emissions in infants and children. *Journal of the Acoustical Society of America, 102,* 2860–2870.

Prieve, B. A., Fitzgerald, T. S., Schulte, L. E., & Kemp, D. T. (1997). Basic characteristics of distortion product otoacoustic emissions in infants and children. *Journal of the Acoustical Society of America, 102,* 2871–2879.

Probst, R., Coats, A. C., Martin, G. K., & Lonsbury-Martin, B. L. (1986). Spontaneous, click- and toneburst evoked otoacoustic emissions. *Hearing Research, 21,* 261–275.

Probst, R., & Harris, F. P. (1993). Transiently evoked and distortion-product otoacoustic emissions—comparison of results from normally hearing and hearing-impaired human ears. *Archives of Otolaryngology, 119,* 858–860.

Probst, R., Harris, F. P., & Hauser, R. (1993). Clinical monitoring using otoacoustic emissions. *British Journal of Audiology, 27,* 85–90.

Probst, R., & Hauser, R. (1990). Distortion product otoacoustic emissions in normal and hearing-impaired ears. *American Journal of Otolaryngology, 11,* 236–243.

Probst, R., Lonsbury-Martin, B. L., Martin, G. K., & Coats, A. C. (1987). Otoacoustic emissions in ears with hearing loss. *American Journal of Otolaryngology, 8,* 73–81.

Probst, R., Lonsbury-Martin, G., & Martin, G. (1991). A review of otoacoustic emissions. *Journal of the Acoustical Society of America, 89*(5), 2027–2067.

Proschel, U., & Eysholdt, U. (1993). Evoked otoacoustic emissions in children in relation to middle ear impedance. *Folia Phoniatrica (Basel), 45,* 288–294.

Psarommatis, I., Tsakanikos, M., AD, K., Ntouniadakis, D., & Apostolopoulous, N. (1997). Profound hearing loss and presence of click-evoked otoacoustic emissions in the neonate: A report of two cases. *International Journal of Pediatric Otorhinolaryngology, 39,* 237–243.

Puel, J.-L., Bobbin, R. P., & Fallon, M. (1990). Salicylate, mefenamate, meclofenamate, and quinine on cochlear potentials. *Otolaryngology—Head and Neck Surgery, 102,* 66–73.

Puel, J. L., Bonfils, P., & Pujol, R. (1988). Selective attention modifies the active micromechanical properties of the cochlea. *Brain Research, 447,* 380–383.

Puel, J.-L., & Rebillard, G. (1990). Effect of contralateral sound stimulation on the distortion product 2f1–f2: Evidence that the medial efferent system is involved. *Journal of the Acoustical Society of America, 87,* 1630–1635.

Pujol, R. (1994). Lateral and medial efferents: A double neurochemical mechanism to protect and regulate inner and outer hair cells functions in the cochlea. In L. Collet & F. Grandori (Eds.), *Suppression effects of otoacoustic emissions* (Vol. III, pp. 1–8). Milan, Italy: Casa Editrice G. Sefanoni-Lecco.

Pujol, R., Carlier, E., & Lenoir, M. (1980). Ontogenetic approach to inner and outer hair cell function. *Hearing Research, 2*, 423–430.

Pujol, R., Lavigne-Rebillard, M., & Uziel, A. (1991). Development of the human cochlea. *Acta Otolaryngologica (Stockh)*, Suppl. 482, 7–12.

Purcell, D., Kunov, H., Madsen, P., & Cleghorn, W. (1998). Distortion product otoacoustic emissions stimulated through bone conduction. *Ear & Hearing, 19*, 362–370.

Puria, S., & Allen, J. B. (1998). Measurements and model of the cat middle ear: Evidence of tympanic membrane acoustic delay. *Journal of the Acoustical Society of America, 104*, 2462–2471.

Qian, J., & Jiang, W. (1997). Distortion product otoacoustic emissions on neonates. *Lin Chuang Erh Pi Yen Hou Ko Tsa Chih, 11*, 3–5.

Quaranta, A., Portalatini, P., Camporeale, M., & Sallustio, V. (1999). Effects of salicylates on evoked otoacoustic emissions and remote masking in humans. *Audiology, 38*(3), 174–179.

Quinonez, R. E. (1999). Distortion-product otoacoustic emissions (DPEs) in neonates: Frequency ratio (F2/F1) and stimulus level differences (L1–L2). *Acta Otolaryngologica (Stockholm), 119*(4), 431–436.

Rabinowitz, W. M., & Widin, G. P. (1984). Interaction of spontaneous otoacoustic emissions and external sound. *Journal of the Acoustical Society of America, 76*, 1713–1720.

Raffin, M. J. M., Blank, C. R., & Hotaling, A. J. (1995). *Criteria for DPOAE.* Paper presented at the Annual Convention of the American Academy of Audiology, Dallas, TX.

Rahko, T., Kumpulainen, P., Ihalainen, H., Ojala, E., & Aumala, O. (1997). A new analysis method for the evaluation of transient evoked otoacoustic emissions. *Acta Otolaryngologica (Stockholm)*, Suppl. 529, 66–68.

Rajan, R. (1988a). Effect of electrical stimulation of the crossed olivocochlear bundle on temporary threshold shifts in auditory sensitivity. I. Dependence on electrical stimulation parameters. *Journal of Neurophysiology, 60*, 549–568.

Rajan, R. (1988b). Effect of electrical stimulation of the crossed olivocochlear bundle on temporary threshold shifts in auditory sensitivity. II. Dependence on the level of temporary threshold shifts. *Journal of Neurophysiology, 60*, 569–579.

Ramotowski, D., & Kimberley, B. (1998). Age and human cochlear traveling wave delay. *Ear and Hearing, 19*, 111–119.

Rance, G., Beer, D. E., Cone-Wesson, B., Shepherd, R. K., Dowell, R. C., King, A. M., Rickards, F. W., & Clark, G. M. (1999). Clinical findings for a group of infants and young children with auditory neuropathy. *Ear & Hearing, 20*, 238–252.

Rasmussen, A. N., & Osterhammel, P. A. (1992). A new approach for recording distortion product oto-acoustic emissions. *Scandinavian Audiology, 21*, 219–224.

Rasmussen, A. N., Osterhammel, P. A., Johannsen, P. T., & Borgkvist, B. (1998). Neonatal hearing screening using otoacoustic emissions elicited by maximum length sequences. *British Journal of Audiology, 32*, 355–366.

Rasmussen, A. N., Popelka, G. R., Osterhammel, P. A., & Nielsen, L. H. (1993). Clinical significance of relative probe-tone levels on distortion product otoacoustic emissions. *Scandinavian Audiology, 22*, 223-229.

Rasmussen, G. L. (1946). The olivary peduncle and other fiber projections of the superior olivary complex. *Journal of Comparative Neurology, 84*, 141–218.

Ravazzani, P., Tognola, G., & Grandori, F. (1996). "Derived nonlinear" versus "linear" click-evoked otoacoustic emissions. *Audiology, 35*, 73–86.

Ravazzani, P., Tognola, G., & Grandori, F. (1999). Optimal band pass filtering of transient evoked otoacoustic emissions in neonates. *Audiology, 38*, 69–74.

Raveh, E., Mount, R. J., & Harrison, R. V. (1998). Increased otoacoustic-emission amplitude secondary to cochlear lesions. *Journal of Otolaryngology, 27*, 354–360.

Rebillard, G., Klis, J. F. L., Lavigne-Rebillard, M., Devaux, P., Puel, J. L., & Pujol, R. (1993). Changes in 2f1–f2 distortion product otoacoustic emission following alterations of cochlear metabolism. *British Journal of Audiology, 27*, 117–121.

Reddell, R. R., Kefford, R. F., Grant, J. M., Coates, A. S., & Fox, R. M. (1992). Ototoxicity in patients receiving cisplatin: importance of dose and method of drug administration. *Cancer Treatment Research, 66*, 19-23.

Reiter, E. R., & Liberman, M. C. (1995). Efferent-mediated protection from acoustic overexposure: Relation to "slow effects" of olivocochlear stimulation. *Journal of Neurophysiology, 73*, 506–514.

Resef (Haran), I., Attias, J., & Furst, M. (1993). Characteristics of click evoked otoacoustic emissions in ears with normal hearing and with noise induced hearing loss. *British Journal of Audiology, 27*, 387–395.

Reuter, G., Bordgen, F., Dressler, F., Schafer, S., Hemmanouil, I., Schonweiler, R., & Lenarz, T. (1998). Neonatal hearing screening with the Echosensor automated device for otoacoustic emissions: A comparative study (in German). *Hals-Nasen-Ohren (HNO), 46*, 932–941.

Rhoades, K., McPherson, B., Smyth, V., Kei, J., & Baglioni, A. (1998). Effects of background noise on click-evoked otoacoustic emissions. *Ear & Hearing, 19*, 450–462.

Rhode, W. S. (1971). Observations of the vibration of the basilar membrane using the Mossbauer technique. *Journal of the Acoustical Society of America, 49*, 1218–1231.

Rhode, W. S. (1978). Some observations on cochlear mechanics. *Journal of the Acoustical Society of America, 64*, 158–176.

Rhode, W. S., & Robles, L. (1974). Evidence from Mossbauer experiments for nonlinear vibration in the cochlea. *Journal of the Acoustical Society of America, 55*, 588–596.

Rhodes, M. C., Margolis, R. H., Hirsch, J. E., & Napp, A. P. (1999). Hearing screening in the newborn intensive care nursery: Comparison of methods. *Otolaryngology—Head and Neck Surgery, 120*, 799–808.

Richards, S. H., O'Neill, G., & Wilson, F. (1982). Middle ear pressure variations during general anesthesia. *Journal of Laryngology and Otology, 96*, 883–892.

Richardson, H. C., Elliott, C., & Hill, J. (1996). The feasibility of recording transiently evoked otoacoustic emissions immediately following grommet insertion. *Clinical Otolaryngology, 21*, 445–448.

Richardson, M. P., Williamson, T. J., Lenton, S. W., Tarlow, M. J., & Rudd, P. T. (1995). Otoacoustic emissions as a screening test for hearing impairment in children. *Archives of Diseases in Childhood, 72*, 294–297.

Richardson, M. P., Williamson, T. J., Reid, A., Tarlow, M. J., & Rudd, P. T. (1998). Otoacoustic emissions as a screening test for hearing impairment in children recovering from acute bacterial meningitis. *Pediatrics, 102*, 1364–1368.

Richter, B., Hauser, R., & Lohle, E. (1994). Dependence of distortion product emission amplitude on primary-tone stimulus levels during middle-ear pressure changes. *Acta Otolaryngologica, 114*, 278–284.

Roberts, D., Johnson, C., Carlin, S., Turczyk, V., Karnuta, M., & Yaffee, K. (1995). Resolution of middle ear effusion in newborns. *Archives of Pediatric and Adolescent Medicine, 149*, 873–877.

Robertson, D. (1985). Brainstem location of efferent neurons projecting to the guinea pig cochlea. *Hearing Research, 20*, 79–84.

Robinette, M., & Glattke, T. (Eds.). (1997). *Otoacoustic emissions: Clinical applications.* New York: Thieme.

Robinette, M. S. (1992). Clinical observations with transient otoacoustic emissions with adults. *Seminars in Hearing, 12*(1), 23–26.

Robinshaw, H. M. (1995). Early intervention for hearing impairment: Differences in the timing of communicative and linguistic development. *British Journal of Audiology, 29*, 315–334.

Robinson, P. M., & Haugton, P. M. (1991). Modifications of evoked oto-acoustic emissions by changes in pressure in the external ear canal. *British Journal of Audiology, 25*, 131–133.

Robles, L., Ruggero, M. A., & Rich, N. C. (1980). Two-tone distortion in the basilar membrane of the cochlea. *Nature*, 413–414.

Rogowski, M., Gindzienska, E., & Chodynicki, S. (1998). Evoked otoacoustic emissions in the neonatal hearing screening (Polish language). *Klinika Otolaryngologii, 52*, 441–445.

Rosanowski, F., Hoppe, U., Hies, T., & Eysholdt, U. (1998). Johanson-Blizzard syndrome: A complex dysplasia syndrome with aplasia of the nasal alae and inner ear deafness (in German). *Hals-Nasen-Ohren (HNO), 46*, 876–878.

Ross, M. D. (1973). Autonomic components of the VIII nerve. *Advances in Otorhinolaryngology, 20*, 316–336.

Rothenberg, M. B., & Sills, E. M. (1968). Iatrogenesis: The PKU anxiety syndrome. *Journal of the American Academy of Child Psychiatry, 7*, 689–692.

Roush, J., Bryant, K., Mundy, M., Zeisel, S., & Roberts, J. (1995). Developmental changes in static admittance and tympanometric width in infants and toddlers. *Journal of the American Academy of Audiology, 6*, 334–338.

Royster, J. D., Royster, L. H., & Killion, M. C. (1991). Sound exposures and hearing thresholds of symphony orchestra musicians. *Journal of the Acoustical Society of America, 89*, 2793–2803.

Ruah, C. B., Schachern, P. A., Zelterman, D., Paparella, M. M., & Yoon, T. H. (1992). Age-related morphologic changes in the human tympanic membrane: A light and electron micropscopic study. *Archives of Otolaryngology—Head and Neck Surgery, 117*, 627–634.

Ruan, R. S., Leong, S. K., & Yeoh, K. H. (1997). Ototoxicity of sodium nitroprusside. *Hearing Research, 114*, 169–178.

Rubel, E. W., Popper, A. N., & Fay, R. R. (Eds.). (1998). *Development of the auditory system.* New York: Springer.

Ruggero, M. A., & Rich, N. C. (1991). Furosemide alters organ of Corti mechanics: Evidence for feedback of outer hair cells upon the basilar membrane. *Journal of Neuroscience, 11*(4), 1057–1067.

Ruggero, M. A., Rich, N. C., & Freyman, R. (1983). Spontaneous and impulsively evoked otoacoustic emissions: Indicators of cochlear pathology? *Hearing Research, 10,* 283–300.

Ruggero, M. A., Robles, L., & Rich, N. C. (1992). Two-tone suppression in the basilar membrane of the cochlea: Mechanical basis of auditory nerve rate suppression. *Journal of Neurophysiology, 68,* 1087–1099.

Rupp, K., & Hall, J., III. (1998). Pediatric auditory brainstem response assessment: The cross-check principle twenty years later. *Seminars in Hearing, 19*(1), 41–60.

Russell, A. F. (1992). *Heritability of spontaneous otoacoustic emissions.* University of Illinois, Urbana.

Russell, I. J., & Murugasu, E. (1997). Medial efferent inhibition suppresses basilar membrane responses to near characteristic frequency tones of moderate to high intensities. *Journal of the Acoustical Society of America, 102,* 1734–1738.

Rutten, W. L. C. (1980). Evoked acoustic emissions from within abnormal human ears: Comparison with audiometric and electrocochleographic findings. *Hearing Research, 2,* 263–271.

Ryan, S., Kemp, D. T., & Hinchcliffe, R. (1991). The influence of contralateral stimulation on otoacoustic emission responses in humans. *British Journal of Audiology, 25,* 391–397.

Rybak, L. P. (1982). Pathophysiology of furosemide ototoxicity. *Journal of Otolaryngology, 11,* 127–133.

Rybak, L. P. (1983). Furosemide ototoxicity: clinical and experimental aspects. *Laryngoscope, 95*(Suppl. 38), 1–14.

Sabin, H. I., Prasher, D., Bentivoglio, P., & Symon, L. (1987). Preservation of cochlear potentials in a deaf patient fifteen months after excision of an acoustic neuroma. *Scandinavian Audiology, 16,* 109–111.

Sachs, M. B., & Kiang, N. Y. S. (1968). Two-tone inhibition in auditory nerve fibers. *Journal of the Acoustical Society of America, 43,* 1120–1128.

Sakashita, T., Kubo, T., Kusuki, M., Kyunai, K., Ueno, K., Hikawa, C., Wada, T., Shibata, T., & Nakai, Y. (1998). Patterns of change in growth function of distortion product otoacoustic emissions in Meniere's disease. *Acta Otolaryngologica (Stockholm), 538,* 70–77.

Sakashita T., Minowa, Y., Hachikawa, K., Kubo, T., & Nakai, Y. (1991). Evoked otoacoustic emissions from ears with idiopathic sudden deafness. *Acta Otolaryngologica (Stockholm), Suppl. 486,* 66–72.

Salamy, A., Eldredge, L., & Sweetow, R. (1996). Transient evoked otoacoustic emissions: Feasibility in the nursery. *Ear & Hearing, 17,* 42–48.

Salamy, A., & McKean, C. M. (1976). Postnatal development of human brain stem potentials during the first year of life. *Electroencephalography and Clinical Neurophysiology, 41,* 418–426.

Salamy, A., McKean, C. M., & Buda, F. B. (1975). Maturational changes in auditory transmission as reflected in human brainstem potentials. *Brain Research, 96,* 361–366.

Salata, J., Jacobson, J., & Strasnick, B. (1998). Distortion-product otoacoustic emissions hearing screening in high-risk newborns. *Otolaryngology—Head and Neck Surgery, 118,* 37–43.

Salomon, G., Groth, J., & Anthonisen, B. (1993). Preliminary results and considerations in hearing screening of newborns based on otoacoustic emissions. *British Journal of Audiology, 27,* 139–141.

Santaolalla Montoya, F., Martinez Ibarguen, A., & Sanchez del Rey, A. (1998). Study of acoustic trauma in hunters using otoacoustic emission recording. *Acta Otorrinolaringology Espanol, 49,* 125–128.

Sato, H., Sando, J., & Takahashi, H. (1991). Sexual dimorphism and development of the human cochlea: Computer 3–D measurement. *Acta Otolaryngologica, 111,* 1037–1040.

Satoh, N. (1992). A study of auditory screening in infant by evoked otoacoustic emissions (EOAE) (in Japanese). *Audiology Japan, 35,* 259–271.

Scates, K. W., Woods, C. I., & Azeredo, W. J. (1999). Inferior colliculus stimulation and changes in 2f–f2 distortion product otoacoustic emissions in the rat. *Hearing Research, 128,* 51–60.

Schacht, J. (1998). Aminoglycoside ototoxicity: Prevention in sight? *Otolaryngology—Head and Neck Surgery, 118,* 674–677.

Scharf, B., Magnan, J., & Chays, A. (1997). On the role of the olivocochlear bundle in hearing: 16 case studies. *Hearing Research, 103,* 101–122.

Scharf, B., Quigley, S., Aoki, C., Peachey, N., & Reeves, A. (1987). Focussed auditory attention and frequency selectivity. *Perceptual Psychophysics, 42,* 215–223.

Schell, M. J., McHaney, V. A., & Green, A. A. (1989). Hearing loss in children and young adults receiving cisplatin with or without prior cranial irradiation. *Journal of Clinical Oncology, 7,* 754–760.

Scherer, A. (1984). Evozierte oto-akustische Emissionen bei der Vor-, Simultan- und Nachverdeckung (pre- and postmasking). *Akustica, 56*, 34–40.

Schloth, E. (1983). Relation between spectral composition of spontaneous otoacoustic emissions and fine-structure of threshold in quiet. *Acustica, 53*, 250-256.

Schmiedt, R. A. (1986). *Effects of asphyxia on levels of ear canal emissions in gerbils.* Paper presented at the Association for Research in Otolaryngology.

Schloth E, et al. (1983). Mechanical and acoustical influences on spontaneous otoacoustic emissions. *Hearing Research,11*, 285-293.

Schneider, B., Morrongiello, B., & Trehub, S. (1990). The size of the critical band in infants, children and adults. *Journal of Experimental Psychological and Human Perceptual Performance, 16*, 642–652.

Schorn, K. (1993). The Munich screening programme in neonates. *British Journal of Audiology, 27*, 143–148.

Schrott, A., Puel, J.-L., & G, R. (1991). Cochlear origin of 2f1–f2 distortion products assessed by using 2 types of mutant mice. *Hearing Research, 52*, 245–254.

Schrott, A., Stephan, K., & Spoendlin, H. (1989). Hearing with selective inner hair cell loss. *Hearing Research, 40*, 213–220.

Schulman-Galambos, C., & Galambos, R. (1975). Brain stem auditory evoked responses in premature infants. *Journal of Speech and Hearing Research, 18*, 456–465.

Schulman-Galambos, C., & Galambos, R. (1979). Brain stem auditory evoked response audiometry in newborn hearing screening. *Archives of Otolaryngology—Head and Neck Surgery, 105*, 86–90.

Schweitzer, V. G. (1993). Ototoxicity of chemotherapeutic agents. *Otolaryngology Clinics of North America, 26*(5), 759–789.

Sellick, P. M., Patuzzi, R. B., & Johnstone, B. M. (1982). Measurement of basilar membrane motion in the guinea pig using the Mossbauer technique. *Journal of the Acoustical Society of America, 72*, 131–141.

Selleck, P. M., & Russell, I. J. (1979). Two-tone suppression in cochlear hair cells. *Hearing Research, 1*, 227–236.

Sequi-Canet, J. M., Plana, B. M., Cencillo, C. P., Solanes, J. B., & Algarra, J. M. (1992). Results of a study of spontaneous otoacoustic emissions in neonates (in Spanish). *Annals Espanol Pediatrics, 37*(2), 121–125.

Sequi-Canet, J. M., Solanes, J. B., Plana, B. M., Cencillo, C. P., & Algarra, J. M. (1992). Evoked otoacoustic emissions versus auditory brainstem response in newborns (in Spanish). *Annals Espanol Pediatrics, 37*(6), 457–460.

Serbetcioglu, M. B., & Parker, D. J. (1999). Measures of cochlear traveling wave delay in humans: I. Comparisons of three techniques in subjects with normal hearing. *Acta Otolaryngologica (Stockholm), 119*(5), 537–543.

Sewell, W. F. (1984a). The effects of furosemide on the endocochlear potential and auditory-nerve fiber tuning curves in cats. *Hearing Research, 14*, 305–314.

Sewell, W. F. (1984b). The relation between the endocochlear potential and spontaneous activity in auditory nerve fibers of the cat. *Journal of Physiology (London), 347*, 685–696.

Shapiro, S. M., & Conlee, J. W. (1991). Brainstem auditory evoked potentials correlate with morphological changes in Gunn rat pups. *Hearing Research, 57*, 16–22.

Sheppard, S., Brown, A., & Russell, P. (1996). Feasibility of acoustic distortion product testing in newborns. *British Journal of Audiology, 30*, 261–274.

Shera, C. A., & Guinan, J. J., Jr. (1999). Evoked otoacoustic emissions arise by two fundamentally different mechanisms: A taxonomy for mammalian OAEs. *Journal of the Acoustical Society of America, 105*, 782–798.

Shera, C. A., & Zweig, G. (1991). Reflection and retrograde waves within the cochlea and the stapes. *Journal of the Acoustical Society of America, 89*, 1290–1305.

Shiomi, Y., Tsuji, J., Naito, Y., Fujiki, N., & Yamamoto, N. (1997). Characteristics of DPOAE audiogram in tinnitus patients. *Hearing Research, 108*, 83–88.

Shivapuja, B. G., Gu, Z.-P., Saunders, S. S., & Quirk, W. S. (1993). Acute effects of cocaine on cochlear function. *Hearing Research, 69*, 243–250.

Shurin, P. A., Howie, V. M., Pelton, S. I., Ploussard, J. H., & Klein, J. O. (1978). Bacterial etiology of otitis media during the first six weeks of life. *Journal of Pediatrics, 92*(6), 893–896.

Sie, K., & Norton, S. (1997). Changes in otoacoustic emissions and auditory brain stem response after cis-platinum exposure in gerbils. *Otolaryngology—Head and Neck Surgery, 116*, 585–592.

Siegel, J. (1994). Ear-canal standing waves and high-frequency sound calibration using otoacoustic emission probes. *Journal of the Acoustical Society of America, 95*(5), 2589–2597.

Siegel, J. H. (1995). Cross-talk in otoacoustic emission probes. *Ear & Hearing, 16*, 150–158.

Siegel, J. H., & Hirohata, E. T. (1994). Sound calibration and distortion product otoacoustic emissions at high frequencies. *Hearing Research, 80*, 146–152.

Siegel, J. H., & Kim, D. O. (1982). Efferent neural control of cochlear mechanics? Olivocochlear bundle stimulation affects cochlear biomechanical nonlinearity. *Hearing Research, 6,* 171–182.

Siegel, J. H., Neely, S. T., & Spear, W. H. (1998). Vector decomposition of distortion-product otoacoustic emission sources in humans. *Association for Research in Otolaryngology, 21.*

Simmons, F. B., & Russ, F. N. (1974). Automated newborn hearing screening: The Crib-O-Gram. *Archives of Otolaryngology, 100,* 1–7.

Simoncelli, C., Molini, E., Capolunghi, B., Ricci, G., Alunni, N., & Trabalza, N. (1992). Evoked otoacoustic emissions during the first 60 hours of life (in French). *Acta Oto-rhino-laryngologica Belgium, 46,* 63–66.

Sininger, Y., Hood, L., Starr, A., Berlin, C., & Picton, T. (1995). Hearing loss due to auditory neuropathy. *Audiology Today, 7,* 10–13.

Skellett, R. A., Crist, J. R., Fallon, M., & Bobbin, R. P. (1996). Chronic low-level noise exposure alters distortion product otoacoustic emissions. *Hearing Research, 98,* 68–76.

Sladen, D., Lamb, M., & Hall, J. W. III. (1996, April 18). *Intra- and intersubject variance for distortion product otoacoustic emission amplitudes.* Paper presented at the American Academy of Audiology, Salt Lake City, Utah.

Slaven, A., & Thornton, A. R. D. (1998). Neonatal otoacoustic emissions recording using maximum length sequence stimuli. *Ear & Hearing, 19,* 103–110.

Slepecky, N. B. (1996). Structure of the mammalian cochlea. In P. Dallos, A. N. Popper, & R. R. Fay (Eds.), *The cochlea* (pp. 44–129). New York: Springer.

Smith, C., & Rasmussen, G. (1963). Recent observations on the olivocochlear bundle. *Annals of Otology, Rhinology, and Laryngology, 72,* 489–497.

Smith, C. A. (1961). Innervation pattern of the cochlea. *Annals of Otology, Rhinology, and Laryngology, 70,* 504–527.

Smoorenburg, G. F. (1972a). Audibility region of combination tones. *Journal of the Acoustical Society of America, 52,* 603–614.

Smoorenburg, G. F. (1972b). Combination tones and their origin. *Journal of the Acoustical Society of America, 52,* 615–631.

Smurzynski, J. (1994). Longitudinal measure of distortion-product and click-evoked otoacoustic emissions of preterm infants: Preliminary results. *Ear & Hearing, 15,* 210–223.

Smurzynski, J., Jung, M., Lafreniere, D., Kim, D., Vasudeva Kamath, M., Rowe, J., Holman, M., &

Leonard, G. (1993). Distortion-product and click-evoked otoacoustic emissions of preterm and full-term infants. *Ear & Hearing, 14,* 258–274.

Smurzynski, J., Jung, M., Leonard, G., & Kim, D. O. (1993). Otoacoustic emissions in full-term newborns at risk for hearing loss. *Laryngoscope, 103,* 1334–1341.

Sorenson, J. R., Levy, H. L., Mangione, T. W., & Sepe, S. J. (1984). Parental response to repeat testing of infants with "false-positive" results in a newborn screening program. *Pediatrics, 73,* 183–187.

Souter, M. (1995). Suppression of stimulus frequency otoacoustic emissions by contralateral noise. *Hearing Research, 91,* 167–177.

Spector, G. J., & Ge, X. X. (1981). Development of the hypotympanum in the human fetus and neonate. *Annals of Otology, Rhinolaryngology, and Laryngology, 88*(Suppl.), 2–20.

Spektor, Z., Leonard, G., Kim, D. O., Jung, M. D., & Smurzynski, J. (1991). Otoacoustic emissions in normal and hearing-impaired children and normal adults. *Laryngoscope, 101,* 965–976.

Spoendlin, H. (1969). Innervation pattern of the organ of Corti of the cat. *Acta Otolaryngologica (Stockholm), 67,* 239–254.

Spoendlin, H. (1981). Autonomic innervation of the inner ear. *Advances in Otorhinolaryngology, 27,* 1–13.

Stach, B., Westerberg, B. D., & Roberson, J. B. J. (1998). Auditory disorder in central nervous system miliary tuberculosis: Case report. *Journal of the American Academy of Audiology, 9,* 305–310.

Stach, B. A. (1997). *Comprehensive dictionary of audiology.* Baltimore: Williams & Wilkins.

Starr, A., McPherson, D., Patterson, J., Don, M., Luxford, W., Shannon, R., Sininger, Y., Tonokawa, L., & Waring, M. (1991). Absence of both auditory evoked potentials and auditory percepts dependent on timing cues. *Brain, 114,* 1157–1180.

Starr, A., Picton, T., Sininger, Y., Hood, L., & Berlin, C. (1996). Auditory neuropathy. *Brain, 119,* 741–753.

Starr, A., Sininger, M., Winter, M., Dereberry, M. J., Oba, S., & Michalewski, H. J. (1998). Transient deafness due to temperature-sensitive auditory neuropathy. *Ear & Hearing, 19,* 169–179.

Stein, L., Clark, S., & Kraus, N. (1983). The hearing impaired infant: Patterns of identification and habilitation. *Ear & Hearing, 4,* 232–236.

Stein, L., Jabaley, T., Spitz, R., Stoakley, D., & McGee, T. (1990). The hearing impaired infant: Patterns of identification and habilitation revisited. *Ear & Hearing, 11,* 201–205.

Stein, L., Tremblay, K., Pasternak, J., Banerjee, S., Lindemann, K., & Kraus, N. (1996). Brainstem abnormalities in neonates with normal otoacoustic emissions. *Seminars in Hearing, 17*, 197–213.

Stengs, C. H. M., Klis, S. F. L., Huizing, E. G., & Smoorenburg, G. F. (1998). Cisplatin ototoxicity. An electrophysiological dose-effect study in albino guinea pigs. *Hearing Research, 124*, 99–107.

Stephen, R. O., & Badham, N. J. (1996). The effects on transient evoked otoacoustic emissions following changes in external auditory canal acoustic impedance. *Audiology, 35*, 180–193.

Stevens, J., Webb, H., Hutchinson, J., Connell, J., Smith, M., & Buffin, J. (1991). Evaluation of click-evoked oto-acoustic emissions in the newborn. *British Journal of Audiology, 25*, 11–14.

Stevens, J. C., & Ip, B. (1988). Click evoked otoacoustic emissions in normal and hearing impaired adults. *British Journal of Audiology, 22*, 45–49.

Stevens, J. C., Webb, H. B., Hutchinson, J., Connell, J., Smith, M. F., & Buffin, J. T. (1989). Click evoked otoacoustic emissions compared with brainstem electric response. *Archives of Diseases in Children, 64*, 1105–1111.

Stevens, J. C., Webb, H. B., Hutchinson, J., Connell, J., Smith, M. F., & Buffin, J. T. (1990). Click evoked otoacoustic emissions in neonatal screening. *Ear & Hearing, 11*, 128–133.

Stevens, J. C., Webb, H. D., Smith, M. E., & Buffin, J. T. (1987). The effects of stimulus level on click evoked oto-acoustic emissions and brainstem responses in neonates under intensive care. *British Journal of Audiology, 24*, 293–300.

Stevens, J. C., Webb, H. D., Smith, M. E., Buffin, J. T., & Ruddy, H. (1987). A comparison of otoacoustic emissions and auditory brainstem electric response audiometry in the newborn and babies admitted to a special care baby unit. *Clinical Physical and Physiologic Measurements, 8*, 95–104.

Stover, L., Gorga, M. P., Neely, S. T., & Montoya, D. (1996). Toward optimizing the clinical utility of distortion product otoacoustic emission measurements. *Journal of the Acoustical Society of America, 100*, 968–977.

Stover, L., & Norton, S. J. (1991). *Comparisons among different otoacoustic emission phenomena.* Paper presented at the International Symposium on Otoacoustic Emissions, Kansas City, KS.

Stover, L., & Norton, S. (1993). The effects of aging on otoacoustic emissions. *Journal of the Acoustical Society of America, 94*, 2670–2681.

Stover, L. J., Neely, S. T., & Gorga, M. P. (1996). Latency and multiple sources of distortion product otoacoustic emissions. *Journal of the Acoustical Society of America, 99*, 1016–1024.

Strickland, E. A., Burns, E. M., & Tubis, A. (1985). Incidence of spontaneous otoacoustic emissions in children and adults. *Journal of the Acoustical Society of America, 78*, 931–935.

Strominger, N. L., Silver, S. M., Truscott, T. C., & Goldstein, J. C. (1981). The cells of origin of the olivocochlear bundle in new and old world monkeys. *Anatomic Research, 199*, 246.

Strouse, A., Ochs, M., & Hall, J., III. (1996). Evidence against the influence of aging on distortion-product otoacoustic emissions. *Journal of the American Academy of Audiology, 7*, 339–345.

Stypulkowski, P. H., & Oriaku, E. T. (1991). A comparison of the otoxic effects of salicylates and quinine [Abstract]. *Association for Research in Otolaryngology, 14*, 79.

Subramaniam, M., Salvi, R., Spongr, V., Henderson, D., & Powers, N. (1994). Changes in distortion product otoacoustic emissions and outer hair cells following interrupted noise exposures. *Hearing Research, 74*, 204–216.

Suckfull, M., & Mees, K. (1998). Hemoconcentration as a possible pathologic factor of sudden hearing loss. *European Archives of Otorhinolaryngology, 255*, 281–284.

Suckfull, M., Schneeweib, S., Dreher, A., & Schorn, K. (1996). Evaluation of TEOAE and DPOAE measurements for the assessment of auditory thresholds in sensorineural hearing loss. *Acta Otolaryngologica (Stockholm), 116*, 528–533.

Sun, X.-M., Kim, D. O., Jung, M. D., & Randolph, K. J. (1996). The performance of distortion product otoacoustic emission test of sensorineural hearing loss in humans: Comparison of unequal- and equal-level stimuli. *Annals of Otology, Rhinology, and Laryngology, 105*, 982–990.

Sutton, G., Gleadle, P., & Rowe, S. (1996). Tympanometry and otoacoustic emissions in a cohort of special care neonates. *British Journal of Audiology, 30*, 9–17.

Sutton, G. J., & Rowe, S. J. (1997). Risk factors for childhood sensorineural hearing loss in the Oxford region. *British Journal of Audiology, 31*, 39–54.

Sutton, L. A., Lonsbury-Martin, B. L., Martin, G. K., & Whitehead, M. L. (1994). Sensitivity of distortion-product otoacoustic emissions in humans to tonal over-exposure: Time course of recovery and effects of lowering L2. *Hearing Research, 75,* 161–174.

Swigonski, N., Shallop, J., Bull, M. J., & Lemons, J. A. (1987). Hearing screening of high risk newborns. *Ear & Hearing, 8,* 26–30.

Tait, M. et al. (1994) Comparison of early communicative behavior in young children with cochlear implants and with hearing aids. *Ear & Hearing, 15,* 352-361.

Takeno, S., Harrison, R. V., Ibrahim, D., Wake, M., & Mount, R. J. (1994). Cochlear function after selective inner hair cell degeneration induced by carboplatin. *Hearing Research, 75,* 93–102.

Takeno, S., Harrison, R., Mount, R. J., Wake, M., & Harada, Y. (1994). Induction of selective inner hair cell damage by carboplatin. *Scanning Microscopy, 8,* 97–106.

Takeno, S., Wake, M., Mount, R. J., & Harrison, R. V. (1998). Degeneration of spiral ganglion cells in the chinchilla after inner hair cell loss induced by carboplatin. *Audiology and Neuro-Otology, 3,* 281–290.

Talmadge, C. L., Long, G. R., Murphy, W. J., & Tubis, A. (1993). New off-line method for detecting spontaneous otoacoustic emissions in human subjects. *Hearing Research, 71,* 170–182.

Talmadge, C. L., Long, G. R., Tubis, A., & Dhar, S. (1999). Experimental confirmation of the two-source interference model for the fine structure of distortion product otoacoustic emissions. *Journal of the Acoustical Society of America, 105*(1), 275–283.

Talmadge, C. L., Tubis, A., Long, G. R., & Piskorski, P. (1998). Modeling otoacoustic emissions and hearing threshold fine structures. *Journal of the Acoustical Society of America, 104,* 1517–1528.

Talmadge, C. L., Tubis, A., Wit, H., & Long, G. R. (1991). Are spontaneous emissions generated by self-functions of evoked and spontaneous otoacoustic emissions distortion products in human subjects. *Journal of the Acoustical Society of America, 89,* 2391–2399.

Tan, K. L., Skurr, B. A., & Yip, Y. Y. (1992). Phototherapy and the brainstem auditory evoked response in neonatal hyperbilirubinemia. *Journal of Pediatrics, 120,* 306–308.

Tanaka, Y., Suzuki, M., & Inoue, T. (1990). Evoked otoacoustic emissions in sensorineural hearing impairment: Its clinical implication. *Ear & Hearing, 11,* 134–143.

Tasaki, I., & Spyropolous, C. S. (1959). Stria vascularis as a source of the endocochlear potential. *Journal of Neurophysiology, 22,* 149–155.

Tavartkiladze, G., Frolenkov, G., & Artamasov, S. (1996). Ipsilateral suppression of transient evoked otoacoustic emission: Role of the medial olivocochlear system. *Acta Otolaryngologica, 116,* 213–218.

Tavartkiladze, G. A., Frolenkov, G. I., Kruglov, A. V., & Artmasov, S. V. (1994). Ipsilateral suppression effects on transient evoked otoacoustic emission. *British Journal of Audiology, 28,* 193–204.

Telischi, F., Widick, M., Lonsbury-Martin, B., & McCoy, M. (1995). Monitoring cochlear function intraoperatively using distortion product otoacoustic emissions. *American Journal of Otology, 16,* 597–607.

Thiringer, K., Kankkunen, A., Liden, G., & Niklasson, A. (1984). Perinatal risk factors in the aetiology of hearing loss in preschool children. *Developmental Medicine and Child Neurology, 26,* 799–807.

Thoma, J., Gerull, G., & Mrowinski, D. (1986). A long-term study of hearing in children following neonatal hyperbilirubinemia. *Archives of Otorhinolaryngology, 243,* 133–137.

Thomas, I. B. (1975). Microstructure of the pure tone threshold. *Journal of the Acoustical Society of America, 57,* 57S.

Thompson, M. D., & Thompson, G. (1991). Early identification of hearing loss: Listen to parents. *Clinical Pediatrics, 30*(2), 77–80.

Thomsen, K. A., Terkildsen, K., & Arnfred, I. (1965). Middle ear pressure variations during anesthesia. *Archives of Otolaryngology, 82,* 609–611.

Thornton, A. (1994). Contralateral and ipsilateral "suppression" of evoked otoacoustic emissions at high stimulation rates. *British Journal of Audiology, 28,* 227–234.

Thornton, A., Kimm, L., Kennedy, C., & Cafarelli-Dees, D. (1993). External- and middle-ear factors affecting evoked otoacoustic emissions in neonates. *British Journal of Audiology, 27,* 319–327.

Thornton, A. R. D. (1993a). Click-evoked otoacoustic emissions: New techniques and applications. *British Journal of Audiology, 27,* 109–115.

Thornton, A. R. D. (1993b). High rate otoacoustic emissions. *Journal of the Acoustical Society of America, 94,* 132–136.

Thornton, A. R. D. (1994). New techniques: Maximum length sequences. In: R. F. Grandori (Ed.), *Advances in otoacoustic emissions: I. Fundamentals and clinical applications.* Milan: Stefanoni Lecco.

Thornton, A. R. D., Folkard, T. J., & Chambers, J. D. (1994). Technical aspects of recording evoked otoacoustic emissions using maximum length sequences. *Scandinavian Audiology, 23,* 225–231.

Thornton, A. R. D., Kimm, L., Kennedy, C. R., & Cafarelli-Dees, D. (1994). A comparison of neonatal evoked otoacoustic emissions obtained using two types of apparatus. *British Journal of Audiology, 28,* 99–109.

Thornton, A. R. D., & Slaven, A. (1993). Auditory brainstem responses recorded at fast stimulation rates using maximum length sequences. *British Journal of Audiology, 27,* 205–210.

Thornton, A. R. D., & Slaven, A. (1994). The effect of stimulus rate on the contralateral suppression of transient evoked otoacoustic emissions. *Scandinavian Audiology, 24,* 83–90.

Thornton, A. R. D., Slaven, A., MacKenzie, I., & Phillips, A. J. (1994). Evoked otoacoustic emissions recorded at very high stimulation rates. In F. Grandori (Ed.), *Advances in otoacoustic emissions. I. Fundamentals and clinical applications.* Milan: Stefanoni Lecco.

Tilanus, S. C., Stenis, D. V., & Snik, A. F. M. (1995). Otoacoustic emission measurements in evaluation of the immediate effect of ventilation tube insertion in children. *Annals of Otology, Rhinolaryngology, and Laryngology, 104,* 297–300.

Tluczek, A., Mischler, E. H., Farrell, P. M., Fost, N., Peterson, N. M., Carey, P., Bruns, W. T., & McCarthy, C. (1992). Parents' knowledge of neonatal screening and response to false-positive cystic fibrosis testing. *Developmental and Behavioral Pediatrics, 13*(3), 181–186.

Tognola, G., Grandori, F., & Ravazzani, P. (1998). Time-frequency distribution methods for the analysis of click-evoked otoacoustic emissions (in Polish). *Technology Health Care, 6,* 159–175.

Tognola, G., Grandori, F., & Ravazzani, P. (1999). Evaluation of click evoked otoacoustic emissions in newborns: Effects of time-windowing. *Audiology, 38*(3), 127–134.

Topolska, M. M., Hassman-Poznanska, E., & Musiatowicz, M. P. (1998). The influence of the middle ear status on the measurement of evoked otoacoustic emissions (DPOAE). *Otolaryngology Poland, 52*(4), 451–455.

Toth, L., Racz, T., Dioszeghy, P., & Repassy, G. (1994). Otoacoustic emission in myasthenia gravis patients and the role of efferent innervation. *Hearing Research, 126,* 123–125.

Trahiotis, C., & Elliott, D. N. (1968). Behavioral investigation of some possible effects of sectioning the crossed olivocochlear bundle. *Journal of the Acoustical Society of America, 47,* 592–506.

Trautwein, P., Hofstetter, P., Wang, J., Salvi, R., & Nostrant, A. (1996). Selective inner hair cell loss does not alter distortion product otoacoustic emissions. *Hearing Research, 96,* 71–82.

Trine, M. B., Hirsch, J. E., & Margolis, R. H. (1993). Effects of middle ear pressure on evoked otoacoustic emissions. *Ear & Hearing, 14,* 401–407.

Trybalska, G., Namyslowski, G., & Morawski, K. (1999). Assessment of otoacoustic emission usefulness for early detection of hearing impairment caused by noise (in Polish). *Otolaryngology Poland, 53*(2), 207–211.

Tsue, T. T., Oesterle, E. C., & Rubel, E. W. (1994). Hair cell regeneration in the inner ear. *Otolaryngology—Head and Neck Surgery, 111,* 281–301.

Tubis, A., & Talmadge, C. L. (1998). Ear canal reflectance in the presence of spontaneous otoacoustic emissions. I. Limit-cycle oscillator model. *Journal of the Acoustical Society of America, 103,* 454–461.

Turner, R. G. (1991). Modeling the cost and performance of early identification protocols. *Journal of the American Academy of Audiology, 2,* 195–205.

Turner, R. G. (1992a). Comparison of four hearing screening protocols. *Journal of the American Academy of Audiology, 3,* 200–207.

Turner, R. G. (1992b). Factors that determine the cost and performance of early identification protocols. *Journal of the American Academy of Audiology, 3,* 233–241.

Tyler, R. S., & Conrad-Armes, D. (1982). Spontaneous acoustic cochlear emissions and sensorineural tinnitus. *British Journal of Audiology, 16,* 193–194.

Ueda, H., Hattori, T., Sawaki, M., Niwa, H., & Yanagita, N. (1992). The effect of furosemide on evoked otoacoustic emissions in guinea pigs. *Hearing Research, 62,* 199–205.

Ueda, H., Yamamoto, Y., & Yanagita, N. (1996). Effect of aspirin on transiently evoked otoacoustic emissions in guinea pigs. *Oto-Rhino-Laryngology, 58,* 61–67.

Upfold, G., & Byrne, D. (1988). Variability of ear canal resonance and its implications for the design of hearing aids and earplugs. *Australian Journal of Audiology, 10,* 97–102.

Uppenkamp, S., Jakel, M., Talartschick, B., Buschwel, J., & Kollmeier, B. (1992). Evoked otoacoustic emissions as screening test for infant hearing? (in German). *Laryngo-Rhino-Otologie, 71,* 525–529.

Uppenkamp, S., & Kollmeier, B. (1994). Narrowband stimulation and synchronization of otoacoustic emissions. *Hearing Research, 78,* 210–220.

Uziel, A. (1990). Les oto-emissions acoustiques. Applications cliniques. *Annals of Otologie & Laryngologie (Paris), 107,* 48–50.

Uziel, A., & Piron, J.-P. (1991). Evoked otoacoustic emissions from normal newborns and babies admitted to an intensive care baby unit. *Acta Oto-laryngologica (Stockholm),* Suppl. 482, 85–91.

van Cauwenberge, P. B., Vinck, B., de Vel, E., & Dhooge, I. (1995,). *Tympanometry and click evoked otoacoustic emissions in secretory otitis media: Are C-EOAE really consistently absent in type B tympanograms?* Paper presented at the Sixth International Symposium on Otitis Media, Fort Lauderdale, FL.

van der Hulst, R. J. A. M., Dreschler, W. A., & Urbanus, N. A. M. (1988). High frequency audiometry in prospective clinical research of ototoxicity due to platinum derivatives. *Annals of Otology, Rhinology, and Laryngology, 97,* 133-137.

van Dijk, P., Maat, A., & Wit, H. P. (1997). Wiener kernel analysis of a noise-evoked otoacoustic emission. *British Journal of Audiology, 31,* 473–477.

van Dijk, P., & Wit, H. P. (1987). Temperature dependence of frog spontaneous otoacoustic emissions. *Journal of the Acoustical Society of America, 82,* 2147–2150.

van Dijk, P., & Wit, H. P. (1998). Correlated amplitude fluctuations of spontaneous otoacoustic emissions. *Journal of the Acoustical Society of America, 104*(1), 336–343.

van Huffelen, W., Mateijsen, N., & Wit, H. (1998). Classification of patients with Meniere's disease using otoacoustic emissions. *Audiology & Neuro-Otology, 3,* 419–430.

van Rijn, P. M., & Cremers, C. W. R. J. (1991). Causes of childhood deafness at a Dutch school for hearing impaired. *Annals of Otology, Rhinology, and Laryngology, 100,* 903–908.

van Zanten, B. G. A., Kok, M. R., Brocaar, M. P., & Sauer, P. J. J. (1995). The click-evoked oto-acoustic emission, C-EOAE, in preterm-born infants in the post conceptional age range between 30 and 688 weeks. *International Journal of Pediatric Otorhinolaryngology, 32*(Suppl.), S187–S197.

Vedantam, R., & Musiek, F. E. (1991). Click evoked otoacoustic emissions in adult subjects: Standard indices and test-retest reliability. *American Journal of Otology, 12,* 435–442.

Veuillet, E., Collet, L., & Duclaux, R. (1991). Effect of contralateral auditory stimulation on active cochlear micromechanical properties in human subjects: Dependence on stimulus variables. *Journal of Neurophysiology, 65,* 724–735.

Veuillet, E., Collet, L., & Morgon, A. (1992). Differential effects of ear canal pressure and contralateral acoustic stimulation on evoked otoacoustic emission in human. *Hearing Research, 61,* 47–55.

Veuillet, E., Duverdy-Bertholon, F., & Collet, L. (1996). Effect of contralateral acoustic stimulation on the growth of click-evoked otoacoustic emissions in humans. *Hearing Research, 93,* 128–135.

Vinck, B., De Vel, E., Xu, Z.-M., & Van Cauwenberge, P. (1996). Distortion product otoacoustic emissions: A normative study. *Audiology, 35,* 231–245.

Vinck, B. M., Van Cauwenberge, P. B., Corthals, P., & De Vel, E. (1998). Multi-variant analysis of otoacoustic emissions and estimation of hearing thresholds: Transient evoked otoacoustic emissions. *Audiology, 37,* 315–334.

Vinck, B. M., Van Cauwenberge, P. B., Leroy, L., & Corthals, P. (1999). Sensitivity of transient evoked and distortion product otoacoustic emissions to the direct effects of noise on the human cochlea. *Audiology, 38,* 44–52.

Vohr, B., Carty, L. M., Moore, P. E., & Letourneau, K. (1998). The Rhode Island Hearing Assessment Program: Experience with statewide hearing screening. *Journal of Pediatrics, 133,* 353–357.

Vohr, B., White, K., & Maxon, A. (1996). Effects of exam procedure on transient evoked otoacoustic emissions (TEOAEs) in neonates. *Journal of the American Academy of Audiology, 7,* 77–82.

Vohr, B., White, K., Maxon, A., & Johnson, M. (1993). Factors affecting the interpretation of transient evoked otoacoustic emission results in neonatal screening. *Seminars in Hearing, 14,* 57–72.

Vohr, B. R., Lester, B., Rapisardi, G., O'Dea, C., Brown, L., Peucker, M., Cashore, W., & Oh, W. (1989). Abnormal brain-stem function (brain-stem auditory evoked response) correlates with acoustic cry features in term infants with hyperbilirubinemia. *Journal of Pediatrics, 115,* 303–308.

von Békésy, G. (1960). *Experiments in hearing* (Wever, E.G., Trans.). New York: McGraw-Hill Book Co.

von Békésy, G. V. (1970). Traveling wave as frequency analyzers in the cochlea. *Nature, 225,* 1207–1209.

Wable, J., & Collet, L. (1994). Can synchronized otoacoustic emissions really be attributed to SOAE? *Hearing Research, 80,* 141–145.

Wable, J., Collet, L., & Chery-Croze, S. (1996). Phase delay measurements of distortion product otoacoustic emissions at 2f1–f2 and 2f2–f1 in human ears. *Journal of the Acoustical Society of America, 100,* 2228–2235.

Wada, H., & Kobayashi, T. (1990). Dynamical behavior of middle ear: Theoretical study corresponding to measurement results obtained by a newly developed measuring apparatus. *Journal of the Acoustical Society of America, 87,* 237–245.

Wada, H., Kobayashi, T., Suetake, M., & Tachizaki, H. (1989). Dynamic behavior of the middle ear based on sweep frequency tympanometry. *Audiology, 28,* 127–134.

Wada, H., Kobayashi, T., & Tachizaki, H. (1992). Diagnosis of middle ear disease with eardrum perforation by a newly developed sweep frequency measuring apparatus. *Audiology, 31,* 132–139.

Wada, H., Metoki, T., & Kobayashi, T. (1992). Analysis of dynamic behavior of human middle ear using a finite-element method. *Journal of the Acoustical Society of America, 92,* 3157–3168.

Wada, H., Ohyama, K., Kobayashi, T., Koike, T., & Noguchi, S.-I. (1995). Effect of middle ear on otoacoustic emissions. *Audiology, 34,* 161–176.

Wada, H., Ohyama, K., Kobayashi, T., Sunaga, N., & Koike, T. (1993). Relationship between evoked otoacoustic emissions and middle-ear dynamic characteristics. *Audiology, 32,* 282–292.

Wake, M., Anderson, J., Takeno, S., Mount, R. J., & Harrison, R. V. (1996). Otoacoustic emission amplification after inner hair cell damage. *Acta Otolaryngologica, 116,* 374–381.

Wake, M., Takeno, S., Ibrahim, D., & Harrison, R. (1994). Selective inner hair cell ototoxicity induced by carboplatin. *Laryngoscope, 104,* 488–493.

Wake, M., Takeno, S., Ibrahim, D., Harrison, R., & Mount, R. (1993). Carboplatin ototoxicity: An animal model. *Journal of Laryngology and Otology, 107,* 585–589.

Walsh, E. J., & McGee, J. (1987). Postnatal development of auditory nerve and cochlear nucleus neuronal responses in kittens. *Hearing Research, 28,* 97–116.

Ward, W. D. (1955). Tonal monaural diplacusis. *Journal of the Acoustical Society of America, 27,* 365–372.

Warr, W. B. (1975). Olivocochlear and vestibular efferent neurons of the feline brain stem: Their location, morphology and number determined by retrograde axonal transport and acetylcholinesterase histochemistry. *Journal of Comparative Neurology, 161,* 159–182.

Warr, W. B. (1986). Organization of the efferent fibers: The lateral and medial olivocochlear systems. In R. A. Altschuler, D. W. Hoffman, & R. P. Bobbin (Eds.), *Neurobiology of hearing: The cochlea* (pp. 333–348). New York: Raven Press.

Warr, W. B. (1992). Organization of olivocochlear efferent systems in mammals. In D. B. Webster, A. N. Popper, & R. R. Fay (Eds.), *Mammalian auditory pathway: Neuroanatomy* (pp. 410–448). New York: Springer-Verlag.

Warr, W. B., & Guinan, J. J., Jr. (1979). Efferent innervation of the organ of Corti: Two separate systems. *Brain Research, 173,* 152–155.

Warren, E. H., & Liberman, M. C. (1989). Effects of contralateral sound on auditory-nerve responses. I. Contributions of cochlear efferents. *Hearing Research, 37,* 89–104.

Waters, G. S., Ahmad, M., Katsarka, A., Stanimir, G., & McKay, J. (1991). Ototoxicity due to cis-diamminedi-chloroplatinum in the treatment of ovarian cancer: Influence of dosage and schedule of administration. *Ear and Hearing, 12,* 91–102.

Watkin, P. (1996). Outcome of neonatal screening for hearing loss by otoacoustic emission. *Archives of Diseases in Children, 75,* 158–168.

Watkin, P. M. (1996). Neonatal otoacoustic emission screening and the identification of deafness. *Archives of Diseases in Children, 74,* f16–25.

Watkin, P. M., Baldwin, M., Dixon, R., & Beckman, A. (1998). Maternal anxiety and attitudes to universal neonatal hearing screening. *British Journal of Audiology, 32,* 27–37.

Watkin, P. M., Baldwin, M., & McEnery, G. (1991). Neonatal at risk screening and the identification of deafness. *Archives of Diseases in Childhood, 66,* 1130–1135.

Waun, J. E., Swietzer, R. S., & Hamilton, W. K. (1967). Effect of nitrous oxide on middle ear mechanics and hearing acuity. *Anaesthesiology, 28,* 846–850.

Weatherly, R. A., Owens, J. I., & Catlin, F. I. (1991). Cis-platinum ototoxicity in children. *Laryngoscope, 101,* 917–924.

Webb, H. D., & Stevens, J. C. (1991). Auditory screening in high risk neonates: Selection of test protocol. *Clinical Physical and Physiologic Measures, 12,* 75–86.

Weber, R., & Mellert, V. (1975). On the non-monotonic behavior of cubic distortion products in the human ear. *Journal of the Acoustical Society of America, 57,* 77–80.

Wegel, R. L., & Lane, C. E. (1924). The auditory masking of one sound by another and its probable relation to the dynamics of the inner ear. *Physiological Review, 23,* 266–285.

Weir, C. C., Norton, S. J., & Kincaid, G. E. (1984). Spontaneous narrow-band otoacoustic signals emitted by human ears: A replication. *Journal of the Acoustical Society of America, 76,* 1248–1250.

Weir, C. C., Pasanen, E. G., & McFadden, D. (1988). Partial dissociation of spontaneous otoacoustic emissions and distortion products during aspirin in humans. *Journal of the Acoustical Society of America, 84,* 230–237.

Welch, D., Greville, K. A., Thorne, P. R., & Purdy, S. C. (1996). Influence of acquisition parameters on the measurement of click evoked otoacoustic emissions in neonates in a hospital environment. *Audiology, 35*, 143–157.

Welzl-Muller, K., & Stephan, K. (1994). Confirmation of transiently evoked otoacoustic emissions based on user-independent criteria. *Audiology, 33*, 28–36.

Welzl-Muller, K., Stephan, K., & Stadlmann, A. (1993). Click-evoked otoacoustic emissions in a child with unilateral deafness. *European Archives of Otorhinolaryngology, 250*, 366–368.

Wennberg, R. P., Ahlfors, C. E., Bickers, R., McCurty, C. A., & Shetter, J. L. (1982). Abnormal auditory brainstem response in a newborn infant with hyperbilirubinemia: Improvement with exchange transfusion. *Journal of Pediatrics, 100*, 624–626.

Wenner, C. H. (1968). Intensities of aural difference tones. *Journal of the Acoustical Society of America, 43*, 77–80.

Werner, L. A., & Rubel, E. W. (Eds.). (1992). *Developmental psychoacoustics.* Washington, DC: American Psychological Association.

Westbrook, G. F. S., & Bamford, J. M. (1992). Probe-tube microphone measurements with very young infants. *British Journal of Audiology, 26*, 143–151.

Westwood, M. L., & Bamford, J. M. (1992). Probe-tube microphone measurements with very young infants. *British Journal of Audiology, 26*, 143–151.

White, D. R. et al. (1998). Effectiveness of intermittent and continuous acoustic stimulation in hearing and hair cell loss. *Journal of Acoustical Society of America,103*, 1566–1572.

White, K. R. (1996). Universal newborn hearing screening using transient evoked otoacoustic emissions: Past, present, and future. *Seminars in Hearing, 17*, 171–183.

White, K. R., & Behrens, T. R. (Eds.). (1993). The Rhode Island Hearing Assessment Project: Implications for universal newborn hearing screening *Seminars in Hearing, 14.* New York: Thieme Medical Publishers.

White, K. R., Behrens, T. R., & Strickland, B. (1995). Practicality, validity, and cost-efficiency of universal newborn hearing screening using transient evoked otoacoustic emissions. *Journal of Childhood Communication Disorders, 17*, 9–14.

White, K. R., Culpepper, B., Maxon, A. B., Vohr, B. R., & Mauk, G. W. (1995). Transient evoked otoacoustic emission-based screening in typical nurseries: a response to Jacobson and Jacobson. *International Journal of Pediatric Otorhinolaryngology, 33*, 17–21.

White, K. R., & Maxon, A. B. (1995). Universal screening for infant hearing impairment: Simple, beneficial, and presently justified. *International Journal of Pediatric Otorhinolaryngology, 32*, 201–211.

Whitehead, M., Kamal, N., Lonsbury-Martin, B., & Martin, G. (1993). Spontaneous otoacoustic emissions in different racial groups. *Scandinavian Audiology, 22*, 3–10.

Whitehead, M., Lonsbury-Martin, B., & Martin, G. (1992). Evidence for two discrete sources of 2f1–f2 distortion-product otoacoustic emission in rabbit: II. Differential physiologic vulnerability. *Journal of the Acoustical Society of America, 92*, 2662–2682.

Whitehead, M., Lonsbury-Martin, B., & Martin, G. (1993). The influence of noise on the measured amplitudes of distortion-product otoacoustic emissions. *Journal of Speech and Hearing Research, 36*, 1097–1102.

Whitehead, M., Stagner, B., McCoy, M., Lonsbury-Martin, B., & Martin, G. (1995). Dependence of distortion-product otoacoustic emissions on primary levels in normal and impaired ears. II. Asymmetry in the L1, L2 space. *Journal of the Acoustical Society of America, 97*, 2359–2377.

Whitehead, M., Wilson, J. P., & Baker, R. J. (1986). The effects of temperature on otoacoustic emission tuning properties. In B. C. J. Moore & R. D. Patterson (Eds.), *Auditory frequency selectivity* (pp. 39–48). New York: Plenum Press.

Whitehead, M. L. (1991). Slow variations of the amplitude and frequency of spontaneous emissions. *Hearing Research, 53*, 269-280.

Whitehead, M. L., Jimenez, A. M., Stagner, B. B., McCoy, M. J., Lonsbury-Martin, B. L., & Martin, G. K. (1995). Time-windowing of click-evoked otoacoustic emissions to increase signal-to-noise ratio. *Ear & Hearing, 16*, 599–611.

Whitehead, M. L., Stagner, B. B., Martin, G. K., & Lonsbury-Martin, B. L. (1996). Visualization of the onset of distortion-product otoacoustic emissions, and measurement of their latency. *Journal of the Acoustical Society of America, 100*, 599–611.

Whitworth, C., Morris, C., Scott, V., & Rybak, L. P. (1993). Dose-response relationships for furosemide ototoxicity in rat. *Hearing Research, 71*, 202–207.

Widick, M. P., Telischi, F. F., Lonsbury-Martin, B. L., & Stagner, B. B. (1994). Early effects of cerebellopontine angle compression on rabbit distortion-product otoacoustic emissions: A model for monitoring cochlear function during acoustic neuroma surgery. *Otolaryngology—Head and Neck Surgery, 111*, 407–416.

Wiederhold, M. L. (1992). *Frequency-dependent effect of tympanic membrane loading on reverse middle-ear transmission.* Paper presented at the Association for Research in Otolaryngology, St. Petersburg, Florida.

Wiederhold, M. L., & Kiang, N. Y. S. (1970). Effects of electrical stimulation of the crossed olivocochlear bundle on single auditory nerve fibers in cat. *Journal of the Acoustical Society of America, 48,* 950–965.

Wier, C. C., Norton, S. J., & Kincaid, G. E. (1984). Spontaneous narrow-band otoacoustic signals emitted by human ears. *Journal of the Acoustical Society of America, 76,* 1248–1250.

Wier, C. C., Pasenen, E. G., & McFadden, D. (1988). Partial dissociation of spontaneous otoacoustic emissions and distortion products during aspirin use in humans. *Journal of the Acoustical Society of America, 84,* 230–237.

Williams, D., & Darbyshire, J. (1982). Diagnosis of deafness: A study of family responses and needs. *Volta Review, 84,* 24–30.

Williams, E., Brookes, G. B., & Prasher, D. K. (1993). Effects of contralateral acoustic stimulation on otoacoustic emissions following vestibular neurectomy. *Scandinavian Audiology, 22,* 197–203.

Williams, E. A., Brookes, G. B., & Prasher, D. K. (1994). Effects of olivocochlear bundle section on otoacoustic emissions in humans: Efferent effects in comparison with control subjects. *Acta Otolaryngologica (Stockholm), 114,* 121–129.

Wilson, J. L., Henson, M. M., & Henson, O. W. (1991). Course and distribution of efferent fibers in the cochlea of the mouse. *Hearing Research, 55,* 98–108.

Wilson, J. P. (1980a). Evidence for a cochlear origin for acoustic re-emissions, threshold fine structure and tonal tinnitus. *Hearing Research, 2,* 233–252.

Wilson, J. P. (1980b). Recording of the Kemp echo and tinnitus from the ear canal without averaging. *Journal of Physiology, 298,* 8–9.

Wilson, J. P. (1985). The influence of temperature on frequency-tuning mechanisms. In J. B. Allen, J. L. Hall, A. Hubbard, S. T. Neely, & A. Tubis (Eds.), *Peripheral auditory mechanisms* (pp. 229–236). New York: Springer-Verlag.

Wilson, J. P., & Evans, E. G. (1983). Effects of furosemide, flaxedil, noise, and tone over-stimulation on the evoked otoacoustic emissions in the ear canal of the gerbil. *Proceedings of the International Union of Physiological Science, 15,* 100.

Wilson, J. P., & Sutton, G. J. (1981). Acoustic correlates of tonal tinnitus. In D. Everedm & G. Lawrenson (Eds.), *Tinnitus* (pp. 82-107). London: Ciba Pitman Books,Ltd.

Wilson, J. P., & Sutton, G. J. (1983). A family with high-tonal objective tinnitus—An update. In R. Kinke & R. Hartmann (Eds.), *Hearing: Physiological bases and psychophysics* (pp. 97-103). Berlin: Springer-Verlag.

Winslow, R. L., & Sachs, M. B. (1988). Single-tone intensity discrimination based on auditory-nerve rate responses in backgrounds of quiet, noise, and with stimulation of the crossed olivocochlear bundle. *Hearing Research, 35,* 165–190.

Winton, A., Smyth, V., Kei, J., McPherson, B., Latham, S., & Loscher, J. (1998). Infant hearing screening: a comparison of two techniques. *Australia and New Zealand Journal of Public Health, 22*(2), 261–265.

Wit, H., & Ritsma, R. (1990). Evoked acoustical responses from the human ear: Some experimental results. *Hearing Research, 2,* 253–261.

Wit, H. P. (1985). Diurnal cycle for spontaneous otocoustic emission frequency. *Hearing Research, 18,* 197–199.

Wit, H. P., Langevoort, J. C., & Ritsma, R. J. (1981). Frequency spectra of cochlear acoustic emissions (Kemp-echoes). *Journal of the Acoustical Society of America, 70,* 437–445.

Wit, H. P., & Ritsma, R. J. (1979). Stimulated acoustic emissions from the human ear. *Journal of the Acoustical Society of America, 66,* 911–913.

Wit, H. P., van Dijk, P., & Avan, P. (1994). On the shape of (evoked) otoacoustic emission spectra. *Hearing Research, 81,* 208–214.

Wood, S., Mason, S., Farnsworth, A., Davis, A., Curnock, D. A., & Lutman, M. E. (1998). Anomalous screening outcomes from click-evoked otoacoustic emissions and auditory brainstem response tests. *British Journal of Audiology, 32,* 399–410.

Worthington, D. W., & Peters, J. F. (1980). Quantifiable hearing and no ABR: Paradox or error? *Ear & Hearing, 1,* 281–285.

Wright, A., Davis, A., Bredberry, G., Ulehlova, L., & Spencer, H. (1987). Hair cell distribution in the normal human cochlea: A report of a European working group. *Acta Otolaryngologica, 106,* 15–24.

Wysocki, S., Graunaug, A., O'Neill, G., & Hahnel, R. (1981). Lipids in forehead vernix from newborn infants. *Biology of the Neonate, 39,* 300–304.

Xu, L., Probst, R., Harris, F. P., & Roede, J. (1994). Peripheral analysis of frequency in human ears revealed by tone burst evoked otoacoustic emissions. *Hearing Research, 74,* 173–180.

Xu, Z. M., Vinck, B., De vel, E., & van Cauwenberge, P. (1998). Noise-induced hearing loss has a dynamic progression. *Journal of Laryngology and Otology, 112,* 1154–1161.

Yamamoto, E., Tagaki, A., Hirono, Y., & Yagi, N. (1987). A case of "spontaneous otoacoustic emission." *Archives of Otolaryngology—Head and Neck Surgery, 113*, 1316-1318.

Yardley, M. P. J., Davies, C. M., & Stevens, J. C. (1998). The use of transient evoked otoacoustic emissions to detect and monitor cochlear damage caused by platinum-containing drugs. *British Journal of Audiology, 32*, 305–316.

Yates, G. K. (1990). Basilar membrane nonlinearity and its influence on auditory nerve rate-intensity functions. *Hearing Research, 50*, 145–162.

Yoshinaga-Itano, C., Sedey, A. L., Coulter, D. K., & Mehl, A. L. (1998). Language of early- and later-identified children with hearing loss. *Pediatrics, 102*, 1161–1171.

Zapala, D. A. (1998). A probabilistic approach to quantifying DPOAE detection. *Journal of the American Academy of Audiology, 9*, 332–341.

Zenner, H. P. (1986). Motile responses in outer hair cells. *Hearing Research, 22*, 83–90.

Zenner, H. P. (1988). Motility of outer hair cells as an active, actin-mediated process. *Acta Otolaryngologica (Stockholm), 105*, 39–44.

Zenner, H. P., Arnold, W., & Gitter, A. H. (1988). Outer hair cells as fast and slow cochlear amplifiers with a bidirectional transduction cycle. *Acta Otolaryngologica (Stockholm), 105*, 457–462.

Zenner, H. P., Zimmerman, U., & Gitter, A. H. (1990). Cell potential and motility of isolated mammalian vestibular sensory cells. *Hearing Research, 50*, 289–294.

Zhang, M., & Abbas, P. J. (1997). Effects of middle ear pressure on otoacoustic emission measures. *Journal of the Acoustical Society of America, 102*, 1032–1037.

Zhao, F., Meredith, R., & Stephens, S. D. G. (1996). Transient evoked otoacoustic emissions with contralateral stimulation in King-Kopetzky syndrome. *Journal of Audiological Medicine, 6*, 36–44.

Zhao, F., & Stephens, D. (1998). Analyses of notches in audioscan and DPOAEs in subjects with normal hearing. *Audiology, 37*, 335–343.

Zhao, F., & Stephens, D. (1999). Test-retest variability of distortion-product otoacoustic emissions in human ears with normal hearing. *Scandinavian Audiology, 28*(3), 171–178.

Zheng, Y., Ohyama, K., Hozawa, K., Wada, H., & Takasaka, T. (1997). Effect of anesthetic agents and middle ear pressure application on distortion product otoacoustic emissions in the gerbil. *Hearing Research, 112*, 167–174.

Zizz, C. A., & Glattke, T. J. (1988). Reliability of spontaneous otoacoustic emission suppression tuning curve measures. *Journal of Speech and Hearing Research, 31*, 616–619.

Zorowka, P., Schmitt, H. J., Eckel, H. E., Lippert, K. L., Schonberger, W., & Merz, E. (1993). Serial measurements of transient evoked otoacoustic emissions (TEOAEs) in healthy newborns and in newborns with perinatal infection. *International Journal of Pediatric Otorhinolaryngology, 27*, 245–254.

Zorowka, P., Schmitt, H., & Gutjahr, P. (1993). Evoked otoacoustic emissions and pure tone threshold audiometry in patients receiving cisplatinum therapy. *International Journal of Pediatric Otorhinolaryngology, 25*, 73–80.

Zorowka, P. G. (1993). Otoacoustic emissions: a new method to diagnose hearing impairment in children. *European Journal of Pediatrics, 152*, 626–634.

Zurek, P. M. (1981). Spontaneous narrow-band signals emitted by human ears. *Journal of the Acoustical Society of America, 69*, 514–523.

Zurek, P. M., Clark, W. W., & Kim, D. O. (1982). The behavior of acoustic distortion products in the ear canals of chinchillas with normal or damaged ears. *Journal of the Acoustical Society of America, 72*, 774–780.

Zurek, P. M., & Leshowitz, B. H. (1976). Measurement of the combination tones $f2-f1$ and $2f1-f2$. *Journal of the Acoustical Society of America, 61*, 155–168.

Zweig, G., & Shera, C. A. (1995). The origin of periodicity in the spectrum of evoked otoacoustic emissions. *Journal of the Acoustical Society of America, 98*, 2018–2047.

Zwicker, E. (1979). Different behaviour of quadratic and cubic difference tones. *Hearing Research, 1*, 283–292.

Zwicker, E. (1980). Nonmonotonic behavior of (2f1, f2) explained by saturation-feedback model. *Hearing Research, 2*, 513–516.

Zwicker, E. (1983). Delayed evoked oto-acoustic emissions and their suppression by Gaussian-shaped pressure impulses. *Hearing Research, 11*, 359–371.

Zwicker, E. (1986). "Otoacoustic" emissions in a nonlinear cochlear hardware model with feedback. *Journal of the Acoustical Society of America, 80*, 154–162.

Zwicker, E. (1990). On the influence of acoustical probe impedance on evoked otoacoustic emissions. *Hearing Research, 47*(3), 185–190.

Zwicker, E., & Scherer, A. (1987). Correlation between time functions of sound pressure, masking, and OAE suppression. *Journal of the Acoustical Society of America, 81*, 1043–1049.

Zwicker, E., & Schloth, E. (1984). Interrelation of different otoacoustic emissions. *Journal of the Acoustical Society of America, 75,* 1148–1154.

Zwicker, E., & Schorn, K. (1990). Delayed evoked otoacoustic emissions—an ideal screening test for excluding hearing impairment in infants. *Audiology, 29*(3), 241–251.

Zwislocki, J. J. (1980). Theory of cochlear mechanics. *Hearing Research, 2,* 171–182.

I

Index

W

Waardenburg syndrome, 406
Watkin, Peter, 403
Widen, Judy, 143

Y

Yoshinaga-Itano, Christine, 400–401, 402

Z

Zoological Laboratory, Cambridge University, 4, 6
Zwislocki, J. J., 4, 8